Textbook of
Community
Dentistry

Public Health Dentistry

List of Contributors

Acharya Shashidhar
Associate Professor and Head
Department of Community Dentistry
Manipal College of Dental Sciences
Manipal University, Manipal

Deepti Shyam Sunder
Professor
Department of Community Medicine
Govt. Medical College, Amritsar

Goel Pankaj
Professor and Head
Department of Community Dentistry
People's College of Dental Sciences, Bhopal

Grewal Navneet
Professor and Head
Department of Pedodontics and
Preventive Dentistry
Punjab Govt. Dental College and Hospital, Amritsar

Gupta Nidhi
Professor and Head
Department of Community Dentistry
Genesis Institute of Dental Sciences
Firozpur

Sharma Sujata
Professor and Head
Department of Obstetrics and Gyneacology
Govt. Medical College
Amritsar

Sikri RK
General Manager
National Thermal Power Corporation
New Delhi

Sikri Vimal K
Principal
Punjab Govt. Dental College and Hospital
Amritsar

Textbook of Community Dentistry

Public Health Dentistry

Poonam Sikri MDS PDES (Ex)

Professor and Head
Department of Periodontics
Seema Dental College
Rishikesh (Uttarakhand)

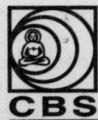

CBS

CBS Publishers and Distributors Pvt Ltd

New Delhi • Bengaluru • Chennai • Kochi • Kolkata • Mumbai
Hyderabad • Nagpur • Patna • Pune • Vijayawada

Textbook of
Community Dentistry
Public Health Dentistry

ISBN: 978-93-86310-83-5

First Edition: 2017

Published by Satish Kumar Jain and Produced by Varun Jain for
CBS Publishers & Distributors Pvt Ltd
4819/XI Prahlad Street, 24 Ansari Road, Daryaganj, New Delhi 110 002, India.
Ph: 23289259, 23266861, 23266867   Fax: 011-23243014   Website: www.cbspd.com
e-mail: delhi@cbspd.com; cbspubs@airtelmail.in.

Corporate Office: 204 FIE, Industrial Area, Patparganj, Delhi 110 092, India
Ph: 4934 4934   Fax: 4934 4935   e-mail: publishing@cbspd.com; publicity@cbspd.com

Branches

* Bengaluru: Seema House 2975, 17th Cross, K.R. Road,
  Banasankari 2nd Stage, Bengaluru 560 070, Karnataka, India
  Ph: +91-80-26771678/79   Fax: +91-80-26771680   e-mail: bangalore@cbspd.com
* Chennai: 7, Subbaraya Street, Shenoy Nagar, Chennai 600 030, Tamil Nadu, India
  Ph: +91-44-26260666, 26208620   Fax: +91-44-42032115   e-mail: chennai@cbspd.com
* Kochi: Ashana House, No. 39/1904, AM Thomas Road, Valanjambalam, Ernakulam 682 016, Kochi, Kerala, India
  Ph: +91-484-4059061-65   Fax: +91-484-4059065   e-mail: kochi@cbspd.com
* Kolkata: No. 6/B, Ground Floor, Rameswar Shaw Road, Kolkata-700014 (West Bengal), India
  Ph: +91-33-2289-1126, 2289-1127, 2289-1128   e-mail: kolkata@cbspd.com
* Mumbai: 83-C, Dr E Moses Road, Worli, Mumbai-400018, Maharashtra, India
  Ph: +91-22-24902340/41   Fax: +91-22-24902342   e-mail: mumbai@cbspd.com

Representatives

* Hyderabad   0-9885175004   • Nagpur   0-9021734563   • Patna   0-9334159340
* Pune   0-9623451994   • Vijayawada   0-9000660880

Printed at   India Binding House, Noida, UP, India

A Living Legend

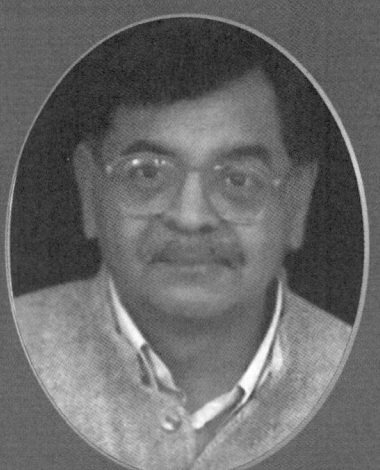

Dr Shyam Sunder Deepti

A Genius
with the supernatural virtue
of humility in the domain of thought

Foreword

Professional books in any discipline are the contemporary thoughts that enrich the body of knowledge in the chosen subject of an author.

I am delighted to know Dr Poonam Sikri, Professor and Head, Department of Periodontics, Seema Dental College, Rishikesh, has authored a book *Public Health Dentistry*.

Dental health with preserved strength and vigour by its very nature is a complicated entity, undoubtedly an inseparable part of total health. It requires a constant effort in trying to update one's own knowledge, record, explain, and present the subject in the best way possible before the students. The work is demanding. In such circumstances writing a book is an additional task with the regular work. Dr Sikri has mirrored her scholarship in this book.

The most daunted challenge in writing a book lies in selecting the subject. She has selected a subject that encompasses almost each speciality and has given a flavour that generates zest for reading. Though the subject encompasses many specialties, she has maintained continuous lucidly in her expression that might make this book stable and unwavering. I had an opportunity to see pre-publication of this book. As a Vice-Chancellor of a large University it was impossible for me to go through sentence by sentence, page by page.

I had a cursory glance. I found the author has clarity over the subject. The chapters on "Nutrition", "Environment and Health" and "Prevention of Oral Diseases" have been written exhaustively keeping in view the importance in public health. She has made every effort to wrap her knowledge comprehensively. This book may vividly establish her credentials in dental fraternity, academics and professionals while being also helpful to the student community.

S Ramananda Shetty
Vice-Chancellor
Rajiv Gandhi University of Health Sciences
Karnataka

Preface

The writing of a book needs blessings of Almighty God coupled with motivation of friends, teachers and family members and also focusing your achieve-a-goal attitude.

It was my long cherished dream to write a book on *Public Health Dentistry*, ever since I started teaching community dentistry along with periodontology at Government Dental College, Amritsar. The present book is presented in such a language and such a format that it will be welcomed by all dental students and teachers. Keeping in view the importance of day-to-day necessities, the chapters of 'Nutrition', 'Prevention of Oral diseases' and 'Environment and Health' have been given special emphasis. Chapter of 'Research Methodology and Biostatics' is written in an extraordinary simple way so that the students can easily understand the subject. I am wholeheartedly thankful to Dr Shyam Sunder Deepti and my brother-in-law, Mr R K Sikri, for making the chapter so simple and lucid.

I am thankful to all the contributors who shared their experiences in the form of text in this book.

My sincere thanks to Dr Gupta ji, a great soul of Rishikesh, for his soft and polite encouragement. I vividly remember the kind advice of late madam Seema ji.

I am thankful to Mrs Sahani of Seema Dental College, Rishikesh, for her friendly help and motivation. I am thankful to Mr. Anirudh's parents for their saintly blessings.

I am indebted to Dr Pulkit, Dr Ruchika, Dr Luxmi, Dr Amrit, Dr Payal, Dr Garima, Dr Ibadat, Dr Meenu, Dr Preeti, Dr Shalini, Dr Mandeep and Dr Monica for checking and rechecking the manuscript. Mr Vipul of Vipul's Ocean of Art deserves special thanks for his sincere and ready-to-help attitude.

I assure that the book in your hands is a refreshing breath of new air for dental professionals. It is the outcome of my experiences with the students and colleagues undertaking Public Health as a subject. The book covers syllabi as prescribed by Dental Council of India and the other universities as well.

I am thankful to Mr Satish Jain, Managing Director, Mr Vinod Jain, Production Director, and Mr YN Arjuna, Publishing Director, CBS Publishers & Distributors, for their constant efforts to reshape the format and outlook of the book.

The completion of the book would have never been possible without the support of my husband, Dr Vimal Sikri, and sons, Ankit and Arpit, who are also pursuing dentistry as a career.

Last but not the least, I am thankful to all those who helped me directly or indirectly in compiling the manuscript of this book.

Poonam Sikri

Contents

1   *Sociology and Health*

Society is a main concern of sociology, which deals with the organizations or structure of social groups. Society is the unique feature of man, which differentiated him from animals. Society is not simply a collection of people in groups, as understood by a layman. It is not only awareness of each other at a physical level and acknowledging each other's physical presence; communication at the psychic or mental level is a must to establish them as a society. For example, a group of people standing in a queue cannot be called a society. They are aware of the presence of others, but know nothing of their aims, aspirations, ideas and needs. The mutual awareness or reciprocal recognition at the psychic level is pre-requisite to the formation of society. Community can be defined as *the group of people living together in a particular area may be because of ethnic, religious or geographical togetherness.*

Let us see how a link can be established at the psychic level. For such a linkage to develop, the factor of commonness has to come into action. As an example, patients from different places come and get admitted in a hospital ward. They are unknown to each other, yet the common factor that brings them together is their suffering. Thereby they change from individual to group, from 'I' to 'WE' when they share their sufferings. This 'WE', the factor of 'likeness', is the essence of society. This is also known as 'consciousness of kind' or 'we feeling'. In short, society may be understood as an organization of member agents having social relationships amongst themselves. The strength of relationship decides the nature of group. The relationship may be primary, secondary or tertiary in nature.

ORIGIN OF SOCIETY

One could say that the micro-organisms do live in a group, e.g. on a culture plate. However such group is only of a biological nature. Higher animals have their own sensory system, enabling them to have an instinctive approach. The two basic instincts: hunger and sex are the manifestations of single broad driving force or motive, i.e. the urge for survival. If an animal eats, it does so in order to survive as an individual. If it reproduces, it does so in order to survive as a species.

It can be seen that biological multiplication and living together in the same environment, with similar activities gives rise to a biological social network. In this context, the family (father, mother, brothers and sisters) is also a form of biological social network. Animals also move in groups called herds. Group activity provides a sense of security, since the group moves in surroundings that are similar structurally (with reference to figure and frame-work) and functionally (with reference to physiology and biochemistry).

Now the question arises how a human society is different from animal society? In the process of evolution, physical framework, physiological and biochemical function and group activity kept on changing and kept on influencing each other. The change from plants to animals, invertebrates to vertebrates and pisces to mammalians was always the product of environment and sense of survival.

External Environment × Sense of Survival = Required Change (Transformation)

1

The milestones in the way of origin of human society are enumerated as:

1. Man, amongst the mammals, transformed himself structurally by standing on his feet and adopting an upright posture and making his hands free.
2. Development of thumb, provided extra strength to the hand in form of a clenched fist. The circumscribed movement of thumb helped the hand to perform finer and complex movements.
3. Development of brain helped man to keep on manipulating his environment.
4. As regards to physiological changes, they started nourishing their offsprings by their milk through mammary glands. This again fostered group life physically as well as mentally.
5. Human female has a menstrual cycle as compared to estrous cycle present in higher mammals. These regular menstrual cycles are helpful in two ways. Firstly, conception can take place during any period of life, secondly, it can be prevented also. Thus in human beings, there is a controlled fertilization.

These five elements can be identified in many animals in varying degree. But man has added one more component to above milestones, namely, the elements of *Culture*. It can be simply understood as, *An art of adding Experience*. This addition can be done by telling something to next generation. So, with this extra element, man has given himself the name—Social Animal.

In contrast, animals either inherit certain instincts or gain experience through hit and trial approach, which however remain limited to their own lifetime. Man on the other hand, learns from the experience of others as well; and can plan for the future through cumulative experience of generations.

STRUCTURAL ASPECTS OF SOCIETY

In order to understand the structure of society, we must acquaint ourselves with its institu-

tions, which not only fit individual members into different positions but also prescribe the ways of doing things or behaving in the society.

Social Institution

It is a social structure and machinery through which human society organizes, directs and executes the multifarious activities required to satisfy human needs. Institutions may be economical, political, educational, religious and recreational in nature. Examples are, a school, hospital or parliament. Family is also a social institution or we can say it is a basic and nuclear institution of society.

Community

It is defined as the group, small or large, living together in a way that the members share not one or more specific interests (like occupational, educational, etc.), but rather the basic conditions of a common life. The hallmark of a community is that one's life may be wholly lived within it. One cannot live a whole life within a club or a business group. However, one can live wholly within a tribe or a village or city.

Associations

Associations are group of people united for a specific purpose or a limited number of purposes and are based on utilitarian interest, e.g. Junior Doctor's Association.

When an association serves a broad interest and does so in an accepted, orderly and enduring way, it may be called an *Institution*, i.e. an established way of doing things. An example would be the Indian Dental Association.

Having gone through the concept of society, let us try to define it in this back-ground. Sociologists define society as, *A system of uses and procedures of authority and mutual aid of many groups coupled with division of control of human behaviour and liberty*. This is a web of social relationships and is always changing. In other words, society is an organization created by man for himself. Individuals in a society are expected to play a number of roles through their relationships. These relationships and groups, may be primary or secondary, are described in Table 1.1.

FUNCTIONAL ASPECTS OF SOCIETY

It is established that society is an organization made by man for himself. So he has also framed the procedures. Every living organism has same basic requirements and tries to satisfy them. These needs give rise to the basic desires or instincts, which the animal tries to satisfy without inhibition. In man, the biological forces trigger the desires, but contrary to animals, there are social standards, which guide man. The resultant of these two forces is the actual behaviour, which is performed in society. Thus, a newly born child is equivalent to an animal.

The day to day teaching and learning constitutes an important functional aspect of society.

SOCIAL NORMS

Every society specifies certain rules of conduct to be followed by its members in certain situations. These specified rules of conduct are technically known as Social Norms. Various social norms and their origins are explained in the Flow chart 1.1.

Types of Norms

Various types of norms, can be considered according to:
- Range of Acceptance
- Range of Enforceability

Folkways

They refer to customary ways of behaviour. People conform to these ways not out of fear

Table 1.1: Relationships in a society	
Primary groups *(Primary relationships)*	*Secondary groups* *(Secondary relationships)*
• Relationship is spontaneous, continuous and informal.	• Relationship is non spontaneous, non-continuous and formal.
• No specific date to start and no specific end of relationship.	• The relation starts on a specific date and ends with a specific date.
• It is a permanent group. There is a contract.	• It is a temporary group. There is no contract.
• The basis of group is 'Emotion'.	• Underlying basis is 'Business'
• Relation is first, Motive is secondary.	• Motive is first, Relation secondary.
• It is 'face to face' or related with 'We' feeling.	• No such feeling.
• The relation is present, even if the group is not physically there.	• No relation or group feeling after the contract is over.
• The relation is not transferable. It cannot be replaced by any one else.	• It is a transferable relation. Any person can come and replace the first one as in business deals.
• There is unique sense of satisfaction attached with the particular person.	• No such feelings are present
• Example: Family friends.	• Example: Business deals.

Flow chart 1.1: Social norms and their origin

```
Person x Situation ────────────────────►  Action
                                             │
      Experience +                           │
      perceptions +                          ▼
      likes and dislikes               Useful action
                                             │
                                             ▼
                                     Approved by society
                                             │
                                             ▼
 Informal expectations ◄───────────── Repetition of action
      (folkways)
         │
         │                           Action becomes part of personality
         ▼                                   │
 Formal prescription                         ▼
      (mores)                        Internalisation of action
         │                                   │
         │                    ◄───────────────
         ▼                                   │
 Written and codified rules          ▼
      (laws)                    Externally mandatory action
```

of being penalized but because it is obligatory in the proper situation. They are enforced by informal social controls like gossip and ridicule. Their origin is usually unplanned and obscure. Examples of such expected forms of behaviour include the ways of greeting, dressing, eating, etc. Folkways vary from culture to culture and society to society. Certain folkways may be common, but otherwise they lend uniqueness to a culture. They are necessary for the group solidarity. Vitality of a group is indicated by the extent to which people follow or abide by folkways.

Mores

Mores are socially acceptable ways of behaviour that involve moral standards. There are greater feelings of horror about violating mores and greater unwillingness to see them violated. While each folkway is not considered tremendously important and is not supported by an extremely strong sanction, each more is believed to be essential for social welfare. Sanctions are informal and the reactions of the group are spontaneous rather than official action.

This is transformation of informal expectation (*folkways*) to formal prescriptions (*mores*)

Folkways are, so to speak, the protoplasm of the cell, the bulky part, while the mores form the nucleus, the essential part.

Taboos

These are the specific types of mores expressed in negative. Examples are abstinence from beef, pork and smoking in Hindus, Muslims, and Sikhs respectively; and also from marrying outside one's own ethnic, caste or religious group.

Laws

Some important mores are converted into laws in order to ensure implementation. This is the last step in the formulation of rules of conduct in a society. Laws are not only prescribed in the written form but are enforced through specific machinery created by society for this purpose.

Let us illustrate the concept of folkways, mores and laws through the example of marriage. The institution of marriage involves several obligations such as:

1. Barat or the marriage party.
2. Performance of garlanding ceremony.
3. Bridal dress.
4. Seven rounds around the fire, i.e. septapadi in Hindu marriage.
5. Some form of dowry, etc.

These obligatory ways are all expected to be performed. Some of these may be violated, such as those relating to the number of persons in the marriage party, garlanding ceremony, dowry, etc. However, this is condemned only at whispering level. On the other hand, it is never expected that a boy may come alone to the bride's house asking the parents to send their daughter with him. Some witnesses, at least, must be present and saptapadi must be performed. Without these rituals marriage may be nullify in law. Thus, if the society feels that its vital or organic essence is in danger due to violation at some conduct or mores, these are written and codified, e.g. Marriage Act, Anti-dowry Act, etc.

Customs and Habits

Custom is a broad term embracing all the norms classified as folkways and mores. It refers primarily to practices that have been repeated by a number of generations, practices that tend to be followed simply because they have been followed in the past. Customs have a traditional mass character. On the other hand, a *Habit* is a purely personal affair, not entailing any obligation. Examples are: having a cup of bed tea, smoking a cigarette after dinner, eating two meals a day, bathing daily, etc. When habits are shared for their necessity and are sanctioned by the society, they are converted into customs in due course of time.

Etiquettes and Conventions

Etiquettes are concerned with choice of the proper form for doing something in relation to other people. Convention is merely an agreed upon procedure. Thus, entering a bus from the rear with exit from front is a convention. When a procedure is adopted and repeated time and again, it may become a rule.

Social Values

Like social norms, values also constitute an important part of the selective behaviour of man. Values refer to those standards of judgment by which things and actions are evaluated as good or bad, moral or immoral, beautiful or ugly. Thus, values are directive principals of human action and serve as criteria for selection. Norms and values are not the same things. It is said that norms are enactment of social values. Every society lays down certain rules of conduct to support its value system. Norms are repeated, sanctioned pattern of behaviour and their philosophical facet is the value. For Example, it is a norm that no man should be differentiated in terms of sex, caste, colour or creed while practising the art of medicine. The value behind it is that "all men are born free and equal".

Culture

Culture means socially inherited characteristics of human groups. It comprises everything, which one-generation can tell, convey or hand down to the next. In other words, it has non-physically inherited traits. Man is distinguished from animals by virtue of the fact that he possesses culture, i.e. he can speak, can frame ideas and has manners, customs, etc. He is a humanist, has sympathy towards others and understands his fellow beings. Man learns from his fellow beings and the society regarding how to behave towards others. Ways of life are cultivated or cultured in an individual by others in the group and the individual becomes social or civilized as a result.

The Oxford English dictionary defines culture as *the training and refinement of mind, tastes and manners, the condition of being thus trained and refined*. Culture is a dynamic force of society. It is the cumulative experience of mankind's history from the origin to the present. Animals are usually more strong and resistant than man. They can often fight natural disasters in a better manner. But man has the power to control nature through his culture. Culture is the total way of life from birth to death, from day to night, at home and work. It embraces all modes of thought and behaviour.

Culture has three parts. It is an experience, which is "learned, shared and transmitted." It is said that Culture is a social heritage, a product of specific and unique history. It is the distinctive way of life of a group of people, their complete design for living. Civilization on the other hand, is the whole machinery or system of devices developed by man.

HEALTH AND VARIOUS INSTITUTIONS

Health and Economics

Economics studies the production, distribution and consumption relationship of man in the society. There are three levels at which economics operate in relation to man and society. These are:
• Individual level
• Individual community interface level
• State level

Individual Level

In economic term, health is more or less a purchasable commodity, even though the government has strived to provide health services to the people. The three basic essentials for human living, namely food, shelter and clothing are directly related with purchasing power of an individual and these are, in a way, directly or indirectly related with health and disease of man.

Individual Community Interface Level

The relation between economic development and health has been well recognized even though poverty is never mentioned as a cause of disease in medical records. The following facts are obvious in this connection.
a. Physical health of poor people is unsatisfactory.
b. Communicable diseases are related to low standard of living in a community.
c. Social ill health is commoner in low socioeconomic groups. Examples are drug abuse, childhood delinquency, sexually deviant behaviour, etc.

State Level

Allotment of budget and public health are very closely related. If the people are not healthy, they cannot contribute to progress and economic upliftment of the country.

Politics and Health

Politics is the institution of governing and administration. It is becoming more and more important in relation to health. Health is a state responsibility, as laid down in the constitution of India. *The state shall, within the limits of its economic capacity and development, make effective provisions for securing right to work, to education and to public assistance in cases of unemployment, old age, sickness and disablement. The state shall regard the raising of the level of nutrition and standard of living of its people and improvement of public health as among its primary duties.*

It is important to realize that the politician can play a crucial role in health since, within the limited resources, it is he who fixes the priority. It has been said that, "the solution of many of today's, problems will not be found in the research laboratories of our hospital, but in our parliaments."

FAMILY AND HEALTH

Family is the basic unit of society. It is the germinal cell from which the society at large develops. In a family, the man and woman may be going to work and children may be going to school. The man may be member of some political party, the woman may be attending religious gathering and the children may be enjoying a picnic party. But, ultimately they all come back to one dwelling under one roof. The inference is that all other institutions are peripheral to the family. One can be a member of several institutions, but one cannot spend his whole life in those institutions. Family is the nuclear unit upon which the life of the society depends.

The origin of family, the basic social unit, is primarily biological. Sex is a basic need, the sexual impulse being related to the instinct of self-preservation of mankind. Breast feeding serves to enhance parental attachment and affection. Pregnancy, delivery and lactation are, no doubt, physiological processes, but woman needs help and co-operation during these periods. This help and co-operation adds the sense of sociality to the biological unit.

In view of the foregoing, the family is defined as *a group characterized by a sex relationship sufficiently precise and enduring for the procreation and upbringing of children.*

Fundamental Features of Family

Universal Nature

It is the most universal and found in all societies. Everyone is or has been a member of a family.

Emotional Basis

It is based on two types of instincts and emotions.
a. Primary instincts of organic nature, i.e. of procreation, mating, maternal devotion and parental care.
b. Secondary type of emotions, e.g. romantic love, pride of race, jealousy, personal possession.

Economic Unit

It is the most important feature of the family and it represents the best example of socia-lized pattern, i.e. work according to capacity and maintenance according to need.

Responsibility of Members

It is a form of active co-operation amongst various members. Everybody is assigned a responsibility. Elders look after the children, nourish and educate them. Males busy them-selves mainly with outdoor activity and physical protection. Females maintain the house, etc. In this way infants, pregnant women, parents and grand parents, all members in the family look after sick and the needy.

Formative Influence

The family has the highest formative influence on children born in the family. A very well known proverb that ' Civilization starts from the home', seems true.

Education

The family is the most effective agency for transmission of the cultural heritage from generation to generation. From sex education to business techniques, all are taught in the family.

Limited Size and Nuclear Position

It is a necessary group of very limited size, defined by biological relationship.

Functions of Family

The five basic functions of family are:
1. Sexual gratification
2. Procreation
3. Socialization of birth of children
4. Economically viable production consumption unit.
5. Caring of vulnerable individuals like infants, elders, pregnant women, etc.

Types of Family

Family of Orientation

The family in which the individuals are born is called the family of orientation.

Family of Procreation

The family that the individual creates after marriage is called the family of procreation.

There are three basic types of families according to arrangement of members of the family.
a. Nuclear family
b. Joint family
c. Extended Nuclear family

a. Nuclear Family

It is the simplest form of family where husband, wife and unmarried children residing under the same roof. In this type, these members form the nucleus and all other relatives are present around the nucleus. The major decision in the family is taken by this nucleus. Even the old parents are outside the nucleus. Thus, there is a conjugal arrangement in this type.

b. Joint Family

It is the lateral extension of the nuclear family, in which the families of siblings live together. It can be pictured as the nucleus of blood relatives surrounded by fringe of spouses. Daughter-in laws, Son-in laws and relatives from the maternal side are not included while taking major decision in the family.

c. Extended Nuclear Family

It is a linear extension of the nuclear family and consists of husband, wife and their married children or nuclear family with old parents.

CHANGING CONCEPT OF HEALTH IN THE SOCIETY

Health remains a matter of concern to man, since time immemorial. It can be traced back to superstitious or magic medicine and traditional medicine. But with the development of scientific concept of health and disease has been redefined. Apart from agents of diseases, like bacteria, viruses, chemical and nutritive elements, social factors in health and disease are very well recognized.

Primitive Medicine

Henry Siegerist, the medical historian has stated that every *culture* had developed a system of medicine and medical history is nothing but one aspect of the history of *culture*. Since, there is an organic relationship between medicine and human advancement, any account of medicine at a given period should be viewed against the civilization and human advancement at that time.

Since, the knowledge of primitive man was limited, he attributed disease and infact all human suffering and other calamities to the wrath of God and the invasion of body by evil spirits. The concept of disease in which ancient man believed is known as the supernatural theory of disease. In a logical sequence, the medicine he practised consisted in appeasing God, by prayers, rituals and sacrifices. He practised the ways to drive out, 'Evil Spirits' from the human body by witchcrafts and other crude means.

The rudiments of primitive medicines still persist in many parts of the world. The supernatural theory of disease is not obsolete.

For example, in India, one may still talk of worshiping Goddess during outbreak of Measles. Leprosy is still considered a sin of past and many more. A class of 'traditional healers' is present everywhere to carry out the supernatural phenomenon of diseases.

Various Systems of Medicine

Ayurveda and Siddha are the medical systems of Indian origin. Ayurveda is practised throughout India and has a state sponsorship, may be a meagre one. Atreya, Charaka, Susruta, and Vaghbatta are celebrated authorities in Ayurvedic medicine. A classic Susruta samihita is treasure of surgical knowledge of that time.

Chinese medicine claims to be the world's first organized body of medical knowledge dating back to 2700 BC. They were also early pioneers of immunization.

Egypt had one of the oldest civilizations, about 2000 BC. A lot is known about ancient Egypt because they invented picture writing and recorded their work on papyrus. In realm of public health, the Egyptians excelled. They built planned cities; the public baths and underground drains that even the modern might envy.

The Greeks enjoyed the reputation - 'the civilizers of the ancient world.' They taught man to think in terms of 'Why' and 'How'. By far the greatest physician in Greek medicine was *Hippocrates*, who is often called the, *Father of Medicine*. He was infact the first true epidemiologist, who was constantly seeking the causes of disease. His book, *Air, Water and Places* is considered a great treasure of social medicine and hygiene. His concept of 'Health and Disease' stressed the relation between man and environment. In the first century BC, Rome became the centre of civilization and they adopted the concept of Greeks in the field of medicine. The fall of Roman empire lead the civilization to Dark Age.

Origin of Scientific Medicine

This period can be traced from 1453 to 1600 AD when Fracstorious, an Italian physician put forward the 'The Theory of Contagion'. He found that syphilis is a sexually transmitted disease and became the founder of Epidemiology.

The 17th Century brought out new discoveries. The discoveries of microscope by Leeuwenhoek opened a new channel in the field of medicine.

In 18th Century, Jenner's vaccination against small pox was another milestone in this direction. Another progress in the field of medicine was sanitary awakening, which took place in England in the mid-nineteenth century.

Louis Pasteur, for the first time disproved the theory of spontaneous generation, on the basis of his demonstration of bacilli in the air. He put forward the 'Germ Theory of Diseases'. Robert Koch confirmed the Germ theory when he demonstrated bacilli of Anthrax. After that one after the other Bacilli were discovered.

History of Public Health

Concept of public health emerged in England around 1840. Peter Franck, a health philosopher, conceived public health as 'good health laws' enforced by the police and also postulated that the health of people is state responsibility. All his views were translated into practice, when Public Health Act of 1848 came into force in England. The early phase of public health is often called the 'disease control phase' when more stress was given towards general cleanliness and disposal of waste.

One of the leading public health men, Winslon defined public health as the science and art of preventing disease, prolonging life and promoting health and efficiency through organized community effort.

With the advance of preventive medicine and practice of public health, a new concept, the concept of 'Risk Factors' as determinants of the diseases especially non-communicable diseases, came into existence. Social and behavioral aspects of disease and health were given a new priority, and the public health moved into the preventive and rehabilitative aspects. Currently, the public health is marching towards the philosophy of 'Health For All'.

CONCEPT OF PREVENTIVE, SOCIAL AND COMMUNITY MEDICINES

Preventive Medicines

It came into picture with the discovery of vaccines and antisera, which lead to prevention of many diseases in specific.

By definition, it applies to healthy people as distinct from public health. It is the science of preventing disease and promotion of health by the action affecting large number of people.

Now the new advances like insecticides, drugs like antimalarial, antileprosy, antitubercular have given boost to preventive medicine in the field of chemoprophylaxis. Screening of diseases is another chapter added to preventive medicines. Today, its canvas is very wide and it has four levels.

1. *Primordial prevention:* Changing life stye and minimizing risk factors.
2. *Primary prevention:* Prevent diseases among healthy.
3. *Secondary prevention:* Early diagnosing the diseases by screening and routine checkups.
4. *Tertiary prevention:* Reduce chronic disability.

Social Medicine

In the beginning of 20th century, the concept made its appearance, with the philosophy that, "Man is not only a biological animal, but also a social being and disease has social causes, social consequences and social therapy."

It got attention especially in non-communicable disease where germ theory of disease was not explainable. But once it set up its influence, than each and every aspect of health and disease came into its preview.

Its precise definition is the study of man as social being in his total environment. All the external factors, which influence man, must be taken into consideration while studying the medicine. These external factors are economical, educational, cultural beliefs, housing, standard of living, etc.

Community Medicine

This is a new concept in medicine. It is an evolutionary step, which has been studied in public health, preventive health, social health, etc.

All these share the concept of promotion of health and preventing the disease, but community medicine finds the solution to health or disease problems not only in the setting of a clinic or hospital, but also in the community setting with an active community participation.

Philosophy of Health for All

With the birth of the WHO (World Health Organization), a revolution in the field of health took place at an International level.

In the sequence of events, the 30th World Health Assembly resolved in May 1977 that, 'the main social target of governments and WHO in the coming decades should be the attainment by all citizens of the world by the year 2000 of a level of health that will permit them to lead a socially and economically productive life.' This culminated in the international objective of *Health for All by the year 2000* as the social goal for all governments.

Health for all means that health is to be brought within the reach of every one in a given community.

Health for all implies the removal of obstacles to health. Health for all depends on continued progress in medicine and health.

PRIMARY HEALTH CARE

This approach to health care came into existence in 1978. The *Alma-Ata conference* defined primary health care as *Essential health care made universally accessible to individuals and acceptable to them.* It is affordable to the families with their full participation.

It was described as a best approach to achieve the goal of health for all.

Elements of Primary Health Care

1. Education concerning prevailing health problems and the methods of preventing and controlling them.
2. Promotion of food supply and proper nutrition.
3. An adequate supply of safe water and basic sanitation.
4. Maternal and child health care, including family planning.
5. Immunization against major infectious diseases.
6. Prevention and control of locally endemic diseases.
7. Appropriate treatment of common diseases and injuries
8. Provision of essential drugs.

Principles of Primary Health Care

Equitable Distribution

The key principle in primary health care strategy is equity or equitable distribution of health services, i.e. health services must be shared equally by all people irrespective of their ability to pay and all must have access to health services.

Community Participation

There must be a continuing effort to secure meaningful involvement of the community in the planning, implementation and maintenance of health services, besides maximum reliance on local resources such as manpower, money and materials.

One approach that has been successfully tried in India is the use of Village Health Guides (VHG) and Trained Birth Attendants (TBA).

Inter-sectoral Co-ordination

The declaration of *Alma Ata* states that,"Primary health care involves in addition to the health sector, all related sectors and aspects of national and community development; in particular agriculture, animal husbandry, food industry, education, housing, public works, communication and other sectors."

Appropriate Technology

This has been worded as 'the technology that is scientifically sound, adaptable to local needs and acceptable to those who apply it and those for whom it is used and that can be maintained by the people themselves in keeping with the principles of self reliance with the resources the community and country afford.'

This signifies a new dimension in the primary health care. It has been described as 'Health by the people; placing people's health in people's hands.'

DENTAL CARE AND HEALTH

An increasing amount of attention is presently being focused on the study of health services in general. Health services research is mainly concerned with the organization, staffing, financing, utilization, and evaluation of health services. It produces knowledge that will contribute to improved delivery of health care. It is also concerned with understanding the psychological, social, cultural, and economic factors that contribute to the availability and utilization of services.

According to a WHO Expert Committee, dental health services may be defined as *those services, which are designed to promote, maintain or restore dental health.* Public or community dental health services are those dental health services, which have an educative, preventive or curative nature, which are organized by governments (central, regional or local), with government resources only or with participation from other individuals or agencies. Dental health may also be defined as *a state of complete normality and functional efficiency of the teeth and supporting structures and also of the surrounding parts of the oral cavity and of the various structures related to mastication and the maxillofacial complex.*

The general objectives of the health services system are often expressed as health promotion and the prevention and treatment of disease. Analogically, the general goals of dental care could be expressed as dental health promotion, and the prevention and treatment of dental disease.

The objective can be analyzed at different levels. Most researchers dealing with program evaluation agree that clarification of a program's ultimate goal is one of the most difficult phases of the evaluation. Studies of intermediate goals are often easier to carry out, but the information gained is always limited. These are justified only when the relationship between intermediate and ultimate goals has already been demonstrated or will be tested in subsequent studies. When analyzing goals in dentistry a distinction should be made between dental care and dental health. The relationship between them is more complex than is generally realized.

Providers of medical care have long been aware of a health paradox: the more care given, the more care is needed. Saved life and cured disease often imply further care for a long time in future. This paradox applies in dentistry, too. Teeth that would have been lost a few decades ago, can now be saved. The more the treatment given today, the more treatment will be needed tomorrow. Dental treatment alone does not guarantee good dental health.

The planners are becoming increasingly aware that additional expenditure for medical services will not in itself guarantee a favourable return in health. Investments in dentistry, for instance, training more dentists, do not as such guarantee better dental health. Before considering dental care, for instance, in the form of increased utilization of dental health services, as a goal for community dentistry, it should be made certain that maximizing this care also maximizes dental health. Programmes and plans should be carefully evaluated in this respect. There can be special goal for dental health services such as equity of access, moderation of costs and assurance of quality. Many communities may wish to alter the present pattern of utilization of dental health services to promote equality between different socioeconomic groups. A change of this kind may result in greater social justice but not necessarily better dental health in the long run.

GOALS OF COMMUNITY DENTISTRY

The procedure of 'goal-setting' for health care starts with some value judgement, either explicit or implicit. The goal to be formulated is then derived from this value. In dentistry the value could be : it is good to have healthy natural teeth. There can be several alternatives for formulating goals from this value.

Perfect dental health for each person is an unrealistic goal. Philosophically, the goal of complete freedom from disease and struggle is almost incompatible with the progression of life. Giving the present generation all the dental treatment it needs according to prevailing dental treatment standard is also economically unrealistic.

Reducing the goal to 'good dental health for most people' implies a choice. What is good dental health and who should have it? For planning purposes there is no universal answer. Health planning must be related to the community and period of time in question. A large number of measurements and standards must be defined such as, health status and needs of the community resources, activities and attitudes of staff and clients, standards of practice and impacts of effects of the programs. This also applies to community dentistry.

The assessment of priorities is a difficult task. Most often it is conducted by a series of informed guesses, value judgements, and percentage additions or subtraction from past efforts.

The ultimate goals of health services are almost similar in all countries. They are derived from basic ethical norms and social values. Very different methods and immediate objectives can be used to achieve them. For instance, the role the society plays in organizing health services varies from country to country.

Most people agree that dental care should be provided at least to the extent that everybody can get relief in case of toothache and that everybody is able to chew properly. Consideration of these basic wishes may constitute a reasonable goal in some communities.

The dental profession is becoming more and more aware that good dental health, no matter how generously it is defined, will never be gained for a whole community by means of restorative dentistry. Instead, prophylaxis has long been considered to be the right way of achieving dental health. Having accepted that prophylaxis is a rational way to reduce dental disease, the next step for the planner is to investigate how this can be achieved and how long it will take at the community level.

Changing Dental Health Habits

The thrust of the present researches is to find the more traditional ways of fighting dental disease. In recent years, increasing number of social and behavioral scientists have been devoting their attention to dental problems. They, as well as many dentists, are trying to answer questions like: Which factors, psychologic, social, etc. determine the overall dental behaviour; can people be motivated to change their behaviour in favour of better dental habits? It is true in medical sociology, where

the approach is mostly been practical and not theoretical. To date, dental sociology lacks practicability. It only consists of collection of theoretical facts and statistics.

A striking feature of dental behaviour is its strong association with socioeconomic factor. Nearly all studies, national as well as international, give evidence of this correlation. Various authors have analyzed the attitude, beliefs, and behaviour at the community level. Personal and social characteristics such as age, education, sex, race, income and size of community were related to positive action and beliefs about preventing oral diseases. They concluded that income and education have the greatest influence on preventive behaviour. The majority of well-to-do, educated people usually take the advice of dentist in all preventive procedures. Beliefs in the efficacy of dental visits and tooth brushing were almost universally accepted, but these attitudes seem to have relatively little effect on the actual behaviour. However, studies have indicated that even those well informed do not take appropriate action to improve or maintain their dental health status. Dental knowledge is not necessarily translated into action.

Customarily, all major social and psychologic concepts relative to dental health behaviour have been combined. Almost every factor considered in the social - psychologic theory of preventive medicine explained at least some of the difference between who did and did not go to the dentist frequently and those who did and did not go for preventive reason. It is stated that changing dental behaviour involves a composite of interrelated factors and that the use of the dentist for preventive care is related to a complex of factors, each of which may be thought of as predisposing or motivating, but none of which explains everything.

It has been observed that dental health is a habit and part of a person's style of living that is not easily influenced by a dentist. Chambers proposed a concept of dental susceptibility, both to disease and to its management, and one of his hypothesis is that the number of people who are susceptible to prevention is a small fraction of those who need it. The American Dental Association presented data from a national survey showing that a person with low socioeconomic status shows the least concern for their teeth, considers them to be less important and often feels that losses are inevitable. This finding suggests that these people are the ones whose lifestyles and orientation to health makes them the least susceptible to preventive programs. Chambers gives a warning when talking about motivation in dental care. What dentists mean by motivating patients to better care at home is not motivation but persuasion or an attempt to change attitudes. Motives refer to a very small set of general needs that are shared by all human beings, e.g. food and water, love and self-respect. Preventive dentistry is not one of them.

Preventive action has been compared in dental health and disease and it was found that people who took one preventive action were the ones most likely to take the other preventive actions. People of higher socioeconomic status consistently took more preventive actions than people of lower socioeconomic level. The general population is not eagerly awaiting and acquiring preventive measures, which may increase the probability of improving their health.

Most studies which have indicated some change in the dental behaviour are characterized by highly enthusiastic dentist or dental educators and good material resources (for instance, free toothbrushes and toothpaste to participants, and free dental examination at regular intervals) and a selected group of participants. The lowest socioeconomic group is usually not included.

Studies with other than purely dental orientation also indicate that the public's concern about dental health is not what dentists might wish. When comparing teeth with other body parts, such as the nose, ear, thumb, etc. People consistently ranked teeth last.

Forming Dental Health Habits

During the past two decades much time, effort, and research throughout the world have been devoted to the study of the school dental health education. School dental health programs as such do not guarantee better dental health. Few school health administrators bother to evaluate their programs. Knowledge of dental health facts is often the central theme in dental education. Measurement of dental conditions and practices after these programs usually show negative result. Dental health facts may be learned after childhood but his knowledge does not alter performed habits. If a child has not learned proper dental health habits during his early years, it is very unlikely that any education will substantially change his habits.

Learning dental health habits does not seem to follow the traditional sequel of the 'Knowledge-> belief-> temporary action-> habit' model. It is pointed out that children learn best from activity. According to Piaget's theory, learning is doing and the child makes substantial progress when he has opportunities for sensory motor activities; cognitive knowledge with which educators are primarily concerned may not develop until behaviour, i.e. activity has occurred. The children are usually interested to know how to brush their teeth. Children are more likely to retain ideas obtained in a practical way rather than what has been taught theoretically. In order to take up the brushing habit it is not necessary to know which are your bicuspids.

It has also been found that children's dental practices are closely related to their mother's dental practices. The dental health values are family affairs. If parents go to the dentist for preventive treatment, a high percentage of teenagers children also do so in high and low income groups.

In some countries free dental treatment is offered to school children. Treatment alone when not combined with any educational/ motivational effort, does not give long term relief from caries and other ailments. Children once motivated for prophylaxis, fluoride applications and other preventive measures always show their interest and there is a good reason to believe that they will continue good dental habits even after school age.

Children who do not respond to education and show a high caries incidence can be identified at the age of 7 years. Identification at the age of 9–10 years is almost too late; the risk is then that the children will need more and more treatments. Short-term goals are usually considered as those to be attained within one or two years and long-term goals in 5–10 years. Keeping in mind that it is easier to form a habit than to change it, it might be suggested that the planning for long-term goals should be done keeping in view the overall personality.

Long term planning for better health services is to face difficulties. There is serious danger of planning on assumption, which in a few years may become obsolete. The pace of change in scientific and social development is such that rigid planning may restrict future capacity to respond to new opportunities. This is true in dentistry too.

2 Dental Public Health Administration

Public health is defined as a science, which deals with the determinants and defense of health at the population level, clinical medicine deals with diseases and their remedies at the individual level. The difference is partly marginal; the ambit of public health covers large numbers across a population, while clinical medicine renders its services to smaller number of individuals. The difference is also qualitative; the public health aims to elucidate and influence the social determinants of health, while clinical medicine focuses on the biological manifestations of health. As India experiences rapid health transition, it is confronted by an unfinished agenda of infectious diseases, nutritional deficiencies and unsafe pregnancies, as well as the rapidly escalating epidemics of non-communicable diseases.

Evolution of the concept and practice of health care in India can be traced back to the Vedic age. Health practices in India, like other countries, were integrated with the entire medical care system. In fact, in the absence of clear understanding of the causes of diseases, the emphasis was always on maintenance of health and preventive modalities. The idea about prevention and control was actually crystallized following the discovery of microbes as the causative agents of certain diseases.

In the eighteenth century, Royal Commission was appointed to look into the causes of high morbidity and mortality among army and civil population. The Commission recommended appointment of Sanitary Commissioner in each province. Later, health services were formed in India. This gave further impetus to develop research laboratories and establishment of Indian Research Fund Association. This was beginning of public health administration.

The landmarks in the development of public health services in India were:

1. The recommendation of the Government of India in 1912 to appoint health officers in each district and municipality. This necessitated the arrangement of training in public health in India and its multidisciplinary status.
2. A special postgraduate diploma course, namely Diploma in Public Health (DPH) was started at the School of Tropical Medicine, Calcutta in 1920, the year of starting the school.
3. Establishment of a institute of public health (All India Institute of Hygiene and Public health, Calcutta) to train medical graduates and other health personnel. The Rockefeller Foundation provided the grant.
4. Establishment of health survey and development committee by the Government of India, popularly known as the Bhore Committee, to prepare a plan for entire health services in India.
5. Acceptance of the recommendation of the committee to introduce primary and subsidiary health centres all over India as the most practical way of providing rural health services in India.
6. Appointment of an Environmental Sanitation Committee, under the chairmanship of Dr. B.C. Dasgupta, Director of Health Services, Govt of West Bengal, in 1952.

7. Establishment of a Central Committee for the control and eradication of Cholera and smallpox, under the auspices of the Indian Council of Medical Research in 1958.

DEVELOPMENT OF THE HEALTH SYSTEM

Health Policies and Strategies

The national health policy was concerned keeping in view the current needs of the society. The main goal of this policy was to evolve a policy structure to reduce the inequalities among the different sections of the society and to see that public health services are provided to all sections of the people.

The main objective is to achieve an acceptable standard of good health among the general population of the country. The approach would be to increase access to the decentralized public health system by establishing new infrastructure in deficient areas, and by upgrading the infrastructure in the existing institutions. Emphasis will be given to increase the aggregate public health investment through a substantially increased contribution by the Central Government.

Further, the rational use of drugs within the system will also be emphasized. Increased access to tried and tested systems of traditional medicine will be ensured. The objectives of the health policy are to achieve the goals of eradicating Polio and Yaws by 2005, eliminate leprosy by 2005, kala azar by 2010, lymphatic filariasis by 2015, achieve a zero level growth of HIV/AIDS by 2007, reduce mortality on the account of TB, Malaria and other vector borne diseases by 2010, reduce prevalence of blindness by 0.5 percent by 2010, reduce Infant Mortality Rate to 30/1000 and Maternal Mortality Ratio to 100/100,000 by 2010, increase utilization of public health facilities from less than 20 to more than 75 percent by 2010, and establish an integrated system of surveillance.

The public health administration at the State level is to render effective service delivery. The contribution of the private sector in providing health services would be much enhanced, particularly for the population group, which can afford to pay for services. Priority will be given to preventive and first-line curative initiatives at the primary health level through increased sectoral share of allocation.

National Health Accounts and Health Statistics by 2005 show increase in the expenditure by the government as a percentage of the GDP from the existing 0.9 percent to 2 percent by 2010, increase share of the central grant to constitute at least 25 percent of the total spending by 2010, increase State sector health spending from 5.5 percent to 7 percent of the budget by 2005 and further increase it by 8 percent by 2010. The policy places great reliance on the strengthening of primary health structure for the attaining of improved public health outcomes on an equitable basis.

Inter-sectoral Cooperation

Inter-sectoral cooperation is essential for the betterment of health services in India. Public health mainly depends on adequate nutrition, safe drinking water, sanitation, a clean environment, primary education, etc. which are all interconnected. There is a need to have interrelated policies. The Expert committee on Public Health System, the Bajaj committee (1996) has emphasized the need for coordination with other sectors for better health outcomes. It has suggested to set two committees, one is cabinet committee on health and the other committee of secretaries comprising all departments concerned with activities influencing health outcomes, like education, sanitation, drinking water, environment, nutrition, etc.

Organization of the Health System

The healthcare services in the country are organized in such a way that the facilities be extended from the national level to the village level. The organization structure of the healthcare system is provided at national, state, district, community, primary health centres and sub-centre levels.

National Level

The organization at the national level consists of the Union Ministry of Health and Family Welfare. The Ministry has three departments, viz. Health, Family Welfare, and Indian system of medicine and Homeopathy, headed by two Secretaries, one for Health and Family Welfare and the other for Indian system of medicine and homeopathy. The department of Health is supported by a technical wing, the Directorate General of Health Services, headed by the Director General of Health Services (DGHS).

State Level

The organization at the State level is under the State Department of Health and Family Welfare in each State headed by the Minister and with a Secretary. By and large, the organizational Structure adopted by the State is in conformity with the pattern of the Central Government. The State Directorate of Health Services, as the technical wing, is an attached office of the State Department of Health and Family Welfare and is headed by a Director. However, the organizational structure of the State Directorate of Health Services is not uniform throughout the country. For example, in some states, the Programme Officers below the rank of Director of Health Services are called Additional Director of Health Services, while in other states they are called Joint/Deputy Director, Health Services. But regardless of the job title, each programme officer below the Director of Health Services deals with one or more subject(s). Every State Directorate has supportive categories comprising of both technical and administrative staff.

The area of medical education which was integrated with the Directorate of Health Services at the State, has once again shown a tendency of maintaining a separate identity as Directorate of Medical Education and Research. Some states have created the posts of Director (Ayurveda) and Director (Homeopathy). These officers enjoy a larger autonomy in day-to-day work, although sometimes they still fall under the Directorate of Health Services of the State.

Regional Level

In certain states, regional or divisional set-ups have been created between the State Directorate of Health Services and District Health Administration. Each regional/divisional set-up covers three to five districts and acts under authority delegated by the State Directorate of Health Services. The status of officers/in-charge of such regional/divisional organizations may differ, however, they are designated as Additional/Joint/Deputy Directors.

District Level

Many states have reorganized their health services structures in order to bring all healthcare programs in a district level. The district level structure of health services is a link between the State/regional structure on one side and the peripheral level structures such as primary health centre/sub-centre on the other side. It receives information from the State level and transmits the same to the periphery by suitable modifications to meet the local needs. It brings out various issues of general, organizational and administrative nature in relation to the management of health services. The district officer with the overall control is designated as the Chief Medical Officer or Chief Health Officer. These officers are in-charge of the health and family welfare programs in the district. They are responsible for implementing the programs according to policies laid down and finalized at higher levels, i.e. State and Centre. The number of such officers, their specialization and status in the cadre of state civil medical services differ from state to state. Due to this, the span of control and hierarchy of reporting of these programme officers vary from state to state.

Sub-divisional/Taluka Level

At the taluka level, healthcare services are rendered through the office of Assistant District Health and Family Welfare Officer (ADHO). Some specialities are made available at the taluka hospital. The ADHO is assisted by Medical Officers. These hospitals are being gradually converted into Community Health Centres.

Community Level

For a successful primary healthcare programme, effective referral support is to be provided. For this purpose, one Community Health Centre (CHC) has been established for every 80,000 to 1, 20,000 population, and this centre provides the basic speciality services in general m1edicine, pediatrics, surgery, obstetrics and gynecology. The CHCs are established by upgrading the sub-district/taluka hospitals or some of the block level Primary Health Centres (PHCs) or by creating a new centre wherever absolutely needed.

Primary Health Centre Level

At present, there is one Primary Health Centre covering about 30,000 (20,000 in hilly, desert and difficult terrains) or more population. Many rural dispensaries have been upgraded to create these PHCs. Each PHC has one medical officer, two health assistants (one male and one female) and the supporting staff. For strengthening preventive and promotive aspects of healthcare, a post of Community Health Officer (CHO) was proposed to be provided at each PHC, but most states could not provide the same.

Sub-centre Level

The most peripheral health institutional facility is the sub-centre manned by one male and one female multi-purpose health worker. At present, in most places there is one sub-centre for about 5,000 population (3,000 in hilly and desert areas and in difficult terrain). The constitutional amendments have given powers to the local bodies in some states of India. In the process, different states have adopted different stakeholders for the benefit of health services with the help of community participation, which gives stress on safe drinking water and sanitation at village level. The Panchayats are given the power to look after the welfare of the people.

Health Information System

Census

The census in India started on regular basis from the year 1891 and the last one was conducted in the year 2001. The data represents the situation as on 1st March (except 1971 census when it was 1st April). It normally provides age and sex structure and spatial distribution of population. In addition, it also provides information on some socio-economic factors. Occasionally, some additional information is also obtained like mortality, disability, etc. Among all sources of information, census information reaches maximum accuracy.

Civil Registration System

It is a continuous permanent systematic activity of enlisting vital events countrywide. Considering its utmost importance, this activity is given legal status through a special Act, "Birth and Death Registration Act 1969." Authorities like local registrar, registrar general under the act in different areas like rural, urban have been designated from various sectors. Normally, the local registrar is from local self-government or from health department. General apathy leads to gross under-registration from time to time and differs from place to place. There is often a considerable time gap between collection of data and its compilation and publication.

Sample Registration System

The government of India introduced the Sample Registration System (1964) for improving reliability of data pertaining to vital events in the states as well as the country. The system also helps in segregating urban and rural data. A government servant, usually a teacher, is selected and trained to function as enumerator. A baseline survey of sample units is conducted to obtain information about usual resident population of the same sampling areas. The enumeration of births and deaths is continuously carried out. Every six months, a supervisor makes a visit and independently checks all the households in the area of enumerator. Thus, it functions as a continuous process and is also superimposed by periodic retrospective surveys. Unmatched or partially matched events after verification are added. Sometimes, additional information is also collected through sub samples. Presently, this is supposed to be most accurate data source providing information about birth rate, death rate, age specific death rates, infant mortality rate, age and sex composition, and seasonal and spatial variations in these statistics. It has been decided to collect data pertaining to causes of deaths on regular basis.

National Sample Surveys

The National Sample Survey Organisation regularly conducts nation-wide surveys collecting information regarding social, economical, demographic, industrial and agricultural conditions. The organisation has many wings. One wing holds the charge of designing the sample survey and improving quality of data, etc. Another wing consists of well trained full time personnel who actually conduct surveys. The organisation also obtains support from state statistical organizations. Normally, the surveys collect multi-sectoral information. The surveys are conducted in the form of rounds stretched over a specific period, generally one year. The first round was carried in the year 1951 and 55th round in the year 1999-2000. The organisation has published extensive information. Health information is also a part of such surveys.

Service Statistics

Information generated from sub centre level is fed to the health information system on specifically designed reporting formats submitted monthly. The health and family welfare information is compiled at the district level and submitted to the state level from where it goes to the central level.

Ministry of Health and Family Welfare brings out two publications yearly, i.e. Family Welfare Yearbook and Health Information Yearbook. These yearbooks compile all information available from various sources and present by districts, states and country.

In addition, all India surveys are also conducted such as National Family Health Survey, etc.

National disease surveillance is also conducted. This surveillance exists only for polio and HIV/AIDS. However, there is a need for a strong disease surveillance network in the whole country for better information on diseases and health initiatives.

Community Action

A considerable change has happened in the last two decades towards implementation of the government's action plans through the institutions of civil society and NGOs. It is to be recognized that a widespread debate on various public health issues has, in fact, been initiated and sustained by NGOs and other members of the civil society. Also, an increasing contribution is being made by such institutions in the delivery of different components of public health services. Certain disease control programmes require close interaction with the beneficiaries for the regular administration of drugs, periodic carrying out of pathological tests, dissemination of information regarding disease control, and other general health information.

Health Research and Technology

Research in the private sector has assumed some significance only in the last decade. In our country, where the aggregate annual health expenditure is of the order of Rs. 80, 000 crores, the expenditure on research, in both public and private sectors in 1998-99, was only of the order of Rs. 1150 crores. It would be reasonable to infer that with such low expenditure on research, it is virtually impossible to make any dramatic breakthrough within the country, by means of new molecules and vaccines; also, without minimal backup of applied and operational research, it would be difficult to assess whether the health expenditure in the country is being incurred through optimal applications and appropriate public health strategies.

NATIONAL RURAL HEALTH MISSION

The National Rural Health Mission (NRHM) was launched in April 2005 by the Government of India. It seeks to provide effective healthcare to rural population throughout the country with special focus on 18 states, which have weak public health indicators and/or weak infrastructure. These states are Arunachal Pradesh, Assam, Bihar, Chhattisgarh, Himachal Pradesh, Jharkhand, Jammu and Kashmir, Manipur, Mizoram, Meghalaya, Madhya Pradesh, Nagaland, Orissa, Rajasthan, Sikkim, Tripura, Uttaranchal and Uttar Pradesh. The Government of India would provide funding for key components in these 18 high focus states.

The NRHM will cover all the villages in these 18 states through approximately 2.5 lakh village-based "Accredited Social Health

Activists" (ASHA) who would act as a link between the health centers and the villagers. One such activist will be raised from every village or cluster of villages, across 18 states. The ASHA would be trained to advise village populations about sanitation, hygiene, contraception, and immunization to provide primary medical care for diarrhea, minor injuries, and fevers. These activists also escort patients to medical centers. They are also trained to give folic acid tablets and chloroquine to patients and to alert authorities to unusual outbreaks. ASHA will receive performance-based compensation for promoting universal immunization, referral and escort services for reproductive and child health programs (RCH), construction of household toilets, and other health care delivery programs.

Goals and Strategies

The goals of the NRHM include:
   a. Reduction in Infant Mortality Rate (IMR) and Maternal Mortality Rate (MMR).
   b. Universal access to integrated comprehensive public health services.
   c. Child health, water, sanitation and hygiene.
   d. Prevention and control of communicable and non-communicable diseases, including locally endemic diseases.
   e. Population stabilization, gender and demographic balance.
   f. Revitalize local health traditions like Ayurvedic, Yoga, Unani, Siddha and Homeopathy Systems (AYUSH).
   g. Promotion of healthy life styles.

The strategies to achieve the goals include:
   a. Train and enhance capacity of Panchayati Raj Institutions (PRIs) to own, control and manage public health services.
   b. Health plan for each village through Village Health Committee of the Panchayat.
   c. Strengthening sub-centers through an untied fund to enable local planning and action (each sub-center will have an

Untied Fund for local action at Rs. 10,000 per annum). This Fund will be deposited in a joint Bank Account of the ANM and Sarpanch and operated by the ANM, in consultation with the Village Health Committee, and other Multi Purpose Workers (MPWs).

d. A provision of 24 hour service in 50% PHCs by addressing shortage of doctors, especially in high focus states, through mainstreaming AYUSH manpower.

e. Preparation and implementation of an intersectoral district health plan prepared by the District Health Mission, including drinking water, sanitation and hygiene and nutrition.

f. Integrating vertical Health and Family Welfare programs at national, state, block, and district levels.

Constraints in NRHM

The constraints in NRHM are:

1. The technical, operational and administrative feasibility of NRHM implementation in any state of the country has not been established. There is no corrective action plan in case of failures.

2. To provide health services to the common man, it would require availability of all weather roads and transport facilities from the villages to the hospital. However, in reality, it would not be uncommon to find the SC/PHC/CHC tangentially located in a rural area because of the political consideration rather on population needs. Beneficiaries still have to travel long distances to reach these health centers to avail facilities. The new mission is being launched without taking stock of failures with previous programs.

3. The currently available regular village level health functionary is frequently not available. It is envisaged that this lacunae will be bridged by ASHA, who being a local resident would be available in the village and act as a link in the provision of primary health care services to the community. Infact, the introduction of ASHA rather than enhancing the ANMs performance, may actually increase the existing indiscipline amongst the regular village level health functionaries. There appears to be some ambivalence in the role and location of the ASHA. She is to act as a bridge between the ANM and the village and, at the same time, she is to be accountable to the panchayat. When the ANM (who is a functionary of the Health Department) herself is not accountable to the panchayat, how is the ASHA supposed to do the balancing act between the ANM and the panchayat?

4. ASHA and Voluntary Health Guide (VHG) scheme launched in 1977 are almost similar in characteristics and philosophy (people's participation in the care of their own health). The scheme was not successful. The areas of family have not been taken into consideration while planning NRHM.

5. For village level health functionaries, a better vigil with inbuilt mechanism for prompt disciplinary action is urgently required. The views of local population should be heard and necessary remedial actions should be instituted.

6. The NRHM ignores the urban population, which constitutes more than 30% of the population. The health parameters in the urban population are usually similar to the rural areas.

7. The mission has a high priority on training, especially as new components have been added. According to the projections made, for a unit of 100 ASHAs which would be in each block of 100,000 population, the total cost of training would be Rs. 741,500. In a district with 12–15 blocks, about one crore of rupees will be available for training of ASHA, which might be practically difficult.

This NRHM aims to improve rural health by targeting phased increase in the funding for the health budget up to 2–3% of the Gross Domestic Product (GDP). The mission also tries to correct most of the shortcomings of previous programs, i.e. inappropriate training, lack of technical guidance, supervision and co-ordination and poor community participation. The mission also plans to cover capacity building, public private partnership and induction of management and public health and financial personnel.

The NRHM has a central functionary named Accredited Social Health Activist (ASHA). The experts have called ASHA, a resurrection of earlier Community Health Worker (CHW) or Village Health Guide (VHG), both almost 30 year old schemes. Agreeably, ASHA is a newer and modified version of CHW but lessons learned from older scheme or causes attributed to her failure, i.e. improper selection, inadequate training, demand of fee for service, has been incorporated in the selection. At the same time, ASHA is an activist and not a worker in the health system as the previous CHW or VHGs. Besides, ASHA is more similar to the very successful and the world famous concept of 'barefoot doctors' in China.

Finding a women educated to up to 8th standard to function as ASHA will not be very difficult, as apprehended by some people. In the last two decades, the literacy rate of women has improved significantly. The selection procedure has some relaxation in exceptional cases to facilitate the mechanism.

ASHA would not be drawing any fixed salary and would be given performance based compensation, a concept which matches closely with recruitment pattern in private organizations. This may start a new era of accountability in the health system. Without even a fixed salary, if she performs, she would get more than Rs 10,000 per annum from courses such as Tuberculosis completion incentive or Allowance in Janani Suraksha Yojana (this scheme is the modification of the earlier National Maternity Benefit scheme, where women from below the poverty line community are given monitory assistance to improve the nutritional status and to encourage routine ante-natal checkups, Tetanus Toxoid immunisation and, to go for institutional delivery). Besides, there is a provision for non monetary compensation in form of recognition, awards and also state level meetings of selected ASHAs. This way, success of ASHA also depends upon the successful implementation of the other national programs.

The success of any program requires a system in place where no link is missing. Functioning from the level of ASHA, sub-centres, PHC has to be improved to bring people to a referral facility. This period in improving the health system at lower levels can be utilised for the implementation of IPHS standards at CHCs, so the raised expectations are not marred by below par facilities at CHC. As some experts have suggested, a system of concurrent evaluation should be in place and the generated data may be utilized for ongoing corrective measures at all levels.

It would be too early to predict its outcome in terms of success or failure. The necessary political will, commitment at all levels, financial support and budgetary allocations, good supporting and monitoring system, efficient scientific and political leadership and, working in coherence holds the ability to make this program successful. The doctors can play a major role by providing good scientific leadership. Maybe, the NRHM is the much dreamt program which can make 'Health for All' and 'Placing people's health in their hand' a reality.

DENTAL PUBLIC HEALTH ADMINISTRATION AND ITS SCOPE IN INDIA

Dental Public Health is a branch and speciaility of dentistry that is concerned with the diagnosis, prevention and control of dental diseases and the promotion of oral health through organized community efforts. Dental Public Health serves the community through research, health promotion, education, and group dental care programs. More broadly, dental public health has been defined as 'the science and art of preventing and controlling dental diseases and promoting dental health through organized community efforts'. It is that form of dental practice which serves the community as a patient rather than the individual. It is concerned with the dental health education of the public, with applied dental research, and with the administration of group dental care programs as well as the prevention and control of dental diseases on a community basis.

It is imperative that the dental public health specialist should have an in-depth understanding in the field of public health administration, research methodology, and the control and prevention of oral diseases. The goal of dental public health is directed towards the protection and improvement of oral health of the whole population. This goal can only be accomplished by the cooperation and understanding of public and the private sectors.

From a patient care perspective, there are many similarities between a private practitioner and the public health specialist. Instead of examining an individual, a *survey* will be conducted in the community. Like the examination of a patient, a survey is often initiated; for example, lack of access to care, high caries rate, and higher prevalence of oral cancer. The survey can be a statistical assessment of oral health problems or it can be a reflection of the attitudes and behaviors of the public. The general health history normally performed on the individual is known as the *situational analysis*, which is defined by the World Health Organization as the 'assessment of population demographics, mobility, economic resources, and infrastructure.'

In public health, the diagnosis made after the examination is represented by the *analysis of the survey*. Treatment planning for a patient is paralleled by *program planning* for a community. When a patient is presented the treatment options, he or she has the ultimate say whether or not to accept the treatment plan. Similarly, the public health specialist must remember that the communities decide which program(s) is to be accepted or rejected.

PRIMARY ORAL HEALTH CARE (POHC)

The primary oral health care is the basic need of the society; however, there are certain challenges facing the oral health, which need a public health approach.

1. Oral diseases and disorders affect oral health and well-being throughout life.
2. Use of safe and effective measures to prevent the most common dental diseases.
3. Lifestyle behaviors that affect general health (such as tobacco use) also affect oral health.
4. The mouth reflects general health and well-being.
5. Oral diseases and conditions are associated with other health problems.
6. Scientific research is key to further reduction of oral diseases and disorders.
7. There are profound oral health disparities.
8. More information is needed to improve oral health.

The 'framework for action' (US Surgeon General's Report on Oral Health) highlighted the principal components of a plan to address those issues, which were:

1. Change public perceptions regarding oral health and disease so that oral health becomes an accepted component of general health.
2. Accelerate the building of the scientific base and apply this science effectively to improve oral health.
3. Build an effective health infrastructure that meets the oral health needs of every person in the society, integrates oral health effectively into overall health.

4. Remove known barriers between people and oral health services.
5. Use public-private partnerships to improve the oral health of those who need them the most.

The American Dental Association's Future of Dentistry report adopted a vision of *Improved health and quality of life for all through optimal oral health*, and laid out seven broad recommendations to help achieve that vision, which are:

1. Establish and support partnerships and alliances among dental, other health care professional, public health organizations as well as business and social service groups in order to address common goals.
2. Aggressively address the oral health needs of the public.
3. Strengthen and expand research and education capabilities in dentistry.
4. Ensure the development of a responsive, competent, diverse, and 'elastic' workforce.
5. Develop strategies to address the fiscal needs of the practice, education and research sectors of dentistry to ensure their viability and vitality.
6. Utilizing the combined resources of the dental profession and dental industry, emphasis should be placed on the development of highly targeted, collaborative marketing and public relations initiatives.

IMPERATIVE FOR CHANGE

The arguments against primary health centres, like meager resources, poor allocation of existing resources, etc. apply equally to dentistry. It is also seen that there are significant number of people who do not have access to dental services. People living in distant locations, living in slums around large cities may and may not be working are usually dentally neglected. Oral health for them remains a dream as long as it continues to be understood in technical terms like fillings, extractions, etc.

Certain constraints do not allow the oral health to become a reality.

1. Resources for oral health programs are few and may be reduced even further as a result of economic adjustments.
2. Achieving oral health should be the overriding goal; usually it is seen as oral treatment, which should be only one of its strategies.
3. Inadequate training of the professionals.

Health care professionals essentially distrust public involvement in decision making about health care matters.

Defining Primary Oral Health Care

The WHO defines primary oral health care as 'Primary oral health care is personal oral health care, delivered in the context of family, culture and community, whose range of services meet all but the most specialized oral health needs of the individuals and families being served.'

Various attributes of the primary oral health care are:
• First contact
• Continuous
• Co-ordinated
• Comprehensive
• Community-oriented
• Family-centred
• Accessible
• Culturally competent
• Developmentally appropriate
• Accountable.

The Primary Health Care principles do apply in Primary Oral Health Care also. These are:

EQUITABLE DISTRIBUTION

• *Inequity* refers to differences that are unnecessary and unavoidable, those are also unfair and unjust.
• *Equity* is concerned with creating equal opportunities for overall health and bringing health differences to the lowest possible levels.

- It would be logical that disadvantaged people have poor oral health because they have fewer healthy alternatives and few opportunities for care. **Inverse Care Law** states that the deprived communities suffer the most.
- It is repeated that people who are poor and with limited education, minorities and older people who live in different circumstances, all continue to be dentally neglected.
- Even in rich countries like Germany, etc. which might have dental insurance system covering more than 90% of the population, extreme differences in oral health is evident.
- POHC (auxiliaries) workers, make equity a realistic goal as they provide equal access to available programs.
- In Peru, health care workers carry out simple dental measures establishing links with primary schools. The small scale oral health programs are supported by public health personnels.

Community Involvement

- Community participation means involving every member of the community.
- In Brazil, a community analyzed its own oral health problems and is struggling to include ORAL HEALTH as a human right and pressing policy makers to accept the same.

FOCUS ON PREVENTION AND HEALTH PROMOTION

- Prevention in dentistry is limited to certain services like placing a sealant, applying fluoride and providing formal dental education.
- Health promotion, a component of prevention is totally forgotten. Health promotion is defined as 'the process of enabling people to increase control over and to improve health'.

- The prevention should focus on personal and community growth supplemented with resources and to create awareness among the population. They will use that awareness to challenge the unhealthy context that surrounds them.

Appropriate Technology

- The challenge is to treat oral diseases appropriately but at a cost that individuals and communities can afford.
- The objective is not the production of cheap, second class materials and equipment, rather helping dental workers cope with economic and technological constraints. Easily available materials and techniques should be adopted.

Multisectoral Approach

- The major reason for lack of success of many oral health programs is the fact that they operate in isolation, separate from general health care structure *(WHO 1989)*.
- Oral health can be integrated into general health programs, by including oral health in general health education.

  For examples, tobacco smoking affects heart disease, respiratory diseases and oral diseases; therefore dental workers must actively participate to support programs aimed at reducing tobacco smoking.
- Oral hygiene should be included in general hygiene teaching and actions carried out by parents, teachers and health workers.
- Brushing of teeth becomes less of an isolated practice and a more important part of body grooming.
- Attention must be given to population as a whole through policies and strategies that require multi-sectoral cooperation and action.

  For example, increase availability of fluoride and promoting sugar less products.

Barriers to Primary Oral Health Care

- Inherent commitment to individuals rather than communities.
- Lack of resources.
- Lack of social and behavioral knowledge.
- Improper training of health personnels.

INTEGRATION OF PRIMARY ORAL HEALTH CARE IN EXISTING PRIMARY HEALTH CARE SYSTEMS

In accordance with essential activities of primary health care, primary oral health care should be restricted to promotional and preventive aspects along with emergency curative aspects.

The non-dental personnels, particularly primary health care personnels are the main force for the success of primary oral health care because of the following reasons:

- The demand for oral health care at primary health centres is mainly of emergency care, which does not require employment of trained dentists.
- Health care personnel (certified nursing assistants and Pediatric primary care providers (dental screening and referral) can successfully carry out emergency oral health care.
- Health personnels usually being taught behavioral and social aspects of counseling and health education. Integration of their training will cut off extra cost and save time. Integration will further remove oral health care from direct competition for funds allocated for overall health services.

Most of the countries have adopted this type of integration, whereby health assistants and even physicians take care of the oral health education.

Implementation

To pursue oral health care as a philosophy and strategy for action, four categories are proposed:

Pursue Partnerships

- Equity cannot be achieved by dentists and related personnel in isolation.
- Linkages are needed with sectors that influence oral health determinants like education, nutrition, etc.
- The dental personnel keen to pursue primary oral health care need a medical partner for the overall development of their communities.

Evaluation and Research

- Evaluating the local people helps to ensure that visible action occurs as a result of information gained.
- Such evaluation and research make dental personnel accountable to their communities.

Reform Existing Theory of Teaching

To have a clear concept,

- The oral health is to be achieved and not to be delivered.
- The present training of professionals does not prepare them to adapt easily with the local people.
- If dental personnel is to practice primary oral health care, their preparation has to be radically different.
- A reaffirmation of goal revised and different set of values are required. The values required include caring for people and being humble enough to recognize the problems and expectations of local people.

Begin with the Self

- For an effective strategy, re-examine the causes which lead to the high levels of disease process.
- Time, temperament and trust are the ingredients for initiating and sustaining community work.
- Time is needed for community empowerment.

- With the passage of time, people are capable of analyzing their own problems deciding what best can be done.

PLANNING AND DELIVERY OF A PRIMARY PREVENTIVE DENTAL SERVICE

The developed and the developing countries are undergoing a social revolution in community health. This revolution can be considered under four headings (STEP – Social, Technical, Economic and Political).

1. *Social:* The community must take the lead in dental health care activities. Each community must be educated about
   - The benefits of fluoride in reducing dental caries.
   - Validity of various oral hygiene measures for removal of dental plaque.
   - Correct food habits (restriction of eating sweets to not more than three times a day and suggesting alternatives to in between snacks).
   - Harmful affects of smoking and chewing paan or tobacco, etc.
   - Early recognition of precancerous and cancerous lesions (e.g. Ulcer in the mouth not healing for 2-3 weeks should consult dentist/medical specialist for further investigation and treatment).
   - The importance of regular visits to the dentist and the auxiliary for routine examination.
2. *Technical:* Dental health is not a specific entity but an integral part of National development.
3. *Economic:* Dental Health care must be equitably spread.
4. *Political:* Primary oral health care cannot be developed without the full support of national resources.

The philosophy of Primary Health Care (PHC), with its leading principle of 'basic oral care for all' and emphasis on prevention and affordable and sustainable services, was a guideline in framing priorities in oral health care for deprived communities.

The document outlines three key components that constitute the basic package of Oral Care.
- Oral Urgent Treatment (OUT)
- Affordable Fluoride Toothpaste (AFT)
- Atraumatic Restorative Treatment (ART).

It suggests that the package should be financed predominantly by public funding and implemented by competently trained primary (oral) health care workers.

ORAL HEALTH CARE IN INDIA

Oral Health Care Program

Oral Health Education
- Training of trainers
- Oral health care set up
- Oral health education
- School dental health programme
- Education through media
- Manpower requirement
- Equipment requirement.

Preventive Programs
- Promotion of Fluoride toothpaste
- Legislation against tobacco products
- Sugar free chewing gums
- Sugar substitutes in medicinal syrups.

LEVELS OF DENTAL SERVICE IN DENTAL PUBLIC HEALTH

Level I (Emergency Dental Services)

All public health dental clinics should provide treatment for dental emergencies. Dental emergency include an acute episode of pain, swelling, hemorrhage, or trauma. Treatment modalities for all these problems must be available at the centre.

Level II (Primary Prevention)

All public health dental clinics should provide primary preventive services appropriate for the target population. The primary preventive dental services include:

1. Oral Health Education
   a. Oral hygiene instructions
   b. Dietary counseling
   c. Prevention of traumatic injuries (seat belts and mouth guards, etc.)
   d. Effectiveness of fluoride
   e. Preventive modalities for oral cancer
2. Topical application of fluoride to include the use of fluoride varnish
3. Supplemental fluoride therapy (tablets or drops) as indicated
4. Physical, medical, and dental examinations
5. Prophylaxis
6. Pit and fissure sealants

Level III (Basic Dental Services)

The basic dental services, which eliminate oral diseases should be provided. The examples of such services include:

- Comprehensive oral diagnostic procedures.
- Facilities for dental restorations.
- Basic endodontic, periodontal procedures and oral surgery procedures.

DENTAL PUBLIC HEALTH CLINIC

The dental public health clinic should be located in a facility that provides for adequately sized clinical operatories and proper lighting to provide dental treatment in optimal conditions. It is the responsibility of the dentist to assure that the public health dental clinic is maintained in a manner that provides dental staff and patients with a clean and orderly place to work and receive dental care. The dentist is responsible for assuring that the clinic has the necessary equipment and supplies.

Every dental public health clinic must have a written protocol for management of medical emergencies. Every dental clinic must be equipped with or have ready accessibility to an emergency kit containing devices and drugs that the dentist is trained to use to support life in an emergency situation. The dentist should communicate with the appropriate medical personnel to assure that the kit is maintained with required drugs.

GENERAL TREATMENT INFORMATION

1. The parents and children should be informed concerning their role in the maintenance of good oral health. Each patient should be given home care instructions, which include oral hygiene care and dietary information.
2. Treatment of dental caries and major esthetic defects should be given the highest priority after relief of pain and infection. Treatment should follow a logical sequence. Normally, with minor variations, this is:
   - Relief of pain and suffering
   - Elimination of infection and traumatic conditions
   - Caries control
   - Prophylaxis, oral hygiene instructions
   - Restoration of teeth
   - Endodontic therapy
   - Periodontal therapy
   - Extractions
   - Replacement of teeth
   - Maintenance therapy.
3. Preventive and restorative dentistry should be emphasized.
4. A child should not be physically forced to accept treatment. If reasonable persuasion does not result in the cooperation, it is suggested that the child be referred to a pediatric dentist.
5. Respect and dignity of all patients should be maintained during interactions between patients and the dental auxiliaries.

6. Records must be kept in order to have data available on each patient's dental needs, treatment rendered, and also the effectiveness of the program.

EMERGENCY SERVICES

The dental emergency services should be immediately provided to the patients on a priority basis. If the tooth is restorable and restorative procedures cannot be accomplished at the time of the emergency, palliative care should be rendered. The time of a patient visit and the treatment given is to be recorded.

In *no* instance should a patient be sent home or referred without any measures taken to relieve his/her distress. If the patient is unable to pay the requisite fee, palliative treatment should still be provided. Patients not eligible for additional services should be referred to other dental providers for treatment.

Public health dental clinics usually operate on an appointment system. In general, parents should accompany all minors to the dental clinic and be available in the reception area. When treating minors, no treatment should be rendered without a signed consent from the parent or guardian. The emergency dental treatment must be rendered even if the consent is not signed because of any reason. Patients who qualify for additional comprehensive dental care should be scheduled for dental treatment at the public health facility. A periapical radiograph of diagnostic quality must be made prior to extracting any tooth (except in the case of primary teeth near exfoliation). Periapical radiographs reveal the preoperative condition of the hard and soft tissues. If the patient rejects radiographs being taken, written confirmation must be recorded.

The emergency condition should be treated by the most appropriate method depending upon the available resources and time. The guidelines can be:

- If the tooth can be restored, but time does not allow for a permanent restoration, a temporary or sedative filling can be placed.
- If root canal therapy is indicated, initial endodontic treatment should be performed to relieve pain. The patient should be scheduled to further treatment.
- Patients with acute conditions should receive palliative treatment and be scheduled for more definitive treatment when the acute conditions subside.
- Appropriate antibiotics and/or analgesics are prescribed, if necessary.
- If the emergency is of complex nature and is beyond the ability of the dentist, it should be referred to other appropriate dental surgeon.

PREVENTIVE SERVICES

The majority of dental caries in school-aged children is located in pits and fissures. Numerous clinical studies have demonstrated that sealants are a safe and long-term method of preventing pit and fissure caries. The use of dental sealants is a logical approach for further improvement in children's oral health. Pit and fissure sealants should be applied routinely in public health dental clinics. Indications include:

- Recently erupted teeth
- Individual history of past caries experience
- Children at high caries risk

Studies specifically designed to measure caries progression under small sealed lesions have shown minimal or no caries progression. It is recommended that sealants be placed over incipient caries because it is extremely effective in arresting this type of decay. If there is no gross oral hygiene problem or periodontal disease, the dentist should perform the operative procedures. If a patient has no restorative or surgical needs, a prophylaxis should be carried out to complete the treatment.

The use of dietary fluoride supplements is an alternative method of providing fluoride protection to the teeth of children. Dietary fluoride supplements, in the form of daily tablets, drops, or vitamin-fluoride combinations, provide systemic benefits to developing teeth as well as topical benefits to erupted teeth.

When used appropriately, fluoride supplements provide benefits similar to those obtained from ingesting optimally fluoridated water over the same period of time. When improperly used, fluoride supplements may cause enamel fluorosis. Therefore, systemic fluoride supplements should never be prescribed to children in fluoridated communities who are receiving optimally fluoridated water (0.7–1.2 ppm fluoride). Because of an increase in the milder forms of dental fluorosis associated with fluoride ingestion in excess to what is necessary to prevent tooth decay, a conservative approach to fluoride supplementation should be used.

Restorative Services

The small carious lesions or the black spots should be evaluated thoroughly. The restorative procedure should be carried out following necessary precautions.

Sedative fillings (zinc oxide eugenol) are to be used after removing the caries. In all deep cavity preparations, the pulp should be protected with a cavity liner and base. Pulp exposures and all near exposures should be indicated on the patient's record.

Defective restorations or restorations with recurrent caries should be completely removed and replaced.

Endodontic Services

Endodontic services can be provided in the public health clinic if resources are available, otherwise should be referred to another dental provider for endodontic treatment.

The patient and the parent/guardian should be made aware of the consequences of extraction and the subsequent cost of prosthetic replacement. If there is no other alternative and the parent/guardian insists, then extraction of the tooth may be considered. Informed consent *must* be obtained before extracting any tooth.

Periodontic Services

If there are problems related to periodontal services, viz. gingivitis or periodontal disease, the dentist should inform the patient and parent/guardian before initiating the treatment. Routine scaling and root planning can be carried out. Moderate and severe periodontal disease should be referred to the periodontist.

Oral Surgery Services

Teeth that cannot be restored should be extracted. Deciduous teeth that are indicated for extraction *and* are near exfoliation, asymptomatic, and causing no apparent pathology can be utilized as space maintainers. When any tooth is extracted, all portions of the tooth should be removed, except under circumstances if it is necessary to leave a root tip, the patient should be informed accordingly and all information should be recorded.

Patients who have had oral surgical procedures should be scheduled for a postoperative evaluation. The oral surgery procedures, complications, quantity and type of anesthesia, post-operative instructions, medications and referrals must be recorded.

Referrals

Dental public health facilities should provide comprehensive oral diagnosis, oral disease preventive services, and routine dental treatment. However, it is recognized that in certain instances, children may be referred to pediatric dentists. Also, referrals should be made for services not offered in the dental facility. All referrals for medical/dental consultation or treatment should be documented in the patient's dental record.

Patient Recall

Each patient undergoing dental treatment should be placed on a recall, based on the individual patient's needs. The customary recall period is six months after the last operative visit unless special conditions exist that indicate a need for a more frequent recall schedule.

BIBLIOGRAPHY

1. Armfield, J.M.: Socio-economic inequalities in child oral health: A comparison of disease and composite area-based measures. *J. Public Health Dent*: 2007;67:119.
2. Banergy D. Politics of rural health in India. *Indian J of Public Health* 2005;49:113-22.
3. Chen LC. Philanthropic partnership for public health in India. *Lancet* 2006;**367**:1800–1.
4. Isman R: Integrating primary oral health care into primary care. *J Dent. Educ.* 1993;57:846-52.
5. Jamieson, L.M. and Thomson, W.M. : The dental neglect and dental indifference seeks compared. Comm. Dent. *Oral Epidem* 2002;30:168.
6. Kapil U, Choudhary P. National Rural Health Mission, will it make a difference. *Indian Paed.* 2005;42:783.
7. Locker D, Clarke M and Payne B: Self perceived oral health status, psychological well being and life satisfaction in an older adult population. *J.D.R.*: 2000;79:970.
8. Locker D: Deprivation and oral health: *A review.* Comm. Dent. Oral Epid.: 2000;28:161.
9. McGrath C and Bedi R: Can dental attendance improve quality of life? *B.D.J.*: 2001;190:262.
10. Ragnarsson E, Eliasson ST and Gudnason V: Loss of teeth and coronary heart disease. *Int. J. Prosthodont*: 2004;17:441.
11. Reddy KS. Establishing schools of public health in India. In: Matlin S (ed). *Global Forum update on research for health. Volume 2. Poverty, equity and health research.* Geneva:Global Forum for Health Research; 2005:149–53.
12. Richards W and Ameen J: The impact of attendance pattern on oral health in a general dental practice. *B.D.J.*: 2002;193:697.
13. Richmond S, Chestnutt I, Shennan J and Brown R: The relationship of medical and dental factors to perceived general and dental health. *Comm. Dent. Oral Epidem.*: 2007;35:89.
14. Sachs JD, McArthur JW. The millennium project: a plan for meeting the Millennium Development Goals. *Lancet* 2005;365:347-53.
15. Sanders AE, Spencer AJ and Slade GD: Evaluating the role of dental behaviour in oral health inequalities. Comm. *Dent. Oral Epidem.*: 2006; 34:71.
16. Tewari A, Gauba K and Goel A. Alternate oral health care delivery system. Primary preventive model for rural India, utilizing existing health and educational infrastructure. *J Ind Soc Pedo Prev Dent* 2003; spec issue:1-162.
17. World Health Organization. Planning Oral Health Surveys. WHO Offset Publication No. 53. Geneva: *The Organization*, 1980.

3 *Nutrition and Oral Diseases*

Good nutrition, like good health, is difficult to define. As good health is judged by the absence of disease, Good nutrition is judged by the absence of nutritional deficiencies. Good nutrition can be described as a state where the nutrients are supplied to the body in adequate amount to meet the body needs, with a margin of safety to cover stress situations. Although good health cannot be maintained without good nutrition, good nutrition is not a guarantee for good health. Let us discuss the manifestations of nutritional deficiencies on the oral structures and also the importance of nutrients in our diet.

DEFINITIONS

Food

It is defined as any material, usually of plant or animal origin, that contains or consists of essential body nutrients, such as carbohydrates, proteins, fats, vitamins or minerals and is ingested and associated by an organism to produce energy, stimulate growth and maintain life.

Nutrition

It is defined as the science of food and nutrients, their action and interaction for health and disease, and the ways by which the organs ingest, digest and excrete.

Diet

The sum total of food taken by an individual is called as his diet.

Nutrients

The substances that enable cells and tissues to carry out vital functions are called nutrients.

BALANCED DIET

The human body can be divided into three components:
- Cell mass (55% of the body weight).
- Extracellular supporting tissues (30% of the body weight).
- Energy reserve held in the adipose tissue (15% of the body weight).

The structural components of the body are composed of combinations of six nutrients:- proteins, carbohydrates, fats, minerals, vitamins and water.

Table 3.1 shows the nutrients that are essential for human growth and development. Each nutrient has a specific function; however, proteins are involved in many functions, whereas others may be involved in one or two functions.

A diet is the food and drink which an individual normally takes in his routine. A balanced diet is the one which contains different types of food in such quantities and proportions that the need for energy, amino acids, vitamins, minerals is adequately met for maintaining health, vitality and general well being. It also makes a provision for extra nutrients required during difficult periods.

An adequate diet is one that supplies all the nutrients in amount sufficient for growth and development, maintenance, repair and reproduction. Nutrients are derived from food with

Table 3.1: Nutrients essential for human growth and development

Carbohydrates	Minerals	Vitamins
Monosaccharides	Calcium	**Fat soluble vitamins**
Disaccharides	Phosphorous	Vitamin A
Polysaccharides	Sodium	Vitamin D
Fats or lipids	Potassium	Vitamin E
Linoleic acid		Vitamin K
Linolenic acid		**Water soluble vitamins**
Arachidonic acid	Magnesium	Vitamin B
Proteins	Iron	Thiamine
Essential Amino acids	Selenium	Riboflavin
Leucine	Zinc	Niacin
Lysine	Copper	
Methionine	Cobalt	
Isoleucine	Molybdenum	Pyridoxine
Phenylalanine	Iodine	Cyanocobalamin
Threonine		Pantothenic acid
Valine	Fluorine	Vitamin C
Tryptophan		

various compositions. There is no single food that contains all the nutrients in the required amount and proportion. Therefore, it follows that there is no single diet which can be considered adequate for health.

The Recommended Dietary Allowance (RDA) is a guideline for the nutrient intake setup by the Food and Nutrition Board. RDA is the recommendation for the average daily amounts of nutrients which should be consumed over a period of time. Certain physical conditions like premature birth, inherited metabolic disorders, infections, chronic diseases and the use of medications require special dietary and therapeutic measures.

The following seven major food groups should be consumed in a balanced form.

• Cereals
• Pulses
• Vegetables and Fruits
• Milk and milk products
• Sugar
• Ghee/Oil
• Meat, Egg and Fish for Non-Vegetarian.

Cereals and sugar are the main sources of carbohydrates and are consumed for requirement of energy need. The protein requirement of body is met with pulses in vegetarian and with meat, egg, etc. in non-vegetarian. Pulses are also known as 'poor-man's meat'. Vegetables and fruits are consumed mainly due to their vitamin and mineral value.

The combination of the following makes a balanced diet.

• Energy from carbohydrate (60–65%), which must includes refined carbohydrates (5%).
• Energy from dietary fat (20–30%).
• Ratio of cereal protein to pulse protein: 4:1 or 5:1.
• A minimum intake of milk: 100 ml.
• Salt intake in case of tropical countries like India 10–15 gm daily.
• A minimum level of leafy vegetables (80 gm) and all vegetables (150 gm).

ENERGY REQUIREMENTS OF THE BODY

A kilo calorie (Kcal) or 1000 calories is the unit of energy used in nutrition. It is 1 food calorie or 1000 energy calories. It is the energy necessary to raise the temperature of 1 litre of water by 1° celsius. A kilocalorie is synonymous with large calorie or food calorie. Work energy is measured in Joules (1 Kcal = 4.184 K joules). The average daily requirement of energy is given in Table 3.2.

Humans derive energy by oxidizing carbohydrates, proteins and fats in foods. If no food is available as in starvation, the body tissues particularly fat, is utilized for energy. Oxygen is essential for the biological oxidation reactions that occur in our body.

The release of energy depends not only on the oxygen but also on the availability of vitamins, minerals, enzymes and hormones. Enzymes catalyze the reactions forming-Adenosine triphosphate (ATP), which is used to carry out all the functions of the cells.

For estimating the energy needs, the concept of Reference Man and Reference Woman should be clearly understood. The characteristics of these are:

Reference Man

Age	20–39 years
Weight	60 kg
Body surface area	1.62 sq. meter
BMR	38.1 Kcal/sq.m/hr.

Reference Woman

Age	20–39 years
Weight	50 kg
Body surface area	1.40 sq. meter
BMR	32.9 Kcal/sq.m/hr.

Table 3.2: Average daily requirement of energy (for Indians)		
Age	*Activity*	*K Cal/day*
Man	Light work; moderate work; heavy work	2,4252; 8753; 800
Woman	Light work; moderate work; heavy work	1,8752; 2252; 925
Pregnancy	2nd and 3rd trimester	+300 Extra
Lactation	First 6 months	+550 Extra
	6-12 months	+400 Extra
Infants	Under 3 months	120/kg body weight
	3 to 5 months	115/kg body weight
	6 to 8 months	110/kg body weight
	9 to 11 months	105/kg body weight
	Average 1st year	112/kg body weight
Children	1 to 3 years	1,240 body weight
	4 to 6 years	1,690 body weight
	7 to 9 years	1,950 body weight
	10 to 12 years (males)	2,190 body weight
	10 to 12 years (females)	1,970 body weight
	13 to 15 years (males)	2,450 body weight
	13 to 15 years (females)	2,060 body weight
	15 to 18 years (males)	2,640 body weight
	16 to 18 years (females)	2,060 body weight

Source: Indian Council of Medical Research

Both should be free from systemic diseases.

The total energy requirement in an individual is divided into two components that are: (i) energy required for basic metabolic activities like respiration, digestion, circulation, etc. (ii) energy required for actual physical activities like walking, talking, running, etc. Additionally, energy is also required even when we are off-the-work and also for specific dynamic action.

The energy requirement is directly related to energy expenditure, which is in turn governed by the following factors:
a. Basal metabolism or Basal metabolic rate
b. Physical activity
c. Energy expenditure 'off-the-work'
d. Specific dynamic action

Basal Metabolism or Basal Metabolic Rate

It is the amount of energy while at rest. Basal metabolism is that metabolism which is required to furnish the energy needed for different physiological activities. This energy is used to perform the basic internal functions of the body such as respiration, circulation and glandular activities. The Basal Metabolic Rate (BMR) is expressed as the heat expressed per hour per unit surface of the body. BMR is the amount of energy expended while at rest in neutral temperature environment, in past absorptive state (meaning that digestive system is inactive, which requires 12 hrs. of fasting in humans). The release of energy in this state is sufficient only for the functioning of vital organs, such as heart, lungs, brain and rest of nervous system. The factors that affect the BMR of an individual are:
- *Surface area:* Larger the surface area, more the heat dissipated, i.e. the BMR is less.
- *Body composition:* More lean is an individual, higher is the BMR. Thus, thin people have higher BMRs.

Measurement of BMR: BMR is measured under very restrictive circumstances, when a person is awake but at complete rest. An accurate BMR measurement requires that the person's sympathetic nervous system should not be stimulated. A more common and related measurement, used under less strict conditions is known as Resting Metabolic Rate (RMR).

Calculation of BMR: BMR is calculated by the Katch-Mc Ardle formula, i.e.

$$BMR(P) = 370 + (21.6 \times LBM)$$

where LBM = Lean body mass, in kilograms.
- *Age:* BMR decreases with age, i.e. more is the age less is the BMR.
- *Hormones:* Thyroxine, is the major BMR regulating hormone. More the thyroxine, more the BMR.
- *Growth periods:* BMR value increases during active growth periods while it decreases when growth decreases.
- *Nutritional status:* Malnourished or undernourished people have less BMR while well nourished people have high BMR (due to increased cellular activity).

Physical Activity

Physical activities do need energy. Such energy expenditure depends upon the weight of the individual, the kind and the duration of his activity. To estimate the caloric needs of a person performing an activity, it is necessary to keep a record of activities carried out during the day and the duration of each activity. The caloric cost of each type of activity is then calculated and the sum of the costs of all activities is determined. A rough estimate of caloric cost of light, moderate and heavy activity is given by ICMR to be 1.7, 2.5, 5.0 k cal/kg/hour.

Energy Required 'Off-the-Work'

Certain amount of energy is spent during sitting, standing and walking, etc. It is estimated that an Indian Reference Man may spend 1220 Kcal and an Indian Reference Woman about 826 Kcal for 8 hours off-the-work.

Specific Dynamic Action (SDA)

Specific Dynamic Action (SDA) is defined as the extra amount of heat produced over and above the caloric value of the food stuffs. The SDA of proteins is 30%, carbohydrates is 5% and of fat is 13%.

Consumption Unit

The energy requirement of an average man is considered as 1.0 coefficient, which is known as consumption unit. One consumption unit is equal to 2425 Kcal. The Table 3.3 illustrates the consumption unit of individuals according to their age, sex and activity.

Table 3.3: Energy requirement according to consumption unit

Age	Physical activity	Coefficient
Adult male	(sedentary worker)	1.0
Adult male	(moderate worker)	1.2
Adult male	(heavy worker)	1.6
Adult female	(sedentary worker)	0.8
Adult female	(moderate worker)	0.9
Adult female	(heavy worker)	1.2
12 to 21 years		1.0
9 to 12 years		0.9
7 to 9 years		0.7
5 to 7 years		0.6
3 to 5 years		0.5
1 to 3 years		0.4

One consumption unit is supposed to be of a reference man, who is sleeping for 8 hours (using energy for BMR), remaining 8 hours off the work (using energy for sitting, walking, bathing, etc.) and doing 8 hours light work (using 1.7 kcal/Kg/hr.)

NUTRITIONAL ASSESSMENT

Various methods used to assess the nutritional status of individual, family and community are:
  a. Clinical examination
  b. Anthropometry
  c. Laboratory examination
  d. Diet survey
  e. Vital statistics
  f. Ecological studies

a. Clinical Examination

The individuals are examined clinically for the presence of signs indicating nutritional deficiencies such as conjunctivae for Bitot's spot, keratomalacia, lips for angular stomatitis, nails (koilonychia) for sun deficiency, etc.

Depending upon the conglomeration of signs, the specific disease (and its severity) is diagnosed. If no sign is seen, then the individual may be declared clinically nutritionally healthy.

b. Anthropometry

• *Weight and height:* Weight and height of an individual is compared with the normal 'weight for age' and 'height for age' of normal individuals prescribed by WHO/ICMR.

Normal weight and height from birth to 5 year is tabulated in Table 3.4:

Table 3.4: Normal weight and height

Period	Weight	Height
At birth	2.8 kg	50 cm
1 year	8.4 kg	75 cm
2 years	11.2 kg	87 cm
3 years	13.5 kg	94 cm
4 years	16.0 kg	100 cm
5 years	18.5 kg	107 cm

• There is another index depicting nutritional status called the 'Quetlet index' or 'Body mass index'. It is usually used for screening at the community level.

This is calculated as:

$$\text{Body mass index (BMI)} = \frac{\text{Weight in Kilogram}}{\text{Height in cm}^2} \times 100$$

A person is said to be nutritionally healthy if his BMI is between 0.15 and 0.25.

c. Laboratory Examination

Simple investigations for detection of nutritional diseases are:

* Haemoglobin level
* Total RBC count
* Haematocrit readings
* Total serum proteins

Advanced investigations include:
* Serum Vitamin A
* Blood cholesterol
* Lipidogram, i.e. HDL, LDL
* Serum essential amino acids
* Urinary urea and creatinine, etc.

d. Diet Survey

The diet survey includes quantitative and qualitative adequacy of food taken by any individual. The various methods are:

Oral Questionnaire Method

A questionnaire is prepared regarding consumption of food, i.e. rice, wheat, vegetable, milk, etc. by the family. Total calories consumed by the family are divided by number of *consumption units* present in the family. It gives a fairly good picture of nutritional status of the family and individual. Weight of cooked food and uncooked food can also be calculated.

Stock-investment Method

A balance sheet is prepared comparing the purchase of food items for a month and number of consumption units in the family.

e. Vital Statistics

Vital statistics is the informational data maintained by a government, having records of birth and death of individuals within that government jurisdiction. This data is used in public health programs to evaluate how effective the program is. This is the cornerstone of public health systems.

It is related to malnutrition, especially among younger children. The rate of low birth weight babies and life expectancy of people provide the requisite nutritional status of a population.

Morbidity data like number of cases of anaemia, vitamin deficiencies, endemic goitre can give additional information.

f. Ecological Studies

The ecological studies include per capita supply of food and other socio-economic factors. The health and educational services provided in the community is also included in ecological studies.

FOOD

We eat different types of food. The intake of food varies with climate, regions, environment and religious factors. Food performs several functions in our body. On the basis of performing functions it can be classified as:

a. Energy giving food: Carbohydrates and fats.
b. Body building food: Proteins.
c. Protective food: Vitamins, minerals and proteins.

a. Energy Giving Food

Carbohydrates and fats are chief among energy giving foods.

Carbohydrates

Carbohydrates are the main component of food. These are also the ready source of energy. Carbohydrates provide approximately 85% to 90% energy. They are classified into following three types:

* *Monosaccharides:* Glucose, Fructose, Mannose
* *Disaccharides:* Sucrose, Lactose, Maltose
* *Polysaccharides:* Starches, glycogen

Sources

The sources of carbohydrates are exhibited in Table 3.5. The dietary requirement according to age, sex and different physical activities is given in Tables 3.6 and 3.7.

Diseases associated with intake of Carbohydrates

*   Systemic diseases
    *   i. Obesity
    *   ii. Diabetes
    *   iii. Cardiovascular disease
    *   iv. Glycogen storage disease
    *   v. Fructosuria, galactosemia
    *   vi. Pentosuria
*   Oral diseases

Carbohydrates increase the incidence of caries and periodontal diseases in the oral cavity. The exposure to refined diets, i.e. fermentable carbohydrates, e.g. bread, sugar etc. produce enough acid within 24 hours sufficient to decalcify enamel and dentin. The caries index increases in population having such food habits. Polysaccharides are less easily fermented by plaque bacteria than monosaccharides and disaccharides. Both cane sugar and cooked starches produced acid; however, little acid was formed when raw starches were substituted. Cariogenic carbohydrates are dietary in origin, since uncontaminated human saliva contains only negligible amounts of carbohydrates. Salivary carbohydrates are bound to proteins and other compounds and are not readily available for microbial degradation. Cariogenicity varies with the frequency of ingestion, physical form, chemical composition and route of administration. Meals high in

Table 3.5: Composition of some common foods			
Food	*Carbohydrates (%age)*	*Fat (%age)*	*Protein (%age)*
Bread (Roti)	52.0	3.0	9.0
Rice (cooked)	23.0	0.1	2.2
Banana	20.0	0.5	1.0
Potato	20.0	0.5	1.0
Peas	16.7	0.5	5.2
Apples	12.8	0.5	0.3
Cabbage	5.5	0.3	1.2
Spinach	3.2	0.3	1.6
Eggs	0.7	12.0	13.0
Milk	4.0	4.0	3.0
Butter	0.4	81.0	0.6
Cheese	2.0	32.0	25.0
Meat	0	30.0	22.0
Chicken	0	11.0	20.0
Fish	0	0.4	17.0
Groundnut (roasted)	19.0	50.0	25.8
Honey	85.0	0	Traces
Carrot (raw)	9.7	Traces	0.38
Onion	8.2	Traces	1.7
Orange	12.2	Traces	0.8
Guava	17.1	0.6	1.0

Table 3.6: Recommended dietary requirements (in gms) for adults with different physical activities

Food items	Adult man			Adult woman		
	Sedentary work	Moderate work	Heavy work	Sedentary work	Heavy work	Moderate work
Cereals	460	520	670	410	440	570
Pulses	40	50	60	40	45	50
Leafy vegetables	40	40	40	100	100	50
Other vegetables	60	70	80	40	40	100
Milk	150	200	250	100	150	200
Oils and fats	40	45	65	20	25	40
Sugar and Jaggery	30	35	55	20	20	40
Fruits	25	30	30	25	30	30

Source: Indian Council of Medical Research

Table 3.7: Recommended dietary requirements (in gms) for children in different age groups

Food items	1-3 years	4-6 years	10-12 years (Boys)	10-12 years (Girls)
Cereals	175	270	420	380
Pulses	35	35	45	45
Leafy vegetables	40	50	50	50
Other vegetables	20	30	50	50
Roots and tubers	10	0	30	30
Milk	300	250	250	250
Oils and fats	15	25	40	35
Sugar and Jaggery	30	40	45	45
Fruits	25	40	50	40

Source: Indian Council of Medical Research

fat, protein or salt reduce oral retentiveness of carbohydrates.

Fats

Fat is a necessary ingredient in the diet. Fat is a concentrated source of energy and it supplies approximately double the energy furnished by either protein or carbohydrate. Animal fat such as butter and ghee contains vitamin A, which may be lost to varying degrees during the process of cooking. The vegetable oils, which provide essential fatty acids, play a role in several metabolic reactions. Some fats like groundnut oil, sesame oil or sunflower oil which contain a high proportion of polyunsaturated fatty acids, do not increase blood cholesterol levels. On the other hand, fats like butter, ghee, coconut oil and hydrogenated fats which contain a high proportion of saturated fatty acids cause elevation in the blood cholesterol levels. A total of 40–60 gms of fat can be consumed daily so that it contributes 15-20% of the calories in diet. 1.0 gm of fat yields 9 calories.

The sources and percentage of fat contents in common foods is given in Table 3.5.

The fatty acids active in the promotion of growth as well as in the maintenance of dermal integrity are known as essential fatty acids. These are linoleic, linolenic and arachidonic acids. The essential fatty acid content of certain edible fats and oils is given in Table 3.8.

Fats such as ghee, butter etc. are known as 'visible fats' because it is easy to estimate their intake in the daily diet. Fat present in food such as cereals, pulses and nuts etc. are not visible and it is difficult to estimate their intake. These are called 'invisible fats'.

Table 3.8: Essential fatty acid content of certain edible fats and oils	
Fats	**Linoleic acid (grams per cent)**
Butter fat (ghee)	2
Coconut oil	3
Vanaspati	6
Mustard oil	20
Groundnut oil	28
Sesame (Gingelly) oil	45
Cottonseed oil	50
Corn (Maize) oil	51
Safflower (Kardi) seed oil	75

Source: India Council of medical research

Diseases associated with intake of Fats

The fat contents in the diet must be balanced both quantitatively and qualitatively. If ingested in excess, fats will be deposited in the adipose tissue. On the other hand, fat free diet produces an essential fatty acid deficiency. This stage is called pure deficiency state. The other deficiency state is termed as relative deficiency in which there is low ratio of essential fatty acids to non essential fatty acids. Abnormal intake of fats may lead to:

 i. *Atherosclerosis:* Food rich in animal fat raises serum cholesterol, which is deposited in walls of arteries causing atherosclerosis. However, certain fats have quality of decreasing the serum cholesterol, e.g. marine fish oils.

 ii. *Obesity:* Extra fat results in obesity, which may lead to diabetes mellitus, arterial hypertension, arteriosclerosis and many other diseases.

b. Body Building Food

Proteins are the chief body building food.

Proteins

The term Protein is derived from Greek word 'Protos' which means primary or of first importance. This group of compounds is the most important constituent of a cell. They are present in cytoplasm and the cell membrane of all cells. The enzymes, many hormones regulating body functions and antibodies are proteins in nature. Proteins are formed by the smaller components known as amino acids. These amino acids are twenty in number and are classified as:

1. Essential amino acids

2. Non-essential amino acids

Proteins are also classified into two types considering the health of public:

• Animal proteins (eggs, milk, meat etc.). These are the complete proteins that contain all the essential amino acids in the right proportion (with the exception of gelatin that lacks tryptophan).

• Vegetable proteins (pulses, cereals, nuts, beans etc.) Plant proteins in general are incomplete proteins as they may be lacking in one or more of essential amino acids.

Functions of Protein

1. Proteins are required for growth and maintenance of body.

2. They are required for formation of enzymes, antibodies and hormones.

3. They also serve as precursors of important compounds.

4. They help maintain the fluid balance
5. They play a role in nutrient transport.

Evaluation of Quality of Proteins

Previously the presence of amino acids, essential, semi-essential, non-essential, were used to be the criteria of evaluating proteins in routine. However, their digestibility and availability to the body should also be evaluated.

i. *Digestibility coefficient (DC):* It is the percentage of proteins absorbed into the blood stream after the process of digestion.

ii. *Biological value (BV):* It is the percentage of absorbed nitrogen that is retained by an organism, i.e.

$$BV = \frac{\text{Retained nitrogen}}{\text{Absorbed nitrogen}} \times 100$$

iii. *Net protein utilization (NPU):* It is the percentage of nitrogen in food that is retained by the body, i.e.

$$NPU = \frac{\text{Retained nitrogen}}{\text{Nitrogen in food}} \times 100$$

Also, it is the product of the digestibility coefficient and the biological value divided by 100.

$$NPU = \frac{\text{Digestibility coefficient} \times \text{Biological value}}{100}$$

iv. *Protein efficiency ratio:* It is determined as follows:

$$\text{Protein efficiency ratio} = \frac{\text{Increase in weight in grams of an organism}}{\text{Grams of protein consumed by that organism}}$$

Daily Requirements

The sources and percentages of proteins in common food is given in Table 3.9. Protein requirement varies from one individual to another depending upon age, sex and other physiological needs. The protein requirement varies with net protein utilization (NPU) of dietary food. If NPU is low, the protein requirement is high and vice-versa.

Usually, the protein requirements are expressed in terms of body weight. 1.0 gm protein per kg of body weight is recommended for an Indian Reference Man assuming that NPU is 65%. Daily recommendations are given in Table 3.10.

Protein Deficiency

Protein deficiency usually occurs in age of 1-5 years. In early infancy, breast milk meets the protein requirements adequately. Early weaning and poor socio-economic status are the common causes of protein deficiency in children. Severe protein malnutrition in children can manifest in two forms, i.e. Marasmus and Kwashiorkor, the characteristics of which are given below:

Marasmus: It occurs if protein deficiency occurs in infancy (generally from 0-1 year) and manifests as:

- Wasting, nearly complete loss of body fat.
- Retarded development.
- Mental changes.
- Changed texture of hair.
- Frequent diarrhoea.

Kwashiorkor: It occurs if protein deficiency occurs during 1-5 years of age and has following features:

- Hypoalbuminemia
- Edematous fatty liver
- Dermatosis, skin may show diffuse pigmentation.
- Gastrointestinal disturbances, poor appetite
- Psychic changes
- Often have sparse and silky hair (flag signs)

Protein deficiency in adults is frequently seen in hospitalized patients such as:

Table 3.9: Protein content, Digestibility coefficient (DC), Biological value (BV), Net protein utilization (NPU), of some foods

Name of food	Protein content (%)	DC (%)	BV (%)	NPU (%)
Animals foods				
Hen's egg	13.3	98	98	96
Cow's milk	3.5	95	85	81
Meat	19.8	96	82	79
Fish	21.5	96	80	77
Cereals				
Maize	11.1	85	50	43
Milled Rice	7.0	93	70	65
Whole Wheat	11.8	85	60	51
Pulses				
Bengal gram dal	22.5	84	62	52
Black gram dal	24.0	82	54	45
Green gram dal	24.0	85	58	49
Red gram dal	22.3	83	56	46
Nuts and Oil seeds				
Groundnut	26.7	92	54	50
Coconut fresh	4.5	82	67	56
Soyabean	40.0	86	64	55
Sesame	18.3	80	60	48

- Chronic alcoholics and other drug addicts as they may have irregular food habits and a protein deficient diet.
- Patients suffering from gastrointestinal disorders as they may not be able to eat, digest or absorb the protein.
- Surgical patients with severe injuries or burns have increased nitrogen loss and are unable to feed normally.
- Patients with chronic renal disease lose large amount of protein through their urine that cannot be replaced by diet.
- Patients with hepatic disease are unable to synthesize specific proteins from amino acids.

c. Protective Food

The nutrients in food protect the body from various diseases.

These include vitamins and minerals.

VITAMINS

The name vitamin was derived from two words - vital (latin 'life') and amine (a class of chemical compounds). Unlike the three major food components, the vitamins do not liberate energy by being metabolized. However, some of them are essential in the metabolic sequences in which energy is released from the major dietary components. Others take part in the regulation of various metabolic and cellular activities. The biochemical function of certain vitamins is still under research.

Classification

Traditionally, the vitamins have been divided into two groups on the basis of their solubility.

The fat soluble vitamins —A, D, E and K. They are found in foods in association with lipids

Table 3.10: Recommended protein allowances

Age (Years)	Daily allowance in terms of dietary protein	
	gm/kg body weight	total requirements (gm)
Man (60 kg)	1.0	60
Woman (50 kg)	1.0	50
Pregnancy (2nd and 3rd trimester)		+14
Lactation (0-6 months)		+25
Infants		
0 to 3 months	2.3 (a)	
3 to 6 months	1.8 (a)	
6 to 9 months	1.8 (b)	
9 to 12 months	1.5 (b)	
Children		
1 to 3 years	1.83	22
4 to 6 years	1.56	29
7 to 9 years	1.35	36
Males		
10 to 12 years	1.24	43
13 to 15 years	1.10	52
16 to 18 years	0.94	53
Females		
10 to 12 years	1.17	43
13 to 15 years	0.95	43
16 to 18 years	0.88	44

(a) in terms of milk protein   (b) partly vegetable protein

Source: Indian Council of Medical Research

and are absorbed along with dietary fats. Hence, deficient fat intake impairs their absorption. They are not normally excreted in urine and tend to be stored in the body in moderate quantities.

The water soluble vitamins—B and C. These are the vitamins that are not associated with dietary lipids and are normally excreted in the urine. Thus, they are not stored in the body in appreciable sources and quantities and a constant dietary supply of these vitamins is required in order to avoid their depletion, which subsequently effect normal physiologic functions (as most of these are proven components of essential enzyme systems).

Requirement

The daily requirement of all the vitamins is briefly given in Table 3.11.

Vitamin A

Vitamin A was given the alphabetical designation 'A' because this organic substance was discovered first and was considered as an 'accessory food factor' that is essential for growth and well-being of an individual. It is

Table 3.11: Vitamins, their sources and daily requirements for an adult

Vitamin	Daily requirement	Sources
Vitamin A (retinol)	750-100 mg	green leafy vegetables, carrot, fish, liver oil, liver
Vitamin D (calciferol)	10 mg	milk, fish, liver oil, egg, (on exposure to sunlight the body produces it)
Vitamin E (tocopherol)	10 mg	green leafy vegetables, milk, butter, tomato
Vitamin C (ascorbic acid)	80-100 mg	citrus fruits, especially amla, lime, lemon, orange, gooseberry, guava
Vitamin B1 (thiamine)	1.4 mg	milk, seafood, soyabean, whole cereals
Vitamin B2 (riboflavin)	1.6 mg	milk, peas, beans, yeast, meat, egg
Vitamin B3 (niacin)	15-18 mg	meat, fish, fowl, potato, wholegrain
Vitamin B6 (pyridoxine)	2.0 mg	liver, whole grains, milk, eggs
Vitamin B12 (cyano-cobalamin)	0.5-1.0 mg	meat, liver, fish
Biotin	150-300 mg	liver, egg yolk, nuts, fresh green vegetables
Pantothenic acid	8-10 mg	egg yolk, nuts, whole grains
Folic acid	400 mg	fresh green vegetables, fish, poultry
Vitamin K	50-100 mg	green leafy vegetables, fruits, pork, liver (vit. K is also synthesized in the body)

established that carotene is the precursor of vitamin A.

Forms of Vitamin A

There are several forms of vitamin A. The common form is vitamin A1 (retinol), other forms are A2 (Dehydroretinol) and neo-vitamins A-a and A-b. The dietary Beta-carotene has only a half of the biologic value of vitamin A.

Sources of Vitamin A

The various sources of Vitamin A are:
  i. Yellow vegetables such as carrots, corn, sweet potatoes. Fruits such as apricots, bananas, yellow peaches, papayas etc. are also good sources of the vitamin A.
 ii. Red palm oil is particularly a potent source of carotenoids.
iii. Foods stored in the frozen state retain their vitamin A content. Dried and dehydrated foods have lesser amount of vitamin A.

Functions

The functions of vitamin A are:
  i. It maintains normal vision.
 ii. It has the potential of differentiating specialized epithelial cells (mainly the mucus secreting cells).
iii. It helps in skeletal growth.
 iv. It helps in enhancement of immunity, though this function is controversial.

In addition, beta carotene performs the following functions:
  i. Singlet oxygen quenching: Beta-carotene prevents cellular damage by 'quenching' or inactivating singlet oxygen. Beta-carotene interacts with singlet oxygen, and absorbs the molecule's excess energy.
 ii. Antioxidant: Beta-carotene also reacts directly with free radicals as a 'scavenger' that neutralizes their molecules.
iii. Role in cancer: Oral leukoplakia is thought to be a precursor of oral cancer. It is established that beta carotene supplementation, alone or in combination with

vitamin A, causes partial or complete regression of these lesions and also suppresses the formation of new lesions.

iv. Immune function: Beta carotene helps in enhancement of immunity.

Vitamin A and Systemic Diseases

Hypovitaminosis A: It is the deficiency state due to decreased intake or impaired absorption or excessive loss of vitamin A. Its systemic manifestations are:

a. *In eyes:* Xerosis (dryness of the eye), 'Bitot spots' (build up of keratin debris in small opaque plaques), keratomalacia (softening of cornea), corneal opacities and night blindness occur that may progress to total blindness.

b. *Skin:* Skin becomes dry and rough with hyperkeratinization, atrophy of sweat glands and formation of papules occurs.

c. *Respiratory tract:* Keratinization of bronchopulmonary epithelium, which increases susceptibility to infection.

d. *GIT:* Unhealthy gastrointestinal mucosa which may lead to recurrent diarrhoea.

e. *Urinary tract:* Increased tendency to urinary stone formation due to shedding of epithelial lining which acts as a nidus.

f. *Reproductive system:* Sterility due to faulty spermatogenesis, abortions and foetal malformations.

g. *General:*

　i. Growth retardation and impairment of special senses.

　ii. Immune deficiency causing higher mortality due to common infections.

Vitamin A is responsible for the differentiation of epithelial cells. The primary effect of vitamin A deficiency is on ectodermal tissues, particularly the epithelial cells lining the mucosa of the mouth and salivary glands. These cells are replaced by keratinized epithelium.

Hypervitaminosis A: Increased intake of Vitamin A may be:

i. Acute: Acute poisoning has also been reported (though very rare) and is characterized by headache, drowsiness, irritability, rise in intracranial tension, vomiting, liver enlargement and shedding of skin.

ii. Chronic: Regular ingestion of excess of retinol for longer periods can lead to weight loss, nausea, vomiting, dryness of mucosa of the lips, bone and joint pain, hyperostosis and hepatomegaly.

Vitamin A and Oral Diseases

Hypovitaminosis A: The effects of deficiency of vitamin A in the oral cavity are discussed below:

i. Oral Mucosa: Hyperkeratotic or follicular keratotic changes in oral epithelium.

ii. Gingival epithelium: The gingival epithelium becomes hyperplastic and hyperkeratotic.

iii. Enamel organ: there is atrophy and degeneration of the odontoblasts, which leads to poor matrix formation and calcification resulting in enamel hypoplasia. The odontoblasts are also damaged resulting in atypical dentin formation. Atrophy of the salivary glands leads to reduction in salivary flow, subsequently increasing the incidence of dental caries.

iv. Cementum: Irregular cemental resorption and ankylosis of teeth may be seen.

v. Eruption rate: The eruption rate may be retarded.

vi. Alveolar bone: The alveolar bone is atrophied in severe cases.

Hypervitaminosis A: The mesenchymal tissues are sensitive to hypervitaminosis A. The rate of formation of alveolar bone is greatly reduced, as a result of which the bone becomes abnormally thin.

Vitamin D

Types of Vitamin D

Vitamin D is of three types:

D1: Mixture of antirachitic substances found in food (only of historic interest)

D2: Calciferol: Present in irradiated food (ergocalciferol)

D3: Cholecalciferol: Synthesized in the skin under the influence of ultraviolet rays.

Sources of Vitamin D

Human beings have two possible sources of vitamins D:

- *Endogenous:* It is synthesized in the skin by the action of UV rays.
- *Exogenous:* It is obtained from the diet, like milk and eggs. Vitamin D is rarely found in vegetables. About 20% of the dietary needs is to be taken exogeneously in the diet. About 80% of the body's need can be endogenously derived in a country like India, where adequate sunlight is available round the year.

Requirement

A daily intake of 10 mg is recommended for children, which can be provided by milk.

For adults 2.5 mg/day is the recommended dose, especially for those who are deprived of sunlight for long periods. Intake of more than the recommended levels is potentially dangerous and should be avoided.

Fish liver contains large amounts of the vitamin D. Milk and eggs provide sufficient amount of vitamin D. Vitamin D is rarely found in vegetables.

Functions

The essential function of vitamin D is maintenance of normal plasma levels of calcium and phosphorus by:

- Increasing intestinal absorption of calcium and phosphorus.
- Collaborating with parathyroid hormone in the mobilization of calcium from bone when there is hypocalcemia.
- Stimulating the PTH dependent reabsorption of calcium in the renal tubules.

Also, Vitamin D is required for normal mineralization of epiphyseal cartilage and osteoid matrix.

Causes of Deficiency of Vitamin D

In our country deficiency state generally does not occur due to decreased dietary intake as there is adequate availability of sunlight for whole year. Deficiency occurs if there is:

- Decreased endogenous synthesis of vitamin D.
- Decreased absorption of vitamin D in the intestine.
- Enhanced degradation of vitamin D by certain enzymes and drugs like phenytoin, phenobarbital, rifampicin etc.
- Impaired synthesis, especially in liver disease.
- Decreased synthesis of cholecalciferol in renal disease.
- Resistance of target organ to cholecalciferol.

Diseases due to Deficiency of Vitamin D

Deficiency of vitamin D causes rickets in children and osteomalacia in adults. In rickets there is:

- Overgrowth of epiphyseal cartilage.
- Persistence of distorted, irregular masses of cartilage, many of which project into the marrow cavity.
- Deposition of osteoid matrix in inadequately mineralized cartilaginous remnants.
- Disruption of orderly replacement of cartilage by osteoid matrix with enlargement of osteochondral junction.
- Deformation due to loss of structural rigidity of developing bones.

In osteomalacia, the contours of the bone are not affected. The bone is weak and vulnerable to gross fractures, which are most likely to affect the vertebral bodies and femoral necks.

Oral Manifestations of Vitamin D Deficiency

- The eruption of teeth is retarded.
- Enamel hypoplasia can occur in developing enamel. (The ameloblasts do not function normally)
- Osteoporosis of alveolar bone. The relevant features are:
  - osteoid forms at a normal rate but remains uncalcified, failure of osteoid to resorb.
  - reduction in width of the periodontal space.
  - normal rate of cementum formation but defective calcification and cemental resorption.
  - distortion of the growth pattern of alveolar bone.

Hypervitaminosis D

Vitamin D, if taken excess (100,000 IU in adults and 40,000 IU in children) will induce a very intense calcification of the bone. In addition, the formation of renal calculi and adrenal dysfunction are often seen. When ingested in excess, vitamin D is one of the most toxic of all vitamins.

Effect of Hypervitaminosis D on Teeth and Periodontium

- Hypervitaminosis leads to irregular dentin formation and pulp stones in teeth.
- The alveolar bone, periodontal membrane and gingivae become hypercalcified. The cementum deposition increases, subsequently ankylosis may result.
- Excessive amount of calculus may also be found.
- Rampant caries, thinning of the enamel, dentin and alveolar process and rarefaction of molar roots may be evident. Areas of resorption repaired by irregular dentin and pulpal calcification can be observed.

Vitamin E

Vitamin E, chemically known as alpha-tocopherol is essential to protect against the oxidative destruction of vitamin A. The diseases which interfere with the absorption of vitamin A and vitamin D effect the absorption of vitamin E also.

Sources

Vitamin E is widespread in nature. The richest sources are vegetable and seed oils, butter and liver. Wheat germ oil is a particularly potent source of alpha-tocopherol.

Requirement

The average daily intake is about 10-12 mg.

Deficiency of Vitamin E

Causes: Deficiency of vitamin E can be because of the following factors:
- *Malabsorption:* If the absorption of fat is impaired, then that of vitamin E is also impaired.
- Genetic blood disorders may lead to vitamin E deficiency.
- Immature liver and Gastrointestinal tract.

Deficiency effects:
- *Nervous system:* Anatomic changes in the nervous system. The clinical manifestations depend upon the severity and distribution of neurologic lesions. The most consistent ones are depressed tendon reflexes, ataxia, dysarthria and loss of pain sensation.
- *Blood:* Hemolytic and hypoplastic anaemia.
- *Mesenchymal tissues:* Degenerative lesions in skeletal muscles and heart.

Hypervitaminosis E

Hypervitaminosis E has not been described. Adults taking one gram a day for months do not develop signs of toxicity. Vitamin E is thought to be one of the least toxic of all vitamins.

Vitamin K

Types

The vitamin is available in two varieties - K1 and K2. Synthetic compounds have also been produced and are labelled as K3.

K1 (from plants, fat soluble): Phytodione
K2 (produced by bacteria): Menaquinones
K3 (Synthetic) Fat soluble: Menadione, Acetomenaphthone

Sources

Vitamin K is widely distributed in nature. The richest food sources are green leafy vegetables, pork liver, soyabean and spinach. Milk and eggs contain small amounts.

Man's most important source of vitamin K appears to be his intestinal flora.

Requirement

The total requirement of an adult has been estimated to be 50-100 g/day. The synthetic vitamin may be administered to mothers in labour or to their newborn infants.

Functions

Vitamin K is a cofactor for the synthesis of four proteins which participate in blood coagulation viz. factor II, factor VII, IX and X in the liver.

Deficiency of Vitamin K

The deficiency usually occurs in the following circumstances.

Causes of Deficiency

- In fat malabsorption syndrome, particularly with biliary tract disease.
- Subsequent to ingestion of broad spectrum antibiotics as the endogenous vitamin K synthesizing flora is destroyed.

- In the neonatal period, when liver reserves are less and the bacterial flora has not yet developed.
- The liver diseases interfere with the synthesis of vitamin K.

Deficiency Features

The deficiency leads to:
- Development of a bleeding diathesis characterized by haematomas, hematuria, malena and ecchymoses.
- In neonates the most serious manifestation is intracranial hemorrhage, but bleeding may occur at any site, including skin, umbilicus and viscera.

Vitamin K and Oral Diseases

The most common oral manifestation of vitamin K deficiency is gingival bleeding. Prothrombin levels below 35% will result in bleeding after tooth brushing; however, when prothrombin levels fall below 20% spontaneous gingival hemorrhage will occur.

Hypervitaminosis

There is evidence that excessive use of menadione in the newborn will produce hemolytic anaemia, hyperbilirubinaemia and kernicterus.

Water Soluble Vitamins: These are vitamin B complex and vitamin C that are discussed below:

Vitamin B1 (Thiamine)

Requirement

There is a relationship between the utilisation of Thiamine and the amount of carbohydrate in the diet. The WHO recommends a daily intake of 1.4 mg for all individuals.

Sources

Thiamine is widely available in diet, although refined foods such as polished rice, white flour and white sugar contain very little. The chief sources are cereals, pulses and nuts. Egg yolk contains a fair amount.

As Thiamine is readily soluble in water, large amounts may be lost when rice or vegetables are cooked in an excess of water which is discarded afterwards. If baking soda is added to the vegetables, almost all the vitamin is lost. Normally, about 25% Thiamine is lost in cooking.

Functions

Thiamine has the following functions:

- It regulates appetite and normal digestion.
- Thiamine is helpful for utilization of carbohydrates in the body.
- It maintains neural membranes and normal nerve conduction (chiefly peripheral nerves).

Deficiency of Thiamine

Systemic Manifestations

The thiamine deficiency mainly hits the peripheral nerves, the heart and the brain. A disease known as Beri Beri was known for centuries among population groups whose diet was composed largely of polished rice with a minimum of meat and fresh vegetables. The persistent thiamine deficiency gives rise to three distinctive syndromes.

- **Dry Beri Beri (polyneuropathy):** It is of a non specific peripheral neuropathy with myelin degeneration and disruption of axons, involving motor, sensory and reflex arcs.
  It first appears in the legs, and it may extend to the arms. Classically, the patients present with toe, foot and wrist drop.
- **Wet Beri Beri:** It leads to peripheral vasodilation, and subsequently more rapid arteriovenous shunting of blood. Peripheral oedema has also been noticed. The heart may be normal or markedly enlarged.
- **Wernicke-Korsakoff syndrome:** It is most often encountered in chronic alcoholics with severe deficiency. It is marked by ophthalmoplegia, nystagmus, ataxia of gait and stance, derangement of mental function characterized by confusion, restlessness and disorientation.

Thiamine and Oral Diseases

There are no specific lesions in oral cavity due to thiamine deficiency; however, hypersensitivity of oral mucosa may be seen. Oral and facial neuralgias and pain, herpes simplex and aphthous stomatitis have been treated with thiamine. Edematous swelling of the gingiva and lingual papilla and impairment of taste sensation may be seen.

Hypervitaminosis

Thiamine is non-toxic when taken by mouth even in large doses. However, the parenteral administration has caused reactions resembling anaphylactic shock in hypersensitive individuals.

Contact dermatitis has also been reported in patients allergic to thiamine.

Vitamin B2 (Riboflavin)

Requirement

The WHO recommends an intake of 1.6 mg in the diet regardless of age and sex.

Sources

The best sources of riboflavin are milk products and animal proteins. Also found in eggs, green leafy vegetables and grains. Riboflavin and Thiamine are both synthesized by colonic bacteria but this does not become available to the host.

Functions

Riboflavin participates in a wide range of oxidation-reduction reactions, helping in respiration and metabolism of carbohydrates, fats and proteins.

Deficiency of Riboflavin

The deficiency of riboflavin leads to:

1. *Ariboflavinosis:* It occurs as a primary deficiency state, especially in economically deprived and developing countries.
2. Riboflavin deficiency causes angular stomatitis, cheilosis and nasolabial seborrhoea.
3. *In eyes:* It also causes circumcorneal vascularisation. This ocular lesion is accompanied by lacrimation and photophobia.
4. *In skin:* A fine scaly dermatitis may also occur on the hands, vulva, anus and perineum.

Riboflavin and oral diseases: Following are the oral manifestations of Riboflavin deficiency:

i. *On lips:* The characteristic lip lesions in ariboflavinosis are cheilosis and angular stomatitis. The chronic lesions may develop a yellow crust. The early subjective symptoms are dryness and a slight burning sensation. Both angles are usually involved although they may differ in degree.

ii. *On tongue:* The lingual papillae are swollen, flattened and mushroom shaped, giving the dorsum a granular appearance. Atrophy of the papillae has also been reported. In severe cases, the tongue may turn purplish red or magenta coloured due to dilation and proliferation of capillaries with slowing of the circulation. The tongue may be painful and sensitive to food. Loss or diminution of the taste sensation may occur.

Hypervitaminosis

In humans, riboflavin is nontoxic in amounts far in excess of therapeutic dosage.

Vitamin B3 (Niacin/Nicotinic Acid)

It is distributed practically in all tissues, predominantly as a coenzyme. The greatest quantity is contained in the liver. It is excreted principally in the urine, however small amounts are also excreted in the faeces, sweat and milk of lactating women.

Requirement

The WHO recommends an intake of 15-18 mg nicotinic acid equivalents in the diet.

Sources

It is widely available in grains, legumes, seed oils. The richest sources are lean meats, liver, yeast, peanuts. In some grains it is present in bound form and therefore not absorbable; e.g. maize. Ordinary cooking does not destroy the vitamin. If milk is left exposed to sunlight, niacin is lost.

Functions

Niacin is an essential component of two co-enzymes, nicotinamide adenine dinucleotide (NAD) and nicotinamide adenine dinucleotide phosphate (NADP), both of which have certain roles in cellular intermediary metabolism. NAD functions as a coenzyme in the metabolism of fat, carbohydrate and amino-acids.

Deficiency of Niacin

It usually occurs in alcoholics, persons suffering from chronic debilitating diseases and also protracted diarrhoeal states, with diets that are grossly deficient in proteins. During the prodromal stage of nicotinic acid deficiency, the patient may complain of loss of appetite and vague gastrointestinal symptoms, general weakness, lassitude, mental confusion and forgetfulness.

The systemic manifestation of Niacin deficiency presents as – Pellagra, a syndrome identified by the three D's.

i. *Dermatitis:* Usually bilaterally symmetrical, found mainly on exposed areas of the body.

ii. *Diarrhoea:* Caused by atrophy of columnar epithelium of GI tract.

iii. *Dementia:* Results from degeneration of neurons in the brain accompanied by degeneration of corresponding tracts in the spinal cord.

Now a fourth 'D'—Death has also been added according to latest research as the disease is usually fatal if not treated.

Hypervitaminosis

The untoward side effects of nicotinic acid are attributable to its action as a vasodilator. These include reddening and flushing of the skin, increased skin temperature, dizziness, headache, nausea, vomiting and abdominal pain.

Niacin and Oral Diseases

i. *Oral Mucosa:* The entire oral mucosa becomes fiery red and painful.

ii. *Tongue:* There occurs desquamation of the epithelium of the tongue leaving a scarlet, smooth, dry, beefy tongue. Burning sensation of the tongue is a common feature. Initially, the tip and lateral borders of the tongue are swollen. Later on, the swelling involves whole of the tongue producing indentations along its margins. The tongue is extremely painful and sensitive to food and drinks.

iii. *Gingiva:* Tenderness, pain, redness and ulcerations begin at the interdental papillae and spread rapidly. Salivation becomes excessive and there is a diminution in taste sensation. Superimposed acute necrotizing ulcerative gingivostomatitis or vincent's infection is a common complication.

iv. *Dental caries:* The incidence of dental caries is reduced in nicotinic acid deficiency probably because nicotinic acid acts as an essential growth factor for the oral flora and is an important part of the enzyme system concerned with the degradation of fermentable carbohydrates.

Vitamin B4 (Adenine)

It is a nucleobase, synthesized by the human body. It doesn't have much nutritional value.

Vitamin B5 (Pantothenic acid)

Pantothenic acid is an integral part of coenzyme A, which along with a specific protein enzyme, functions in many reversible acetylation reactions. It participates in the synthesis of fatty acids, steroids and cholesterol.

Requirement

For adults, 8–10 mg is an adequate daily dose and 1.0 mg daily is sufficient for infants.

Sources

Pantothenic acid is available in liver, kidneys, yeast, wheat bran and peas. Milk, meat, eggs, and fruit contain moderate quantities. Mostly, pantothenic acid exists in bound form. Significant loss occurs during the milling of grains but during cooking loss is not much.

Deficiency of Pantothenic Acid

Pantothenic acid deficiency is very rare. Systemic manifestation as 'burning feet syndrome' seen only in severe cases.

Panthothenic Acid and Oral Diseases

There are no specific oral manifestations of pantothenic acid deficiency; however, pantothenic acid has curative value in the treatment of glossitis and cheilitis.

Vitamin B6 (Pyridoxine)

Pyridoxine is a water soluble, white crystalline compound, stable to heat and sensitive to ultraviolet light. It participates in the conversion of tryptophan to nicotinic acid, the utilization of essential fatty acids, the synthesis of haemoglobin and the maintenance of proper neural function and activity. It is excreted in urine.

Requirement

The recommended intake for adults is 2.0 mg/day.

Sources

The best sources are wheat, whole grain, cereals, beef, leafy vegetables, milk, yeast, legumes, meat and certain vegetable fats. Milling of grains in the production of flour results in a loss of approximately half the vitamin B6 content. Other losses are incurred during cooking in an open vessel.

Deficiency of Vitamin B6

Clinically, deficiency of vitamin B6 is rare in humans; however, subclinical deficiency conditions are common.

Clinical findings in B6 deficient patients resemble those of riboflavin and niacin deficiency. Patients may have seborrheic dermatitis, cheilosis, glossitis, peripheral neuropathy and sometimes convulsions.

Pyridoxine and Oral Diseases

The deficiency of vitamin B6 leads to following changes:

  i. *On lips:* bilateral angular cheilosis occurs.
 ii. *On tongue:* glossitis occurs that presents with slight pain, edema, papillary atrophy and purple hue. The glossitis begins with a scalding sensation of the tongue followed by redness and hypertrophy of the filiform papillae at the tip, margins and the dorsal surface. Later on the tongue becomes swollen and fungiform papillae stand out as hypertrophied red knobs.
iii. *Dental caries:* Pyridoxine deficiency increases the incidence of dental caries because it alters the oral flora to more cariogenic organisms.

Vitamin B9 (Folic Acid)/Vitamin M

Folic acid participates in amino acid metabolism and in the production of purine and pyrimidine compounds required for the formation of nucleoproteins.

Requirement

The daily requirement for an average adult is 300 mg.

Sources

Folic acid is particularly abundant in deep green leafy vegetables, liver, kidney and yeast. Moderate amounts are contained in lean beef and wheat cereals. Folic acid loss on cooking and on storage of food at room temperature are fairly high. Refrigerated foods contain considerable folic acid for periods upto two weeks.

Deficiency of Folic Acid

Systemic Diseases

The most notable effect is a macrocytic anaemia associated with a megaloblastic erythropoiesis. In addition, glossitis, stomatitis, diarrhoea and malabsorption may appear. The gastrointestinal defects are particularly prominent in sprue, a syndrome in which steatorrhoea represented by foul smelling, copious, greasy appearing, light, liquid to semiliquid stools is a conspicuous feature.

Folic Acid and Oral Diseases

The effects of folic acid deficiency occur on:

  i. *Tongue:* Folic acid deficiency causes glossitis, seen as swelling and redness along the tip and lateral margins of the tongue. Later on minute, whitish aphthous ulcers with fiery red borders may emerge. The filiform papillae are the first to disappear, the fungiform papillae remaining as prominent spots. In severe cases, the fungiform papillae are lost and the tongue becomes slick, smooth and fiery red.
 ii. *Lips:* Stomatitis, chelitis and cheilosis with ulcerative lesions may also be seen.

Vitamin B12 (Cyanocobalamin)

Vit B12 participates in biochemical reactions in the form of B12 coenzyme. Like folic acid it is involved in nucleic acid synthesis. It influences folic acid metabolism either by effecting the release of free folic acid from the conjugated forms or by catalyzing the formation of folinic acid enzyme.

The human body is capable of storing relatively large amounts of vitamin B12.

Requirement

The human requirements of vitamin B12 have not been established. Studies indicate that a diet containing 3.0 to 5.0 µg of vitamin B12 daily is sufficient.

Sources

It is mainly found in foods of animal origin, most abundant in liver and kidney; along with its presence in muscle tissues and foods derived from milk. Plant sources—carrots and beans though contain small amount of Vitamin B12. In man, microbial synthesis occurs in the colon but relatively little is achieved from this source.

Deficiency of Vitamin B12

Systemic manifestations: The most severe form of vitamin B12 deficiency is pernicious anaemia. The disease is characterized by weakness, glossitis, numbness and tingling of the extremities. It may lead to severe psychosis and extensive mental deterioration. The deficiency of vitamin B12 may also lead to macrocytic anaemia and homocysteinuria.

Vitamin B12 and Oral Diseases

The oral manifestations are:

On Tongue: Pernicious anaemia affects oral cavity characterized by recurrent attacks of sore tongue. The tongue becomes exceedingly painful and fiery red in colour, which is usually confined to the anterior half of the tongue. The lingual papillae may completely disappear, leaving a bald, glazed tongue and diminished taste sensation.

On Lips: Cheilosis, cheilitis and painful mucous membrane lesions affect the buccal mucosa, gingiva and pharynx.

Vitamin B7 (Biotin) Also known as Vitamin I

Biotin is an important constituent of vitamin B complex.

Free biotin is absorbed from both the upper and lower intestine. It is excreted mainly in urine and faeces.

Requirement

The biotin requirement of human beings is not known exactly. Amount available in diet ranges from 150–300 µg, and together with that synthesized by intestinal flora is apparently sufficient.

Sources

Most foods contain biotin in free and protein bound forms. Especially abundant in liver, kidney and yeast. Peanuts, chocolate and mushrooms are good sources. It is synthesized by intestinal bacteria to an extent sufficient to meet normal requirements of body.

Deficiency of Biotin

Systemic Manifestations: Biotin deficiency leads to a scaly dermatitis, greyish pallor of skin and mucosa, muscle pains, depression and lassitude.

Biotin and Oral Diseases

Biotin deficiency results in pallor of tongue and a patchy or generalized atrophy of the lingual papillae.

Vitamin B8 (Inositol)
Also known as the Mouse Factor

Inositol is vital for hair growth. It reduces blood cholesterol and prevents hardening of the arteries. It also removes fat from the liver and aids in redistribution of body fat.

Requirement

The average balanced diet contains about 1.0 gm of inositol, which is sufficient to meet all necessary requirements.

Sources

Fruits, fruit juices and cereals are good sources. In animals, inositol occurs in combination with a protein.

Deficiency of Inositol

Deficiency of inositol leads to high blood cholesterol, constipation, eczema and hair loss.

Choline

Choline is required for proper transmission of nerve impulses from brain through central nervous system. It is used to treat liver damage caused by alcoholism.

Requirement

The choline requirement for human beings has not been documented.

Sources

Large amounts of choline are present in most foods. Egg yolk, meat, fish, cereals and cereal products are particularly rich sources. Green leafy vegetables and legumes contain moderate amounts.

Deficiency of Choline

Deficiency of choline may result in cirrhosis and fatty degeneration of liver, heart problems, high blood pressure, etc.

Vitamin B10 (Para-Amino Benzoic Acid-PABA)

Para-Amino Benzoic acid helps in the maintenance of healthy intestinal flora. It also acts as coenzyme in the breakdown of proteins.

Requirement

25 mg is a dietary reference intake or recommended dietary allowance.

Sources

It occurs in foods in free state, as part of folic acid, and in combination with proteins, amino-acids and polypeptides. The best food sources are yeast, liver, cereals and vegetables. It is also synthesized by intestinal bacteria.

Deficiency of PABA

Deficiency of PABA leads to extreme fatigue, irritability, constipation, digestive disorder and headache, etc.

Amygdalin (Laetrile) Vitamin B17

It is present in almonds, peach, apricot and apple seeds.

It has come into prominence recently because of claims of its effectiveness in treatment of cancer. Its use in anaemia is being studied.

Certain authors don't consider Amygladin as vitamin B component. No specific disease has been associated with its deficiency and more so it has never been shown to promote vital physiological processes.

Bioflavinoids (Also known as Vitamin P)

Bioflavinoids are associated with maintenance of normal capillary permeability and fragility. The chief sources are Apricots, Cherries, Grapes, etc.

The deficiency may results in a syndrome characterized by increased capillary permeability and fragility. They have been used in the treatment of diseases occurring due to vascular abnormality. 150–200 mg daily intake is recommended. Currently used in preventing breast cancer.

Four varieties of Bioflavinoids are:
- Proanthocyanidins (PCO)
- Quercatin
- Citrus bioflavinoids
- Green tea polyphenols

Lipoic Acid

Lipoic acid is used as a coenzyme with several other coenzymes. Since lipoic acid is widely distributed in all natural foods, deficiency symptoms have not been well established.

Vitamin C

Vitamin C isolated from natural sources, has been named L-ascorbic acid, which is water soluble, slightly soluble in alcohol but insoluble in fats. It is readily and rapidly absorbed in the small intestine and little or none is lost in the faeces with a normal diet.

Requirement

The daily requirement of an adult is 80–100 mg which increases in case of pregnancy and lactation.

The usual requirement also increases in cases of trauma, infections and stress conditions.

Sources

The best source of vitamin C are amla and citrus fruits viz. orange, lemon, etc. Additional sources are cabbage, spinach, peas, beans, tomatoes, carrots, bananas, potatoes. It is assumed that 80–85% of vitamin C is lost during cooking. Freezing has no deleterious effect.

Functions

- Vitamin C is concerned with the metabolism of extracellular connective tissue especially collagen.
- It helps in wound healing.
- It reduces ferric iron to ferrous iron, thus helping in absorption of iron.
- High concentration of ascorbic acid in the adrenals has role in stress conditions.
- Vitamin C has been tried to decrease episodes of common cold and flu.

Deficiency of Vitamin C

Severe vitamin C deficiency (Scurvy), once prevalent among sailors, can be seen in malnourished infants, children, elderly, alcoholic and drug addicts.

Hemorrhages constitute one of the most striking features. The defect in collagen synthesis results in purpura and ecchymoses in the skin. Extensive subperiosteal hematomas and bleeding into joint spaces can follow minimal trauma.

Skeletal changes may also appear in children and infants. The primary disturbance is in the formation of osteoid matrix, rather than in mineralization. Both membranous and endochondral bone formation may be affected. Wound healing and localization of focal infections are impaired because of the derangement in collagen synthesis.

Toxicity

Ascorbic acid in large doses is considered as one of the safest drugs; however, it can be dangerous to those with a liability to urinary stones or to iron - storage disease because it increases the urinary output of oxalic acid and uric acid.

Vitamin C and Oral Diseases

Vitamin C deficiency in oral cavity affects:

Gingival and periodontal tissues: The interdental and marginal gingiva is bright red with swollen, smooth, shiny surfaces. The patients have the typical foul breath similar to fusospirochetal stomatitis.

The severe cases of scurvy lead to hemorrhages and swelling of the periodontal membranes followed by loss of bone and loosening of the teeth.

MINERALS AND TRACE ELEMENTS

In addition of carbohydrates, lipids, proteins and vitamins, body also needs small amounts of a number of inorganic substances called minerals and trace elements. Elements, whose daily requirement is more than 1.0 mg are grouped as minerals (calcium, phosphorous, iron, etc.). Certain other elements which are required in traces are grouped as trace elements (cobalt, copper, manganese, etc.) Table 3.12.

Table 3.12: Minerals, their sources and daily requirements for an adult		
Minerals	*Daily requirement*	*Sources*
Calcium	0.6–0.8 gm	Dairy products, green vegetables, whole gram, beans
Phosphorous	1.0–1.5 gm	Dairy products, beans, peas, cereals, nuts
Magnesium	300 mg	Nuts, cereals, legumes, coca, almonds
Zinc	10–15 mg	Meat, whole grain, legumes
Iron	2.0 gm	Meat, meat products, cereals, leguminous plants and leaves
Selenium	50–200 mg	Fish, meat and cereals
Copper	2.0 mg	Green leafy vegetables, legumes and meat
Cobalt	1.0–2.0 mg	Widely distributed in plants and animal tissues
Iodine	0.10–0.14 mg	Fruits, vegetables, cereals and meat

The absorption of these elements requires presence of the specific carrier protein whose synthesis is controlled by the concentration of the corresponding mineral. The dietary deficiency as well as excess of these minerals is harmful to the body.

Calcium

Calcium is the fifth most common inorganic element of the body. Essentially, 99% of the body calcium is present in bones and teeth, the remaining 1.0% in the soft tissues and body fluids.

The level of calcium in normal blood serum ranges from 9–11 mg percent.

Sources

Calcium is found abundantly in milk (including skimmed milk and butter milk), cheese and green leafy vegetables. Amaranth and drumstick leaves are particularly rich in calcium. Nuts and legumes represent the richest sources of calcium. Most cereals contain some amounts of calcium but rice is deficient in calcium.

Requirement

Children need relatively more calcium to meet the needs of the growing bones. Expectant and nursing mothers also require higher amount of calcium.

The daily requirement for an adult is about 0.6-0.8 gm. In the case of growing children, pregnant and lactating woman, a daily allowance of 1.0 gm of calcium is suggested. A part of calcium in cereal based diet remains unavailable because of the presence of Phytin, which interferes with the absorption of calcium. Likewise, part of the calcium present in some leafy vegetables and oil seed cakes may not be available due to its association with oxalic acid.

Functions

- Calcium controls the permeability of all cell membranes in competition with sodium and potassium. Lecithin is the substance which binds calcium in the cell membrane.
- It regulates muscle and nerve irritability. Irritability of nervous tissue increases as the blood calcium level decreases. Low blood

calcium level causes tetany with convulsions. High levels of blood calcium depress nerve irritability.

- An optimum level of blood calcium is required for normal cardiac functions, contraction, etc.
- It plays an important part in the clotting of blood. The formation of fibrin from fibrinogen requires thrombin, and calcium is an essential part of the prothrombin complex.
- Calcium is an activator of enzymes lipase, alkaline phosphatase, etc.
- It is essential for the absorption of vitamin B12 from the intestinal tract.
- It helps in calcification of bones and teeth.

Deficiency

Systemic Manifestations

Abnormal calcium metabolism may result in one of the following abnormalities.

Rickets: In rickets, there is poor mineralization of organic cartilagenous matrix. Unlike normal bone formation, the epiphyseal cartilage cells do not degenerate and there is no continuation of the expansion of capillaries followed by mineralization. New cartilage forms and the epiphysis becomes irregularly widened. Retarded or inadequate mineralization in combination with gravitational and mechanical stresses may lead to skeletal malformations.

Rickets can be due to:

- Inadequate intake of calcium.
- Inadequate absorption of calcium.
- Developmental defects in cell metabolism.

Osteomalacia: The generalized rarefaction and demineralization of the bone are common features of osteomlalacia. It occurs in adults and is due to calcium and vitamin D deficiency.

Osteoporosis: Osteoporosis infers increased porosity of bone. It is the most common disorder of the skeletal system, seen commonly in elderly patients.

Acidosis: This causes an increased excretion of calcium in the urine which may result in rarefaction of the skeleton.

Steatorrhoea: In steatorrhoea, the excretion of calcium in faeces is increased and the absorption of vitamin D is impaired.

Hypocalcemia: Hypocalcemia may occur if too much parathyroid tissue is removed, causing diminished mobilization of calcium from bone. It is usually due to impaired alimentary absorption. It may also occur in patients with malabsorption syndrome.

When plasma calcium is reduced, nerves and muscles become more readily excitable. Tingling sensation or numbness may be present. Twitching of muscles, known as tetany, may be followed by spasm. The face, hands and feet are mainly effected. Characteristically the wrist and metacarpophalangeal joint are flexed and the interphalangeal joints are extended. The larynx may get affected causing a coarse stridor.

Calcium Deficiency and Oral Diseases

The oral manifestations are:

- *Effect on alveolar bone:* Alveolar bone being cancellous is sensitive to calcium deficiency. Marrow spaces of alveolar bone become haemorrhagic and get filled with fibro-osteoid tissue. As a result of alveolar bone resorption, the teeth become loose. Destruction of the periodontal ligament may occur.
- *Effect on teeth:* The serum calcium level, when falls as low as 6–8mg/100ml, results in enamel hypoplasia in developing teeth.

Hypocalcification appears as opaque chalky white spots on the surface of the enamel. Dietary stresses cause injury to the functioning ameloblasts, resulting in faulty maturation. The mottled appearance of the tooth is because of these isolated white spots.

Clinically, hypoplasia is characterized by pitting caused by damage of ameloblasts. The pits are arranged in horizontal rows, extending into the enamel may be as far as the dentino-enamel junction.

Calcium and Dental Caries

A positive correlation has been reported between hypoplastic enamel and the incidence of caries. It has also been suggested that the hyperplasia in deciduous teeth is different from that in permanent teeth. The erupting hypoplastic deciduous tooth is smooth, soft, chalky and lacks density. The hyperplastic permanent tooth is pitted, grooved and of normal density. Susceptibility to decay is greatly dependent on the presence of pit and fissures on the enamel surface which serve to retain food.

This condition develops due to the following reasons.

• Increased dietary intake of calcium.
• Hyperparathyroidism
• Hypervitaminosis D
• Idiopathic hypercalcemia in infants

It causes loss of appetite, vomiting, constipation, weakness of muscles and sluggish reflex activities of the central nervous system.

Phosphorus

Phosphorus is widely distributed in most of the tissues in the body. A normal adult body contains about 600–800 gm of phosphorus, of which 80 to 90% is present in the bones and teeth and 10 to 20% in the soft tissue. In the hard tissues most of the phosphorous is present as phosphate or hydroxyapatite. Some of the soft tissue phosphorus is in the striated muscles as orthophosphates and pyrophosphates. A small amount of soft tissue phosphorus is in brain tissue in the form of nucleoprotein, lecithin and cephalin. The blood contains less than 2.0 gm phosphorus. The average biological life span of phosphorus in the animal body is only 30 days. The turnover of phosphorus in hard tissue requires months, while that in soft tissue takes only minutes.

About 10–40% of the dietary phosphorus is absorbed as inorganic phosphates in the small intestine. Absorption of phosphorus also depends upon the dietary contents of phosphorus, calcium and vitamin D. It is mainly excreted in urine and faeces.

Requirement

The daily requirement varies from 1.0 to 1.5g/day.

Sources

Calcium rich diets are rich sources of phosphorous also. Phosphorus is widely distributed in foods from plant and animal sources, e.g. wheat germ, nuts, walnuts, cheese, almonds, beans, wheat, fish, chicken, eggs, white bread and milk.

Functions

• Essential for the mineralization of bones and teeth along with calcium.
• Phosphorus, in the form of phospholipids, is essential for the transport and metabolism of lipids and also forms an integral part of the cell membrane.
• It is an integral part of the nucleus of the cell in the form of nucleic acids and thus is essential for protein synthesis and cell multiplication.
• It is necessary for the metabolism of carbohydrates and production of energy.
• It also plays an important role in the maintenance of acid-base balance and pH of the body fluids.

Deficiency of Phosphorus

Phosphorus deficiency seldom occurs in human populations because the common food is rich in phosphorus contents. Low serum phosphorus concentration may cause defective bone calcification.

Phosphorus and Dental Caries

Phosphorous deficiency leads to increased caries incidence.

Magnesium

Magnesium is one of the major minerals in animals and plant tissues. Human body contains approximately 20–30gm of magnesium. About 55% of magnesium is present in the bones. Liver, heart and pancreas also contain good amount of magnesium. 6.4% magnesium is in enamel and 0.9% in dentin.

Nearly 50% of the dietary magnesium is absorbed from the small intestine. High dietary intake of fat, calcium and phosphorus reduces magnesium absorption. An alkaline food also diminishes its absorption.

Magnesium is excreted both through faeces and urine.

Requirement

Average recommended daily intake by an adult is about 300 mg.

Sources

The food rich in magnesium are nuts, cereals and legumes, coca, cashewnuts, almonds, peanuts, oatmeal, walnuts, corn and brown rice.

Functions

- Magnesium is especially regarded as catalyst for many intracellular enzymatic reactions particularly those related to carbohydrate metabolism.
- Magnesium effects muscles and nervous tissues. In large amount it has anticonvulsion effect. In low concentration it causes hyperirritability and convulsions.
- It serves as a cofactor in several enzyme systems, which may be involved in growth and development of teeth and bones.

Deficiency of Magnesium

Magnesium deficiency can occur due to following causes:

- Diarrhoea, even for a few days in infants
- In adults, prolonged diarrhoea with malabsorption syndrome.

- Increased urinary loss due to renal disorder, diabetic ketoacidosis, hyperthyroidism and hyperparathyroidism.
- In chronic alcoholics.

Systemic Manifestations

Deficiency of magnesium leads to alopecia, tropic skin lesions, hematomas and hyperaemic gums. Magnesium also interferes with protein synthesis. Magnesium deficiency also causes depression, hyperirritablility, cardiac arrythmias, muscular weakness and convulsions. Low levels of magnesium may also produce tetany.

Oral Manifestations

The effects of magnesium deficiency occur as follows:

1. *On Enamel Organ*
   a. The pre-dentin becomes two to three times wider, causing the dentin-pre-dentin junction to be in a different level known as 'Predentinstep' - a unique feature of magnesium deficiency.
   b. The dentin in the labial portion of the tooth is seriously affected. When magnesium deficiency is continued for 6 months, the enamel organs of the incisal area become completely atrophied and the cells are replaced by a noncellular structure. The enamel organ completely disappears from the apical portion and the connective tissue comes in direct contact with the outer dentin.
2. *On gingival tissues:* There is gingival hypertrophy with chronic destructive periodontitis and subsequently loosening the teeth.
3. *On enamel:* The deficiency affects tooth solubility thus indirectly helping caries development.

Zinc

The total body content of zinc in an adult is over 2.0 gm. The choroid of the eye and the prostate contain the highest concentration of zinc. Relatively high concentration is also present in the skin and bones

Only about 20% of zinc is absorbed. The main route of excretion is the faeces.

Requirement

Daily adult intake is about 10–15µgm.

Sources

Green leafy vegetables are excellent sources of zinc, e.g. lettuce, cabbage, peas, beans, asparagus, spinach, amaranth leaves, coriander leaves, mint and raddish leaves, etc. The greener the leafy vegetable, the higher is its carotene content.

Functions

- It plays an important role in nucleic acid and protein synthesis.
- It plays an important role in alcohol metabolism.
- It forms complex with insulin and helps in its storage.
- It is necessary for maintaining plasma concentration of vitamin A by stimulating its release from liver into blood.
- It stabilizes the structure of RNA and DNA.
- Since protein metabolism is of fundamental importance in aging, zinc plays an important role in aging.

Zinc Deficiency

Zinc deficiency may either be due to consumption of a diet deficient in zinc or malabsorption as in inflammatory bowel diseases. Because zinc remains bound to albumin, considerable amount of zinc may be lost in cases of nephropathy, dialysis, uraemia, alcoholism and patients with excessive burns.

Zinc deficiency leads to:

- Poor growth
- Loss of Appetite
- Hypogonadism
- Altered taste and smell
- Delayed wound healing
- Alopecia

Oral Manifestations

Concentration of zinc in enamel and dentin is about 0.02%. It has not been established whether zinc affects tooth mineralization and dental caries development.

Iron

Iron is an essential nutrient because it permits oxygen and electron transport. The total quantity of body iron varies with weight, haemoglobin concentration, sex and size of the storage component. The iron content of adult human beings varies between three and five grams. Two functional compartments of body iron are recognized:

- *An essential component:* It comprises about 70% of the total iron of body in the form of haemoglobin, myoglobin, haemoenzymes, cofactor and transport iron.
- *Non-essential components:* The remainder non-essential storage iron, found predominantly in liver, spleen and bone marrow as ferritin and haemosiderin.

The level of iron in the serum ranges from 0.09 to 0.18 mg/100 ml for men and from 0.07 to 0.15 mg/100 ml for women. The total amount of Iron in circulating plasma of an adult amounts to only 3–4 mg. It is important to note that sufficient haemoglobin is broken down each day to release about 20 to 25 mg of iron. Since the actual requirement of a normal man each day is only 1.0 mg, it is evident that essentially all the iron required for haemoglobin synthesis is recovered from discarded haemoglobin molecules.

The consumption of common beverages may affect iron absorption. It is decreased by tea. This may be due to binding of iron by tannin. Alcohol may promote absorption.

Calcium and phosphorus may interfere with iron absorption, since iron and phosphorus have low solubilities and calcium reduces the acidity of aqueous mixtures.

Iron is excreted both in the faeces and urine.

Requirement

An adult man requires approximately 1.0 mg of iron daily, while a woman of menstrual age requires a total of about 2.0 mg of iron daily.

Sources

Meat, meat products, cereals, vegetables and fruits all contain iron. Leguminous plants and green leafy vegetables have excellent concentration of iron.

Functions

The essential iron or the functional iron is involved in the normal metabolism of the cells. This is a component of several proteins such as haemoglobin, myoglobin, peroxidases and catalases, cytochromes and also iron requiring enzymes, e.g. xanthine oxidase, dehydrogenase, etc.

Iron Deficiency

Systemic Manifestations

Iron deficiency results in hypochromic microcytic anaemia. A common mild form of iron deficiency syndrome is characterized by chronic fatigue, depleted iron stores and slightly depressed blood haemoglobin.

Patients with iron deficiency anaemia feel exhausted and are pale.

Oral Manifestations

Iron deficiency anaemia or plummer-vinson disease is characterized by fissures in the labial commissures and superficial glossitis. The papillae of the tongue are atrophied, thus giving the tongue a smooth, shiny and red appearance. The affected oral tissues become more susceptible to carcinoma.

- *Tongue:* The tongue has been described as a 'patchy irregular denudation of the papillae'. The epithelial tufts of the filiform papillae are absent.
- *Dental caries:* The effect of iron on caries development has not been fully established. However, iron has both a stimulatory and inhibitory effect upon the growth of oral bacteria.

Selenium

Selenium is an essential nutrient. Selenium is widely distributed in all tissues especially renal cortex, pancreas, pituitary and liver. Selenium is absorbed mainly in the duodenum and is excreted in the faeces and expired air.

Requirement

The daily required intake of selenium for an adult is about 50–200 µg.

Sources

Fish, meat and cereals are rich sources of selenium. Selenium is also available in milk, vegetables and fruits. The food content of selenium depends upon the selenium content of the soil.

Functions

- Selenium is closely related to vitamin E. It is postulated that vitamin E and selenium together have a protective effect in certain cancers because of their antioxidant properties.
- It prevents Keshon disease, which is characterized by multi-focal myocardial necrosis and reduced serum selenium contents.
- Selenium binds cadmium, mercury and other metals and masks their toxic effects.
- It plays a critical role in the control of oxygen metabolism, particularly in catalyzing the breakdown of hydrogen peroxide.
- It is required for the growth of human fibroblast and other cells.

Deficiency of Selenium

The deficiency of selenium is rare. In animals, deficiency may result in liver necrosis, degenerative changes in all parenchymal organs, muscular dystrophy, degeneration of heart muscles, endocardial calcification and pancreatic atrophy. It may result in cardio-myopathy and congestive heart failure.

Effect on Dental Tissue

Low concentration of selenium exerts a significant antibacterial effect on Streptococcus mutans. So it decreases the cariogenicity of plaque. Combination of selenium and fluoride may be more effective as a preventive agent for dental caries.

Chromium

Chromium is an essential micro nutrient required for the maintenance of normal glucose tolerance. The total body content of chromium in an adult man is 5–10 mg.

Chromium is absorbed in the small intestine and is excreted in urine.

Requirement

The required intake is about 2.0–5.0 mgm.

Sources

The sources are yeast, meats, whole grains and cheese.

Functions

Chromium is important in the regulation of blood glucose and acts as a potentiator of insulin secretion. The organic component of chromium is termed as glucose tolerance factor. It is also important in the metabolism of lipoprotein and has been shown to maintain normal levels of cholesterol in blood.

Deficiency

It causes impairment of glucose tolerance.

Manganese

The total body content is 11–20mg. It is found in the skin, muscles, bone and blood (RBC contains two third of the total body content). Manganese absorption occurs in duodenum and it is excreted through the biliary system.

Requirement

Daily requirement is about 50–100 mg.

Sources

It is widely distributed in nuts, whole grain, cereals, legumes and leafy vegetables. Tea is a rich source of Manganese.

Functions

- Proper synthesis of collagen and muco-polysaccharides.
- Stimulation of cholesterol synthesis.
- Auto-oxidation of melanin granules.
- Nutrition of brain.

Deficiency

Manganese deficiency is rare. Marked hypo-cholesteraemia, transient dermatitis, change in colour, slow growth of hair and weight loss has been noted.

Copper

The healthy adult human body contains about 100–150 mg of copper, out of which nearly 50% is found in muscles and 25% in bones. It is stored in liver, spleen and bone marrow.

Copper is absorbed from the upper section of the small intestine and is normally excreted in the bile, sweat and by desquamation.

Requirement

Daily requirement is 2.0 mg/day for adults.

Sources

Green leafy vegetables, legumes and meat are good sources while milk is a poor source of copper.

Normal adult diet provides about 1.0–3.0 mg of copper/day.

Functions

The main role of copper is in cellular oxidation reduction reactions. It also helps in synthesis and maintenance of structure and function of central nervous, cardiovascular and skeletal system.

Causes of Deficiency

Copper deficiency is less common in adults. In children, Kwashiorkor, recurrent diarrhoea, proteinuric states and diet consisting exclusively of milk are relatively common causes of deficiency.

Systemic Manifestations

Two definite disorders due to copper deficiency have been identified.

* Microcytic hypochromic anaemia: Copper is essential for iron absorption, transport and synthesis of haem. Anaemia due to copper deficiency is usually seen in children.
* Menke's Kinkyhair Syndrome is a progressive brain disease in infants. The features are:
  * Severe mental deficiency
  * Steel hair
  * Long metaphyseal abnormalities
  * Micrognathism
  * Neonatal ataxia
  * Hypothermia
  * Abnormal elastic tissue in arteries leading to fragmentation of endothelium, tortuous cerebral arteries, arterial occlusion and even early death.

Oral Manifestations

Copper salts have been shown to decrease plaque formation in human thus affecting the pathogenesis of caries.

Cobalt

An adult human body contains only about 1.0–2.0 mg of cobalt, which is mainly concentrated in liver and kidneys.

Cobalt is poorly absorbed from the gut and most of the endogenous cobalt is excreted in urine.

Requirement

Daily adult requirement is about 1.0–2.0 µg/day.

Sources

Cobalt is widely distributed in plants and animal tissues.

Functions

It is an important constituent of vitamin B12. It is also an activator of many enzymes.

Deficiency

Cobalt deficiency has not been observed in human body. It's deficiency may cause nutritional type of anaemia.

Cadmium

Calcium is mostly concentrated in the kidneys. The kidneys of hypertensive individuals have more cadmium levels than normal subjects.

Certain foods, particularly shell fish and mammalian liver, may contain more than 100 mg/gm. Usually the daily amount ingested is approximately 50 mg.

A diet deficient in calcium or protein may permit increased cadmium absorption from the gut. A cigarette contains 2.0 µg of which 5–10% may be inhaled. It is established that cadmium is cariogenic.

Strontium

Strontium is widely distributed in food and skeleton, however, it is not essential for human life.

Most of the intake is excreted in faeces and urine.

Dietary Sources

It is present in foods rich in calcium especially milk and fresh vegetables.

Strontium and Dental Caries

Effect of strontium on dental caries varies according to its salt. Low caries incidence is reported with use of strontium fluoride than strontium chloride.

Strontium is more effective after the teeth have started erupting.

Iodine

About 50 mgm of iodine is present in adult human body. Nearly two third is present in thyroid glands. Iodine is absorbed through alimentary canal. Most of the iodine in blood is in plasma. It is required for the synthesis of thyroid hormones and thyroxine.

Requirement

0.14 mg/day is sufficient for an average adult man and 0.10 mg/day for an adult woman. Iodine requirements are mostly fulfilled by drinking water.

Sources

Fruits, vegetables especially spinach, cereals and meat are good sources.

Deficiency

Deficiency of iodine results in enlargement of thyroid gland causing hypothyroidism, goitre and myxoedema. Iodine toxicity may results in throtoxicosis.

Molybdenum

Molybdenum is present in all tissues but liver and kidney contain maximum amount. It is essential part of several flavoprotein containing enzyme systems. For example, xanthine oxidase, aldehyde oxidase, etc. About 50% dietary molybdenum is absorbed and absorption occurs in small intestine.

Requirement and Sources

Daily requirement is 0.5–2.0 mg for an average adult. Pulses, cereals, green leafy vegetables and meat are good sources.

Fluorine

It is an essential nutrient for mineralization of bones and formation of enamel. For details see Chapter 4.

Water

Water is an important constituent of diet, comprising intracellular and extracellular component of our body. It cannot be labelled as food as it does not give energy like other nutrients. It constitutes about two thirds of the man's body weight.

As water constitutes two third of human body, a normal man of 65 kg contains approximately 40 liters of water. About 28 liters of this is intracellular and 12 liters is extracellular. Almost all membranes of the body are permeable to water. It passes easily into all the cells and fluid compartments. The final distribution between the compartments is determined by osmotic and the hydrostatic pressure. Under normal conditions, total amount of water remains constant in the body.

Water acts as solvent for all the salts helping in digestion and absorption by the body. It also dissolves the waste materials providing good medium for excreting body wastes. Another important role of water in our body is regularizing the body temperature by sweating and evaporation. The volume and the composition of the body fluids are regulated with water. An adequate intake of water and electrolytes is essential for the maintenance of the volume and composition of the body fluids.

Life is beyond imagination without water. Water requirements are dependent on age of the patient, body temperature, temperature of the surroundings, renal solute load and extra renal loss. The total fluid intake increases with age. The total body fluid requirement is 1200 ml for 1 year olds and 1500 ml for 5 years age group. It exceeds to 3000 ml per day for adults.

Water is an essential nutrient to surgical patients. The intracellular and extracellular fluid balance must be maintained for them. Water retention is largely dependent on body sodium and sodium excretion is dependent on body water. A surgical patient with normal kidney should receive 1500 to 2500 ml. of water daily.

For geriatric patients, drinking water in smaller amounts at frequent intervals is recommended. This will relieve them from constipation.

Sources and Distribution of Water

We get water from many sources like vegetables, fruits, meat, fish, tea, coffee, milk, juices and even plain drinking water. The amount of water needed depends on age, type of work and climate. In our body some of the water is a by-product of oxidation of glucose (carbohydrate).

Consequences of Water Depletion in Human Body

Physiologically water is lost from urine, skin, during expiration, sweating and faeces. Water is also lost from the human body due to excessive bleeding, vomiting and diarrhoea leading to dehydration so the extracellular fluid becomes hypertonic and the concentration of plasma sodium rises. Water then migrates extracellularly from the cells until osmotic equilibrium is re-established and intracellular dehydration occurs. Patient exhibits mental confusion, vertigo and difficulty in swallowing. In severe cases the skin and tissues become doughy in consistency. Ultimately renal blood flow is reduced and blood urea concentration rises.

Regulation

Since water contributes two third of body weight in adults, an adequate intake of water and electrolytes is essential for maintenance of volume within normal limits. Any change in osmotic pressure will stimulate the hypothalamus which has neural connections with post pituitary. This stimulation will release antidiuretic hormone (ADH) into general circulation and ultimately reaches the renal tubules, where it increases the reabsorption of water and thus decreases urine volume. Ingestion of fluids in excess decreases plasma osmotic pressure, suppresses ADH release and increases urine volume to re-establish fluid equilibrium.

Water and Health

The quality of life is expressed in terms of cleanliness. The health of an individual, a community or a nation is determined by the environment. Any disturbance in the balance between the man and the environment will lead to disease. The environment must be clean in order to control or prevent the occurrence of a disease. Sanitation is a way of life which is expressed in terms of cleanliness of an individual and his surroundings and it must come from within the people. The WHO defines environmental sanitation as "the control of all those factors in man's physical environment which exercise or may exercise a deleterious effect on his physical development, health and survival". For the environmental sanitation, services of public health qualified doctor, the epidemiologist, the public health engineer, the town planner, the sociologist, the economist and the health inspector are required.

In India, 80% of the population live in rural areas. These areas must be supplied by safe and wholesome water and the human excreta must be disposed off properly. The standard of living vis-a-vis the public health can be improved by controlling a number of factors like food, water, housing, clothing and sanitation.

Water being the most important needs of the human body should not only be safe for drinking but also agreeable to use. It should be free from pathogens, free from harmful chemical substances, pleasant to taste and useable for domestic purposes. Water gets polluted or contaminated by various agents viz. micro-organisms, poisonous chemical substances, industrial and other wastes or sewage.

Other Aspects of Nutrition

Food Hygiene

It implies to the hygiene in the production, handling, distribution and serving of all types of food. Its main aim is to prevent food poisoning and other food borne diseases.

Food Borne Diseases

It is defined as a disease either infectious or toxic in nature caused by an agent that enters the body through the ingestion of food. The possible diseases are:

a. Due to intoxication
   • Lathyrism
   • Endemic ascitis
   • Botulism
   • Ergot
b. Due to infection
   • *Bacterial:* Typhoid, Paratyphoid, Salmonellosis.
   • *Viral:* Viral hepatitis, Gastroenteritis.
   • *Parasitic:* Amoebiasis, Taeniasis.

Among the *food borne diseases,* milkborne and meatborne diseases are of special importance.

Milkborne diseases are Tuberculosis, Brucellosis, Q fever, Cow pox, Anthrax, etc.

Meatborne diseases are Tapeworm infections like Taenea solium and bacterial infections like anthrax, tuberculosis, etc.

Food Additives

These are non-nutritious substances which are added intentionally to improve appearance, flavour, texture or storage properties of food. There are:
• Colouring agents such as Saffron, Turmeric.
• Flavouring agents as Vanilla.
• Sweeteners such as Saccharin
• Preservatives such as Sodium benzoate, Sorbic acid.
• Imparting activity such as Acetic acid.

Food Fortification

It is the process whereby nutrients are added to foods to maintain or improve the quality of food. For example, Vanaspati which is a vegetable ghee, is deficient in vitamin A and D as compared to animal fat (Desi Ghee), so vanaspati is fortified with vitamin A and D. Similarly common salt, i.e. Sodium Chloride is fortified with Iodine.

Food Adulteration

It is defined as the process of mixing, substituting, concealing, putting up decomposed foods for sale, misbranding or giving false labels and addition of food additives more than recommended doses. Examples are:
• Mixing water in milk or mustard oil with argemone oil.
• Subtracting cream from milk.
• Non-permitted colours used by sweet makers, green dye used in green peas packing.

BIBLIOGRAPHY

1. Bendich Adrianne: Vitamins and Immunity. J. Nutr. : 122, 601, 1992.
2. Blackburn, G.L. : Standards for nutritional assessment. Clin. Consult. Nutr. Suppl. : 1, 10, 1981.
3. Bray, G. and Atkinson, R.L. : Factors affecting basal metabolic rate. Food Nutr. Sci. : 2, 395, 1977.
4. Grande, F. and Keys, A. : Body weight, body composition and calorific status. Mod. Nutr. Hyg. Dis. : 6, 297, 1980.

5. Maki, A. Patricia and Newberne, M. Paul: Ditary lipids and immune function. J. Nutr. : 122, 610, 1992.

6. Prabhu, P. : Geriatric nutrition. Res. and Dev. J. : 4, 3, 1997.

7. Rao, N. Pralhad: Monitoring nutrient intake in India. Ind. Pedia. : 54, 495, 1987.

8. Reddy Vinodini: Child nutrition in India; Priorities for the coming decade. Ind. Pedia. : 30, 289, 1993.

9. Rogers, J. Peter: How important is breakfast? Brit. J. Nut. : 78, 197, 1997.

10. Ruxton, C.H.S. and Kirk, T.R. : Breakfast: a review of associations with measures of dietary intake, physiology and biochemistry. B. J. of Nut. : 78, 199, 1997.

11. Saini, A.S., Kaur, J., Lal, H. and Kumar, N. : Nutritional requirements in infancy. Ind. Pedia. : 29, 203, 1992.

12. Waterlow, J.C. : Protein turnover in the whole body. Nature: 253, 157, 1975.

13. Young, V.R., Skeffee, W.P. and Pencharz, P.B. : Total human body protein synthesis in relation to protein requirements at various ages. Nature: 253, 192, 1975.

4 Fluorides

Inventions and discoveries, mostly, are accidental. Fluoride was also accidently discovered by *Mckay* of Colorado in 1901. He discovered that many of his patients were suffering from discolouration of teeth—a unique type of staining, which he termed *Colorado stain*. Later, it was found to be related with the fluoride content of drinking water. Thereafter the pathology was named *mottled enamel*. By that time it was established that the causative factor was definitely the fluoride present in drinking water. Various authors confirmed the role of fluoride in mottling, as some children who were kept on drinking water free of fluoride did not show such discolouration of teeth. Till that time, the exact percentage of fluoride present in water or the percentage of fluoride which was responsible for mottling, etc. was not known to the profession. Later, a few authors noted stains resembling mottled enamel in experimental animals kept on high fluoride drinking water. Further, it was established that the severity of mottling of enamel was related to the concentration of fluoride in drinking water. Dean established that upto 1 ppm fluoride is not injurious to public health. He also presented the Mottling Index or classification of mottling.

Mckay also observed that there might be an inverse association between level of mottling and prevalence of caries. Mottled enamel was found to be less susceptible to decay than normal enamel. Studies were conducted to determine the concentration of fluoride which could inhibit caries without having any systemic side effects. *Dean*, in his study, observed that children taking water containing 0.6 ppm to 1.5 ppm fluoride, exhibited only 4–5% caries free incidence whereas children who had used water containing 1.7–2.5 ppm fluoride showed 22% caries free incidence. Many other authors confirmed that the caries prevalence was lower in high fluoride areas compared to low fluoride areas. In the light of all these studies, fluoride and dental caries entered a new phase in Public Health Dentistry.

After prolonged studies and deliberations, important milestone was reached that at 1 ppm fluoride near maximum caries reduction can be achieved. Only the mildest form of mottling may appear which can be practically insignificant. All these findings paved the way for implementation of water fluoridation as a public health measure worldwide. World Health Organization accepted that water fluoridation is a simple and inexpensive measure to reduce the prevalence of dental caries in public.

FLUORIDATION AS A PUBLIC HEALTH MEASURE

Water fluoridation can be defined as *the adjustment of the concentration of fluoride ion in public water supply in such a way that the concentration of fluoride ion in water may be consistently maintained at 1 ppm by weight*. In hot climate countries where water consumption is more, slightly less than 1 ppm fluoride level is maintained. In very cold climate, level of 1.2 ppm fluoride is recommended and in very hot climates 0.7 ppm fluoride is recommended. The optimum fluoride concentration for a particular community can be calculated by the following equation.

ppm = (Fluoride concentration by weight)
    = 0.34/K

where K = –0.038 + 0.0062 × Temperature of the area in °F

Defluoridation of water is also taken up for public health where the fluoride concentration is more than 1 ppm.

Why and Where?

Any population with moderate to high prevalence of caries needs fluoridation. Fluoridation requires an efficient public water supply and it must reach the public in every nook and corner. If part of a population consumes water from wells and other sources, the fluoridation scheme is not indicated. Until recently, high prevalence of dental caries was a problem limited to western countries only but this has now inflicted Asian countries as well. Anticipating the trend, most Asian countries have started implementing fluoridation.

The number of dentists with respect to population size is insufficient in almost every country. In India, the dentist-population ratio of 1:80,000 is much more worrisome than the corresponding figure of 1:1200 in Sweden. Every country is planning to expand the horizon of dental services so as to meet the alarming challenge of caries prevalence.

In agreement with the old saying, 'prevention is better than cure', treating caries by whatever means would be practically impossible at the community level. Fluoridation could be the best way to reduce caries prevalence. This is economically more reliable, time saving and avoids the sequelae of caries e.g. pain, abscess formation, extraction etc. Mental and physical trauma to the patients suffering from caries and/or loss of teeth can be avoided by prevention and water fluoridation would be the best method of doing so at the community level.

The United States carried out artificial water fluoridation for the first time in 1945, whereby for six years children were given water containing 1 ppm fluoride. Afterwards it was noticed that caries prevalence was reduced to half. So convincing was the evidence in favour of fluoridation that other cities of the U.S. followed suit and it was confirmed that 1 ppm fluoride in drinking water was the best source to act as a caries inhibitor. Subsequently, many countries in the world started water fluoridation. Certain other countries like Ireland made water fluoridation mandatory for its population. Till date, more than 70 million people all over the world are protected by artificial fluoridation. Unfortunately in India, a water fluoridation project has not started at the Government level even though around 30% people consume pipe water. The dentist-population ratio in India is very low and coupled with a lack of awareness about oral health; community water supply having an optimum fluoride level is therefore considered to be the most effective, practical and economical way of preventing dental decay. At the least, water fluoridation at the school level can be considered. For the communities, different methods can be explored and implemented with the help of the media.

ALTERNATIVE METHODS OF FLUORIDATION

In India, about 70% of the population is deprived of the facility of pipe water. Various other countries also have a similar problem. Keeping in view this dilemma, it becomes imperative to look for other dietary sources which can be safely digested and used systemically, taking advantage of fluorides.

Different dietary components have been tried viz., fluoridated salt, milk, tablets, etc. to provide continuous systemic ingestion.

Salt Fluoridation

Switzerland was the first country to use fluoridated salt for its population. The rationale behind this approach was that if iodised salt can be helpful in reducing goitre incidence, fluoridated salt can be utilized in reducing caries. 20–25% reduction in dental caries was observed when salt containing 90 ppm fluoride was used. Toth reported that after 8 years of salt fluoridation at a level of 250 mg fluoride/kg salt there was a 41% decrease in dmft in 2–6 years old children; 58% decrease in 7–11 years and 36% in 12–14 years old children. Various other studies substantiated that addition of fluoride in salt reduces the prevalence of caries.

Fluoride is usually added to salt by spraying a concentrated solution of sodium fluoride or potassium fluoride on it followed by mixing. There is no international consensus regarding the concentration of fluoride in salt as yet. 90 mg fluoride/kg salt was used in Switzerland, while 200 mg/kg salt is being used in Columbia and Spain, etc. It is estimated that up to 300 mg fluoride/kg salt can be considered safely. Since the addition of fluoride in salt does not alter its colour and taste it is accepted by all.

Milk Fluoridation

Theoretically, milk fluoridation is advantageous, but practically milk consumption is limited, especially in developing countries like India. A majority of children living in rural and urban areas cannot afford milk daily and moreover there is a need for a central milk supply. Various studies have indicated that an addition of 2.5 mg NaF in milk which was served daily to school children resulted in 35% of reduction in caries.

There was a controversy regarding the use of fluoride in milk as opponents of the concept were of the view that fluoride binds with calcium and protein making it unavailable for its anticariogenic activity. However, other authors, using radioactive isotopes proved that the availability of fluoride four hours after consumption of milk was the same as that of water.

Fluoride Tablets

Fluoride tablets result in systemic effects before mineralization of primary and permanent dentitions is completed; whereas after the completion of mineralization, they have topical effects as well. Various studies have shown caries reduction to be in the range of 50–80% when fluoride tablets were administered for a period of 2–3 years. Various other authors have given different percentages of caries reduction, but all were of the view that there was a definite reduction of caries prevalence using fluoride tablets. The dose was kept at 0.5 mg fluoride tablet daily for children below three years of age and 1.0 mg thereafter. Most of the studies were conducted using NaF tablets; however few of them used Acidulated phosphate fluoride (APF) tablets.

The data strongly supports the observations that the use of fluoride supplements during development of the dentition results in caries reduction much better than water fluoridation. It was agreed upon that the critical period during which fluoride must be ingested systemically in order to exert maximum cariostatic effect is during the mineralization of the surface of a crown.

Commercially, fluoride tablets are available as NaF tablets of 2.2 mg, 1.1 mg and 0.55 mg yielding 1 mg, 0.5 mg and 0.25 mg fluoride respectively. The trade name of these tablets are Fluoroday, Tymaflour and Luride. Drops of these dosages are also available for young children who are unable to swallow tablets. Combinations of NaF and vitamins in tablet form are also available and can be given wherever indicated.

Vitamin supplements are indicated in the following situations:

a. Children from deprived families who did not have adequate diet.

b. Children suffering from anorexia, poor appetite, and poor eating habits.
c. Dietary insufficiency in breast-fed infants of malnourished mothers.

Routine use of vitamin supplements is of no use since there is little evidence of mineral insufficiency except that of iron. However, total insufficiency of minerals is the major nutritional problem in children especially amongst lower socio-economic groups.

Fluoride tablets should be chewed and swallowed to obtain dual benefits of topical as well as systemic effects. This dual role of fluoride tablets makes them an important means for dental caries prevention, especially at the community level.

Fluoride Mouth Rinses

Wherever water fluoridation is not feasible, different modalities have been tried using low concentration of fluoride. Mouth rinsing with a fluoride solution twice or thrice a week can be helpful. It has been established that using 0.2% NaF mouth rinse would lead to 40-50% reduction of caries. Various authors in their respective studies have shown a reduction in dental caries using fluoride mouth rinses. Further, it was observed that both APF and NaF were found to be equal as far as cariostatic potential was concerned.

Fluoride rinses daily or weekly can be made compulsory in schools. Alternatively, at homes, daily rinsing with fluoride is feasible. One tablet of 200 mg NaF can be dissolved in approximately 25ml of clean water which is sufficient for rinsing for one family.

Clinically, the frequent use of a low concentration of fluoride (0.05% NaF) is more cariostatic than less frequent use of higher concentration (0.25% NaF). Where water fluoridation is present or fluoride content of water is sufficiently high, rinsing would give a superadded benefit. It has been reported that rinsing with a diluted solution of fluoride results in rapid elevation of plaque fluoride concentration but that level essentially returns to normal within 24 hours. From these findings one can assume that daily rinsing would be superior to once a week rinsing. In case stannous fluoride is used, it provides additional cariostatic action because stannous fluoride exerts an antibacterial effect against some plaque microorganisms and also inhibits plaque formation by reducing the free energy of enamel.

It is reported that very low levels of fluorides in the oral fluids are associated with concentrated level of fluorides in plaque and even low concentrations of fluorides are sufficient to inhibit glycolysis and acid production by plaque organisms. In addition, repeated exposure to low concentration of fluoride effectively promotes remineralization of incipient carious lesions.

Many studies later confirmed and suggested that optimum preventive results with fluoride could be achieved by frequent exposure of plaque to low concentrations of fluoride ions.

Various other fluoride compounds have been tested as mouthrinses, but none of them has shown sufficient cariostatic activity as compared to sodium fluoride and stannous fluoride. One compound, amine fluoride, commonly used as mouthrinse, showed no superiority over neutral sodium fluoride. Similarly, ammonium fluoride mouthrinse was not as effective as sodium fluoride.

Various authors have used rinsing of 200 ppm F as NaF or SnF_2 for two years and noted that rinsing with stannous fluoride continued to have selective suppression of Streptococcus mutans. Many techniques and studies have proved the efficiency of SnF_2 in reducing Streptococcus mutans. Chemically, growth and adherence changes in S. mutans have been associated with the accumulation of tin in these cells. The usual explanation for antimicrobial properties of stannous fluoride is that with mouthrinsing, stannous fluoride inhibits acid production in plaque for several hours and this subsequent increase in plaque pH creates an environment not conducive for Streptococcus mutans.

Stannous fluoride has long been prescribed by dental professionals since long without any known adverse effects. The tin ions are quite safe even when ingested. Staining and metallic taste are some of the reported side effects. A thorough understanding of the appropriate concentration, frequencies and dosage of stannous fluoride will enable the most effective and efficient use of this agent in the prevention of plaque, caries, and periodontal diseases.

Fluoride mouthrinses are relatively safe, as accidental swallowing of even the full volume of the rinse would result in ingestion of 9 mg F or 2.3 mg F on the basis of weekly or daily regime respectively. This is well below the minimum dose of 120 mg F estimated to be safely tolerated by a 5 year old child. Older children have a proportionally greater margin of safety.

Fluoride mouthrising appears to be more cost effective and quite successful as a preventive procedure in reducing caries incidence. It is a simple, safe, well accepted and relatively inexpensive way of preventing caries.

Fluoride Dentifrices

The term dentifrice was derived from a Latin word meaning *by rubbing the tooth*. The most commonly evaluated dentifrices are NaF and SnF_2 and recently sodium monofluorophosphate has also been used.

Earlier studies reported no effect of 0.2% NaF and 0.4% SnF_2 in reducing caries. Certain authors, however, reported reduction in dental caries ranging from 6 to 20 percent with these agents.

Recently, amine fluoride has been shown to have cariostatic potential. It was observed that organic fluorides were better than inorganic fluorides when used as dentifrices. Dentifrices containing monofluorophosphate at a concentration of 0.76% fluoride with sodium metaphosphate have led to variable reduction in caries rates ranging from 17% to 34% depending upon fluoride and non-fluoride areas. Monofluorophosphate dentifrices are considered to be more advantageous than SnF_2 and NaF because MFP has a neutral pH (6.5) compared to SnF_2, which has an acidic pH (4.8).

Fluoride containing tooth pastes generally have approximately 500–1000 ppm fluoride. About 8 to 16 mg fluoride per kg body weight is considered the safe dose of fluorides. The lethal dose of fluoride is 32-64 mg fluoride per kg body weight. It accounts for about 5,000 to 10,000 mg of NaF for a 70 kg adult. So a large sized tube containing 200 gm tooth paste is safe even if its contents are ingested all at once.

The recommended norms for use of fluoride tooth pastes are:

* Below 6 years, no fluoride tooth paste.
* 6-10 years, once daily.
* Above 10 years, twice daily.

The protocol for use of prophylaxis pastes in caries prevention can be one of the following:

a. Caries inhibitory potential of frequent professional prophylaxis with fluoride free and fluoride containing tooth pastes.

b. Caries inhibitory potential of infrequent professional prophylaxis with fluoride free and fluoride containing prophylaxis tooth pastes.

c. Caries inhibitory potential of self applied fluoride containing tooth paste.

d. Routine use of fluoride free or fluoride containing pastes prior to professional topical fluoride treatment.

All these methods with varying periods of observation have been studied by various authors. Annual or biannual dental prophylaxis is routinely used in most of the preventive programmes, but there is no evidence to support that the infrequent use of pastes have any cariostatic results.

Both fluoride containing and fluoride free pastes have been used prior to traditional topical applications. Neither has been shown to impart any beneficial effect. Thus the routine use of prior prophylaxis is not recommended. The conclusion is that prophylaxis pastes play no role in the prevention of dental caries. However, pastes do remove extrinsic stains and help in reducing plaque (an important component of periodontal disease). Whenever teeth are polished, a thin layer of enamel is abraded resulting in the loss of fluoride from the tooth surface. Fluoride containing tooth pastes may replenish the fluoride abraded by the polishing procedures. Prior to its use, the bioavailability of fluoride from the fluoride paste must be assessed. Since dentifrices do not require specific methods and supervision, their use can be considered safe and the best method, provided the fluoride is made available to the enamel.

Professionally Accepted Topical Fluorides

Dean, the pioneer in fluoride research, demonstrated that fluoride ions in a diluted solution when kept in contact with teeth, bind with the enamel surface and render it less soluble than the original enamel surface. This observation led to the idea of topical fluoridation. Since water fluoridation has its own limitations, topical fluoridation can be an effective method at the school level.

In early studies 0.1% NaF solution was used in topical fluoride preparations. Later, various other agents were also tried, e.g. stannous fluoride (SnF_2), acidulated phosphate fluoride (APF) and other fluoride varnishes. Various techniques of fluoride application have also been tried. 0.1% NaF solution when applied for 7–8 minutes, repeating the same at four monthly intervals in the first year and two monthly interval in the second year led to 45% reduction in caries after one year and 33% after two years. In another technique, four applications of NaF at weekly intervals in one year

and booster application of NaF at 7, 10 and 13 years of age were tried. Different regimes of NaF applications for various periods led to 20–40% reduction in caries

Method of Application

The teeth are cleaned and polished. They are then isolated and dried. 0.2% NaF is applied with cotton applicators and is permitted to dry on the teeth. It takes about 4–5 minutes. This procedure is repeated for every quadrant. The patient is instructed to avoid eating and drinking for at least one hour so as to prolong the availability of fluoride ions on the tooth surfaces. Second, third and fourth applications are given at weekly intervals. Using the same technique, 8% SnF_2 is applied once a year. APF is also applied in a similar way. To make APF in a gel form, methyl cellulose or hydroxy ethyl cellulose is added.

The interproximal surfaces with their contacts and protected areas for bacterial colonization are high risk surfaces. Tray application of topical fluorides certainly contacts the buccal and lingual surfaces, but may not cover the interproximal sites. The areas below the contact points are not covered with conventional gels. To achieve fluoridation of these contact areas, flossing of the interproximal surfaces with APF gel is beneficial. This will carry the gel into the interproximal sites. The mean DMFS after topical application of APF gel by various methods is given in Table 4.1.

Fluoride Varnishes

The topical fluoride solutions currently in use, such as NaF, SnF_2 or APF, have a major disadvantage that they remain in contact with teeth only for a short period and then get diluted with saliva. It has also been observed that with a topical fluoride solution much of the acquired fluoride, probably unreacted fluoride, leaches away within the first 24 hours.

Table 4.1: Evaluation of procedures that use prophylaxis paste for caries prevention

Procedure	Comments
• Frequent professional prophylaxis (upto 1 x ½ weeks) with a fluoride containing or fluoride-free paste	• Method impractical
• Infrequent professional prophylaxis (1 x 1 or 2 x 1 year) with a fluoride-free paste	• No evidence of effectiveness
• Infrequent professional prophylaxis (1x1 or 2 x 1 year) with a fluoride containing paste	• Effective in controlled clinical trials
• Self administered prophylaxis with a fluoride containing paste	• Not effective in controlled clinical trials
• Preliminary prophylaxis with a fluoride containing paste prior to professional topical fluoride application	• Does not provide additional benefits to the topical fluoride treatment
• Preliminary prophylaxis with a fluoride free paste prior to professional topical fluoride application	• Does not provide additional benefits to the topical fluoride treatment. Unnecessary as a routine procedure

Courtesy: Wei (1985)

Experiments were carried out aiming at overcoming the disadvantages of topical fluorides and prolonging the contact of fluoride solutions with tooth enamel leading to deeper penetration of fluoride in enamel. Fluoride ions were bound with the tooth surface by using cyanoacrylates which kept saliva away for some more time. *Groneveld et al (1982)* used fluoride lacquer which released fluoride ions to the dental enamel in high concentration for several hours. Consequently, the use of fluoride varnishes in caries prevention became the treatment of choice. The most commonly used varnishes are Duraphat (NaF containing 2.5% F) and Fluorprotector (Silane fluoride with 0.7% F). They have the ability to adhere to the enamel thereby extending the fluoride exposure time to several hours.

Various authors have observed reduction in caries prevalence with the use of fluoride varnishes. Few authors have compared Duraphat and Fluorprotector and have found that caries was significantly reduced by both fluoride varnishes, but Duraphat was found to be more effective than Fluorprotector. However, *Groeneveld (1982)* has reported no difference in caries incidence after an annual application of Fluorprotector and Duraphat. It has been shown that silane fluoride of Fluorprotector reacts with water to produce considerable amounts of hydrofluoric acid (HF), which penetrates enamel more readily than fluoride. Fluorosilanes enhance retention and penetration of fluoride in enamel. Authors were of the view that the acidic condition produced by a reaction between silane fluoride and oral fluids enhances the formation of CaF_2, which leads to slow release of fluoride to the deeper layers. It was proved that if a sufficient amount of CaF_2 is deposited on the enamel surface for a sufficiently long time, the amount of fluoride in enamel can be increased significantly.

The technique of application remains the same. 0.5 ml of fluoride varnish is required for the entire dentition. The varnish sets in 4-5 minutes; till that time complete isolation is maintained. The patient is instructed not to drink for one hour and not to eat for 24 hours after treatment. In order to prevent the deleterious effects of saliva, its flow can be decreased using systemic medicines. A single

Table 4.2: Mean DMFS increments of children receiving biannual professional APF gel-tray topical fluoride treatment

Treatment	Ripa et al 1983 (Two years)	Houpt et al 1983 (Two years)	Katz et al 1984 (2.5 years)	Ripa et al 1984 (Three years)
Prophylaxis + Topical Fluoride	2.12	2.05	2.23	3.33
Self Brush + Topical Fluoride	1.87	2.48	2.33	3.18
Topical Fluoride	2.02	2.14	2.09	3.19

Courtesy : Wei (1985)

application of Duraphat (0.5ml) contains 11.3 mg F and Fluorprotector contains 3.1 mg F. The plasma fluoride level for Fluorprotector has been found to be lower than Duraphat owing to low fluoride content. The plasma fluoride level after 2 hours was found to be 0.180 g/ml after Duraphat application and 0.140 g/ml after Fluorprotector application.

It is an accepted fact that *Streptococcus mutans* is essential in the initiation of caries and it is also reported that if the *Streptococcus mutans* count is more than 6,00,000 (6 lac) per ml of saliva, the individual is at a high risk. Specifically, reducing plaque by antibiotic therapy and/or chlorhexidine rinse may prove to be effective, but suppression or elimination of *Streptococcus mutans* without reducing non-pathogenic bacteria would be superior and more biologically acceptable. Professional application of 8% SnF_2 has been found to be very effective in reducing *Streptococcus mutans*. However, no effect was seen on *Streptococcus sanguis* and Lactobacilli.

PRENATAL FLUORIDES

A discussion of the rationale for the use of prenatal fluorides in preventing dental caries includes several factors, although the efficacy of prenatal fluorides is still a controversial topic. Various authors in their different studies have reported conflicting results.

The permeability of the placenta to fluoride has been questioned due to several observations such as:

a. Lack of literature reporting fluorosis in deciduous teeth.

b. A high concentration of fluoride in placenta.

c. Fluoride concentration of bound tissues of foetus differ in areas with different concentration of fluorides in water.

d. Validity of transfer of fluoride from the maternal circulation to the foetal circulation.

Since primary teeth calcify primarily before birth and few reports exist of fluorotic primary teeth, fluoride is assumed to have limited access to the foetus. However, *Thylstrup (1978)* has observed that primary teeth of all children in areas where water contained 3.5, 6.0 or more ppm fluoride exhibited varying degrees of fluorosis. The severity of fluorosis was positively associated with the concentration of fluoride in water supply. *Thylstrup* is of the view that placenta is permeable to fluoride and the appearance of fluorosis in primary teeth may be affected by enamel thickness.

Fluoride supplements given to pregnant mothers are absorbed primarily in the maternal stomach and to a lesser degree in the small intestine. Fluoride as hydrogen fluoride diffuses across the gastric mucosa and then dissociates in the circulatory system to yield fluoride ions. The maximum plasma fluoride level is achieved within 30–60 minutes, after which the extraction of fluoride from plasma exceeds absorption. Ultimately, most of the fluoride is either taken up by the mineralized tissues or excreted in urine. Unabsorbed fluoride is excreted in the faeces. *Wei (1985)* has quoted various authors who have proposed that fluoride does diffuse across the placenta. High fluoride concentration in the placenta has been observed and also that the placenta acts as a barrier to prevent traces of fluoride from reaching the foetus. Few authors are of the view that fluoride is taken up by the foetal bones and teeth.

Fluoride uptake increases with age of the foetus and is greater in bones than teeth. There is little significant difference between tissues formed at 1 ppm F and 0.5 ppm F.

Studies on pregnant women and animals treated with an intravenous fluoride show rapid maternal clearance with a slight increase in fetal blood fluoride. Generally, fluoride concentration in foetal blood does not exceed 25% of the fluoride concentration of maternal blood. It is agreed that fluoride concentration of foetal blood is greater when the mother either receives a 1.0 mg tablet of fluoride or drinks artificially fluoridated water during pregnancy then when she drink non fluoridated water or receive no fluoride supplement.

Prenatal Exposure to Fluoridated Water

The effect of fluorides on caries reduction when given prenatally has been studied by various authors. In most of the studies, fluoride has been given both prenatally and post natally. Mostly, an insignificant decrease in caries prevalence in deciduous teeth of children whose mothers were exposed to increased amount of fluoridated water during pregnancy has been observed. A 30–35% reduction in caries was noticed when fluorides were given both prenatally and postnatally. Also fluoride given both prenatally and postnatally was found to be more effective as compared to when it was given only post-natally. Since the results were consistent with the studies of fluorides analysis of foetuses, it was concluded that prenatal exposure to fluoride produced pronounced reduction in dental caries rates.

Few authors reported definite caries reduction attributed to the use of prenatal fluoride supplements in optimally fluoridated areas. They were, however, later criticized on several accounts concerning the methodology, size of the population and in the validity of their conclusions.

It can be summarized that there is little amount of clinical evidence to show that prenatal fluoride supplements have cariostatic benefits. Prenatal fluoridated supplements, particularly in fluoridated areas cannot be recommended for public health measures due to problems associated with it.

Remineralization and Fluorides

Remineralization is one of the mechanisms by which fluorides can reduce caries incidence. This is the process by which a small carious lesion can be arrested or reversed. This can be affected by oral fluids and/or exposing the lesions to synthetic calcifying fluids. Various authors have confirmed that the presence of fluoride ions greatly enhances the degree of remineralization achieved and reduces the total time necessary for the same.

Basically, remineralization affects a carious lesion in two ways:

a. The lesion is reduced in size because of fluoride deposition.

b. The remineralized lesion becomes more resistant to progression.

The latter factor predominates in the prevention of caries.

Effect of Oral Fluids and other Synthetic Calcifying Fluids

Oral fluid contains a whole saliva sample and has additional components not found in salivary secretion obtained directly from a gland.

The calcifying fluid is prepared from a synthetic hydroxyapatite with calcium/phosphate ratio of 1:63. Sodium chloride and potassium hydroxide are added to adjust the pH at 7.0.

In the studies conducted, fluoride ions were added to samples of oral fluids and calcifying solution in a concentration of 10 ppm to 100 ppm. Artificial caries like lesions were created on the tooth surfaces by exposure to lactic acid gels (pH 3–4) for a period of 4–6 weeks. Longitudinal sections were obtained and were exposed to either the oral fluids or the calcifying solutions.

The results of these studies showed that when oral fluids were used as calcifying fluid, a very small reduction in lesion size was found, limited to the surface of the lesion. Addition of fluoride ions upto 10 ppm produced no noticeable increase in remineralization. When the fluoride level was increased upto 100 ppm, increase in remineralization was found and the lesion was reduced by upto 10% in size. Tenacious deposits were produced on the enamel surface. The bulk of coating was organic in nature but crystalline deposits were seen scattered all over. These crystalline bodies were precipitated from the oral fluids which were supersaturated with respect to both calcium and phosphate. It is reported that oral fluids containing physiological concentration of either magnesium, zinc, bicarbonate etc. significantly lowers the rate of remineralization.

With the calcifying fluids, a greater degree of remineralization occurred. Mean reduction for ten lesions selected at random was found to be 9%, when a calcifying fluid was used without fluoride ions. When fluoride was added, the body of the lesion showed 24% reduction in area. The greater effect achieved by the addition of fluoride ions occurred irrespective of the level of fluoride added. Similar results were obtained with different fluoride levels (10–100 ppm). No greater degree of remineralization occurred by increasing the fluoride level within the calcifying fluids. Marinelli et al (1997) compared the effectiveness of fluoride mouthrinse (0.05% NaF), fluoride dentifrices and glass-ionomers in remineralizing the adjacent caries lesions and found that the NaF mouthrinse was the most effective method.

The pore volume of the subsurface area is important in determining the fate of the lesion. The subsurface zone acts as a restricting membrane. Even in a very small undetectable lesion, the subsurface body approaches pore volume of about 25%. Therefore, if remineralization is to occur, ions must pass through this barrier.

The remineralized lesion always exhibits a greater degree of resistance to progression of caries. Why this is so remains debatable in literature? Initially it was believed that the increased level of fluoride in the lesion was solely responsible for the same. Recent studies have shown that during lesion formation, submicroscopic crystals are affected and dissolution results in their diminution. The resultant smaller crystals are responsible for increased pore volume in the lesion with increasing demineralization. The presence of large crystal relative to small cyrstal produces a favourable change in the surface area to volume ratio. Also, the new crystals formed are fluoridated hydroxyapatite - all these factors collectively account for the increased resistance of the lesion.

Summarily, it is established that fluorides reduce caries incidence by remineralization. Although the use of fluoride is important in enhancing remineralization, it is not necessary to use a high concentration. Maximum remineralization occurs with even 1 ppm fluoride available at the enamel surfaces. A hundred times increase of fluoride concentration has no added effect on remineralization. In this respect, fluoridated dentifrices are major contributing factors in supplying low fluoride levels so as to enhance remineralization of lesions. The remineralized lesions are resistant to progression of caries thereby preventing caries incidence.

FLUORIDES IN PERIODONTAL THERAPY

Periodontal infections result from a combination of accumulation and growth of specific pathogenic bacteria in the dental plaque. Nine out of ten persons are suffering from one or the other form of periodontal disease and by the age of 60, 1/3rd of the people lose all their teeth because of gum diseases. These facts have created great interest in the diagnosis, treatment and prevention of periodontal diseases. The chronic nature and high prevalence of periodontal diseases creates problems regarding their prevention at the community level. It is now recognized that the targets of therapy are specific pathogenic bacteria. Prevention of the growth of pathogens within plaque by chemotherapeutic agents has been widely used as a treatment modality. The most commonly used agents are chlorhexidine and fluoride compounds.

Fluoride compounds have potential therapeutic and preventive uses in periodontal diseases at community level. It is observed that stannous fluoride is the best amongst available fluorides because it can:

  i. Reduce plaque
 ii. Reduce bleeding during probing in periodontal problems
iii. Reduce enamel solubility
 iv. Reduce dentin hypersensitivity.

Various formulations and many routes of applications have been studied to determine the effect of stannous fluoride and other fluoride agents over a period of time.

Before we study the efficacy of fluorides in periodontal therapy, let us first study the concept of periodontal disease in brief.

Concept of Periodontal Disease

It has been established that various types of periodontal diseases and their severity are associated with different combinations of specific bacterial interactions within the host. This specificity of bacteria leads to formation of plaque. This plaque can be supragingival or subgingival, attached or unattached.

Supragingival Plaque

The plaque occurring coronal to the gingival margin is called supragingival plaque. Plaque accumulation involves the association of gram positive bacteria with the tooth surface. Other factors such as salivary and dietary components, oral hygiene and other local factors influence the nature and pathogenic potential of plaque. Once supragingival plaque is established, qualitative and quantitative changes in it ultimately lead to gingivitis.

Early changes in the gingiva usually include oedema, swelling, an increase in gingival fluid etc. These changes in the gingiva are partly responsible for subsequent plaque formation. These types of changes suggest that specific bacteria are responsible for the observed pathogenic changes.

Subgingival Plaque

Subgingival plaque is primarily associated with anaerobic bacteria, both gram positive and gram negative. These bacteria utilize the proteins and other nutrients provided in the subgingival environment by gingival fluid. Subgingival plaque has been characterized on the basis of its anatomic association with the tooth surface and adjacent soft and hard tissues. Investigators have differentially quantitated the organisms isolated from scrapings of subgingival plaque before and after treatment.

Effect of Fluorides on Periodontal Diseases

Fluorides are used both in periodontal health and disease. In periodontally healthy patients, the main objective is prevention. The major role of fluorides is to prevent the establishment of pathogens within plaque. This can be accomplished by various ways such as:

  i. Reduction in plaque volume and its formation.

ii. Reduction in the effect of pathogens in existing plaque.

iii. Retention of fluoride within the plaque for potentially prolonged beneficial effects.

In such patients, high concentration of fluorides is not required. Only routine use of fluoride toothpastes, rinses etc. can prevent periodontal disease. It is suggested that the fluoride agents may improve the efficiency of oral hygiene and decrease the likelihood of developing periodontitis.

The patients who are suffering from one or another form of periodontal disease can also be benefited by the use of fluorides. While undergoing active treatment, the goal of fluoride therapy is to reinforce the mechanical treatment modalities. This reinforcement can be accomplished by:

i. Eliminating pathogenic bacteria within the plaque.

ii. Preventing or slowing down of the recolonization of bacteria.

iii. Reducing plaque volume.

iv. Decreasing post treatment sensitivity.

v. Decreasing recurrent caries.

The antibacterial potential of fluorides against various pathogens has already been demonstrated. *Yoon et al (1979)* examined the effects of fluoride on *Actinomyces viscosus* and reported that sodium fluoride (NaF), stannous fluoride (SnF_2) and acidulated phosphate fluoride (APF) were all effective in decreasing the percentage of this group of organisms. They further observed that SnF_2 at lower concentrations was also effective against *Bacteroides melaninogenicus*. It was established later that stannous (Sn^{2+}) ions play a major role as an antibacterial agent. It has also been suggested that SnF_2 could effectively reduce the number of bacteria.

Various other authors have used SnF_2 alone or in combination with chlorhexidine as an adjunct to scaling and root planing in perio-dontally involved teeth. They have demonstrated than SnF_2 alone or in combination with chlorhexidine significantly reduces colonization of potential pathogens upto 7 weeks. With the use of SnF_2 there was found to be significant reduction in supragingival plaque and gingival bleeding after 3-6 months of use. The combination of chlorhexidine and SnF_2 dentifrice was found to have a dramatic and sustained effect in decreasing the signs of periodontal problems.

Since all these measures are adjunctive, they must be combined with routine therapeutic measures, which include proper oral hygiene, mechanical removal of plaque and periodic monitoring of the patient's dental health. Further studies are required to ascertain the role of fluorides vis-à-vis its dose and related problems in prevention of periodontal disease. Some of the issues which must be explored are:

i. The identification of optimum doses and agents for individual periodontal needs.

ii. The type of monitoring required to measure the effectiveness of the agents.

iii. The most effective modality for adjunctive treatment regimes.

iv. The possible treatment alternatives where patient compliance is poor.

EFFECT OF FLUORIDES ON ROOT CARIES

One of the major consequences of periodontal disease is the apical migration of the epithelial attachment. This leads to denudation of root surface which is a prerequisite for root caries and dentinal sensitivity. Exact epidemiological data is not available but studies have suggested that root caries is quite prevalent in older adults in India.

Caries preventive programmes in patients with a high risk of root caries involve oral hygiene instructions, dietary advice and fluoride therapy. Two forms of fluoride treatment have been advocated at the community level. One form uses 1.1% NaF (sodium fluoride), which provides 5000 ppm fluoride and is applied for 5–10 minutes/day. The other form uses 0.4% SnF_2 gel (stannous fluoride), which provides 1000 ppm fluoride for 1 minute/day. The effectiveness of 1.1% NaF was originally demonstrated in children but now it is widely used for the high risk adult population. Patients not using NaF gel develop an immediate and pronounced increase in *Streptococcus mutans* in their dental plaque. Daily application of NaF for 5 minutes may not eliminate the cariogenic flora but definitely curbs the increase of *Streptococcus Mutans*, which usually seen after radiation therapy. Further, fluoride therapy significantly reduces acid production in plaque.

For patients whose roots are too sensitive, a neutral NaF gel in the concentration of 10,000 ppm has been used. These high concentration fluoride gels are usually used by professional people and is not allowed for patients' personal use. The treatment schedule consists of two 5 minute applications each day for two weeks followed by one daily application for additional two weeks. After each application, patients are instructed to rinse with a remineralizing mouthwash for two minutes. This remineralizing mouthwash contains 5 ppm calcium, 3 ppm phosphate and 2 ppm fluoride. After the fluoride treatment is over (4 weeks), the mouthwash is continued for the next couple of weeks

NaF mouth rinses in various concentrations (0.2% used for 1 minute weekly, or 0.05% for 1 minute daily) have been reported to be effective in reducing coronal caries in children. The exact relationship of topical fluorides and caries is not clear. In a fluoride dentifrice study in children, using 250, 750 and 1000 ppm fluoride, a marked caries reduction was noted. However, many authors claimed no difference in caries prevention between children who used dentifrice with 250 ppm fluoride and those using dentifrice with 1000 ppm fluoride.

It has been reported that life long residence in a fluoridated community is associated with a highly significant reduction in the prevalence of root caries. *Rosen et al (1984)* have found that topical fluoride swabbed twice a day on the molar teeth of rats significantly inhibited root surface caries. The agents tested were NaF solution (5000 ppm F), NaF dentifrice (500 ppm F) and water (0 ppm F). The corresponding root surface caries scores were 10.4, 15.5 and 24%. *Heilman et al (1997)* have also confirmed that fluorides inhibited root demineralization and the remineralization occurred in previously demineralized root surfaces.

Dentinal Sensitivity

Dentinal sensitivity results from the denudation of the cementum leading to the exposure of dentinal tubules. Such exposures result in pain after thermal, osmotic, chemical or tactile stimulation. Quick exposure of dentin always results in sensitivity, however slower exposure of dentin which occurs from abrasion and/or erosion is less likely to result in sensitivity. The most accepted theory of dentin sensitivity is the hydrodynamic theory, which states that with the application of an external irritant, there occurs a rapid flow of fluid in the tubules either inward or outward, resulting in displacement of the tubular content at the pulpodentinal wall. Pain is produced by these disturbances and activation of mechanoreceptors.

If we follow the hydrodynamic theory, any desensitizing agent must mechanically block the tubules either by precipitation of compounds or by surface coating. The desensitizing agent must be non-irritating to the pulp, relatively painless on application, easily applied, effective for long periods of time, non-staining and rapid in action. Many different agents have been tried to desensitize the root surface. The major ones among these are formaldehydes, potassium nitrates, strontium chloride, sodium fluoride and stannous fluoride. In experimental animals, the dentifrices containing these salts were not significant in reducing the dentinal sensitivity as compared with routine dentifrices. The Council on Dental Therapeutics has accepted dentifrices containing potassium oxalate, stannous chloride and certain chloride compounds. Here we are mainly concerned with fluoride compounds when used as desensitizing agents. Earlier, NaF mixed with clay and glycerine in the form of paste was used as a densensitizing agent.

Iontophoresis is one method by which NaF ions are made to penetrate the tooth surface by the aid of a direct electric current. The sensitive tooth is isolated, 2% NaF solution on a cotton pellet is applied to the exposed dentin by means of a disposable plastic holder placed over an electrode tip. The electrode is then connected to the positive pole, and the current is adjusted so as not to exceed 1 mA of electricity/min/tooth. It has been reported that NaF iontophoresis provides better desensitization than treatment with NaF paste.

Recently, SnF_2 has been found to be superior to NaF in decreasing dentinal sensitivity. It has been reported that SnF_2 with carboxy methyl cellulose and glycerine significantly reduces dentinal sensitivity. However, certain authors reported that 0.4% SnF_2 did not exhibit a significant improvement over the control group using non-fluoride dentifrices. Higher concentration of SnF_2 (upto 3%) when applied for 5 minutes gave a measurable reduction in dentinal sensitivity. With iontophoresis there was a definite improvement in the reduction of dentinal sensitivity. A similar result was obtained when sodium monofluorophosphate was used.

It is certain that fluoride salts alone or in combination or with iontophoresis definitely reduce dentinal sensitivity but whether this effect is due to fluoride or other ingredients of the dentifrice is yet to be established.

FLUORIDE TOXICITY

Fluoride ions are incorporated into tooth enamel layers following eruption. It has been established that fluoride ions results in an anticarious effect depending upon their concentration. The possible optimum concentrations have been defined, and a variety of techniques for achieving these have been studied. The studies include natural fluoride intake, where levels are already above optimum and methods of supplementation to achieve the aforesaid anticariogenic effect.

When fluorides are used as a supplement for achieving optimum levels, the chances of overdosage are always there. The effects of overdosage are multiple. These effects are studied under two subheads:

- Chronic fluoride toxicity
- Acute fluoride toxicity

Chronic Fluoride Toxicity

The recommended optimum levels of fluoride for drinking water is 1.0 ppm (WHO,1963). The average daily intake of fluoride from all sources recommended for adults is 2.0–2.2 mg and in the case of children it is 1.2 mg. This leads plasma fluoride levels within the range of 0.019–0.038 ppm or 19–38 mg F/ml of plasma.

The only known adverse effect associated with the ingestion of relatively low levels of fluoride (1–2 ppm in the drinking water) is dental fluorosis.

Chronic exposure to high levels of fluoride (more than 5 ppm), mainly through drinking water, may result in skeletal fluorosis, which can cause osteosclerosis and increased risk of bone fracture.

The commonly recognized effects of fluoride ingestion through fluoridated water at various levels are given in Table 4.3.

Table 4.3: Effects of fluoride ingestion through fluoridated water at various levels

Concentration of fluoride in drinking water	Effects
0.7-1.2 ppm (Depending upon the temperature of the area)	Prevent dental caries
1.5-3.0 ppm (Consumed over a period of 5-10 years or more)	Dental fluorosis (milder form)
4.0-8.0 ppm (Consumed over a period of 15-20 years)	Dental fluorosis (severe form) Skeletal fluorosis (milder form)
8.0 ppm or more (Consumed over a period of > 5-10 years)	Dental fluorosis and Skeletal fluorosis (severe form)

DENTAL FLUOROSIS

Enamel fluorosis can occur following either an acute or chronic exposure to fluoride during tooth formation, but it usually occurs by chronic intake of water having concentration more than 1 ppm of fluoride, during the tooth-formation period.

Fluoride ingestion in concentration less than or equal to 1 ppm during tooth-formation results in the formation of dental enamel which is more resistant to caries. However, increased levels of fluoride cause the retention of proteins such as amelogenins in the tooth structure, leading to enamel fluorosis. The enamel thus formed is hypomineralized and has a different refractive index than sound, non-fluorotic enamel. As a result, light refraction through this enamel is altered resulting in the appearance of chalky areas. Mildly fluorosed enamel is fully functional and is more resistant to acid attack in vitro than is enamel of individuals from low or optimally fluoridated areas. Exposure to higher levels of fluoride results in porous, pitted, and discoloured enamel, which is more prone to fracture and wear.

Classification of Dental Fluorosis

Various authors have classified dental fluorosis in different ways. The most commonly used classification are given below:

1. *Classification by Dean (1934):* The criteria are given as follows:

Category	Numerical value	Condition
Normal	0	Normal enamel, smooth and glossy
Questionable	0.5	Few white specks or white spots on teeth
Very mild	1.0	Small white opaque areas
Mild	2.0	Proper opaque areas, white in colour
Moderate	3.0	All teeth surfaces affected, brown staining, occlusal surfaces worn out
Moderately severe	4.0	All teeth affected with brown staining and discrete, confluent pitting
Severe	5.0	Enamel worn out with brown mottling

2. *Young (1973)* quoted by *Rugg Gunn and Rahmatulla (1988)* classified enamel fluorosis as:

Type A	White areas less than 2.0 mm in diameter
Type B	White areas of, or greater than 2.0 mm in diameter

Type C   Coloured (brown) areas less than 2.0 mm in diameter irrespective of there being white areas

Type D   Coloured (brown) areas more than 2.0 mm in diameter, irrespective of there being white areas.

Type E   Horizontal white lines, irrespective of there being any white non-linear areas

Type F   Coloured (brown) or white lines associated with pits or hypoplastic areas.

3. *Thylstrup and Fejerskov (1978)* based on clinical appearance of fluorotic enamel, classified fluorosis as follows :

1. Normal translucency of enamel remains after prolonged air-drying.

2. Narrow white lines located corresponding to the perikymata.

3. *Smooth surfaces:* More pronounced lines of opacity which follow the perikymata. Occasional confluence of adjacent lines.

   Occlusal surfaces: Scattered areas of opacity 2.0 mm in diameter and pronounced opacity of cuspal ridges

4. *Smooth surfaces:* Merging and irregular cloudy areas of opacity. Accentuated drawing of perikymata often visible between opacities.

   Occlusal surfaces: Confluent areas of marked opacity. Worn areas appear almost normal but are usually circumscribed by a rim of opaque enamel.

5. *Smooth surfaces:* The entire surface exhibits marked opacities or appears chalky white. Parts of surface exposed to attrition appear less affected.

   Occlusal surfaces: Entire surface exhibits marked opacity. Attrition is often pronounced shortly after eruption.

6. *Smooth and occlusal surfaces:* Entire surface displays marked opacity with focal loss of outermost enamel (pit) 2.0 mm in diameter.

7. *Smooth surfaces:* Pits are regularly arranged in horizontal bands 2.0 mm in vertical extension.

   Occlusal surfaces: Confluent area 3.0 mm in diameter exhibiting loss of enamel. Marked attrition.

8. *Smooth surfaces:* Loss of outermost enamel in irregular areas involving half the entire surface.

   Occlusal surfaces: Change in the morphology caused by merging pits and marked attrition.

9. *Smooth and occlusal surfaces:* Loss of outermost enamel involving half of the surface.

10. *Smooth and occlusal surfaces:* Loss of main part of enamel with change in anatomic appearance of surfaces. Cervical rim of almost unaffected enamel is often noted.

This classification is more sensitive as it relates histological features to macroscopic changes.

4. The classification of *Murray and Shaw (1979)* is as follows: The occlusal, buccal and lingual surfaces of each tooth are examined and scored separately for presence of any enamel opacity according to the criteria given below.

- White opaque spots (flecks) less than 2.0 mm in diameter.

- White opaque spots (or patches) greater than 2.0 mm measured in any direction, well demarcated from the surrounding area.

- Coloured spots, flecks or patches.

- Horizontal white lines, irrespective of there being any white non-linear lines. Not associated with deficiency of enamel substance (hypoplasia).

- Hypoplasia, in association with any of categories 1 to 4.
- Possible early carious lesions.
- Missing.

5. *Horowitz et al (1984)* have also proposed a classification of classified fluorosis, which they named the Tooth Surface Index of Fluorosis (TSIF). The scoring is carried out as follows:

Level	Condition of teeth
0	Enamel shows no evidence of fluorosis
1	Enamel shows definite evidence of fluorosis. The white chalky appearance is in less than 1/3rd of the total area
2	Permanent white spots are in more than 1/3rd of the area and less than 2/3rd of the area
3	Total fluorosis with at least 2/3rd of the area involved
4	Enamel shows staining (usually brown)
5	Discrete pitting of enamel surface
6	Both pitting and staining of the enamel surfaces
7	Large area of enamel missing with confluent pitting all around

Teeth commonly affected are (a) central incisors (b) lateral incisors (c) molars of the permanent dentition.

Skeletal Fluorosis

Chronic exposure to high levels of fluoride (> 5 ppm) in drinking water may result in skeletal fluorosis.

A fluorosed bone shows characteristic structural changes viz.

- Increased bone mass and density.
- Exostosis (bony outgrowth).
- Increased osteoid activity around resorption surfaces.

- Increased trabecular bone volume, cortical porosity and periosteocytic lacunar surface.
- Increased osteon diameter and mottling of the osteon.
- Formation of unmineralized cartilagenous loci within the trabeculae of the cancellous bone but not in the cortical bone.
- Accumulation of glycosaminoglycans especially the isomer dermatan sulphate in the cartilagenous region of the cancellous bone.

Signs and Symptoms

- Severe pain and stiffness in the neck and back bone.
- Severe pain and stiffness in the joints.
- Severe pain and rigidity in the hip region (pelvic girdle).
- Radiographs reveal increased thickening and density of bone. In certain patients, due to the calcium deficiency, osteomalacia type changes may be seen (where bone appears weak, revealing the inner structure).
- Constriction of vertebral canal and intervertebral foramen exerts pressure on nerves, blood vessels leading to paralysis and pain.

Effect on Red Blood Cells

It is established that when fluoride is ingested, it accumulates on the erythrocyte membrane, besides other cells, tissues and organs. The erythrocyte membrane in turn loses its calcium content. The membrane, which is deficient in calcium content, is pliable and is thrown into folds. The RBCs attain the shape of an amoeba with pseudopodia like folds projecting in different directions. Such RBCs are termed Echinocytes.

The echinocytes are found in circulation in large numbers, depending upon the extent of fluoride poisoning and duration of exposure to fluoride. The RBCs in humans have a life span of 120–130 days. However, the echinocytes undergo phagocytosis and are eliminated from the circulation quite early. This means that RBCs in individuals exposed to fluoride poisoning do not live the entire life span, and are likely to be eliminated as echinocytes. This leads to low haemoglobin levels.

Effect on Skeletal Muscles

The patients suffering from fluoride toxicity usually complain of muscle weakness. Other features are:

- In the fluorosed muscle there are widespread changes within a fibre revealing destruction of the actin and myosin filaments.
- The mitochondria lose their structural integrity, thereby providing evidence that muscle energy is likely to be depleted.
- The levels of certain phosphokinases are high in the serum of patients suffering from skeletal fluorosis, which is an indication that muscle mitochondria are destroyed and the muscle membrane is rendered highly permeable.

Effect on Ligaments and Blood Vessels

Tissues, like ligaments and blood vessels tend to harden and calcify. Blood vessels can get blocked by such calcifications.

Neurological Manifestations

Fluoride toxicity adversely affects certain regions of the brain leading to nervousness, depression, tingling sensation in fingers and toes, excessive thirst (polydypsia) and a tendency to urinate frequently (polyuria).

Effect on Kidneys

Fluoridation is by and large safe for persons with normal kidneys. However, fluoride may aggravate pre-existing renal diseases. Renal failure causes fluoride retention, leading to higher tissue fluoride concentration.

No renal pathology ascribed to fluoride has been found in experimental animals maintained for protracted periods on a diet or drinking water containing 50 ppm F or less. The borderline water concentration at which individuals of certain species exhibit changes is about 100 ppm.

Urine may be much less in volume, yellowish red in color and itching may occur.

The acute effect after a heavy single dose of fluorides is taken intentionally or accidentally can be acute toxic nephritis.

Acute Fluoride Toxicity

Acute fluoride toxicity with the accidental or intentional intake of sodium fluoride has been reported, since sodium fluoride is used as a pesticide.

Serious fluoride poisoning has declined, as fluoride compounds are rarely found in homes today, with the exception of dental products. However, the rate of exposure to potentially harmful amounts of fluoride has increased, especially among children.

Toxic Dose for Acute Poisoning

The toxic dose for the acute poisoning differs according to different authors. The range varies from 10–100 mg F/Kg of body weight. The difference was due to the fact that the actual dose taken by the individual was not known. Whitford (1992) after reviewing various studies concluded that the "certainly lethal dose" (CLD) of sodium fluoride for a 70 kg person was 5–10 g when taken orally. This corresponds to a fluoride dose of 32–64 mg F/Kg.

Four deaths have been reported, which were caused by the ingestion of fluoride contained in dental products. The fluoride dose ranged from nearly 4 to 30 mg F/Kg body weight. The probable toxic dose (PTD) as concluded by various studies is 5 mg F/Kg body weight. The PTD was defined as the 'minimum dose that could cause toxic signs and symptoms, including death, and that should trigger immediate therapeutic intervention and hospitalization'.

Shulman et al (1997) have enumerated various dental products which can cause acute fluoride toxicity in children. They have cautioned manufacturers to use child resistant packaging for all fluoride products intended for use at home.

It would be impossible for fluoridated water to cause acute fluoride poisoning. When water is fluoridated at a level of 1 ppm F, one litre of water contains 1 mg F. Thus, in order to receive even 1g F one would have to consume, over a very short period of time, 1000 litres of water.

Signs and Symptoms

Fluoride combines with hydrochloric acid in the stomach to form hydrofluoric acid. The corrosive effect of hydrogen fluoride on the gastric mucosa accounts for gastrointestinal symptoms such as nausea, vomiting, diarrhoea, and abdominal pain.

A more serious consequence of fluoride overdose is hypocalcemia caused by the affinity of fluoride to cations in the serum. Calcium becomes indispensable for the functional integrity of the voluntary and autonomic nervous systems. Hence, hypocalcemia may be associated with symptoms such as paresthesia, paresis, muscle fibrillation, tetany, convulsions, decreased myocardial contractility, etc.

Acute fluoride toxicity has been associated with hyperkalemia leading to ventricular arrhythmias and cardiac arrest. There is also evidence that fluoride intoxication may interfere with enzyme systems, including glycolytic enzymes, cholinesterases and enzymes in which magnesium and manganese are present.

Treatment of Acute Toxicity

Emergency treatment for fluoride overdose is given in the Table 4.4.

Toxicity of Fluoride Due to Dental Products

Fluoride Gels

The fluoride concentration in gels ranges from 0.4 to 1.23%. The gels are applied professionally 2–4 times in one year. Gels can also be used at home by self-application either daily or twice a day. The amount of fluoride used in each application is high enough to warrant care and caution. When 3–5 ml of 1.23% gel is used in a tray the child is exposed to 60mg of fluoride. The acidic nature of gels stimulates salivary secretion and increases the possibility of swallowing an excess of the saliva-gel mixture.

Sufficient documentation exists concerning the systemic ingestion of fluoride by children and adults following self application of topical gels leading to increased plasma fluoride level. It has been reported that after one hour of application of gel containing 1.23% fluoride, the plasma level of fluoride increases to 1443 mg F/ml. In such cases, the plasma fluoride level crosses the nephrotoxic threshold of 950 mg/ml. Thus professional application of APF gel in young children should be done with caution. The stepwise procedure is:

- Limit the amount of gel placed in each stock tray to not more than 2 ml or 40% of the tray capacity.
- Seat the patient in an upright position with the head inclined forward.
- Use suction throughout the procedure.
- Use saliva ejector for 30 seconds after the gel application.
- Keep the container out of the reach of the patient.
- Never leave the patient unattended.

Fluoride Dentifrices

Fluoridated dentifrices generally contain available fluoride in the range of 700–800 ppm. A single session of brushing with a full ribbon of paste on a brush head provides about 1 gm

Table 4.4: Emergency treatment for fluoride overdose

Milligram fluoride ion per kilogram body weight	Treatment
Less than 5.0 mg/kg	1. Give calcium orally (milk) to relieve gastrointestinal symptoms. Observe for a few hours. 2. Do not induce vomiting.
5 mg/kg to 15 mg/kg	1. Empty stomach by induced vomiting with emetics. For infants <6 months old with depressed gag reflex, and individuals with Down's syndrome or severe mental retardation, induced vomiting is contraindicated and endotracheal intubation should be performed before gastric lavage. 2. Give soluble calcium orally in any form (for example milk, 5% calcium gluconate, or calcium lactate solution). 3. Observe for a few hours after hospital admission.
More than 15 mg/kg	1. Admit to hospital immediately. 2. Induce vomiting. 3. Begin cardiac monitoring and be prepared for cardiac arrhythmias. Observe for peaking T-waves and prolonged Q-T intervals (physician/cardiologists should take care). 4. Slowly administer intravenously 10ml of 10% calcium gluconate solution. Additional doses may be given if clinical signs of tetany or Q-T interval prolongation develop. Electrolytes, especially calcium and potassium should be monitored and corrected as necessary. 5. Adequate urine output should be maintained using diuretics if necessary. 6. General supportive measures for shock.

of toothpaste and the individual gets exposed to topical effect of 0.75 mg F.

Children brushing twice daily with a full ribbon of paste or thrice daily with an almost two-thirds ribbon of paste each time on the brush head are exposed to about 1.5 to 2.5 mg fluoride per day. The reports related to fluoride in oral care products are given in the Tables 4.5 and 4.6.

Investigations have been done to study the amount of dentifrice ingested by the children/individuals while brushing. It is reported that children aged 4–5 years who used approximately 0.5 gm dentifrice per brushing ingested 26–33%, while those aged 6–7 years ingested 25–28%, thus ingesting a total of approximately 0.15 mg F per brushing. Even if they brush twice, the total ingestion is 0.3 mg F, which is far less than the amounts which can lead to increased plasma fluoride levels to the extent where dental fluorosis may result.

Although the amount of fluoride ingested while brushing is unlikely to cause dental fluorosis or systemic damage, taking into consideration the risk of ingestion, the recommended schedule for use of fluoride dentifrices in very young children is:

Upto 4 years of age   -   Brushing twice daily without paste

Table 4.5: Reports of the American Association of Poison Control Centres related to oral care products containing fluoride (Chindren under 6 years of age)

Product	#Reports	#Treated in health care facilities	Medical outcome*			
			None	Minor	Moderate	Major
Toothpaste	1999	94	664	387	6	1
Mouthrinse	1090	37	455	64	0	0
Supplements	3788	268	1505	519	8	0
Vitamins**	2860	107	354	99	0	0

* No deaths were reportred   ** with fluoride but without iron

Courtesy: Litovitz et al (1993)

Table 4.6: Fluoride contents of dental products and their relationship to the 'Probably toxic dose'

Product	Concentration			Amount of product and fluoride usually used		Amount containing the PTD for	
	Self	Fluoride					
	percent	%	ppm	Product	Fluoride	10kg child	20kg child
Rinse							
Sodium Fluoride	0.05	0.023	230	10 ml	2.3 mg	215 ml	430 ml
Sodium Fluoride	0.20	0.091	910	10 ml	9.1 mg	55 ml	110 ml
Stannous Fluoride	0.40	0.097	970	10 ml	9.7 mg	50 ml	100 ml
Dentifrice							
Sodium Fluoride	0.22	0.10	1000	1 gm	1.0	50 gm	100 gm
Mono Fluorophosphate	0.76	0.10	1000	1 gm	1.0	50 gm	100 gm
Mono Fluorophosphate	1.14	0.15	1500	1 gm	1.5	33 gm	66 gm
Topical gel/solution							
Sodium Fluoride (APF)	2.72	1.23	12300	5 ml	61.1	4 ml	8 ml
Stannous Fluoride	0.40	0.097	970	1 ml	.97	50 ml	100 ml
Stannous Fluoride	8.0	1.94	19400	1 ml	19.4	2.5 ml	5 ml
Tablet							
0.25 mg F	-	-	-	1/day	0.25	200 tab	400 tab
0.50 mg F	-	-	-	1/day	0.50	100 tab	200 tab
1.0 mg F	-	-	-	1/day	1.00	50 tab	100 tab

The PTD is the threshold for the "probable toxic dose", 5mg/kg. If this amount or more is ingested, the individual should receive emergency treatment and hospitalization. The average body weight of a 1 year old child is approximately 10kg; the average weight of a 5-6 years old child is 20 kg.

4–6 years of age	-	Brushing thrice daily - once with fluoridated paste and twice without any paste
6-8 years of age	-	Brushing thrice daily - twice with fluoridated tooth paste and once without any paste

Usually 5 mg/Kg body weight is considered as the Probable Toxic Dose. If this amount or more is ingested, the individual should receive emergency treatment and hospitalization. The average body weight of a one year old child is approximately 10kg; the average weight of a 5–6 years old child is 20 kg.

The manufacturers should be cautious regarding the product containing fluorides. They should:

- Consider producing dentifrices for children that have a lower fluoride concentration.
- Reduce the diameter of toothpaste tube for use by children and encourage the use of a "pea-sized" amount of the product.
- Equip product containers with tops that are difficult for young children to open.

Further:

i. The parents should regularly assist pre-school children in brushing.

ii. Only a large pea-sized portion of fluoride paste should be put on the child's tooth-brush.

iii. Children should be regularly reminded to rinse and spit out thoroughly while brushing.

A child may swallow the full contents of a family sized (270 mg) fluoride toothpaste but even that is clearly below the lethal dose of 320 mg fluoride for a two year old child. Moreover, it is very difficult for a child to ingest 270 mg of tooth paste. Detergents, flavouring oils etc. present in dentifrices irritate the gastric mucosa and cause vomiting. Also, ingredients such as abrasives in dentifrices interfere with the intestinal absorption of fluoride from ingested toothpaste.

Systemic Fluoride Supplements

Currently, most systemic fluoride supplements such as tablets etc. contain either 1.0 mg of fluoride (2.2 mg NaF), 0.5 mg of fluoride (1.1 mg NaF) or 0.25 mg of Fluoride (0.25 mg NaF). These tablets are safe even when taken twice or thrice; the lethal dose starts at 100 tablets, the ingestion of which is highly unlikely.

Fluoride Mouthrinses

The fluoride mouth rinses are not recommended for pre-school children since at this age, they usually have inadequate control of their swallowing reflexes.

Hence, care should be taken to prevent the toxicity of fluoride by mouthrinses, i.e. they should be used under guidance.

FLUORIDATION AND DEFLUORIDATION

The effectiveness of fluorides in caries reduction has been studied for many years. Since the realization of the efficacy of fluorides in the reduction of dental caries, local water supplied in many communities all around the world has been fluoridated to optimal levels. Research has indicated that there is an inverse relationship between the amount of fluoride in the water supply and the number of carious lesions. Considering that fluoride is a natural constituent of drinking water, the fluoridation of water supplies has been found to be the most practical and effective method of fluoride administration.

Optimal Level

The optimal recommended fluoride level varies with climate because the average consumption of water increases in warmer climates. In cold climates the recommended fluoride level is as high as 1.2 ppm while in extremely hot climates a level of about 0.7 ppm is recommended. In moderate climatic conditions the optimum fluoride concentration has been shown to be 1 ppm. The optimal fluoride level in drinking water is the level that produces the greatest protection against dental caries with the least risk of fluorosis. A formula dependent on temperature has been derived for determining the optimal fluoride level.

ppm fluoride = 0.34/E
E = −0.038 + 0.0062 × average maximum temperature (°F)

Though substitutes for water fluoridation, like fluorides tablets, fluorides salt, fluorides in milk, fluorides in vitamin preparations, fluoride mouth washes and dentifrices etc. are present, water fluoridation is preferred because of the following reasons:

- Water fluoridation makes fluoride available to all the people residing in area served by water supply.
- Water fluoridation requires no conscious and sustained effort on the part of the individual.
- Water fluoridation automatically restricts dosage of fluoride to levels which have been proved to be safe for everyone.

Effectiveness

Water fluoridation prevents dental caries, which is well documented. Other expected benefits from fluoridated water are:

- A 75% decrease in first permanent molar loss
- A decrease in the size and complexity of new carious lesions
- Better appearance of teeth
- Lesser incidence of malocclusion among children

- Continued dental benefits into adulthood

Since fluorides also strengthen bones, there is some evidence that there may be additional health benefits for individuals who live in high fluoride areas, such as:
- A lower rate of osteoporosis in elderly women
- Lower death rates from falls for elderly women
- Less osteosclerotic hearing loss

Fluoridation leads to life long resistance to caries in a fluoridated community. Fluoride becomes a part of the dental enamel while the teeth are developing, providing protection from dental caries and other benefits.

An important shortcoming of water fluoridation is that it can only be implemented in areas with a central pipe water supplying system. In most urban areas where fluoride levels are low, it can be provided. But the rural population, which comprises the majority, especially in a developing country like India, will remain deprived of the benefits of fluoride owing to the absence of a central water supply system.

Implementation and monitoring of fluoridation as part of the regular duties for water treatment are relatively simple procedures for water work engineers. The importance of their role and responsibility in maintaining the fluoride at its optimal level should be reinforced periodically by the dental community and appropriate health authorities.

Water Fluoridation in Schools

School water fluoridation is one of the primary preventive services, provided in the community. School fluoridation may be defined as the 'adjustment of the fluoride content of a school water supply to the optimum level for prevention of dental caries'. Since, children ordinarily do not begin school before 4-5 years of age and as they are in school only 5-6 hours a day, six days a week, school water supplies are fluoridated at a higher concentration than central water supplies in order to obtain adequate amounts of fluoride for them. Care should be taken with regard to the fluoridation of water supplies where children are staying.

The drawback of fluoridation of school drinking water is that only a few affluent schools might be able to afford the initial installation cost, supplies and maintenance. Secondly, it should not be used in schools where some of the children live in areas which have fluoridated water supply.

Artificial Fluoridation of Water

It is reported that when fluoride is present in the domestic water supply (be it natural or added artificially), about 50% reduction in DMF scores results.

In areas where public water supply does not contain sufficient fluorides to have the concentration of 1.0 to 1.2 ppm, artificial fluoridation of water to achieve the optimum level would definitely benefit the community.

It can be concluded that fluoride as a natural constituent of the domestic water supply, or sodium fluoride added artificially will result in a prompt reduction in the incidence of dental caries, especially in children. One of the most important considerations is that the younger the child when he begins consuming water, and the longer he remains in contact with this supply of water, the greater is the overall reduction in caries.

Various fluoride compounds have been used to fortify the community water supply. The different compounds used are:
1. Sodium fluoride
2. Sodium silico-fluoride (Sodium fluoro-silicate)
3. Hydrofluoric acid or Hydrofluorosilicic acid
4. Ammonium silico-fluoride

As regards to the fluoride compound to be used, other factors are to be considered such as cost, ease of handling in addition to the dental caries reducing ability and possible toxic potential.

Some authorities assume that all fluoride compounds soluble to the extent of one part per million behave alike in preventing dental caries. However, sodium fluoride is used most frequently as the fluoridating agent of communal water supplies.

Method

The equipment for feeding the material consists of a hopper (a unit in which the fluoride compound is added). Usually 100 kg bags are added to ensure positive movement of the compound from the lower end of the hopper into the dissolving tank. Following dissociation of the compound, the supernatant fluid is pumped by a proportioning pump into the water line. This proportioning pump is essential to feed a given amount of fluoride solution continually to a proportionate amount of water. Liquid fluoride feeders require only a proportioning pump between the container of the hydrofluorosilicic acid and the point of injection to ensure safety. Daily monitoring occurs with daily adjustment of the fluoride concentration. By adjusting the rate of the feeder pump (stroke of the piston), the fluoride concentration is increased or decreased. The result of adjusting the pump is the introduction into the drinking water of a specific amount of pound equivalents of Hydrofluorosilicic acid or sodium fluoride etc. per gallon that will yield the optimum level of fluoride.

The Safety of Water Fluoridation

Recently, opponents of communal water fluoridation have gained considerable publicity worldwide by claiming that fluoridation increases cancer mortality rates. In the past, water fluoridation was linked with a variety of conditions including allergies, Down's syndrome (mongolism), heart disease and cancer. These data have been found to be misleading as a result of uncontrolled or poorly controlled observations, or of observations made with little regard to known important environmental or social variables.

There is no evidence that water containing optimal concentration (0.7–1.2 ppm) of fluoride impairs general health. Clearly, the most persuasive argument for the safety of water fluoridation is based on the health of communities where, for generations, the inhabitants have been drinking water with natural fluoride at a concentration of 1 ppm.

Water fluoridation may be considered safe, effective, practical and economic measure to reduce one of the most prevalent diseases in our society, i.e. dental caries.

DEFLUORIDATION

Dental fluorosis, a defect of tooth enamel caused by the consumption of high fluoride levels in drinking water during tooth development is the major problem in certain areas of India, Africa, Thailand, the USA and other countries. In India, the high fluoride levels (endemic fluoride belts) include Punjab, Haryana, Rajasthan, Gujarat, Madhya Pradesh, Andhra Pradesh, Tamil Nadu etc. In Punjab, parts of Sangrur district including Barnala, the whole of Bhatinda district, major parts of Faridkot and Ferozepur districts are mainly involved.

If the fluoride concentration is between 1 to 4 ppm, then the result may be a dentition with a poor appearance, but higher concentrations, i.e. more than 4 ppm, especially in a hot climate, have a more damaging effect. In severe fluorosis, the defective enamel is rapidly abraded just after tooth eruption and becomes pitted and misshaped. Unless expensive restorative treatment is performed, the teeth may be functionally impaired. Skeletal fluorosis can result if the water contains fluoride above 4.0 ppm and is consumed regularly over a long period of time.

Ever since the relationship between dental fluorosis and water fluoride concentration was established, many different procedures and agents have been suggested for reducing an excessive concentration of fluoride in drinking water. Basically, the procedure depends on one of the two principles, namely ion adsorption and ion exchange. In the former, fluorine is attracted to the surface of an inert substance, usually an insoluble aluminium salt, while the latter involves the uptake of fluoride in exchange for some other anion. Synthetic calcium phosphate and bone char have been used most commonly for ion exchange in preference to the expensive synthetic resins (e.g. Amberlite IR-4B). Fluoride adsorption methods are found to be better for water defluoridation schemes in large communities whereas ion exchange is used more commonly in small scale or home based units. These possess the added advantage over chemical reagents in that the resin can be reused, whereas calcium based defluoridating agents must be discarded.

Constraints

Both methods of defluoridation have two problems in common. First, competing ions invariably present in water interfere with fluoride uptake, e.g. silica in the case of adsorption, and chloride, sulphate and bicarbonate in case of ion exchange. Special precautions are often required to overcome this effect. Secondly, fluoride is removed efficiently when a new or recently regenerated batch of chemicals is used and thereafter, it gradually decreases. Gradual exhaustion of the adsorbent or ion exchange can be monitored in a large scale project, but is not easily detected in a small home appliance.

Various Methods of Defluoridation

Polystyrene Anion Exchange Resins

Polystyrene anion exchange resins are generally basic quarternary ammonium type resins known to remove fluorides from water alongwith other anions. These resins provide 20–145 bed volume of defluoridated water per cycle but lose their fluoride removal capacity on prolonged use (10–15 cycles) and a total replacement becomes necessary. The anion exchange resin treatment, besides being costly, imparts an unacceptable taste to the treated water.

Fluorapatite Precipitations

Sparingly soluble fluoride salt, fluorapatite has been used to defluoridate drinking water. Water containing high fluoride is saturated with brushite, resulting in a state of super saturation with respect to fluorapatite. Subsequent treatment with hydroxyapatite causes a lowering of calcium, phosphate and fluoride concentration in solution. Repeating the same process can lead to defluoridation.

Use of Magnesium Oxide

This method is usually employed in borehole water which contains 1–10 ppm fluoride. Magnesium oxide and bone meal are used as chemical defluoridation agents to reduce excessive amounts of fluoride from borehole water. The water filtered with magnesium oxide is slightly cloudy, but palatable. Either of the two chemical agents may be used in simple defluoridation procedures in rural or suburbans areas using borehole water. It is an inexpensive and efficient method of defluoridation.

Use of Calcium Hydroxide and Bone Char

The combined use of all of the above mentioned salts leaves a low concentration of phosphate in solution and optimizes the fluoride uptake capacity. Repeated use of the same for 10–20 times consecutive cycles improves the uptake of fluoride, provided that brushite and calcium hydroxide are also added.

Use of Alum

Sulphonated saw dust impregnated with 2% alum solution can also be used. It is prepared by treating 20–40 sieved saw dust with sulphuric acid, washing the excess acid, soaking the sulphonated product in alum solution for 2 hours and finally washing it to remove excess alum.

Carbion and Defluoron II

It is a cation exchange resin of good durability and can be used both in sodium and hydrogen cycles. It has a bulk density of 680 gms/litre. A unit, using carbion and defluoron II in a proportion of 8:1 has been installed at Gangapur (Rajasthan). Filter alum solution of 2, 3, 5, 6 and 10% is used to replenish the mixed medium.

Nalgonda Technique

Although defluoron-II has proved successful in removing fluoride, the regeneration and maintenance of the plant requires skilled operation, which may not be readily available. In order to overcome this problem, a method has been evolved which is so simple and adequate that even illiterate individuals can make use of it (Newlakhe et al, 1975).

The method is named Nalgonda Technique, and involves the addition of two readily available chemicals. The process comprises addition, in sequence of sodium aluminate or lime, bleaching powder, and filter alum to the fluoride water followed by flocculation, sedimentation and filteration. Sodium aluminate or lime hastens settlement of the precipitate and bleaching powder ensures disinfection. Lime is cheaper than aluminate and is preferred since its dose is only 1/20th - 1/28th that of filter aluminium. The fluoride concentration is reduced to about 1 mg/litre and alkalinity of raw water does not become limiting. The technique can be used both for domestic as well as community water supplies.

BIBLIOGRAPHY

1. Addy, M. and Dowell, P: Dentine hyper-sensitivity—a review. Clinical and in vivo

evaluation of treatment agents. J. Clin. Periodont: 10, 351, 1983.

2. Al-Alousi, W., Jakson-D., Crompton-G. and Jenkins, OC: Enamel mottling in a fluoride and non fluoride communtiy Part I and II. BDJ: 138, 9 and 56, 1975.

3. Al-Joburi, W. and Koulourides, T: Effect of fluoride on in vitro root surface lesions. Caries. Res. : 18, 33, 1984.

4. Armfield, JM: The benefits of water fluoridation across areas of differing socio-economic status. Aust. Dent. J: 53, 180, 2008.

5. Baxter, PM: Toothpaste ingestion during tooth brushing by school children. B.D.J. 148, 125, 1980.

6. Cawson, RA. and Stocker, IPD: The early history of fluorides as anti caries agents. B.D.J. 157, 403, 1984.

7. Clark, DC: A review on fluoride varnishes. An alternative topical fluoride treatment. Comm. Dent. Oral Epidem. : 10, 117, 1982.

8. Dean, HT: Classification of mottled enamel diagnosis. JADA: 21, 1421, 1934.

9. Driscoll, W: A review of clinical research on the use of prenatal fluoride administration for prevention of dental caries. J. Dent. Child. : 48, 109, 1981.

10. Duxbury, A.J., Leach, F.N. and Duxbury, JT: Acute fluoride toxicity. BDJ: 153, 64, 1982.

11. Estupium, DY S.R., Bac, Z.R. and Harowitz, H: Salt fluoridation and dental caries in Jamaica community. Dental Oral Epidem. : 29, 247, 2001.

12. Featherstone, JD: Prevention and reversal of dental caries : Role of low level fluoride. Comm. Dental Oral Epidem. : 27, 31, 1999.

13. Groeneveld, A., Thenus, H. and Kwant, G: Effect of a fluoride containing lacquer on dental caries. JDR: 61, 569, 1982.

14. Groeneveld, A., Van Eck, A. and Backer, D: Fluoride in caries prevention: is the effect pre or post eruptive? JDR: 69, 751, 1990.

15. Heilman, J.R., Jordon, R.H., Warwick, R. and Wefel, JS: Remineralization of root surfaces demineralized in solution of differing fluoride levels. Caries Res. : 31, 423, 1997.

16. Horowitz, H.S., Driscoll, W.S., Meyers, R.J., Heifetz, S.B., Kingman, AA: A new method for assessing the prevalence of dental fluorosis - the tooth surface index of fluorosis. JADA: 109, 37, 1984.

17. Horowitz, HS: A review of systemic and topical fluorides for the prevention of dental caries. Comm. Dent. Oral Epidem.: 1, 104, 1973.

18. Horowitz, HS: Review of topical application. Fluorides and fissure sealants. J. Can. Dent. Assoc. : 46, 38, 1980.

19. Kabayashi, S., Kishi, H. and Yushikara, A: Treatment and post treatment effects of fluoride mouth rinse after 17 years. J. Pub. Health Dent. : 55, 229, 1995.

20. Kalsbeek, H., Verrips, G.H. and Backer, D: Use of fluoride tablets and effect on prevalence of dental caries and dental fluorosis. Com. Dent. Oral Epidem. : 20, 241, 1992.

21. Koning, KG: Role of fluoride tooth paste in a caries preventive strategy. Caries Res. : 27, 23, 1993.

22. Koulourides, T: Fluoride and the caries process. JDR: 69, 558, 1990.

23. Kumar, J.V. and Moss, M.E. : Fluorides in dental public health programmes. Dent. Clinic North Am. : 52, 387, 2008.

24. Levy, S.M., Warren, J.J. and Brofitt, B: Patterns of fluoride intake from 36-72 months of age. J. Public Health Dent. ; 63, 211, 2003.

25. Levy, S.M., Warren, J.J., Brofitt, B. and Kanellis, MJ: Association between dental fluorosis of the permanent and primary dentitions. J. Public Health Dent. : 66, 180, 2006.

26. Litovitz, T.L., Holm, K.C. and Clancy, C: The 1992 annual report of the American Association of Poison Control Centres national data collection system. Am. J. Emerg. Med. : 11, 494, 1993.

27. Marinelli, C.B., Donly, K.J., Wefel, J.S., Jokobsen, J.R. and Denehy, GE: An invitro comparison of the fluoride regimes on enamel remineralization. Caries Res. : 31, 418, 1997.

28. Maupome, G., Shulman, J.D., Clark, D.C., Levy, S.M. and Berkowitz, J. : Tooth surface progression and reversal changes in fluoridated and no-longer fluoridated communities over a 3-year period. Caries Res. : 35, 95, 2001.

29. Mc Donagh, M.S., Whiting, P.F. and Wilson, PM: Systematic review of water fluoridation. BMJ: 321, 855, 2000.

30. Mc Guire, S. : A review of the impact of fluoride on dental caries. J. Clin. Dent. : 4, 11, 1993.

31. Murray, J.J. and Shaw, L: Classification and prevalence of enamel opacities in the human deciduous and permanent dentition. Arch. Oral Biol. : 24, 7, 1979.

32. Newbrun, E: Effectiveness of water fluoridation. Journal of Public Health Dent.: 49, 279, 1989.

33. Newlakhe, W.G., Kulkarni, D.N., Pathak, B.N. and Bulusu, KR: Defluoridation of water by Nalgonda technique. Ind. J. Env. Health: 17, 26, 1975.

34. Pendrys, DG: Dental fluorosis in perspective. JADA: 122, 63, 1991.

35. Pendrys, DG: The fluorosis risk index: A method for investigating risk factors. J. Public Health Dent. : 50, 291, 1990.

36. Pessan, J.P., Silva, S.M.B., Lauris, J.R.P., Sampaio, F.C., Whitford, G.M. and Buzalaf, M.A.R. : Fluoride uptake by plaque from water and from dentifrice. JDR: 87, 461, 2008.

37. Riordan, PJ: The place of fluoride supplements in caries prevention today. Aust. Dent. J: 41, 335, 1996.

38. Rolla, G. and Ogaard, B: Clinical effect and mechanism of cariostatic action of fluoride containing tooth paste - A review. Int. Dent. J: 41, 171, 1991.

39. Rosen, S., Beck, F.M. and Beck, E: Efect of NaF dentifrices on root surface caries. JDR: 62, 238, 1984.

40. Rugg Gunn, A.J. and Rahmatulla, M: New frontiers in fluoride studies for health. National University of Singapore. 1988.

41. Shulman, J.D. and Wells, LM: Acute fluoride toxicity from ingesting home-use dental products in children, birth to 6 years of age. J. Pub. Health Dent. : 57, 150, 1997.

42. Slade, G.D., Spencer, A.J., Davies, M.J. and Stewart, JF: The influence of exposure to fluoridated water on socio-economic inequalities in children's caries experience. Community Dental Oral Epidemiology: 24, 89, 1996.

43. Spencer, A.J., Armfield, J.M. and Slade, GD: Exposure to water fluoridation and caries increment. Community Dental Health: 25, 15, 2008.

44. Swango, PA: The use of topical fluorides to prevent dental caries in adults—A review of literature. JADA: 107, 447, 1983.

45. tenCate, J.M., Exterkate, R.A. and Buijas, MJ: The relative efficacy of fluoride toothpaste assessed with pH cycling. Caries Res. : 40, 136, 2006.

46. tenCate, J.M. and Featherstone, JDB: Mechanistic aspects of the interactions between fluoride and dental enamel. Crit. Rev. Oral Biol. Med. : 2, 283, 1991.

47. Thylstrup, A. and Fejerskov, O: Clinical appearance of dental fluorosis in permanent teeth in relation to histologic changes. Comm. Dent. Oral Epidem. : 6, 315, 1978.

48. Thylstrup, A: Distribution of dental fluorosis in the primary dentition. Comm. Dent. Oral Epid. : 6, 329, 1978.

49. Toda, S. and Fatherstone, JD: Effect of fluoride dentifrices on enamel lesion formation. JDR: 87, 224, 2008.

50. Toth, K: A study of 8 years of domestic salt fluoridation for prevention of caries. Comm. Dent. Oral Epid. : 4, 106, 1976.

51. Truman, B.I., Gooch, B.F. and Sulemann, I: Reviews of evidence on intervention to prevent dental caries, oral and pharyngeal cancers and sports related craniofacial injuries. Am. J. Prev. Med. : 23, 21, 2002.

52. Twefman, S., Axelsson, S., Dahlreen, M., Holm, A.K, Kallestal, C. and Lagerlof, F: Caries preventive effect of fluoride toothpastes : a systemic review. Acta. Odont. Scand. : 61, 347, 2003.

53. Vogel, G.L., Shim, D., Schumacher, G.E., Carey, D.M., Chow, L.C. and Takagi, S: Salivary fluoride from fluoride dentifrices or rinses after use of a calcium pre-rinse or calcium dentifrice. Caries Res. : 40, 449, 2006.

54. Vogel, RI: Extrinsic and intrinsic discoloration of the dentition - A literature review. J. Oral Med. : 30, 99, 1975.

55. Warren, .J.J., Levy, S.M. and Kanellis, MJ: Prevalence of dental fluorosis in the primary dentition. J. Public Health Dent. : 61, 87, 2001.

56. Wei, SHY: Clinical uses of fluorides. Lea and Febiger 1985, Philedelphia.

57. Weintraub, J.A., Ramos, G.F. and Jua, B: Fluoride varnish efficiency in preventing early childhood caries. JDR: 85, 172, 2006.

58. Whitford, G.M., Buzalaf, M.A.R., Bijella, M.F.B. and Waller, JA: Plaque fluoride concentrations in a community without water fluoridation: effects of calcium and use of fluoride or placebo dentifrice. Caries Res. : 39, 100, 2005.

59. Whitford, G.M., Wasdin, J.L., Shaffer, T.E. and Aclair, SM: Plaque fluoride concentrations are dependent on plaque calcium concentration. Caries Res. : 36, 256, 2002.

60. Whitford, GM: Acute and chronic fluoride toxicity. JDR: 71, 1249, 1992.

61. Yoder, K.M., Maupome, G., Ofner, S. and Swigonski, NL: Knowledge and use of fluoride among Indiana dental professionals. J. Public Health Dent. : 67, 140, 2007.

62. Yoon, NH: Antimicrobial effect of fluorides on Actinomyces viscosus. JDR: 58, 1824, 1979.

5 *Environment and Health*

The environment is the sum total of influences which interact with man and affect his well-being. It comprises of physical, biological, social and psychological dimensions. All these activities may lead to changes in the environment subsequently affecting human health.

The environmental health include housing, urban and regional population, control of air, and noise pollution, management of transport system, accident prevention, public recreation, water-supplies, waste management, food hygiene, irrigation and sanitation and also radiation control measures.

HOUSING

According to the WHO, housing is defined as the physical structure, which include all necessary services, facilities, equipment, and devices needed or desired for physical, mental and social well-being of the individual and the family.

Criteria for Healthful Housing

An expert committee of the WHO recommended the following criteria for healthful housing

- It should provide physical protection and shelter.
- It should provide adequate space for cooking, eating, washing and excretory functions.
- It should be so designed, constructed, maintained and used as to prevent the spread of communicable diseases.
- It should provide for protection from hazards of exposure to noise and air pollution.
- It should encourage personal and community development, and should be free from unsafe physical arrangements.

House Standards

The Environmental Hygiene Committee (1949) in India defined that a house means a residential house or flat designed for family life. Standards of housing may vary from country to country and from region to region. The committee recommended the following standards as the basis of a national housing code in India.

Site

The site of a house should meet the following criteria:

- The site should be elevated from its surroundings so that it is not subject to flooding during rains.
- It should be in pleasing surroundings.
- The soil should be dry and safe for founding.
- The site should have an independent access to the main street.
- It should be away from the breeding places of mosquitoes and flies.
- It should be away from nuisance such as dust, smoke, excessive noise and traffic.
- The structure should be well drained.
- The subsoil water should be below 10 feet.

Rural Housing

Minimum standards for rural housing are:
- There should be at least two living rooms, ample verandah space may be provided.
- Built-up area should not exceed 1/3rd of total area.
- There should be a separate kitchen with a paved sink or platform for washing utensils.
- The house should be provided with a sanitary latrine.
- The window area should be at least 10% of the floor area.
- There should be a sanitary well or tube well within 250 meters from the house.
- Cattle and other live stock should not be kept inside the dwelling house.
- Cattle sheds should be at least 25 feet away from the dwelling house.

Overcrowding

The degree of overcrowding can be best expressed as the number of persons per room.

Accepted standards are:

1 room	:	2 persons
2 rooms	:	3 persons
3 rooms	:	5 persons
4 rooms	:	7 to 8 persons
5 or more	:	10 persons

A baby under 12 months is not counted; a child between 1 to 10 years may be counted as half person.

Health Hazards Due to Poor Housing

Poor housing lead to health hazards like:
- Respiratory infections, common cold, Tuberculosis, influenza, whooping cough etc.
- Rat infestation leading to plague.
- Infection due to house flies, mosquitoes etc.
- Psychosocial effects viz. feeling of isolation, insecurity, behavioural disorders, delinquency, etc.
- It affects morbidity and mortality.

NOISE POLLUTION

Noise may be defined as a wrong sound in the wrong place, at the wrong time.

Noise has two features:
a. Loudness
b. Frequency

Loudness

Loudness or intensity depends upon the amplitude of vibrations which initiated the noise and is measured in decibels (dB).
- Normal conversation produces a noise of 60–65 dB.
- Whispering produces a noise of 20–30 dB.
- Heavy street traffic produces a noise of 60–80 dB.

Frequency

Frequency is measured in hertz (Hz).

Humans can hear frequencies from 20–20,000 Hz.

Effects of noise exposure are of two types:
a. auditory
b. non-auditory.

Auditory Effects (Fatigue)

Auditory effects start appearing in the 90 dB region. Temporary deafness occurs in the frequency range between 80–90 dB while permanent deafness results from exposure to noise above 100 dB.

Non-Auditory Effects

Non-auditory effects include interference with speech and communication.

The affected persons usually feel annoyed. This is primarily a psychological response. Neurotic people are more sensitive to noise than balanced people.

It affects efficiency of a person and can lead to physiological changes, which include rise in BP, rise in intracranial pressure, an increase in heart rate and breathing and increased stress. It may interfere with sleep.

Noise Control

The basic principles of noise control are:

- *Control of noise at source:* This may be achieved by segregating noisy machines and applying noise reducers to machines.
- *Control of transmission:* This is achieved by building enclosures and covering the room walls with sound absorbing materials.
- *Protection of exposed persons:* Hearing protection is recommended for all the workers who are consistently exposed to noises louder than 85 dB. Using ear plugs and ear muffs is essential. In addition, workers must be regularly rotated between noisy areas and comparatively quiet areas in factories. Periodic audiograms can evaluate the ill effects of noise pollution.
- *Legislation and education:* The community should be educated as regards importance of noise as a health hazard.

One should remove loud horns from one's own vehicles and also protest against such horns being used by others.

LIGHTING

Good lighting is essential for efficient vision.

Requirements of Good Lighting

- **Sufficiency:** The lighting should be sufficient to enable the eye to discern the details of an object as well as the surroundings without strain.

  An illumination of 15–20 foot candles. Foot candle, a unit used for measurement of light, is accepted as a basic minimum for satisfactory vision.
- **Distribution:** The distribution of light should be uniform, having the same intensity all over.

- **Absence of glare:** Glare is excessive contrast. Glare could be a 'direct' glare from a light source or 'reflected' glare from sources such as table-tops and other polished surfaces.
- **Absence of sharp shadows:** Shadows cause confusion to the eye and therefore should not be present in the field of vision.
- **Steadiness:** The source of light should be constant.

Types of lighting

Lighting may be natural or artificial.

Natural lighting

Natural lighting is derived partly from the visible sky and partly from reflection. Day-light factor (Df) is the unit for measuring day light.

$$Df = \text{Instantaneous illumination indoors} \times 100$$

It is recommended that the daylight factor should be at least 10% in living rooms and around 22% in kitchens.

Artificial Lighting

There are five ways of achieving artificial lighting.

a. **Direct lighting:** In direct lighting, 99–100% of the light is projected directly towards the working area.

b. **Semi-direct:** Here 10–40% of light is projected upwards. So that it is reflected back on the object by the ceiling.

c. **Indirect:** Light does not strike a surface directly, because 90–100% of the light is projected towards the ceiling walls.

d. **Semi-indirect:** Here, 60–90% of light is directed upward and the rest downward.

e. **Direct-indirect:** Here, light is distributed equally.

Adverse Effects of Excessive Artificial Lighting

These include effect on biologic rhythms of body temperature, physical activity, the stimulation of melanin synthesis, the activation of precursors of vitamin D and also the food consumption.

POPULATION

Population is a set of individuals in a given area like a village, town, state or community.

According to Census

The census bureau of Population Estimates Programs (PEP) estimates July 1 any year after the last published decennial census. Existing data series such as births, deaths, domestic and international immigration are used to update the decennial census base counts.

Characteristics of Population

Density

- Population density is defined as the number of persons per square kilometer.
- The population density of India in 2001 was 324 persons per square kilometer.
- There is large variation in population density across India. It varies from 13 persons per square kilometer in Arunachal Pradesh to 9294 in Delhi. Among the states West Bengal is the most thickly populated with a population density of 904.

Natality

- The increase in the number of individuals in a population under given environmental conditions is called natality. The number of children born per thousand in a year is called Birth Rate.
- According to the 2001 census, birth rate in India is 26. It means that in India 26 babies are born per thousand person in a year. In

England it is 12 and in USA the birth rate is 18 per thousand per year.

Mortality

- The loss of individuals due to death in a given population under given environmental conditions is termed mortality.

Age Distribution

- Various age groups in a population determine its reproduction status.
- A population with more young members grows rapidly while one that has a large number of older individuals grows slowly.
- Approximately 95% of this growth is occurring in the developing countries.
- Currently one-third of the world's population is under the age of 15 and will soon enter the reproduction bracket, giving a greater boost to population growth.

WORLD POPULATION

World population is the total number of humans on Earth at a given time.

In the 20th century, the world saw the biggest increase in its population in human history due to medical and agricultural advances. In 2000, the United Nations Organization estimated that the world's population was growing at a rate of 1.14% (or about 75 million people) per year. According to CIA's 2005–06 World Factbook, the world human population increased by 203,800 everyday. The 2007 CIA fact book raised this to 211,090 people per day. In February 2008, the world's total population is believed to have reached over 6.65 billion. In line with population projections, the figure continues to grow at rates that were unprecedented before the 20th century, although the rate of increase has almost halved since its peak, which was reached in 1963 (2.2% per year). On its current trajectory, the world's population is expected to reach nearly 9,000,000,000 by the year 2050.

The Most Populous Nations

S.No.	Country	Total population (Percentage of total world population)
1.	China	1.32 billion (about 17%)
2.	India	1.12 billion (about 14.6%)
3.	USA	300 million (about 3.5%)
4.	Indonesia	225 million (about 3.5%)
5.	Brazil	185 million (about 2.8%)
6.	Pakistan	165 million (about 2.5%)
7.	Bangladesh	145 million (about 2.3%)
8.	Russia	143 million (about 2.2%)
9.	Nigeria	135 million (about 2.1%)
10.	Japan	128 million (about 2.0%)
11.	Mexico	108 million (about 1.7%)
12.	Vietnam	87 million (about 1.3%)
13.	Philippines	86 million (about 1.3%)
14.	Germany	82 million (about 1.3%)
15.	Egypt	75 million (about 1.2%)

4.3 billion people live in these 15 counties, representing roughly 2/3rd of the world's population.

Population of India

The total population of India as in census 2008 is, 1, 139, 964, 932.

Rate of increase in Indian population.

Per year	155, 31, 000
Per month	12, 73, 033
Per day	42, 434
Per hour	1768

The 1st Census dates back to 1871. The census work was started in 1860 and was completed in 1871.

The census has been carried out every 10 years, the last was in February-March 2001. It is carried out by the Registrar General and Census Commissioner of India offices under the Ministry of Home Affairs, Govt. of India. February 1 is celebrated as the Census Day.

Density of Population In India (Census of 2001)

Year	Density (/Km²)
1921	81
1931	90
1941	103
1961	142
1971	177
1988	177
1991	274
2001	324

Population estimate				
Rank	State	City	2007	2008
1.	Maharashtra	Mumbai	11, 914, 398	13, 073, 926
2.	Delhi	Delhi	09, 817, 439	11, 505, 196
3.	Karnataka	Bangalore	04, 292, 223	05, 281, 927
4.	West Bengal	Kolkata	04, 580, 544	04, 643, 011
5.	Tamil Nadu	Chennai	04, 210, 268	04, 376, 400
6.	Andhra Pradesh	Hyderabad	03, 059, 262	03, 980, 938
7.	Gujrat	Ahmedabad	02, 966, 312	03, 867, 336
8.	Maharashtra	Pune	01, 702, 376	03, 230, 322
9.	Gujrat	Surat	01, 498, 817	03, 124, 249
10.	Uttar Pradesh	Kanpur	01, 879, 420	03, 067, 663

Population Explosion: Boon or Curse?

Carrying Capacity is defined as the maximum number of individuals of a population that can be sustained indefinitely in a given habitat. Population explosion on the other hand, may be defined as population growth which exceeds the carrying capacity in a year.

The population of the world totalled 1 billion around 1810. Just 120 years later, this doubled to 2 billion people (1930), then 4 billion in 1975. The number of people in the world has risen from 4.4 billion in 1980 to 5.8 billion in 2001. It is estimated that the population would be nearly 1 trillion by 2030.

The change in population can be summarized as:

Population change = (Birth + Inward Migration) – (Death + Outward Migration)

The causes for such changes are:
i. Difference in birth rate and death rate and
ii. Difference between immigration and emigration

Two demographic variables namely fertility and mortality are responsible for the growth of population in the world. Before 1950 there was shortage of food and methods of land cultivation were insufficient and ineffective. But after 1950, due to technical advancements, prevention and control of diseases, and expansion and growth of medical services, the population of the world increased dramatically. The decline in death rates did not keep pace with the rise in birth rate, which still remains high.

Theory of Demographic Transition

The Theory of Demographic Transition is one that throws light on changes in the birth rate and death rate and consequently, the growth rate of a population. In the words of E.G. Dolan, "Demographic transition refers to a population cycle that begins with a fall in the death rate, continues with a phase of rapid population growth and concludes with a decline in the birth rate."

Causes of High Birth Rate

- Natural factors: Tropical countries where girls attain puberty at an early age and achieve motherhood in the age group of 12-15 years.
- Child marriage
- Illiteracy and Poverty
- Joint family system
- Predominance of villages
- Low status of women
- Social taboos
- Lack of recreational activities
- Lack of family planning measures
- Increase in life expectancy

It is established that "India currently faces approximately 33 births a minute, 2000 an hour, 48,000 a day, which calculates to nearly 12 million a year". Unfortunately, the resources do not increase as the population grows. Instead, the resources keep depleting, subsequently the basic necessities like food, clothing and shelter become dearer and even the survival becomes difficult.

Causes of Decline in Mortality

- Decline in epidemics due to availability of vaccines
- Urbanization of population
- Better medical facilities
- Rise in female education
- Balanced diet
- Increase in food production and distribution

Cycle of Poverty

The rise in population helps perpetuate the vicious circle of poverty. People have to spend a large part of their resources on the upbringing of their children. As a result, saving and the rate of capital formation decline. No improvement is made in technology to absorb additional labour power in agriculture.

FAMILY PLANNING

Family planning describes various methods of achieving or avoiding pregnancy based on knowledge of signs and symptoms of human fertility. It requires abstinence from genital contact during the ovulatory (fertile) phase of a woman's cycle to avoid pregnancy. The aims of family planning are to bring down population growth, thereby improving the standard of living and to reduce the mortality rates. The frequent pregnancies and unsafe abortions are also prevented. The family planning methods are divided into two:

A. Natural contraception

B. Barrier methods of contraception

C. Miscellaneous

A. Natural Contraception

The natural contraception methods routinely used are:

1. Calendar (Rhythm) Method
2. Basal Body Temperature (BBT) Method
3. Lactational Amenorrhoea Method (LAM)
4. Coitus Interruptus (Withdrawal method)

1. Calender (Rhythm) Method

The calendar (Rhythm) method is based on three assumptions:

- That ovulation occurs fourteen days before the beginning of menstruation, plus or minus two days.
- That sperm remain alive for three days.
- That the ovum (egg) survives for twenty-four hours.

The couples avoid sex or use barrier or withdrawal during fertile period.

Advantages

- No cost
- Lack of side effects
- Failure rate is reasonable

Disadvantages

- It is difficult to calculate the safe period.
- Compulsory abstinence from sexual act during this period may lead to emotional stress.
- It is not applicable during lactational amenorrhoea or when the periods are irregular.
- Involvement of both the partners is essential.

The fertile period or the safe period can also be calculated by recognizing cervical mucus discharge. The secretions during peak days are most slippery, stretchy and wet. The couples should avoid sex or use barrier or withdrawal method until 4 days after the peak day.

Cervical mucus stages (sample of regular 28 days cycle)	
Day(s) of cycle	*Cervical mucus characteristic*
Day 1–5	Bleeding (normal period)
Day 6–8	Dry days (no cervical mucus)
Day 9–10	Cloudy, thick and little or no stretchability
Day 11	Not as cloudy, thinner and more stretchable
Day 13 (peak day)	Clear, slippery and has consistency of raw egg white; more stretchability
Day 16	Cloudy thick and little or no stretchability

2. Basal Body Temperature (BBT) Method

The basic pattern is that BBT falls by 0.5°C at the time of ovulation and rises by 0.5–1°C after ovulation due to thermogenic effect of progesterones in 2nd half of cycle.

It is not very effective method since it informs only the beginning of late infertile phase and not the end of it.

The women can identify fertile and infertile days by combining BBT, cervical mucus changes and other signs and symptoms of ovulation like abdominal pain, breast tenderness, etc. The failure rate is high since the signs and symptoms can vary.

However, ultrasound follicular study detects correct ovulation time and is fool proof; however, it is costlier and time consuming.

3. Lactational Amenorrhoea Method (LAM)

Lactational amenorrhoea method is effective during the first six months postpartum (post-delivery). The features are:
* Breastfeeding must be the infant's only source of nutrition. Feeding solids reduces the effectiveness of LAM.
* The infant must be breastfed at least every four hours during the day and at least every six hours at night.
* The infant must be less than six months old.
* The mother must not have had a period after 56 days postpartum.

4. Coitus Interruptus (Withdrawal Method)

The withdrawal method implies discharge of semen outside the female genitalia at the end of intercourse.

Advantages
* No appliance is required.
* No cost.

Disadvantages
* Requires sufficient self control by man
* Women develop anxiety neurosis, vaginism or pelvic congestion.
* Chance of pregnancy cannot be ruled out as pre-coital secretion may contain sperm and deposit into vagina.
* Failure rate is reasonable.

B. Barrier Methods of Contraception

The barrier methods prevent sperm deposition in the vagina utilizing certain mechanical/chemical devices which produce sperm immobilization. The methods are:

Mechanical

a. *Male condom:* It is made of latex, polyurethane or tactylon. It is available as dry, lubricated and spermicidal condom. It fits over the erect penis. It is contraindicated for males allergic to latex.

It acts as a physical barrier preventing direct genital contact and exchange of genital fluids.

Advantages
* Cheap
* No side effects
* Simple to use
* Protection against pelvic inflammatory diseases
* Reduces the incidence of ectopic pregnancy
* Protects against cervical cell abnormalities
* Useful where the coital act is infrequent and irregular

Disadvantages
* May accidently break or slip off during coitus.
* To be discarded after each coital act.
* Higher failure rate.
* Inadequate sexual pleasure.

b. *Female condom:* Female condom is also known as Femshield/Femidom. It is a pouch made of polyurethane which lines the vagina and also the external genitalia. It measures 15–17 cm in length. The outer portion lies outside vagina and the inner one having closed end lies inside.

Advantages
* Can be worn well in advance without side effects.
* Does not slip off easily.
* Stronger than male condom, does not burst.
* Protects against sexually transmitted diseases.

- Available without a prescription.
- Can be used with oil-based lubricants.
- Less likely to constrict the penis and decrease sensation.

Disadvantages
- It is expensive.
- Flexible inner ring may cause discomfort.
- Requires proper insertion technique.
- Can make noise during sexual intercourse.
- Failure rate is reasonable.

c. *Diaphragm:* It is a dome shaped intra vaginal device made of rubber with flexible metal or spring at the margin. It's diameter is 50-95 mm. The diameter is the distance between tip of middle finger placed in the posterior fornix and a point over the finger below the symphysis pubis. It should be placed 3 hours before coitus and kept for 6-8 hours after coitus.

Advantages
- Cheap
- Can be used repeatedly
- No side effects
- Can be used during breastfeeding

Disadvantages
- Requires help of a doctor or a paramedical staff
- Risk of vaginal irritation and urinary tract infections
- Does not protect against certain sexually transmitted diseases
- If left for long time may cause toxic shock syndrome
- Failure rate is reasonable

Contraindications
- Cases of Prolapse, cystocele, rectocele because accurate fitting may not be possible.
- Recurrent urinary tract infections
- Allergy to rubber latex
- In anatomical abnormalities

d. *Cervical cap:* It is thimble shaped rubber cap with solid rubber rim. It fits closely to cervix. It is available in 4 sizes (22, 25, 28, 31 mm). The cap provides effective contraception for 48 hours.

Advantages
- Cheap
- Can be used repeatedly
- No side effects
- Can be used during breastfeeding

Disadvantages
- Should not be used during menstruation.
- Causes vaginal odour and discharge.
- May lead to toxic shock syndrome.
- Discomfort during coitus.
- Accidental dislodgement.

Contraindications
- Chronic cervicitis
- Erosion and cervical laceration

Chemical Methods

The chemical method implies use of certain chemical agents which produce sperm immobilization and decreases the viability of sperms. The chemical are available as creams, jellies, foams and tablets.

Creams and Jellies are introduced high in the vagina with the help of an applicator. The tablets can be introduced five minutes prior to coitus. Certain examples are Gossypol, sperm enzyme inhibitor and propranol.

Advantages
- Effective for 1–2 hours.
- When used in conjunction with mechanical barriers, reliable contraceptive effect can be achieved.
- Does not require a prescription.
- May be discontinued at any time.
- Safe.

Disadvantages
- Failure rate is quite high.
- Not effective in isolation.

- Can cause local allergic manifestation.
- May cause irritation in the vagina or on the penis.
- May interrupt sexual activity.

A combination of mechanical and chemical method, routinely used as vaginal contraceptive sponge, also known as *Today*. It is a mushroom shaped polyurethane sponge. It measures 2.0" in diameter, 1.25" thick and contains 1.0g nonoxynol-9. It is placed high in the vagina with concave side facing the cervix. It remains effective for 24 hours. It is mechanical barrier, prevents sperm entry into cervical canal, absorbs semen and releases spermicide. It should not be removed for 6 hours after coitus.

Disadvantages
- Not effective in preventing sexually transmitted diseases
- Produces lesion in the genital tract
- Failure rate is reasonable
- May cause toxic shock syndrome
- Vaginal yeast infection is common

C. Miscellaneous

a. Intrauterine contraceptive devices (IUCD): Intrauterine contraceptive devices are made of plastic or metal meant for insertion into uterine cavity for contraception. It is the 2nd most commonly used family planning method, after voluntary female sterilization. These are particularly suitable for women who want to delay pregnancy or prefer methods that does not require supervision before sexual intercourse.

Both medicated and unmedicated devices are available. Hormonal releasing devices are also used.

Advantages
- Highly effective and economical
- Does not interfere with intercourse
- Easy to use
- Long lasting
- Easily reversible
- Quick return of fertility
- No systemic effects

Disadvantages
- Requires motivation
- Limitation in its use
- Adverse local reactions manifested by menstrual abnormalities, etc
- Risk of ectopic pregnancy
- Failure rate is minimal

Mechanism of action: The primary mechanism is prevention of fertilization by reducing mobility and viability of sperm and inhibiting development of ova.

- Acts by inhibiting the implantation of fertilized ova through enzymatic interference.
- Certain biochemical changes in the endometrium leading to gametotoxic and spermolytic effects.
- Lysosomal disintegration from the macrophage attached to the device with liberation of prostaglandins also has antifertility effect.
- Copper devices release free copper and copper salts which produce alteration in cervical mucus and endometrial secretions.
- Progesterone releasing IUCDs causes inhibition of implantation and survival of sperms. It also decreases menstrual blood loss and dysmennorhoea.
- Levonorgestrol IUCD causes partial inhibition of follicular development and ovulation.

Indications
- Any women seeking a reliable, reversible, coitally independent method of contraception.
- Women seeking long term birth control.
- A method requiring less compliance.
- Breast feeding women.

- Copper-based intrauterine device can be used for post-coital contraception within 5 days.
- Levonorgesterol intrauterine contraceptive device decreases menstrual flow and cramping (suitable for women with mennorhagia and dysmennorhoea).

Contraindications

- Pregnancy
- Current, recurrent or recent (within 3 months) pelvic inflammatory disease or sexually transmitted disease.
- Puerperal sepsis (post-delivery sepsis).
- Immediate postseptic abortion.
- Severely distorted uterine cavity
- Unexplained vaginal bleeding
- Malignant trophoblastic disease
- Allergy to copper

Side effects

- Bleeding: Non-medicated devices may cause irregular menstrual bleeding. There is 65% increase of menstrual bleeding with copper devices. However, Levonorgesterol device decreases menstrual blood loss.
- Pain or Dysmenorrhoea: Levonorgestrol decreases dysmennorhoea.
- Hormonal devices can cause depression, acne, headache, breast tenderness.
- Rarely lead to ovarian cyst.

Complications

- Severe bleeding or abdominal cramping 3-5 days post-insertion (Perforation, infection).
- Irregular bleeding and/or pain in every menstrual cycle (dislocation or perforation).
- Fever, chills, unusual vaginal discharge (infection).
- Pain during intercourse (infection, perforation, partial expulsion).
- Shorter, longer or missing strings (partial or complete expulsion, perforation).

Indications of removal

- Persistent excessive uterine bleeding.
- Perforation of uterus.
- Partial expulsion.
- Pregnancy inspite of the device in situ.
- Women desirous of baby.
- Missing thread.
- One year after menopause.
- When effective life span of the device is over.

b. *Oral contraceptive pills:* The oral contraceptive pills are the commonly used method for contraception. These are tabulated as follows:

Oral	
• Single preparations	• Progestins only pills (mini pill) Oestrogen only (emergency)
• Combined preparations	• Monophasic Biphasic Triphasic Emergency (post coital)
Parenteral	
• Injectables	• DMPA NET-EN Combined (once a month injection)
• Implants	• Morplant Implanon Levonorgesterol Rod Levonorgestrol
• Devices IUCD (LNG-IUS) Vaginal ring	• Intrauterine Contraceptive device LNG ring Combined (oestrogen and progesterone) ring
• Transdermal patches	• Nestorone

Mechanism of action: The main mechanism of action is to suppress gonadotropin secretion, thereby inhibiting ovulation. And also:

- Development of endometrial atrophy, making endometrium unreceptive to implantation.
- Production of viscous cervical mucus that impedes sperm transport.
- Possible effect on secretion and peristalsis within the fallopian tube, which interferes with ovum and sperm transport.

Indications

- Any woman seeking a reliable, reversible, coitally independent method of contraception.
- It is particularly suited for women who wish to take advantage of its non-contraceptive benefits.
- The use of condoms is still recommended in combined oral contraceptive users for protection against sexually transmitted infections and human immunodeficiency virus.

Contraindications

- Less than 6 weeks postpartum if breast feeding
- Hypertensive
- Current or past history of venous thromboembolism
- Ischaemic heart disease
- History of cerebrovascular accident
- Complicated valvular heart disease
- Migraine headache with focal neurological symptoms
- Breast cancer
- Diabetes with retinopathy/neuropathy/nephropathy
- Severe cirrhosis and tumor of lever

The non-contraceptive benefits of these pills are:

- Cyclic regulation
- Decreased menstrual flow
- Increased bone mineral density
- Decreased dysmenorrhoea
- Decreased acne
- Decreased hirsutism
- Decreased endometrial cancer
- Decreased ovarian cancer
- Decreased risk of fibroids
- Less colorectal carcinoma

The use of contraceptive pills has following side effects:

- Abnormal menstrual bleeding
- Nausea
- Weight gain
- Mood changes
- Breast tenderness
- Headache

The main aims of combined oral contraceptives are:

- Effective contraception
- Acceptable cycle control
- The least side-effects

The combined oral contraceptives can be started during the first 5 days of menstrual cycle. If the combined OC is started within the first 5 days of the menstrual cycle, a backup method of contraception is not necessary for prevention of pregnancy. Alternatively, quick start method can be adopted where the first pill is taken in the health care provider's office after ruling out pregnancy. A back-up method of contraception should be used for the first week after combined OC initiation of the quick start method is used. A follow up visit should be scheduled to review the experience, satisfaction and compliance, as well as evaluate the blood pressure. If indicated, a pelvic examination can be performed at the follow up visit.

The contraceptive pills can be used routinely, which decreases incidence of pelvic pain, headache, bloating/swelling and breast tenderness. However, long term safety has not been documented.

Trouble shooting
- Breakthrough bleeding
- Missed pills
- Amenorrhoea
- Chloasma
- Breast Tenderness (mastalgia) and galactorrhoea
- Nausea
- Pregnancy

c. *Vaginal contraceptive ring (NUVA-RING):* The vaginal contraceptive is a flexible transparent ring having 54 mm/4mm cross-sectional diameter. It releases 15 mg Estradiol and 0.12 mg of desogestral (etonorgestrel)/day. The ring is used for 3 weeks continuous followed by one ring-free week.

d. *Combined injectable contraception (LUNELLE):* Monthly injectable contraceptive composed of 5.0 mg estradiol cypionate and 25 mg medroxyprogesteronic acetate. It is administered once a month. It causes less bleeding.

e. *Injectable progestin depot medroxy progesterone acetate (DMPA):* It is highly effective with a failure rate less than 0.3%/year. 150 mg intramuscular injection is given every 12 weeks starting during first five days of menstrual cycle. Usually it is effective within 24 hours of the injection. It inhibits the secretion of pituitary Gonadotropins, thereby suppressing ovulation. It also increases viscosity of cervical mucus.

Indications
- Any women seeking reliable, reversible coitally independent method of contraception
- Women who have difficulty in complying with other methods since it does not require daily attention
- Women with migraine headache
- Women who are breastfeeding
- Women with sickle cell disease

- Women taking anticonvulsant and medications
- Mentally handicapped women

Contraindications
- Pregnancy
- Unexplained vaginal bleeding
- Current breast carcinoma
- Severe liver cirrhosis
- Active viral hepatitis
- Benign hepatic adenoma

Side effects
- Menstrual cycle disturbance:
  - Irregular bleeding
  - Abnormally heavy or prolonged bleeding
- Hormonal side effect: Headache, acne, decrease libido, nausea and breast tenderness.
- Weight gain
- Depressive symptoms.

Risks
- Delayed return of fertility
- Reduction in bone mineral density
- Venous thromboembolism

f. *Oral progestins:* Oral progestins are also known as Minipills. The package contains 28 tablets. The pills can be started on the first day of the menstrual cycle or any day if pregnancy excluded. It must be used at the same time every day within 3 hours. A back up contraception must be used for 7 days. It should be used continuously. No pill free interval. The failure rate is 0.5%. It can be used immediately postpartum with no effect of lactation.

Indications
- It can be used for any women seeking reliable, reversible, coitally independent method of contraception.
- Women with contraindications to estrogen.

- Women having migraine headache with neurological symptoms.
- Women who have unwanted side-effects of combined contraceptive.
- Breast feeding women.

The pills act by decreasing volume and increasing viscosity of cervical mucus or alter its molecular structure that causes little or no sperm penetration.

The sperm motility is also impaired and decrease fertilization. Ovulation is suppressed in 60% of the women. Endometrial changes occur that decrease implantation.

Contraindications

- Pregnancy
- Current breast cancer
- Active viral hepatitis
- Liver tumors

g. *Progesterone Intrauterine System (LNG-IUS):* The system increase thickness of cervical mucus to inhibit sperm migration and endometrial atrophy. It improves menorrhagia and may cause amennorhoea in many users. Failure rate is 0.1%.

h. *Emergency contraception:* Any method used after unprotected or inadequately protected sexual intercourse. Three types are available:

- *High dose progestin only:* 1.5 mg norgestral at one time or in divided doses within 72–120 hours of intercourse.
- *Yuzpe method (Preven):* The dose is 100 mg of ethinyl estradiol and 0.50 mg of levonorgestral. The first dose is given within 72 hours of intercourse and second after 12 hours.
- *Copper intrauterine contraceptive device:* The device is placed within 5 days of unprotected coitus. It interferes with implantation after fertilization.

Indications

- For aged couples who meet very infrequently.

- Following a single act of sexual exposure in young girls.
- When pregnancy is apprehended owing to rupture of condoms, detection of defect in diaphragm after its use or premature ejaculation in couples practicing coitus interruptus.
- In case of rape/incest.

Advantages

- Saves the couples from unwanted pregnancies.
- Avoids unnecessary operative interferences.
- Prevents adolescent pregnancies.
- Helps to reduce unsafe abortion.

Permanent sterilization

- *Female Sterilization:* It interrupts the patency of fallopian tube thereby preventing fertilization. The failure rate is 0.8–3.7%.
- *Male Sterilization:* It is commonly known as Vasectomy, which ligates or cauterize the vas deferens. It prevents passage of sperm into seminal fluid. The failure rate is 0.15%. It is advised to use contraception until completely azoopermic for two consecutive sperm count (usually takes 12 weeks or 10–20 ejaculations). It does not affect ability to have an orgasm.

Sociology of Family Planning

The problem of family planning is essentially the problem of social change. Contraceptive technology is no shortcut to the problem. What is more important is to stimulate social changes affecting fertility such as raising the age of marriage, improving the status of women, education and employment opportunities, old age security, compulsory education of children, accelerating economic changes designed to increase per capita income etc. It is now axiomatic that economic development is the best contraceptive. The examples of all the countries which have controlled population successfully show that the best motivation is economic – a desire to improve the standard of living. The solution to the problem is one of mass education and communication so that people may understand the benefits of a small family.

Voluntary Organizations

Voluntary organizations have played a major role in the population control programs since the beginning. They are involved in every possible way so as to complement government efforts to promote the National Family Welfare Program including running of Family Welfare Centres, Post Partum Centres, the ANM training schools, population research centres and other innovative projects.

Some well known voluntary agencies in India are:
- Family Planning Association of India
- The Family Planning Foundation
- The Population Council of India
- The Indian Red Cross
- The Indian Medical Association
- Rotary Clubs
- Lions' Club
- Citizen Forum

NATIONAL FAMILY WELFARE PROGRAM

The government of India launched a nationwide family planning program in 1952, making it the first country in the world to do so.

- The beginning of the program was done with the establishment of a few clinics and improvement in education material, research and training.
- During the third five year plan, family planning was declared as "the very centre of planned development".
- During the fourth five year plan, the Govt. of India gave 'top priority to the program'. The program was made an integral part of MCH activities of PHCs and their sub-centres.
- During the fifth five year plan (1975-80) there were major changes in April 1976; the county framed its first National Population Policy.
- The sixth and seventh five year plans were accordingly set to achieve the goal of the two child family norm through the attainment of a birth rate of 21 and a death rate of 9 per 1000 of the population.
- The government of India has designed a more detailed and comprehensive National policy in 2000 to promote family welfare.

6   *Air Pollution*

The atmosphere is a complex, dynamic natural gaseous system that is essential to support life on the planet earth. The ozone layer act as shield to protect from very harmful UV rays coming from the sun. The ozone layer absorbs UV rays and prevents most of them in reaching earth's surface. Stratospheric ozone depletion due to air pollution has long been recognized as a threat to human health as well as to the Earth's ecosystems. **Air pollution** is the introduction of chemicals, particulate matter, or biological materials that cause harm or discomfort to humans or other living organisms.

An **air pollutant** is known as a substance in the air that can cause harm to humans and the environment. Pollutants can be in the form of solid particles, liquid droplets, or gases. In addition, they may be natural or man-made.

Pollutants can be classified as either primary or secondary. Usually, 'primary pollutants' are substances directly emitted from a process, such as ash from a volcanic eruption, the carbon monoxide gas from a motor vehicle exhaust or sulfur dioxide released from factories.

'Secondary pollutants' are not emitted directly. Rather, they form in the air when primary pollutants react or interact. An important example of a secondary pollutant is —at the ground level of ozone, reaction of one of the many pollutants that make up photochemical smog.

Some pollutants may be both primary and secondary, since they are emitted directly and also formed from other primary pollutants.

Primary Pollutants Include

- Sulfur oxides (especially sulfur dioxide) sulfur dioxide is produced by volcanoes and in various industrial processes. Since coal and petroleum often contain sulfur compounds, their combustion generates sulfur dioxide. Further oxidation of sulfur dioxide, usually in the presence of a catalyst such as nitrous oxide, forms sulphuric acid, and thus acid rain. This is one of the causes for concern over the environmental impact of the use of these fuels as power sources.

- *Nitrogen oxides (especially nitrogen dioxide):* Nitrogen dioxide is one of the several nitrogen oxides emitted from high temperature combustion. This reddish-brown toxic gas has a characteristic sharp, biting odor. Nitrogen dioxide is one of the most prominent air pollutants.

- *Carbon monoxide:* Carbon monoxide is a colorless, odorless, non-irritating but very poisonous gas. It is a product of incomplete combustion of fuels such as natural gas, coal or wood. Vehicular exhaust is a major source of carbon monoxide.

- *Carbon dioxide:* Carbon dioxide is also emitted from combustion but is vital to living organisms. It is a natural gas in the atmosphere.

- *Volatile organic compounds:* Volatile organic compounds are an important outdoor air pollutant. They are often divided into methane and non-methane categories. Methane is an extremely efficient greenhouse gas which contributes to enhanced global warming. Within the non-methane category, the aromatic compounds benzene, toluene and xylene are suspected carcinogens and may lead to leukemia through prolonged exposure. 1,3-butadiene is another dangerous compound which is often associated with industrial uses.

- *Particulate matter:* The particulate matter are tiny particles of solid or liquid suspended in a gas. In contrast, aerosol refers to particles and the gas together. Sources of particulate matter can be man made or natural. Some particulates occur naturally, originating from volcanoes, dust storms, forest fires, living vegetation, and sea spray. Human activities such as burning of fossil fuels in vehicles, power plants and various industrial processes also increase level of aerosols in environment. Increased levels of fine particles in the air are linked to health hazards such as heart disease, altered lung function and lung cancer. Diesel exhaust is a combustion derived particulate matter contributing to air pollution. The diesel exhaust has been linked to acute vascular dysfunction and increased thrombus formation.
- Toxic metals such as lead, cadmium and copper.
- *Chlorofluorocarbons (CFCs):* They are harmful to the ozone layer and are emitted from certain banned products.
- *Ammonia:* Ammonia is emitted from agricultural processes and it has characteristic pungent odor. Ammonia contributes significantly to the nutritional needs of terrestrial organisms by serving as a precursor to foodstuffs and fertilizers. Ammonia, either directly or indirectly, is also a building block for the synthesis of many pharmaceuticals. Although in wide use, ammonia is both caustic and hazardous.
- Odors from garbage, sewage, and industrial processes.
- Radioactive pollutants produced by nuclear explosions, war explosives, and natural processes such as the radioactive decay of radon.

Secondary Pollutants Include

- Particulate matter formed from gaseous primary pollutants and compounds in smog. The word "smog" is a combination of smoke and fog, a kind of air pollution. The smog results from large amounts of coal burning in an area caused by a mixture of smoke and sulfur dioxide. Modern smog is not because of coal burning but from vehicular and industrial emissions. This may combine with the primary emissions to form photochemical smog. Particulate matter with coarse (particle size between 2.5 and 10 mm) and fine particles (measuring less than 2.5 mm) are considered to contribute to the heath effects observed in urban environments. PM_{10} represents the particle mass that enters the respiratory tract including both coarse and fine particles. According to the Air Quality guidelines by the WHO, recommends long term exposure more than 20 mg/m^3 annual mean and short-term exposure more than 50 mg/m^3. 24 hour mean of PM_{10} represents the lowest end of the range over which significant effects on survival were observed.
- Ground level ozone formed from nitrous oxide and volatile organic compounds. The ozone is a key constituent of the troposphere. Photochemical and chemical reactions involving it drive many of the chemical processes that occur in the atmosphere by day and by night. At abnormally high concentrations brought about by human activities (largely the combustion of fossil fuel), it may at as pollutant. The WHO Air Quality Guidelines (AQG) for ozone levels at 120 mg/m^3 for an 8-hour daily average.
- Peroxyacetyl nitrate also formed from nitrous oxide and volatile organic compounds. WHO Air Quality Guidelines

(AQG) for nitrogen dioxide for long-term exposure is 200 mg/m^3 for 1-hour mean. Similarly long-term exposure for sulfur dioxide is 20 mg/m^3 24-hour mean and short-term exposure for sulfur dioxide is 500 mg/m^3 10-minute mean.

Apart from these pollutants, a variety of persistent organic pollutants, which can attach to particulate matter are also source of air pollution.

Persistent organic pollutants are organic compounds that are resistant to environmental degradation through chemical, biological, and photolytic processes. They persist in the environment for a longer period and bioaccumulate in human and animal tissue, thereby significantly affecting human health.

Sources

Sources of air pollution refer to the various locations, activities or factors which are responsible for the release of pollutants in the atmosphere. These sources can be classified into two major categories.

- Anthropogenic sources
- Natural sources

Anthropogenic Sources (human activity)

These are mostly related to burning different kinds of fuel

- 'Stationary sources' include smoke stacks of power plants, manufacturing units, incinerators, furnaces and other types of fuel-burning heating devices.
- 'Mobile sources' include motor vehicles, aircraft and the collective effect of sound etc.
- Chemicals, dust and controlled burn practices in agriculture and forestry. Controlled burning is used in forest management, since fire is a natural part of both forest and grassland ecology. Controlled burning stimulates the germination of some desirable forest trees, thus renewing the forest.

- Fumes from paint, hair spray, varnish, and other solvents
- Waste deposition generates methane. Methane is non toxic; however, it is highly flammable and may form explosive mixtures with air. Methane is also an asphyxiant and may displace oxygen in an enclosed space. Asphyxia or suffocation may result if the oxygen concentration is reduced to below 19.5%.
- Military tools such as toxic gases and germ warfare.

Natural Sources

- Dust from natural sources, usually large areas of land with little or no vegetation.
- Methane, emitted by the digestion of food by animals.
- Radon, a colorless, odorless, naturally occurring, radioactive noble gas that is formed from the decay of radium. It is considered to be a health hazard. It is the second most frequent cause of lung cancer after cigarette smoking. Radon gas from natural sources can accumulate in buildings, especially in confined areas such as the basement, etc.
- Smoke and carbon monoxide from wildfires.
- Volcanic activity, which produce sulfur, chlorine and ash particulates.

Quantifying Air Pollutants

The quantity of a pollutant released to the ambient air is usually expressed as emission factors. These factors are usually expressed as the weight of pollutant divided by a unit weight, volume, distance or duration of the activity emitting the pollutant (e.g. kilograms of particulate emitted per megagram of coal burned). Such factors facilitate estimation of emissions from various sources of air pollution.

Indoor Air Quality

A lack of indoor ventilation concentrates air pollution. Radon gas, a carcinogen, is exuded from the Earth in certain locations and trapped inside houses. Building materials including carpeting and plywood emit formaldehyde gas. Paint and solvents give off volatile organic compounds as they dry. Lead paint can degenerate into dust is a potential health hazard. Intentional air pollution is introduced with the use of air fresheners and other scented items. Controlled wood fires in stoves and fireplaces can add significant amount of smoke particulates into the air. The pesticides and other chemical sprays without proper ventilation cause air pollution.

Carbon monoxide poisoning and fatalities are often caused by faulty vents and chimneys, or by the burning of charcoal inside the rooms. Traps are built in all domestic plumbing to keep sewer gas, hydrogen sulfide out of interiors. Dry cleaned clothes emits tetrachloroethylene for a prolonged period.

Biological sources also created in door air pollution. People produce dust from minute skin flakes and decomposed hair, carpeting and furniture produce enzymes and micro-metre-sized fecal droppings, inhabitants emit methane, air conditioning systems can incubate Legionnaires' disease and surrounding gardens can produce pollen, dust. The lack of air circulation allows these airborne pollutants to accumulate more than they would otherwise occur in nature. Prevalence of indoor dampners which is estimated to affect 10–50% of indoor environment in Europe, North America, Australia, Japan and India is the most important trigger of growth of micro-organisms including fungi, actinomycetes and other bacteria. Keeping in view of the indoor air pollution, following guidelines were formulated by the WHO:

- Persistent dampness and microbial growth on interior surfaces and in building structures should be avoided or minimized, as they may lead to adverse health effects.
- Microbial growth include the presence of condensation on surfaces or in structures, visible mould, perceived mouldy odour and a history of water damage, leakage or penetration. Thorough inspection and, if necessary, appropriate measurements can be used to confirm indoor moisture and microbial growth.
- As the relations between dampness, microbial exposure and health effects cannot be quantified precisely, no quantitative health-based guidelines values or thresholds can be recommended for acceptable levels of contamination with microorganisms. Instead, it is recommended that dampness and mould-related problems be prevented. When they occur, they should be remediated because they increase the risk of hazardous exposure to microbes and chemicals.
- Well-designed, well-constructed, well-maintained building envelopes are critical to the prevention and control of excess of moisture and microbial growth as they prevent thermal bridges and the entry of liquid or vapour-phase water. Management of moisture requires proper control of temperatures and ventilation to avoid excess humidity, condensation on surfaces and excess moisture in materials. Ventilation should be distributed effectively throughout spaces and stagnant air zones should be avoided.
- Building owners are responsible for providing a healthy workplace or living environment free of excess moisture and mould by ensuring proper building construction and maintenance. The occupants are responsible for managing the use of water, heating, ventilation and appliances in a manner that does not lead to dampness and mould growth. Local recommendations for different climatic region should be updated to control dampness-mediated microbial growth in buildings and to ensure desirable indoor air quality.

- Dampness and mould may be particularly prevalent in poorly maintained housing for low-income people. Remediation of the conditions that lead to adverse exposure should be given priority to prevent an additional contribution to poor health in populations who are already living with an increased burden of disease.

Effects of Air Pollution on Health

The health effects caused by air pollutants may range from subtle biochemical and physiological changes from difficulty in breathing, wheezing, coughing and aggravation of existing respiratory to cardiac conditions. The air pollution principally affect the respiratory system and the cardiovascular system. Individual reactions to air pollutants depend on the type of pollutant, the degree of exposure, the nutritional status and also the immunity.

Sulfur oxides mainly contribute to the incidence of respiratory diseases. Acid rain, a form of precipitation that contains high levels of sulfuric or nitric acids, can contaminate drinking water and vegetation. It has the potential to damage aquatic life and erode buildings. When a weather condition known as a temperature inversion prevents dispersal of smog, inhabitants of the area, especially children and the elderly and chronically ill, are warned to stay indoors and avoid physical stress. Carbon monoxide by driving oxygen out of the bloodstream causes apathy, fatigue, headache, disorientation, and decreased muscular coordination and visual acuity.

Even everyday levels of air pollution may affect health and behaviour. Indoor air pollution is a problem in developed countries. In less developed nations the lack of running water and indoor sanitation can encourage respiratory infections.

Heart and Lung Diseases

There are many factors that can increase the chances of lung diseases. The role of air pollution as the underlying cause remains unclear but is the subject of considerable research. However, it is clear that air pollution, infections and allergies can exacerbate these conditions. An early diagnosis can lead to appropriate treatment and ensure a normal quality of life. The following are the most prevalent diseases:

- The common cold is the most familiar with symptoms including sore throat, stuffy or runny nose, coughing and sometimes irritation of the eyes.
- Bronchitis and pneumonia are common. Symptoms may include cough, fever, chills and shortness of breath.
- **Asthma** is also common chronic disease among children and adults. It causes shortness of breath, coughing or wheezing or whistling in the chest. Asthma attacks can be triggered by a variety of factors including infection, pollen, allergies and stress. It can also be triggered by sensitivity to non-allergic types of pollutants present in the air such as smog.
- **Chronic obstructive pulmonary disease** encompasses two major disorders: emphysema and chronic bronchitis. Emphysema is a chronic disorder in which the walls and elasticity of the alveoli are damaged. Chronic bronchitis is characterized by inflammation of the cells lining inside of bronchi, which increases the risk of infection and obstructs airflow in and out of the lung. Smoking is responsible for approximately 80% of such cases while other forms of air pollution may also influence the development of these diseases. Symptoms include cough, production of mucous and shortness of breath.
- **Lung cancer** is the most common cause of death. Cigarette smoke contains various carcinogens and is responsible for most cases of this fatal disease. The symptoms of lung cancer begin silently and then progress to chronic cough, wheezing and chest pain. Air pollution has also been linked to lung cancer.

Heart Diseases

Inhalation of air deficient in oxygen, coupled with air pollutants are major cause of heart diseases. The common diseases are:

- **Coronary artery disease** includes angina and heart attack which share similar symptoms of pain or pressure in the chest. Unlike angina, the symptoms caused by heart attack do not subside with rest and may cause permanent damage to the heart. Smoking, lack of exercise, excess weight, high cholesterol levels in the blood, family history and high blood pressure are some of the factors that may contribute to this disease.

- **Heart failure** is a condition in which the heart is unable to cope with its work load of pumping blood to the lungs and the rest of the body. The most common cause is severe coronary artery disease. The main symptoms are shortness of breath and swelling of the ankles and feet.

- **Heart-rhythm problems** are irregular rhythms of the heart beat. In some cases heart-rhythm problems are caused by coronary artery disease. The common symptoms of heart-rhythm problems is palpitation.

Pyramid of Health Effects

Air pollution can affect both the respiratory and cardiac systems. The health effects of air pollution can be seen as a pyramid, with the mild effects at the bottom of the pyramid, and the severe ones at the top of the pyramid. The pyramid demonstrates that as severity decreases the number of affected people increases.

The effect of air pollution is slow and takes years to be detected. The research is under way to assess the long-term effects of chronic exposure to low levels of air pollution as well as to determine how air pollutants interact with one another in the body and with physical factors such as nutrition, stress, alcohol, cigarette smoking, and common

medicines. Another subject of investigation is the relation of air pollution to cancer, birth defects, and genetic mutations.

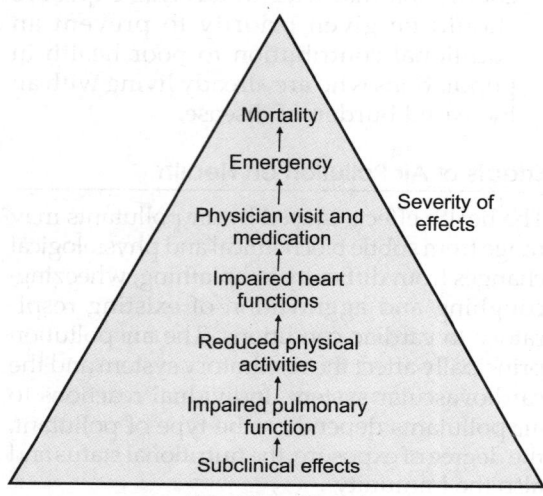

A recently discovered result of air pollution are seasonal 'holes' in the ozone layer in the atmosphere above Antarctica and the Arctic, coupled with growing evidence of global ozone depletion. This can increase the amount of ultraviolet radiation reaching the earth, where it damages crops and plants and can lead to skin cancer and cataracts. This depletion has been caused largely by the emission of chlorofluorocarbons from refrigerators, air conditioners and aerosols.

Effects on Children

The exposure of children to air pollutants may lead to asthma, pneumonia and other lower respiratory infections as well as a low initial birth rate. The World Health Organization has cautioned the greatest concentration of particulate matter particles in countries with low economy and high population rates. Since children move outdoors more and many have minute ventilation are more susceptible to the dangers of air pollution. Use of compressed natural gas could help minimize air pollution, especially due to automobiles.

Control Devices

The following ways are usually recommended as pollution control devices. The contaminants are either destroyed or removed from an exhaust stream before it is emitted into the atmosphere.

Particulate Control

- Mechanical collectors.
- *Electrostatic precipitators:* An electrostatic precipitator or electrostatic air cleaner is a particulate collection device that removes particles from a flowing gas (such as air) using the force of an induced electrostatic charge. Electrostatic precipitators are highly efficient filtration devices that minimally impede the flow of gases and can easily remove fine particulate matter such as dust and smoke from the air stream.
- *Baghouse:* It is designed to handle heavy dust loads. It consists of a dust filter, a filter-cleaning system and a dust receptacle or dust removal system.
- *Particulate scrubbers:* The scrubbers remove air polluttants by continuously contacting the air or other gases. In a wet scrubber, the polluted gas is brought into contact with the scrubbing liquid or by forcing it through a pool of liquid so as to remove the pollutants.

Nitrous Oxide Control

Various devices controlling nitrous oxide are:
- Low Nitrous oxide burners
- Selective catalytic reduction
- Selective non-catalytic reduction
- Nitrous oxide scrubbers
- Catalytic converter.

Miscellaneous

- Continuous emissions monitoring systems
- Sulphur dioxide control by Biofilters and Catalytic oxidizers
- Mercury control by electro-catalytic oxidation
- Dioxin and furon control by other capturing systems.

BIBLIOGRAPHY

1. Azizi, B.H., Zulfkifli, H.I. and Kasim, S.: Indoor air pollution and asthma in hospitalized children in a tropical environment. J. Asthma. : 32, 413, 1995.
2. Boy, E., Bruce, N. and Delgado, H. : Birth weight and exposure to kitchen wood smoke during pregnancy. Environment Health Perspective: 110, 109, 2002.
3. Burge, M.: Bioaerosols: Prevalence and health effects in the indoor environment. J. Allergy Clin. Immunol. : 86, 687, 1990.
4. Ellegard, A. : Tears while cooking : An indicator of indoor air pollution and related health effects in developing countries. Envrion. Res. : 75, 12, 1997.
5. Gray, A. : Lung cancer deaths from indoor radon and the cost effectiveness and potential of pohius to reduce them. B.M.J. : 338, 3110, 2009.
6. Heningson, E.W. and Ahlberg, M.S. : Evaluation of microbiological aerosol samples: a review. J. Aerosol Sci. : 25, 1459, 1994.
7. Kraidman, G. : The microbiology of airborne contamination and air sampling. Drug Cosmetic Ind. J. : 3, 40, 1975.
8. Lal, K., Dutta, K.K., Vachharajani, K.D., Gupta, G.S. and Srivastava, A.K. : Histomorphological changes in lung of rats following exposure to wood smoke. Indian J. Exp. Biol. ; 31, 761, 1993.
9. Leggat, P.A. and Kedjarme, U. : Bacterial aerosols in the dental clinic : a review. Int. Dent. J. : 51, 39, 2001.
10. Lu, D.P. nd Zambito, R.F. : Aerosols and cross infections in dental practice : a historic view. Gen. Dent. : 2, 136, 1981.
11. Mc Kinley, I.B. Jr. and Ludlow, M.U. : Hazard of laser smoke during endodontic therapy. J. Endod. : 20, 558, 1994.
12. Perez, P.J., Perez, G.C., Baez, S.R. and Torres, C.A.: Cooking with biomass stores and tuber-culosis : a care control study. Int. J. Tuberc. Lung. Dis. : 5, 1, 2001.
13. Smith, K., Samet, J., Romein, I. and Burce, N. : Indoor air pollution in developing countries and acute respiratory infections in children. Thorax: 55, 518, 2000.

7   *Water Pollution*

The earth's surface water is undoubtedly the most precious natural resource that exists on our planet. Life without water would be non-existent since it is essential for everything to grow and prosper.

Water is an important constituent of diet, though not labelled as food as it does not give energy like other nutrients. It constitutes about two third of the human's body weight. Out of this, another two third is intra-cellular and one third is extra-cellular. Under normal conditions, total amount of water remains constant in the body. Water acts as solvent for all the salts helping in digestion and absorption. It also dissolves the waste materials providing good medium for excreting body wastes. Another important role of water in our body is to regularize the body temperature by sweating and evaporation. The volume and the composition of the body fluids are regulated with water.

Water requirements are dependent on age, body temperature, temperature of the surroundings, renal solute load and extra renal loss. The total fluid intake increases with age approximately three liters per day for adults.

The importance of water is recognized; even then it is polluted by fellow individuals. The rivers, lakes are becoming unhygienic and the organisms are dying at alarming rate. The menace of water pollution is to be dealt at community level as well as through education from government side.

Potable water: Potable water implies water free of all pathogenic organisms and harmful substances. It should be palatable and be useful for all domestic needs.

Use of Water

Water is commonly used for the following purposes:
- Domestic uses
- Public recreations
- Industrial uses
- Agricultural purpose.

Sources of Water

Water is available from many sources. Water is also available as a by-product of oxidation of glucose (carbohydrate) in the body. The main sources are:
- Surface Water
- Rivers
- Wells
- Streams
- Springs
- Ground Water

WATER AND HEALTH

The standard of public health can be improved by controlling a number of factors like food, water, housing, clothing and sanitation. The environment determines the health of an individual, a community or a nation. Any disturbance in the balance between the man and the environment will lead to disease. The environment must be clean in order to prevent the occurrence of a disease. Sanitation or cleanliness of the surroundings affects individual's health. The WHO defines environmental sanitation as *the control of all those factors in man's physical environment which exercise or may exercise a deleterious effect on his physical development, health and survival.* The services of a qualified doctor, epidemiologist, public health engineer, town planner, sociologist, economist and the health inspector are required for environmental sanitation.

The communities must be supplied by safe and wholesome water. The human excreta must be disposed off properly.

Water should not only be safe for drinking but also clean for other uses. It should be free from all types of pathogens and other harmful chemical substances, pleasant to taste and useable for domestic purposes. Water gets polluted by various agents, viz. organic matters, microorganisms, chemical substances, industrial wastes or sewage.

Water Pollution: According to the dictionary, pollution means foul, unclean or dirty. Water pollution means addition of large amounts of waste materials in the water, making it unfit for its intended use. Inorganic and organic impurities dissolve, get suspended or colloided in water.

Causes of Pollution

The causes of pollution include sewage and fertilizers containing nitrates and phosphates. The excess level of such elements stimulates the growth of aquatic plants and algae. Excessive growth of these types of organisms, consequently clogs the water ways. They block sun-light to deeper water subsequently affecting the metabolic ability of fish and other invertebrates that reside in water. Under natural conditions, lakes and rivers, etc.

undergo putrefaction, a process that slowly fills the water body with sediment and organic matter. Water depth is reduced leading to impaired respiration of water animals and other aquatic organisms.

Pollution in the form of organic matter enters water as sewage, leaves and grass clippings.

Many types of fish and bottom-dwelling animals cannot survive when levels of dissolved oxygen drops low. Low oxygen level kills organisms in large numbers which leads to disruptions in the balance between organisms and food.

Pathogens such as bacteria, viruses, etc. are another type of harmful pollutants. They may cause typhoid and dysentery to minor respiratory and skin disease. These pollutants enter water-ways through sewage, storm drains and septic tanks, etc.

Sources of Water Pollution

The pollution source can be of following two types:
- Point sources
- Non-point sources

The differences are tabulated in Table 7.1.

Point sources can be controlled; however, non-point sources are much more difficult to control. Pollution arising from non-point sources accounts for a majority of contaminants in streams and lakes.

The sources of pollution can also be categorized as:
- Natural sources
- Human sources

Table 7.1: Differences in point and non-point sources of pollution	
Point source	*Non-point source*
When harmful substances are emitted directly into the water	Pollutants are emitted indirectly through environmental changes
For example: Oil spill illustrates a point source of pollution	For example: Fertilizers and other pollutants from field are carried away by air and rain, which in turn are settled in lakes, etc. affecting aquatic life.

Natural Sources

Natural elements that cause pollution are gases, soil, minerals and waste created by living organisms. The presence of minerals like sodium, potassium, calcium, nickel, lead, mercury and cadmium are also responsible for water pollution.

Human Sources

Household Detergents and Sewage

Water is used for drinking, preparation of food, bathing and for cleaning the houses. Domestic waste water when mixed with other wastes such as plastic, detergent, and human faecal material is known as municipal waste.

Many detergents and fertilizers contain phosphates. When phosphate is discharged into water-ways, it promotes rapid growth of algae.

Industrial Waste

Industries dealing with chemicals, pulp and paper, food processing, etc. produce waste material such as heavy metals and synthetic organic compounds. The waste reaches water bodies either through direct discharge or by leaching from waste dumps.

Oil Spills

The consequence of oil spills is of great environmental concern. Crude oil is transported in tankers across oceans. The oil spill has definite impact on the marine ecosystem. Offshore drilling operations also contribute oil spill into sea.

WATER PURIFICATION

Water available in day to day life is generally not pure. Inorganic and organic impurities, in routine, dissolve or get suspended in water. Purification makes the water potable. Potable water implies water free of all pathogenic organisms and harmful substances. It should be palatable and be useful for all domestic needs. To achieve this objective, various water purification methods are employed.

Water Purification is the process of removing contaminants from a raw water source. The goal is to produce water for a specific purpose with a treatment designed to limit the inclusion of specific contaminants. The water after purification is required for many purposes such as medical, pharmacology, chemical and industrial applications.

Pre-Treatment

- *Direct pumping:* Water must be pumped directly into pipes or other source. The physical infrastructure should be made from appropriate materials so that accidental contamination does not occur.
- *Screening:* The large debris such as sticks, leaves and other particles which may interfere with subsequent purification steps are removed.
- *Storage:* Water from rivers may be stored in reservoirs to allow natural biological purification.
- *Pre-conditioning:* Water rich in hardness salts are treated with soda ash to precipitate calcium carbonate.
- *Pre-chlorination:* The water is chlorinated to minimize the growth of organisms in the pipes and tanks.

The purification treatment includes the following:

The pH Adjustment

Distilled water has an average pH of 7 and sea water has pH of 8.3. If the water is acidic, lime or soda ash is added to raise the pH. Lime is more common but often leads to hardness of water. Making the water slightly alkaline ensures that coagulation and flocculation processes work effectively and help minimize the risk of lead being dissolved from lead pipes and lead solder in piping.

Flocculation

Flocculation is a process which starts with removing any turbidity or color so that the water becomes clear from these impurities. It is carried out by forming a precipitate of certain salts in the water. Initially the precipitate is in the form of very small particles but as the water is gently stirred, these particles get stuck to each other to form bigger particles – the process is called flocculation. Iron hydroxide and aluminium hydroxide are widely used flocculating agent.

Sedimentation

Water from flocculation basin is shifted to another basin, called settling basin. It is a large tank, which allows floc to settle to the bottom. The sedimentation basin is located close to the flocculation basin so that the transit remains easy. The minimum time is normally four hours. As the particles settle to the bottom of the basin, a layer of sludge is formed on the floor of the tank. This layer must be removed off and on. The water can be stored for a few days, which decreases the bacterial count and lead to other chemical changes. Storing water for more than two weeks can be harmful since algae start appearing after long storage.

Filtration

Filtration is an important stage of purification of water. It can be slow filtration or fast filtration. The 'Slow Sand Filter' is very effective in removing impurities. The 'Rapid Sand Filter' is an ideal choice because of increasing demand of water.

i. **Slow Sand Filter (Biological filters):** The slow sand filter requires sufficient space as the water is to pass very slowly through the filters. These filters rely on biological processes rather than physical filtration. The filters are carefully constructed using graded layers of sand with the coarsest at the top and finest at the base.

Filtration depends on the development of thin biological layer on the surface of the filter. An effective slow sand filter may remain in service for many weeks or even months. The top layer of sand is scraped off when flow is obstructed by biological growth.

ii. **Rapid Sand Filter:** It is a type of filter commonly used for purifying municipal water. Rapid sand filter use relatively coarse sand to remove particles and impurities that have been trapped during flocculation procedures. Water and the salts pass through the filter medium under gravity (Gravity type filters) or under pumped pressure (Pressure type filter); subsequently, the flocculated material is trapped in the sand matrix. The filters are cleaned frequently by backwashing, which involves reversing the direction of water and adding compressed air.

Advantages

- Flow rate is higher than a slow sand filter.
- Requires relatively small area of land.
- Less sensitive to changes in the raw water quality.
- Large amount of water can be filtered.

Disadvantages

- It is not an adequate treatment on its own.
- It requires greater maintenance than slow sand filter.
- Generally ineffective against taste and odor.

Boiling

Water is heated to high temperatures for sufficient time to kill the microorganisms that normally survive in water at room temperature. In areas where the water is 'hard', boiling decomposes the bicarbonate ions, resulting in partial precipitation as calcium carbonate. The process is not suitable at community level.

Carbon Filtering

Charcoal, a form of carbon absorbs many toxic compounds routinely present in water. Water passing through activated charcoal is common in household water filters and fish tanks.

Advantages

- Removes dissolved organics and chlorine effectively
- Long life

Disadvantages

- May generate carbon fumes

Distillation

Water is heated to boiling and the vapours rise to a condenser where cooling water lowers the temperature so the vapours are condensed, collected and stored. Most contaminants remain behind in the liquid phase vessel. The herbicides and pesticides cannot be removed efficiently at boiling point lower than 100°C and even concentrate in the distilled water.

Advantages

- Removes a broad range of contaminants
- Reusable

Disadvantages

- Some contaminants can be carried into the condenser
- Requires careful maintenance to ensure purity
- Not suitable at community level

Ion Exchange

The ion exchange process percolates water through bead like spherical resin materials. Ions in the water are exchanged for other ions fixed to the beads. Ion exchangers are either 'cation exchangers' that exchange positively charged ions (cations) or 'anion exchanger' that exchange negatively charged ions (anions). There might be 'amphoteric exchangers' that are able to exchange both cations and anions

simultaneously. Typical ion exchangers are polymers, zeolites, clay and soil humus. Ion exchange is a reversible process and the ion exchangers can be regenerated with desirable ions. The most common exchange methods are:

    i. Softening
    ii. Deionization
    iii. Electro-deionization

i. Softening

Softening is used primarily as pretreatment method to reduce water hardness. In this application ion exchange resins are used to replace the magnesium and calcium ions found in the hard water. This method is useful in dish washers.

ii. Deionization

Deionized water, also known as demineralized water, is that water which has had its mineral ions removed such as cations from sodium, calcium, iron, copper and anions such as chloride and bromide. In this process, an ion exchange resin binds to and filter out the mineral salts from water.

iii. Electro-deionization

Water is passed between a positive and negative electrode. Ion selective membranes allow the +ve ions to separate from the water towards the −ve electrode and the −ve ion towards the +ve electrode. The deionized water so produced is highly pure. The water is usually passed through a reverse osmosis unit first to remove non-ionic organic constituents.

Reverse Osmosis

This is the most economical method of removing practically all the contaminants. The membranes used in the procedure are capable of rejecting practically all particles, bacteria and other organic constraints. Natural osmosis occurs when solutions with two different concentrations are separated by a semi-permeable membrane. Osmotic pressure drives through the membrane; the water dilutes the more concentrated solution and the end result is an equilibrium. In these systems, hydraulic pressure is applied to the concentrated solution to counteract the osmotic pressure. It involves an ion exclusion process. Only solvent is allowed to pass through semi-permeable membrane while virtually all ions and dissolved molecules are retained. This is the most efficient method for water bottling plants and also purifying tap water.

Advantages
- Effectively removes all types of contaminants to some extent
- Requires minimal maintenance

Disadvantages
- Flow rates are limited to a certain gallons/ day rating

Ultra-filtration

A microscopic membrane filter removes particles functioning as a molecular sieve. It separates the dissolved molecules on the basis of size by passing a solution through a fine filter. The ultra filter is a tough, thin, selectively permeable membrane that retains most macromolecules above a certain size including colloids, micro-organisms and pyrogens.

Advantages
- Effectively removes particles, pyrogens and micro-organisms
- Regenerable

Disadvantages
- May not remove dissolved inorganic particles

Disinfection

Disinfection is accomplished by filtering out harmful microbes and later by adding disinfectant chemicals. The pathogens which pass through the filters are disinfected. The following methods are in use:

- *Chlorination:* The method utilizes chlorine or its compounds such as chloramines or chlorine dioxide as disinfectant agents. Chlorine is a strong oxidant that rapidly kills any harmful micro-organisms.
- *Ozone:* The free radical of oxygen, an unstable molecule which readily gives up one atom of oxygen, acts as a powerful oxidizing agent. This is toxic to most of the water borne organisms.
- *Ultraviolet radiations:* The radiations are very effective as long as the water has a low level of color turbidity so the radiations can pass through without being absorbed.

WATER QUALITY STANDARDS

The essentiality of pure water is established. Therefore, international standards authorities, viz. The International Organization for Standardization (ISO) and The American Society for Testing and Materials (ASTM) have set water quality standards for general use.

The specification for water for laboratory use covers three grades as follows:

Grade 1

Essentially free from dissolved or colloidal ionic and organic contaminants. It is suitable for the stringent analytical requirements including those of high performance liquid chromatography (HPLC). It should be produced by further treatment of grade 2 water; for example, by reverse osmosis or ion exchange followed by filtration (filter of pore size 0.2 mm) to remove particle matter.

Grade 2

Very low inorganic, organic or colloidal contaminant and suitable for sensitive analytical purpose including atomic absorption spectrometry (AAS) and the determination of constituents in trace quantities. It can be produced by multiple distillation, ion exchange or reverse osmosis.

Grade 3

Suitable for chemistry work and preparation of reagent solutions. It can be produced by single distillation, by ion exchange, or by reverse osmosis. Unless otherwise specified it should be used for ordinary analytical work.

THE WATER (PREVENTION AND CONTROL OF POLLUTION) ACT

The Water Act was enacted by Parliament in 1974 and later modified in 1990. Its purpose is to control and prevent the water pollution and maintaining the wholesomeness of water. It is applicable in all the states of India. A central board at the centre and the state board at the state level were constituted. Joint board can also be constituted under the act.

Composition of Central Board

- A full time chairman having knowledge relating to environment pollution (appointed by center).
- Up to 5 officials to represent central government.
- Up to 5 officials as representing state boards up to 2 to represent local authorities.
- Up to 3 non-officials to represent fisheries, agriculture, industry, etc.
- Up to 2 persons to represent corporate sector (nominated by centre)
- A full time member secretary, having qualification and experience in science, engineering, management, etc.

Composition of State Board

- A full time chairman having knowledge relating to environment pollution (appointed by center).

- Up to 5 officials to represent state government.
- Upto 5 officials as representing local authorities.
- Up to 3 non-officials to represent fisheries, agriculture, industry, etc.
- Up to 2 persons to represent corporate sector (nominated by state)
- A full time member secretary, having qualification and experience in science, engineering, management, etc.

Composition of Joint Board

- Water Pollution Act makes provisions for formation of Joint Boards by two or more Government of contiguous States or Central Government, State Governments and Union Territories.
- A full time chairman having knowledge relating to environment pollution (appointed by center).
- Two officials each from each state to represent states
- One person from each state to represent local authorities
- One non-official from each state to represent fisheries, agriculture, industry, etc.
- Two persons to represent corporate sector (by state government.)
- A full time member secretary having qualification and experience in science, engineering, management, etc.

The relevant provisions of the act are as follows:

Under Section 19

State Government, after consulting with the boards, can declare some areas as water pollution control areas and in such cases, Government may restrict the application of Act to those specified areas, by notification of Official Gazette. The water pollution, prevention and control area may be declared with reference to a map or otherwise can be altered, added or deleted.

Under Section 21

Officials of the board can take samples of the water effluent from any industry stream or well or sewage for the purpose of analysis.

Under Section 23

Officials of the state boards can enter any premises for the purpose of examining any plant, record, register etc. or for any other function of the Board.

Under Section 24

No person shall discharge any poisonous, noxious or polluting matter into any stream or well or sewer or even on land.

Under Section 25

No person shall, without the previous consent, can:

a. Establish or take any step to establish any industry, operation or process or any treatment and disposal system for any extension or addition thereto, which is likely to discharge sewage or trade effluent into a stream or well or sewer or on land.
b. Bring into use any new or altered outlet for the discharge of sewage.
c. Begin to make any new discharge of sewage.

Under this section, the state board may grant consent to the industry after satisfying itself on pollution control measures taken by the unit; or refuse such consent for reasons to be recorded in writing.

Under Section 27

A state board may from time to time review any condition imposed by it on the person under section 25 and may revoke that condition.

Under Section 28

Any person aggrieved by the order made by the State Board under Section 25 may within thirty days from the date on which the order is communicated to him, prefer an appeal to such authority (referred to as the appellate authority) as the State Govt. may think fit to constitute (in case of NCT of Delhi Appellate authority under this section is Financial Commissioner, Delhi Administration).

Under Section 33

The State Board can direct any person who is likely to cause or has caused the pollution of water in street or well to desist from taking such action.

Under Section 33A

The department can issue any direction to any person, officer or authority and such person shall be bound to comply with such directions. The directions include the power to:

i. Closure of any industry.
ii. Stoppage supply of electricity, water or any other services.

Under Section 43

Whoever contravenes the provisions of Section 24 shall be punishable with imprisonment for a term which shall not be less than one year and six months; may extend to six years with fine.

Under Section 45

If any who has been convicted of any offence under section 24, 25 or 26 is again found guilty of an offence involving a contravention of the same proviso shall be on every subsequent conviction be punishable with imprisonment for a term which shall not be less than two years; may extend to seven years with fine.

Under Section 45A

Whosoever contravenes any of the provisions of this act or fails to comply with any order or direction given under this act for which no penalty has been elsewhere provided in this act, shall be punishable with imprisonment which may extend to three months or fine, which may extend to ten thousand rupees or with both.

Under Section 51 and 52

Central Government can establish Central Water Laboratory and specify its functions (section 51). State Government can establish State Water Laboratory or authorize any laboratory for that purpose (section 52).

Under Section 53

Government analysts with requisite qualifications can be appointed by Central Government or State Government. Report of such approved analysts can be used as evidence in Court.

BIBLIOGRAPHY

1. Byoung, H.L., Won Chu, S., Jong, Gyu, H., Hyion, Y. and Young, S.K. : Effect of ozone in treating drinking water by DAF system. Water Science and Technology: 9, 247, 2009.
2. Cavineross, S. : Sanitation in the developing world: Current status and future solutions. Int. J. Environment Health Res. : 135, 123, 2003.
3. Craun, G.F. and Calderon, R.L. : Waterborne diseases outbreaks caused by distribution system deficiencies. J. Am. Water Works Assoc. : 93, 64, 2001.
4. Gleik, P.H. : Basic water requirements for human activities: Meeting basic needs. Water International: 21, 83, 1996.
5. Hattingh, J. and Classen, M.: Securing water quality for life. Int. J. Water Resource Development : 24, 401, 2008.
6. Huang, C.F. and Hsuan, H.Y.: Study on algae coagulation removal. Water Science and Technology: 9, 167, 2009.
7. Jimenez, A. and Perez, F.A. : International investment in the water sector. Int. J. Water Resources Development: 25, 1, 2009.
8. Le Chevallier, M., Gullick, R., Karim, M., Friedman, M. and Funk, J. : The potential for health risk from intrusion of contaminants into the distribution system from pressure transients. J. Water Health: 1, 3, 2003.
9. Moe, C.L. and heingans, R.D.: Global challenges in water, sanitation and heath. J. Water and Health: 45, 41, 2006.
10. Olmstead, S.M. : Water supply and poor communities: What price got to do with it ? Environment: 45, 22, 2003.
11. Postel, S.L. : Water and world population growth. J. Am. Water Works Assoc. : 92, 131, 2000.
12. Rahman, R., Aha, A., Ryu, H. and Abbaszadegem, M.: Identification of microbial fecal sources in the new river in the United States-Mexican border region. J. Water Health : 7, 267, 2009.
13. Storey, .V. and Ashbolt, N.J. : Enteric various and microbial biofilms – a secondary source of public health concern ? Water Sci. Tech. : 48, 97, 2003.
14. Vieira, F. and Ramus, F.M.: Optimization of the energy management in water supply systems. Water Science and Technology: 9, 59, 2009.

8 *Radiations and Health*

Radiation is the transmission of energy through space and matter. Radiations affect human tissues in many ways. The effect may be physical, chemical or both. The radiations affect the mitotic division of the cells. The symptoms only appear if a large number of cells is irreparably destroyed.

There are two types of radiations:

a. Electromagnetic radiations (non-particulate) – X-rays, gamma rays, infrared, UV rays, cosmic rays, TV, radio, etc.
b. Corpuscular radiations (particulate)– alpha, beta rays and cathode rays.

Sources of Radiations

1. Natural
   a. External
      i. Cosmic
      ii. Terretrial
   b. Internal
2. Artificial

Cosmic radiations include energetic sub-atomic particles, photons of extra-terrestrial origin that reaches the earth. The effects of cosmic radiations are primarily a function of altitude, almost doubling with each 2000 meter increase in elevation.

Sea level	exposure= 0.24mSv per year
1600 meter elevation	exposure= 0.50mSv per year
3200 meter elevation	exposure= 1.25mSv per year

Cosmic radiations also include exposure resulting from airline travel.

Terrestrial radiations are the exposures from terrestrial sources; the radioactive nuclides in the soil.

The extent of exposure varies with the type of soil and its contents of the naturally occurring radionuclides k-40 and the radioactive decay product of Uranium is 238 and Thorium is 232.

Internal radiation: Man is subjected to internal radiation from radioactive matter stored in the body tissues that are taken up from the external environment by inhalation and ingestion. Materials include mainly radon and minute quantities of uranium, thorium and related substances and isotopes of potassium, strontium and carbon.

Man-made Sources of Radiation

a. *Medical diagnosis and treatment:* X-rays are the greatest man-made source of radiation exposure. Two distinct groups involved are:
   i. Patient
   ii. Radiologist and technicians: The skin dose to the patient from single X-ray film varies roughly from 0.02–3.0 Rad.
b. *Nuclear explosion/Weapons:* It releases tremendous amount of energy in the form of heat, light and ionizing radiations. The important radioactive substances are isotopes of carbon, iodine, cesium and strontium.
c. *Consumer and industrial products:* Some everyday appliances are radioactive. This group includes TV sets, nuclear and coat fired electric appliances, air-planes, pocket

watches, smoke alarms, dental porcelain etc.

Biological Effects of Radiations

The biological effects of radiations can be classified as:

I. Direct/Indirect
II. Somatic/Genetic
III. Stochastic/Non-stochastic
IV. Short term/Long term

I. *Direct:* There is alteration of biologic molecules when x-ray photons directly strike the cells.

Indirect: is due to formation of free radicals.

II. *Somatic:* Somatic effect is that which occurs in exposed individuals.

Genetic: Genetic effect is that which is manifested in the future generation of the exposed individuals.

III. *Stochastic effects:* For which the probability of an effect occurring rather than its severity is regarded as a function of the dose without threshold.

Non-stochastic effects: For which the severity of the effect varies with the dose for which a threshold may matter.

Examples of stochastic effects are:
- Carcinoma
- Leukaemia
- Hereditary effects

Examples of non-stochastic effects are:
- Cataract
- Shortening of life span
- Infertility.

IV. *Short term:* Short term effects can be nausea, vomiting and alopecia.

Long term: Long term effects can be carcinoma, genetic defects.

Units of Radiations

The units of radiations are tabulated in Table 8.1.

Lethal Dose

The radiation sensitivity or response varies considerably from one species to another. To compare the radiation response the term lethal dose is used. This is designated as LD 50/30. This is the whole body acute dose required to kill 50% of the exposed organisms within 30 days after irradiation. LD 50/30 for humans is 400–600 rem. It is much higher in fish (700 rem) snail (10,000 rem), and amoeba (1,00,000 rem).

SOMATIC EFFECTS

Somatic effects can be classified into acute and chronic effects:

- Acute effect will be manifested within a few hours to a few days of acute irradiation and the severity of the effect will depend on the dose and the dose rate.

Table 8.1: Unit of radiations

Quantity	SI unit	Traditional unit	Importance
Exposure	Coulomb/kg	Roentgen (R)	Measures radiation quantity
Absorbed dose	Gray (Gy)	Rad (1Gy = 100 rad)	Measures energy absorbed by ionizing radiation per unit mass
Equivalent dose	Sievert (Sv)	Rem (1Sv = 100 rem)	Use to compare biologic effects of different types of radiation on tissue
Radioactivity	Becquerel (Bq)	Curie (Ci)	Describes the decay rate of a sample of radioactive material

- Chronic effects are mainly due to low levels of irradiation for longer periods or chronic irradiation.

Dose levels have been established, below which no effect is expected to be observed in persons irradiated. No harmful effect can be seen if patients and operators maintain these doses.

For convenience, effects of radiation, both somatic and genetic, can be studied under two heads:

I. Acute
    i. Large area of the body
    ii. Small area of the body
II. Chronic
    i. Large area of the body
    ii. Small area of the body.

Acute radiations affecting large area of the body: Such types of effects are never seen in dentistry. These are only possible in nuclear accidents and atomic bombardments. With a large amount of the radiations, the following effects are seen.

0–25 rem = no possible effects

25–50 rem = minor blood changes

50–200 rem = vomiting, etc. severity rises with dose. No deaths

200–300 rem = 20% of deaths can occur after six weeks.

400–700 rem = Hematological changes: No survivals.

Above 700 rem = CNS changes—death within few hours

Acute radiations affecting small area of the body: Such types of effects are seen in cases of treatment of malignant tumors. Large doses up to 6000 R are administered in short span of 3–10 days. This results in the death of the irradiated cells. Acute reactions do occur over skin and other parts resulting in skin erythema and even bone marrow depression.

In dentistry, many radiographs are required only in case of root canal therapy. However, skin reactions vary from individual to individual depending upon the threshold. Usually 350 Roentgen is considered as the Threshold Erythema Dose (TED). In dentistry exposures are kept ½ of the TED.

OSTEORADIONECROSIS

The term implies an infection in bone rendered necrotic by ionizing radiation. This is frequent complication in the treatment of cancer of the oral cavity by irradiation. Because of its high mortality rate, it is the duty of the dentist to prevent its occurrence.

Osteoradionecrosis results from either of the following or in combination:

a. Radiation in massive doses

b. Partial necrosis of bone

c. Trauma which causes infection.

Radiation is delivered as a therapeutic measure for cure of malignant tumor of oral cavity in areas such as:

- Tongue
- Floor of the oral cavity
- Salivary glands
- Sinuses and neoplasms, etc.

Sometimes even small, superficial lesions of the face may cause osteoradionecrosis of mandibular and maxillary bones. Necrosis and ulceration of soft tissues occur two to three months after the irradiation.

Bone, because of its histological architecture, is highly susceptible to radiation. Radiation further leads to its vascular damage and interference with its nourishment. Radiation primarily leads to thickening of the periosteum and strangulation of blood vessels, which combine and ultimately lead to the depletion of blood supply to the bone. The chances of necrosis are enhanced by the fact that most of the patients are well past middle age, a stage where a certain degree of osteoporosis and arteriosclerosis are almost always there. The dentist must realize that the patients can function well with undernourished and partly necrotic mandible and maxilla. So infection and trauma should be avoided. Extractions and other procedures are not indicated for such patients.

Poor oral hygiene, periodontal diseases, residual roots, caries, etc. are local factors which must be eliminated prior to irradiation in order to prevent osteoradionecrosis. Systemic diseases, which affect oral health; such as diabetes, anaemia, etc. are also some of the predisposing factors. Questionable teeth, which can cause infection later on, must be removed prior to irradiation. Usually any bone receiving 5000–6000 Rads radiations may not be able to recover from trauma and in case of the mandible, it must not exceed 2500 Rads. The patient should be put on thorough oral hygiene measures, viz. mechanical and chemical plaque control. Preventive measures should be followed until and unless the extraction becomes necessary. If at all extraction is to be executed, it should be carried out under antibiotic cover and thorough sterilization.

It may also be understood that a tooth in a reasonably good condition may deteriorate after irradiation. Saliva is diminished and enzymes are altered. Teeth may become brittle and prone to caries. The dentist must question the patients before extractions regarding their irradiation dose and time.

Radiographic Appearance

The X-ray picture in the case of osteoradionecrosis is very deceptive before infection. Trabecular pattern, size and configuration of medullary spaces show normal appearance. Once the infection gets established, ragged radiolucent areas can be seen. Clinically, the patient experiences excruciating pain and there can be a suppurative discharge from the sequestrated sites.

Chronic Radiations Affecting Large Area of the Body

This type of hazard is seen usually in workers (occupational hazard) or exposure received by a group of population.

In dentistry, occupational hazard is associated with X-ray machine operators. A committee on radiation protection had set a maximum permissible dose (MPD) as 1.2 R/week and 0.6 R/week previously; but now 0.3 R/week is the MPD.

However, the total accumulated dose should not be more than 5 R/year. What matters is the total accumulated dose which is given to the tissues one over the other. Patients feel nervous, apprehensive and tired. Nausea, vomiting and other GIT disturbances follow.

Accumulated MPD over the years is:
MPD = (N − 18) × 5 rems
where N is the age in years.
This is always greater than 18.

Chronic Radiations Affecting Small Area of the Body

Small doses of X-radiations when given to the smaller areas can lead to various types of hazards such as:
- **Radiation burns:** This effect is seen especially in cases where the operator holds the film in the patient's mouth. The small amount of the radiation received today plus the amount received yesterday and so on, until the tissues have received an amount that produces an erythema. Appearance is something like sunburns.
  - Skin becomes dry, slightly discolored and patient feels burning sensations.
  - Nails become friable with ends broken.
  - Cuticle around the nails is also affected.
  - Slight change is evident in blood supply of the sebaceous and sweat glands.
  - In later stages, cracks appear, which may lead to malignant changes.

- **Loss of hair (alopecia):** Loss of hair (alopecia) can result because of too frequent or too long an exposure to the roentgen rays. Although the loss of hair is not permanent, however, one must be vigilant.
- **Cataract:** Cataract can result from chronic exposure of X-radiations in and around the eyes.
- **Effect on oral mucous membrane:** The mucous membrane shows areas of redness and inflammation. With repeated exposures pseudo-membranes are formed because of breakdown of the mucous membrane. Secondary infection by Candida albicans is a common complication. Usually the mucous membrane heals rapidly once the irradiation is over. Otherwise after a few months, the mucous membrane will tend to become atrophic and relatively avascular.
- **Effect on the taste-buds:** Taste-buds are very sensitive to radiation and soon degenerative changes begin. Loss of taste is very common. Alteration in saliva may account for overall reduction of the taste sensitivity.
- **Effect on the salivary glands:** Salivary glands come under exposure during the treatment of cancer in the oral cavity and the oropharyngeal region. There occurs acute inflammation involving serous acini. A marked increase in the serum amylase has been reported. As the exposure progresses, the glands demonstrate degeneration. The salivary changes have a marked influence on oral microflora and even on the dentition. Increase in Streptococcus mutans, Lactobacillus and Candida has been reported. Xerostomia has also been reported.
- **Effect on the teeth:** The growth is retarded when teeth are irradiated during their development. If the radiation precedes calcification, the tooth may be destroyed. After calcification, if irradiation continues, malformation can result. The root development is retarded. In some instances the tooth erupts prematurely. Fully developed teeth are usually very resistant to the X-radiations.
- **Effect on the bones:** In dentistry, mandible is most susceptible among bony tissues to be irradiated frequently during the treatment for the cancers. The predominant change occurs in the marrow, where a progressive loss of vascular and haemopoietic elements may occur. There occurs lack of osteoblastic activities. The lacunae of the compact bone are empty indicating early necrosis. A marked decrease in the vascularity of bone because of irradiation decreases the capacity of bone to resist infection. Osteoradionecrosis is also a complication because of such exposures.
- **Radiation caries:** The decrease in the salivary flow, its pH and buffering capacity coupled with increased viscosity are the complications of radiation exposure which lead to rampant type of carious lesions. The histological features of these carious lesions are similar to those of typical carious lesions; however, they can be distinguished by their rapid attack. Topical application of 1.0% sodium fluoride (1.0% NaF) and proper oral hygiene measures can reduce the radiation caries.

GENETIC EFFECTS

Most of the studies, regarding effect of radiations on the reproductive system have been conducted mainly on animals and rarely on human beings. Gene mutations do occur depending upon the severity of dose. Radiations cause fragmentation of chromosomes and mutation of genes of sex cells, and these mutant genes with altered characteristics pass on to next generation.

From conception to age 30, genetic cells can be given 50R radiations and from 30–40, another 50R can be given. Most of the children are borne when the parent's age is below 30 years.

In case of dentistry, when the patient's teeth are exposed, it is said that 1/10000th of secondary/stray radiations are directed from face to reproductive organs in the males; and 1/7th of this in females. In children, the exposure is much more because of their short stature.

The human embryo is said to be the most sensitive especially during 15–42 days of its life. Therefore, X-radiations in pregnant women must be avoided.

With heavy doses, sterility in human beings has been reported.

RADIATION DETECTION AND MEASUREMENT

Detection and measurement of nuclear radiation must be accomplished by suitable instruments, since these radiations are invisible and their presence cannot be generally sensed by human perception.

All methods of detection of radiations are based on the ability of radiation to cause ionization, i.e. to produce charged particles from originally neutral atoms and molecules.

A detection system consists of two parts:
- A device which responds to nuclear radiation
- A measuring part which indicates this response

Various radiation measurement units are available which differ in the ionization media and the method by which the ionization is directed. Various types of detectors are: (a) Gas filled detectors; (b) ionization chambers; (c) photographic emulsions; (d) solid state dosimeters.

a. Gas Filled Detectors

It is generally of a cylindrical shape with a central rod electrode. The central electrode and the outer sheath are separated by an insulator.

A variable positive voltage is applied to the central electrode with respect to the outer sheath. On exposure to radiations ion pairs are formed (ionization). The numbers of ion pairs collected at different voltages are measured and five distinguishable regions of response can be noticed. They are:

i. *Region of recombination:* The applied voltage being low, some of the ion-pairs recombine to form neutral atom. Recombination usually decreases as the voltage is increased.

ii. *Ionization chamber region:* All the ion pairs are collected as there would be no recombination. The number of ion pairs produced and collected depends upon the energy spent by the radiation inside the detection volume.

iii. *Region of proportionality:* The negative ions towards the central electrode are accelerated because of higher electrical fluid in the vicinity of central electrode. The electrons gain sufficient energy to produce secondary ionization when they interact with gas molecules. This results in an increase in the number of ion pairs collected, which is proportional to the energy dissipated by the incident particles inside the detector.

iv. *Region of limited proportionality:* The amplification is not constant and depends upon the energy dissipated by the incident particles.

v. *Geiger-Mueller region:* The sensitive region spread over the entire length of the chamber and there will be no difference in pulse heights for particles of different ionizing abilities.

vi. *Region of continuous discharge:* Ionization chamber region, proportional region and Geiger-Mueller region are regions commonly used for radiation detection.

b. Ionization Chamber

In the measurement of radiation exposure, the ionization chambers are filled with air generally at atmospheric pressure. The effective atomic number of the wall material should be close to that of the air. Materials such as graphite, bakelite, etc. satisfy this requirement. Ionization chambers are also used for personal monitoring. They are called pocket dosimeters. It has a built-in capacitance which can be charged by the external potential. The reduction in voltage across the capacitance is a measure of the amount of ionization and hence the quantity of radiation exposure. In the self-reading type of pocket dosimeter, a fiber electrometer with an eyepiece graticules is incorporated in the ionization chamber capacitance unit. Total dose accumulated at a given date is mR, which can be measured. It indicates the total exposures as well as exposure in between. A pocket dosimeter can be recharged.

c. Photographic Emulsions

Photographic film consists of the sensitive emulsion layer which on exposure to radiations forms a latent image. The radiations cause ionization of silver bromide crystals. The films when processed show blackening and the amount of blackening is related to the quantity of radiations recorded. The amount of the blackening is in terms of the measured optical density and is defined as $\log_{10}(I_o/I_t)$ where:

I_o = Intensity of incident light

I_t = Intensity of transmitted light

The optical density is measured using an instrument known as dosimeter.

d. Solid State Thermoluminescent Dosimeters

Many thermolucent materials like LiF, Al_2O_3, $CaSO_4$, etc. are available. $CaSO_4$ is useful for dosimetry. These materials have the property of emitting light when exposed to radiations. The emitted light is proportional to the exposure to the radiations. These are used as personal monitoring services. Thermoluminescent dosimeters can measure gamma dose as low as 1R and as high as 10^5R.

PERSONAL MONITORING

Monitoring is the physical measurement of X-radiations. Personal monitoring is the evaluation of radiation doses received by the persons working in the department concerning radiation. A commonly used device is the film badges, which can be of different types. Films badges and thermoluminescent badges are commonly employed. With a film badge, a wide range of doses from 10 mR to 1000R of different types of radiations can be measured. This is worn on the chest and measures the whole body radiations under normal conditions. X-rays, β-rays, γ-rays, etc. are all measured with the film badges.

Cadmium can be used to detect the radiations of higher penetrating wavelengths.

Advantages

- Permanent record can be kept
- All types of radiations can be differentiated

Disadvantages

- It cannot be read immediately
- It is not very accurate
- It cannot record accidental exposures

The second type of badge is the thermo-luminiscent dosimeter. This consists of three $CaSO_4$ discs embedded in a metallic frame work and enclosed in a multifilter casette. This can be used to monitor β, γ and X-radiations. This can cover wide range of doses from 10 m rem to 1000 rem.

Film badges can also be formed with the gradation of only copper over the film. Stepwise increased thickness of copper is placed over the film.

AREA MONITORING

Area monitoring is the assessment of radiation levels at different locations in the vicinity of radiation sources. On the basis of this measurement, protection measures are taken. The most commonly used area monitoring device is the survey-meter based on the ionization chambers. The chamber is provided with a window and by opening the window β-radiations can be measured. This meter usually does not function at the high radiation levels.

RADIATION PROTECTION

The philosophy of radiation protection follows the principle of ALARA (as low as reasonably achievable). Even with a single periapical film, the exposure to the patient is 217 mR. According to the ALARA principle, the exposure to X-radiation is to be reduced as far as possible. The three basic parameters which affect radiation doses are described below:

i. **Shielding:** Various shielding materials are used such as iron, lead, concrete wall and hard plastic, etc. As the thickness of the shielding interposed between X-ray beams and the point of interest (e.g. location of the operator) is increased the exposure rate decreases exponentially. The thickness of the shielding material, which reduces the intensity of the radiations to half its original value (50%) is defined as the half value thickness (HVT) of the material. Exponential attenuation is seen in the case of X-rays and γ-rays and not for electrons as such. This implies that even a very large thickness of the shielding material will not completely attenuate the radiations to have zero intensity. It is pointed out that the X-radiations have a spectrum of energies and that the low energy or soft X-rays are preferentially attenuated than the hard ones. The basic rule is, larger the shielding thickness, lower the exposure rate.

ii. **Distance:** The exposure rate from a point source of radiations at a specified location varies inversely as the square of the distance. The exposure rates E_1 and E_2 at distances D_1 and D_2 are related as:

$$\frac{E_1}{E_2} = \frac{D_2^2}{D_1^2}$$

The practice of being as far away from the machine as possible should be encouraged. Basic formula is larger the distance from the source, lesser is the radiation dose.

iii. **Time:** For a uniform distance and shield, the exposure from a source at a point will be directly proportional to the time during which the exposure was on. Other things remaining constant, the exposure time must be kept to the minimum possible. Lower the exposure time; lower the radiation dose to patients and personnel.

PROTECTION OF THE PATIENT AND THE OPERATOR

Unless and until the lead apron or proper shielding is provided to the operator, the installation should be so arranged that the operator should stand as far away from the source as possible. Minimum of six feet distance is recommended.

The recommendation is that the walls of the operatory room should be sufficiently thick or covered with black paper so that someone occupying the adjacent room should not receive radiations greater than 10R/week.

- The rule of six feet distance and the proper angle of the operator with respect to X-ray tube must be followed. An angle of 90–135° to the central ray is recommended as a safer zone.
- The operator should never hold the film in the patient's mouth.
- The tube should never be held by the operator during exposure.
- Personal monitoring devices should be used and checked every week.

- Protective guards, especially around gonads should be used both by operator and the patient.
- Personnel working in X-ray department should be kept informed of various newer materials and equipment and also the various protective devices.
- Avoid the use of a pointed cone and use an open-ended cone. Pointed cone produces more stray radiations (Fig. 8.1).

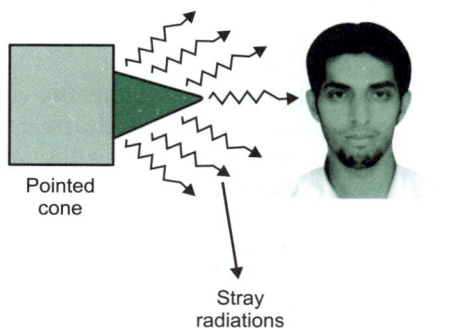
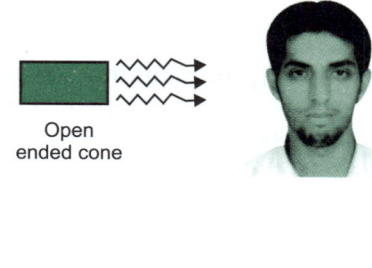

Fig. 8.1: Stray radiations using pointed cone and open ended cone

BIBLIOGRAPHY

1. Alcox RW: Biological effects and radiation protection in the dental office. Dent Clin North Am : 22, 517, 1978.

2. Colquitt, W.N. and Richards, A.G. : An old/new idea for reducing exposure to X-rays. O Surg, O Med, O Path: 54,597, 1982.

3. Coucke ME, Dermant LR: Radiation dose in temporomandibular joint zonography. O Surg, O Med, O Path: 71(B);756, 1991.

4. Farman AG, Farmann TT: A comparison of 18 different X-ray detectors currently used dentistry. O Surg, O Med, O Path: 99, 485, 2005.

5. Marx, R.E. : A new concept in the treatment of osteoradionecrosis. J. Oral Max Surg. : 41, 351, 1983.

6. Marx RE, Johnson RP: Studies in the radio-biology of radionecrosis and their clinical significance. O Surg, O Med, O Path : 64, 379, 1987.

7. Nowak AJ, Creedon RL, Musselman RJ and Troutman, KC: Summary of the Conference on Radiation exposure in pediatric dentistry. JADA : 103, 426, 1981.

8. Payton HG: The effects of radiation on teeth. O Surg, O Med, O Path : 26, 639, 1968.

9. Richards AG, Colquitt WN: Reduction is dental X-ray exposure during the past 60 years. JADA : 103, 713, 1981.

10. Stenstrom B, Hebrikson CO, Holm B, Richter S : Absorbed doses from intraoral radiography with special emphasis on collimator dimenensions. Swed. Dent. J. : 10, 59, 1986.

11. Underhill T, Chilvarquer I, Kimura K, Langlais PR: Radiobiologic risk estimation from dental radiology I. Absorbed doses from critical organs. O Surg., O Med, O Path : 111, 66, 1988.

12. Underhill T, Kimura K, Chilvarquer I, McDavid, DW: Risk estimation from dental radiology II. Cancer incidence and fatality. O Surg, O Med, O Path : 261, 66, 1988.

13. Weyman J. The effect of irradiation on developing teeth. O Surg, O Med, O Path : 623, 25, 1968

9 *Waste Management*

Since its beginning, humankind has been generating waste. With the progress of civilization, the waste generated became of a more complex nature. At the end of the 19th century the industrial revolution saw the rise of the world of consumers. Not only did the air get more and more polluted, the earth too became more polluted with the generation of non-biodegradable solid waste. The increase in population and urbanization was also largely responsible for the increase in solid waste.

Each household constantly generates garbage or waste. There are different types of solid waste depending on their source. Segregation is an important method of handling solid waste. Segregation of waste at the source can be understood clearly by schematic representation.

As the cities are growing in size and in problems such as the generation of plastic waste, various waste treatment and disposal methods are now being used to try and resolve these problems.

Hospital Waste Management

Hospital waste management means the management of waste produced by hospitals using such techniques that will help to check the spread of diseases through it.

The management of hospital waste poses a major problem in most of the countries. It is an ongoing problem for many countries. In recent years, medical waste disposal has posed even more difficulties with the appearance of disposable needles, syringes, and other similar items. Around 250,000 tonnes of medical waste is annually produced from all

sorts of health care facilities in the country. This type of waste has a bad affect on the environment by contaminating the land, air and water resources.

According to a report, 15 tonnes of waste is produced daily in Punjab. The rate of generation is 1.8 kilograms per day per bed. The province houses 250 hospitals with a total capacity of 41,000 beds.

Guidelines

There are guidelines for hospital waste management in India since 1998 prepared by the Environmental Health Unit, of the Ministry of Health, Government of India, giving detailed information and covering all aspects of safe hospital waste management in the country, including the risk associated with the waste, formation of a waste management team in hospital, their responsibilities, plan, collection, segregation, transportation, storage, disposal methods, containers, and their colour coding, waste minimization techniques, protective clothing, etc.

Improper Disposal

Hospitals and public health care units are supposed to safeguard the health of the community. However, the waste produced by the medical care centres, if disposed of improperly, can pose an even greater threat than the original disease themselves.

India is also facing such problems. Most health care centres have no systematic approach to medical waste disposal. Hospital wastes are simply mixed with the municipal waste in collecting bins at roadsides and disposed off similarly. Some waste is simply buried without any appropriate measure. The reality is that while all the equipment necessary to ensure the proper management of hospital waste probably exists, the main problem is that the staff fails to prepare and implement an effective disposable policy. Some patients, who routinely use syringes at home, do not know how to dispose off them properly. They just throw them in a dustbin or other similar places, because they think that these practices are inexpensive, safe, and an easy solution to get rid of a potentially dangerous waste item.

Hazards Posed by Hospital Waste

If hospital waste is not managed properly it proves to be harmful to the environment. It not only poses a threat to the employees working in the hospital, but also to the people residing in the area where it is dumped. Infectious waste can cause diseases like Hepatitis A and B, AIDS, Typhoid, Boils etc.

The hospital staff should dispose off syringes properly, by cutting the needles of the syringes with the help of a cutter, so that the needle cannot be reused. When waste containing plastics is burnt, dioxin is produced, which can cause cancer, birth defects, decreased psychomotor ability, hearing defects, cognitive defects and behavioural alterations in infants. Flies also sit on the uncovered piles of rotting garbage. This promotes mechanical transmissions of fatal diseases like diarrhea, dysentery, typhoid, hepatitis and cholera. Under moist conditions, mosquitoes transmit many types of infections, like malaria and yellow fever. Similarly, dogs, cats and rats also transmit a variety of diseases, including plague and flea borne fever, as they mostly live in and around the refuse. A high tendency of contracting intestinal, parasitic and skin diseases is found in workers engaged in collecting refuse.

Solution

Some steps should be taken for the minimization of hospital waste. Before any clear improvement can be made in medical waste management, consistent and scientifically based definitions must be established as to what is meant by medical waste and its components, and what the goals are. Plans and policies should be laid down for this purpose. Then the waste should be segregated. Imposing segregating practices within hospitals to separate biological and chemical hazardous waste will result in a clean solid waste stream, which can be recycled easily. If proper segregation is achieved through training, clear standards, and tough enforcement, resources can be turned to the management of the small portion of the waste stream needing special treatment. New emphasis should be put on the reduction of waste, workers' safety should be ensured through education, training and proper personal protective equipment.

Categories of Medical Waste

Cat 1: Human anatomical waste: includes tissues, organs, body parts, human flesh, etc.

Cat 2: Animal waste: animal tissues, organs, fluids, etc.

Cat 3: Microbiology waste and biotech: waste from lab. cultures, live or attenuated vaccines.

Cat 4: Waste sharps: needles, syringes, blade, scalpel, etc.

Cat 5: Discarded medicines and cytotoxic drugs

Cat 6: Soiled waste: items contaminated with blood e.g. dressings, cotton, linen, etc.

Cat 7: Solid waste: tubes, catheters, disposable tubings, etc.

Cat 8: Liquid waste

Cat 9: Incineration ash

Cat 10: Chemical waste

Biomedical waste should be segregated into containers/bags at the point of generation in accordance with **Schedule II** of Biomedical Waste (Management and Handling) Rules 1998.

Color coding	Type of container	Waste categories
Yellow	Plastic bags	Cat 1
		Cat 2
		Cat 3
		Cat 6
Red	• Disinfected container·	Cat 3
		Cat 6
	• Plastic bags	Cat 7
Blue/White	• Plastic Bag·	Cat 4
	• Puncture proof containers	Cat 7
Black	• Plastic Bag	Cat 5
		Cat 9
		Cat 10

General waste like garbage, garden refuse, etc. should join the stream of domestic refuse. Sharps should be collected in puncture proof containers. Bags and containers for infectious waste should be marked with Biohazard symbol. Highly infectious waste should be sterilized by autoclaving. Cytotoxic wastes are to be collected in leak proof containers clearly labeled as cytotoxic waste. Needles and syringes should be destroyed with the help of needle destroyer and syringe cutters provided at the point of generation. Infusion sets, bottles and gloves should be cut with curved scissors.

Disinfection of sharps, soiled linen, plastic and rubber goods is to be achieved at point of generation by usage of sodium hypochlorite with minimum contact of 1 hour. Fresh solution should be made in each shift. On site collection requires staff to close the waste bags when they are three quarters full either by trying the neck or by sealing the bag. Kerb side storage area needs to be impermeable and hard standing with good drainage. It should provide an easy access to waste collection vehicle.

Biomedical waste should be transported within the hospital by means of wheeled trolleys, containers or carts that are not used for any other purpose. The trolleys have to be cleaned daily. Off site transportation vehicle should be marked with the name and address of carrier. Biohazard symbol should be painted. Suitable system for securing the load during transport should be ensured. Such a vehicle should be easily cleanable with rounded corners.

All disposable plastic should be subjected to shredding before disposing off to vendor. Final treatment of biomedical waste can be done by technologies like incineration, autoclave, hydroclave or microwave.

Incineration

Incineration is a waste treatment technology that involves the combustion of organic materials and/or substances. Incineration and other high temperature waste treatment systems are described as "thermal treatment". Incineration of waste materials converts the waste into incinerator bottom ash, flue gases, particulates, and heat, which can in turn be used to generate electric power. The flue gases are cleaned for pollutants before they are dispersed in the atmosphere.

Incineration with energy recovery is one of several waste-to-energy (WtE) technologies such as gasification, pyrolysis and anaerobic digestion. Incineration may also be implemented without energy and material recovery. There are many medical concerns about air emissions, and local communities still have worries with modern incinerators.

In some countries, incinerators built just a few decades ago often did not include materials separation to remove hazardous, bulky or recyclable materials before combustion. These facilities tended to risk the health of the plant workers and the local environment due to inadequate levels of gas cleaning and combustion process control. Most of these facilities did not generate electricity.

Incinerators reduce the volume of the original waste by 95–96%, depending upon composition and degree of recovery of materials such as metals from the ash for recycling. This means that while incineration does not completely replace landfilling, it reduces the necessary volume for disposal significantly.

Incineration has particularly strong benefits for the treatment of certain waste types in niche areas such as clinical wastes and certain hazardous wastes where pathogens and toxins can be destroyed by high temperatures. Examples include chemical multi-product plants with diverse toxic or very toxic waste water streams, which cannot be routed to a conventional waste water treatment plant.

Types of Incinerators

An incinerator is a furnace for burning waste. Modern incinerators include pollution mitigation equipment such as flue gas cleaning. There are various types of incinerator plant designs: moving grate, fixed grate, rotary-kiln, fluidized bed.

The typical incineration plant for municipal solid waste is a moving grate incinerator. The moving grate enables the movement of waste through the combustion chamber to be optimized to allow a more efficient and complete combustion. A single moving grate boiler can handle up to 35 tons of waste per hour, and can operate 8,000 hours per year with only the scheduled stop for inspection and maintenance of about one month's duration. Moving grate incinerators are sometimes referred to as Municipal Solid Waste Incinerators (MSWIs).

The waste is introduced by a waste crane through the "throat" at one end of the grate, from where it moves down over the descending grate to the ash pit in the other end. Here the ash is removed through a water lock.

Municipal solid waste in the furnace of a moving grate incinerator capable of handling 15 tons of waste per hour. The holes in the grate elements supplying the primary combustion air are visible.

Part of the combustion air (primary combustion air) is supplied through the grate from below. This air flow also has the purpose of cooling the grate itself. Cooling is important for the mechanical strength of the grate, and many moving grates are also water cooled internally.

Secondary combustion air is supplied into the boiler at high speed through nozzles over the grate. It facilitates complete combustion of the flue gases by introducing turbulence for better mixing and by ensuring a surplus of oxygen. In multiple/stepped hearth incinerators, the secondary combustion air is introduced in a separate chamber downstream the primary combustion chamber.

According to the European Waste Incineration Directive, incineration plants must be designed to ensure that the flue gases reach a temperature of at least 850°C for two seconds in order to ensure proper breakdown of organic toxins. In order to comply with this at all times, it is required to install backup auxiliary burners (often fueled by oil), which are fired into the boiler in case the heating value of the waste becomes too low to reach this temperature. The flue gases are then cooled in the superheaters, where the heat is transferred to steam, heating the steam to typically 400°C at a pressure of 40 bar for the electricity generation in the turbine. At this point, the flue gas has a temperature of around 200°C, and is passed to the flue gas cleaning system.

At least in Scandinavian countries, scheduled maintenance is always performed during summer, where the demand for district heating is low. Often incineration plants consist of several separate 'boiler lines' (boilers and flue gas treatment plants), so that waste reception can continue at one boiler line while the others are subject to revision.

Research Methodology and Biostatistics

In early days **Statistics** was the by-product of administrative activity of the State (being regarded as the 'Science of Statecraft'). In India, an efficient system of collecting official and administrative statistics existed as early as the reign of Chandragupta Maurya (324–300 BC). The most of the statistical work can be attributed to Sir Ronald A. Fisher (1890–1962) who applied Statistics to a variety of diversified fields such as genetics, biometry, psychology, education, agriculture etc. Later, the subject of statistics earned the status of full fledge science subject.

Definition

The word Statistics has been used to convey different meanings in singular and plural sense. When used as plural, statistics means **numerical set of data** and when used in singular sense it means the science of **statistical methods** embodying the theory and techniques used for collecting, analyzing and drawing inferences from the numerical data.

The most accepted definition of statistics is *the aggregate of facts affected to a marked extent by multiplicity of causes, numerically expressed, enumerated or estimated according to a reasonable standard of accuracy, collected in a systematic manner, for a predetermined purpose and placed in relation to each other.*

The other definitions based on 'Numerical Data' and 'Statistical Methods' are as follows:

Statistics are the classified facts representing the conditions of the people in a State....specially those facts which can be stated in number or in tables of numbers or in any tabular or classified arrangement.

Statistics are numerical statement of facts in any department of enquiry placed in relation to each other.

By Statistics we mean quantitative data affected to a marked extent by multiplicity of causes.

Importance of Statistics in Biology and Medical Science

It is hypothesized that the whole theory of heredity rests on statistical basis. This hypothesis indicates that *the whole problem of evolution is a problem of longevity, of fertility, of health, of disease and it is impossible for the evolutionist to proceed without statistics as it would be for the Registrar General to discuss the rational mortality without an enumeration of the population, a classification of deaths and a knowledge of statistical theory.*

In medical sciences, the statistical tools for collection, presentation and analysis of observed data relating to the causes and incidence of diseases always plays a significant role. For example, the patient's data relating to pulse rate, body temperature, blood pressure, gingival bleeding etc. aid in proper diagnosis of the disease. Biostatistics is the term used when tools of statistics are applied to the data which are derived from the biological science such as medicine, dentistry etc. In dentistry also, all parameters, viz. research, diagnosis or treatment need counting or measurement. For example, the periodontal pocket depth has no meaning unless it is expressed in figures.

Research Methodology

It is defined as a highly intellectual human activity used in the investigation of nature or matter and deals specifically with the manner in which data is collected, analyzed and interpreted.

Types of Research Design

- Descriptive
- Exploratory

Parts of Research Design

- Sample design
- Observation design (condition under which observation is to be made)
- Statistical design
- Operational design (techniques)

The objective of the research design is to produce a sufficiently clear and detailed written protocol which can be used by all, submitted to committee for approval and submitted for grant, if any and also for discussion with others.

Designing a Written Protocol

This written protocol consists of the followings:

- Introduction — background and need for study
- Problem — definition, significance, place and time of study, likely duration.
- Review of past research — significant achievements, gaps and justification of present study.
- Aims and objectives — conceptual model for specific and anticipated outcomes.
- Operational definition of concept
- Scope and limitation — for measurement
  — marking the boundary to make it manageable.
- Expected utility of the research
- Methodology
- Sampling technique
- Data collection methods
- Time schedule
- Budget
- End of protocol (references)

Note: The above components will be explained subsequently.

Comparison between Research Designs

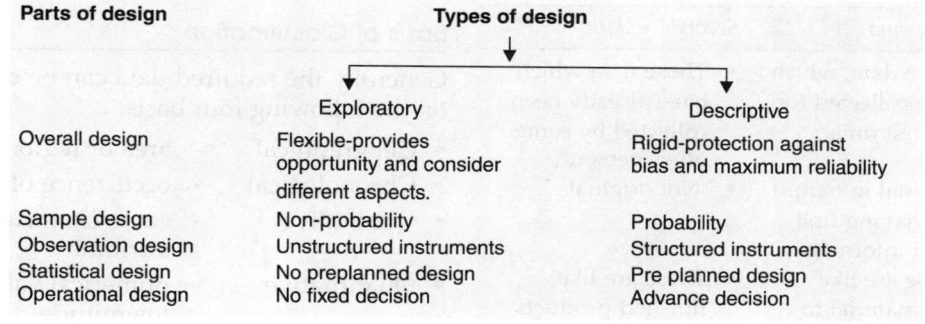

Parts of design	Types of design	
	Exploratory	Descriptive
Overall design	Flexible-provides opportunity and consider different aspects.	Rigid-protection against bias and maximum reliability
Sample design	Non-probability	Probability
Observation design	Unstructured instruments	Structured instruments
Statistical design	No preplanned design	Pre planned design
Operational design	No fixed decision	Advance decision

Collection of Data

Raw material of statistics always originates from the operation of counting or measurement. For any statistical study in dentistry, the basic problem is to collect facts and figures relating to particular phenomenon under study. The objective of collection of data depends upon the scope of study with respect to degree of accuracy aimed at the final results. The required data can be classified as **Primary Data** and **Secondary Data**. The data which are originally collected by a person for the first time for any statistical study are termed as "Primary Data". On the other hand, the data which have already been collected and processed by a person and used by another person for his statistical study are termed as "Secondary Data".

Source of Collecting Primary Data

- Direct personal investigation
- Indirect oral investigation
- Information received through local agencies.
- Information received through mailed questionnaire.

Source of Collecting Secondary Data

- Published
- Unpublished

Comparison between Primary and Secondary Data

Primary data	Secondary data
• Those data, which were collected for the first time.	• Those data which have already been collected by some other person.
• Original in nature and having first hand information.	• Not original
• These are like raw material to	• These are like finished products

Contd...

Primary data	Secondary data
which statistical methods are applied.	as they have already been statistically applied
• These have been collected for a definite purpose.	• These are used for a variety of purpose as per requirement.

Classification

Classification is the process of arranging data into sequences and groups according to their common characteristics, or separating them into different but related parts.

Thus classification impresses upon the arrangement of the data into different classes which are to be determined depending upon the objective of the study. For example number of students registered in Punjab University during academic year 2009–10 may be classified on the basis of sex, age, religion, height, weight, etc.

Classification is one of the most important techniques for any statistical study, therefore it should have the followings guiding principles:

- It should be un-ambiguous
- It should be exhaustive and mutually exclusive
- It should be stable
- It should be suitable for the objective of the study

Basis of Classification

Generally the required data can be classified on the following four basis:

- Geographical   - area or region wise
- Chronological   - occurrence of time
- Qualitative   - some character or attribute
- Quantitative   - numerical value or magnitude

Geographical Classification

Geographical Classification is based on the locations. For example, density of the population (per square kilometer) in different States of India; or number of patients with oral cancer in different cities of Punjab.

Density of population (per square km)	
Punjab	482
Himachal Pradesh	109
Haryana	477
Uttar Pradesh	689
Bihar	880

Source: www.iloveindia.com

Number of patients with oral cancer	
Amritsar	200
Jalandhar	150
Ludhiana	250
Moga	90
Barnala	100

Source: Indicative

Chronological Classification

Chronological Classification is based on the differences in time. For example population of any country over the different years or number of patient with oral cancer in a particular city over the different years.

Total population of India (in thousands)	
1971	548160
1981	683329
1991	846421
2001	1028737

Source: www.indiabudget.nic.in

Number of patients with oral cancer in a particular city	
1950	20
1970	29
1990	36
2009	88

Source: Indicative

Qualitative Classification

Qualitative Classification is based on some qualitative phenomenon which is not capable of quantification such as honesty, beauty, occupation, etc. For example intelligence attribute of a given population can only be classified such as genius, dull, etc.

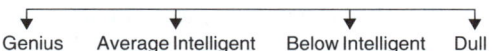

Intelligence in a given population

Genius   Average Intelligent   Below Intelligent   Dull

Quantitative Classification

If data can be classified on the basis of quantitative measurement, like age, height, weight, etc. then it is termed as 'Quantitative Classification'. The quantitative phenomenon under study is also known as "Variable". For example, annual income of employees in a particular institution can be grouped as follows and known as variable:

Annual income (Variable)	No. of employees (Frequency)
Upto 50,000	100
50,000 to 10,00,000	150
1,00,000 to 5,00,000	80
5,00,000 to 10,00,000	40
10,00,000 and above	10

Variable and Frequency

The quantitative phenomenon under study such as annual income of employees, marks in a test, height of student in a college etc is termed as "variable". These variables are of two types:

- Continuous variable
- Discontinuous variable or discrete variable

Those variables which can take all the possible values in a given specified range are termed as "continuous variable". For example, age of students in a college; because age can take all possible values in years, months, days, etc. On the other hand, those variables which cannot take all the possible values within a given specified range are termed as "discontinuous or discrete variable". For example, members in a family, population of a city etc., because members of a family cannot take all possible values (four and a half).

In the above example, annual income of each employee has been grouped in five classes. Annual income is termed as **variable** and number of employee in each class is termed as **frequency**.

Frequency Distribution

The organization of the data pertaining to quantitative phenomenon involves the following four stages:

a. Unorganized (raw) or organized (array) data
b. Ungrouped (discrete) frequency distribution
c. Grouped frequency distribution
d. Continuous frequency distribution

The above stages can be explained by means of marks obtained by fifty (50) students.

70	45	33	64	51	26	65	70	33	20
55	60	65	59	53	36	45	42	33	42
51	47	39	60	53	59	49	42	15	53
42	65	78	65	45	60	54	52	48	46
57	53	55	42	45	39	65	36	26	18

a. The data in the above form is called unorganized (raw) data. If the same data can be arranged in an ascending or descending order, then it is called organized (array) data.
b. If we count the number of times each value of marks (variable) occurs in the above data, then it is known as discrete or ungrouped frequency distribution.

Marks	Frequency	Marks	Frequency
78	1	47	1
70	2	49	1
65	5	59	2
60	3	46	1
55	2	42	5
57	1	45	4
53	4	39	2
51	2	33	3
48	1	36	2
52	1	20	1
54	1	18	1
64	1	15	1
26	2		

Total frequency, i.e. number of students = 50

c. If the entire range of marks (variable) obtained can be grouped as a class of marks, i.e. 21–40 then it is termed as 'grouped frequency distribution'. For example:

Marks (x)	Number of students (f)
0–20	3
21–40	9
41–60	26
61–80	12
81–100	0
Where '*x* 'is variable and '*f*' is frequency	Sum of frequency = $\Sigma f = 50$

The various group into which value of marks (variable) are classified is termed as 'class intervals'. The length of the class interval (difference between 21–40, i.e. 20 in the above example) is called the width or magnitude of the classes.

d. In the above example, marks are always rounded to the nearest integer, i.e 19.25 marks obtained by a student are rounded to 19 marks and so on. But if we consider the age of students in a college then grouped frequency distribution into the classes of age 16–20, 21–25, etc will not be correct because this does not count the students with age between 20 and 21 years. In such situation we form continuous class interval such as age in years:

0–16   = below 16 years
16–20 = 16 or more but less than 20
20–25 = 20 or more but less than 25

The presentation of data into continuous classes of the above type alongwith correspondence frequency is termed as "continuous frequency distribution".

Presentation of Data

There are two main methods of presenting the data, i.e. tabulation and drawing.

Tabulation

Tabulations are devices for presenting data from a mass of statistical data such as shown in Tables I and II.

Table I: Class wise distribution		
1	Oral Medicine and Radiology	315
2	Oral and Maxillofacial Surgery	280
3	Paedodontics and preventive dentistry	105
4	Orthodontics and dentofacial orthopaedics	85
5	Conservative Dentistry and Endodontics	235
	Total	**1020**

Table II: Group wise distribution	
Age in years	*Number of persons suffering from caries*
0–5	2
5–10	5
10–15	10
15–20	15
20–25	3
25–30	4

Drawing

After class wise or group wise tabulation, the frequencies of a variable can be presented by two kinds of drawings, i.e. graphs and diagrams.

Presentation of quantitative (continuous) data through the following graphs

- Histogram
- Frequency polygon
- Frequency curve
- Line chart or graph
- Cumulative frequency curve or ogives
- Scatter or dot diagram

Presentation of qualitative (discrete) data through the following diagrams

- Bar diagram
- Pie diagram
- Picture diagram
- Map diagram

Difference between diagrams and graphs

The differences between diagram and graph are depicted in Table 10.1.

- In the construction of a graph, generally graph paper is used which helps us to study the mathematical relationship between the two variables. On the other hand, diagrams are generally constructed on a plane paper and are used for comparisons only and not for studying the relationship between the variables.

Table 10.1: Differences between graph and diagram

Graph	Diagram
Graph paper is used for construction	Plane paper is used for construction
Used to study the mathematical relations between the two variables	Used for comparison only
Different lines or points are used to present data	Data is presented by rectangle, bars, circles, etc.
Furnish accurate and precise information	Furnish only approximate information
Useful for presenting time series and frequency distribution	Useful only in depicting categorical and geographical data
Construction is easier	Construction is comparatively difficult

- In diagrams, data are presented by devices such as bars, rectangles, squares, circles, cubes, etc. while in graphs, points or lines of different kinds are used to present the data.

- Diagrams furnish only approximate information. They do not add anything to the meaning of the data, therefore are not much of use for further statistical study. On the other hand, graphs are more obvious, precise, and accurate than the diagrams and are quite helpful for statistical study such as slopes, rates of change and estimation (interpolation and extrapolation) etc. In fact, graphs are one of the important tool for any research analysis of statistical data.

- Diagrams are useful in depicting categorical and geographical data but they fail to present data relating to time series and frequency distributions. In fact, graphs are used for the study of time series and frequency distributions.

- Construction of graph is easier as compared to the construction of diagrams.

Presentation of Quantitative Data

The periodontal pocket depth in millimeter (mm) of 200 patients was measured and grouped to understand the presentations through histogram, frequency polygon and frequency curve.

Depth in mm (x)	Number of patients (f)
0–2	24
2–4	52
4–6	48
6–8	42
8–10	26
10–12	8

Total frequency, i.e. number of patients = 200

Histogram: Histogram is a graphical presentation of frequency distribution. Variable (x) of different group are indicated on the horizontal line (x-axis) while frequency (f) is marked on the vertical line (y-axis). Frequency of each group will form a rectangle and such graph is called "histogram" (Fig. 10.1).

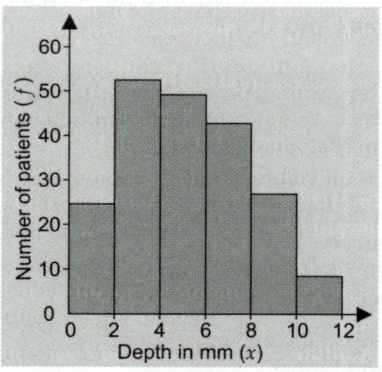

Fig. 10.1: Histogram indicating periodontal pocket depth of 200 patients

Frequency polygon: Frequency polygon is another device of graphical presentation of a frequency distribution. This can be developed over a histogram by joining the mid points of class intervals at the height of frequencies by straight line. It gives a polygon which means a figure with many angles (Fig. 10.2).

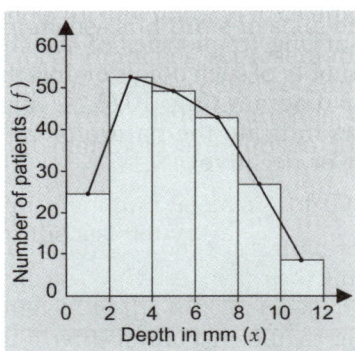

Fig. 10.2: Frequency polygon indicating periodontal pocket depth of 200 patients

Frequency curve: Frequency curve is a smooth free hand curve drawn through the vertices of a frequency polygon. The objective of frequency curve is to eliminate the random or erratic fluctuation that might be present in the data. The area enclosed by the frequency curve is same as that of the histogram or frequency polygon (Fig. 10.3).

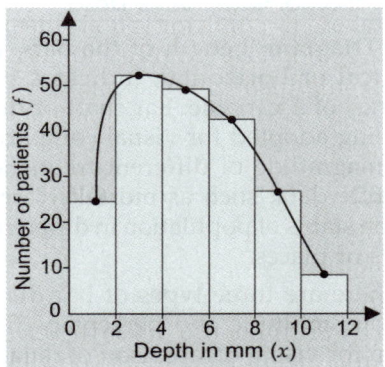

Fig. 10.3: Frequency curve indicating periodontal pocket depth of 200 patients

Line chart or graph: This is a frequency polygon presenting variations by line. It shows the trend of an event occurring over a period of time. It may be rising, falling or showing fluctuations. The events can be population, infant mortality rate, birth rate, death rate, etc. The trend of population in India over a period of 1971 to 2001 is indicated in Fig. 10.4 as line chart.

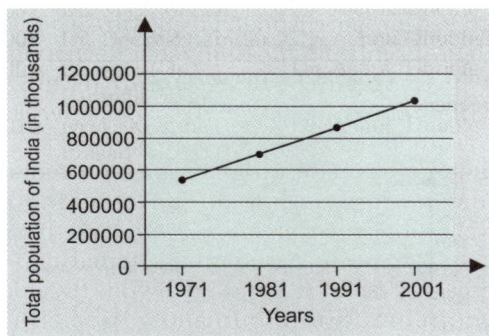

Fig. 10.4: Line chart indicating population trend in India

Cumulative Frequency Curve or Ogive

Ogive is a graphic presentation of the cumulative frequency distribution of continuous variable. Variable (x) are indicated on the horizontal line (x-axis) while cumulative frequency (c.f.) is marked on vertical line (y-axis). Since there are two types of cumulative frequency distributions, i.e. less than cumulative frequency and more than cumulative frequency, therefore ogives are also of two types, i.e. less than ogive and more than ogive. For drawing "less than ogive" we plot less than cumulative frequency against the upper limit of variable; whereas "more than ogive" is obtained by plotting more than cumulative frequency against lower limit of the variable.

Example

Distribution of yearly income (rupees in thousand) for 600 employees of an institution is shown in Fig. 10.5.

Yearly income (x)	No. of employees (f)	Less than c.f.	More than c.f.
Below 75	60	60	600
75–150	170	230	540
150–225	200	430	370
225–300	60	490	170
300–375	50	540	110
375–450	40	580	60
450 and over	20	600	20

Note: x = variable, f = frequency, c.f. = cumulative frequency

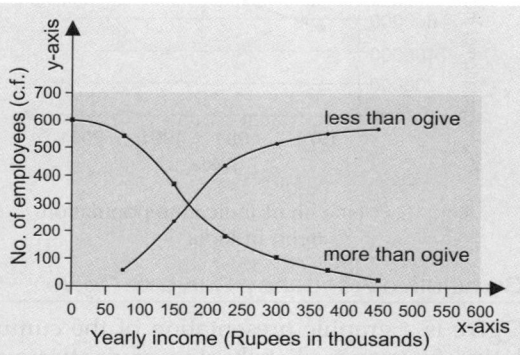

Fig. 10.5: Cumulative frequency curve (ogive) indicating yearly income of employee(s)

Coordinates for 'ogive'

x-axis	y-axis (less than c.f.)	x-axis	y-axis (more than c.f.)
75	60	0	600
150	230	75	540
225	430	150	370
300	490	225	170
375	540	300	110
450	580	375	60
>	600	450	20

Note: Value of median (app. 176) is the intersection point between less than ogive' and 'more than ogive' and perpendicular on x-axis.

Scatter or Dot Diagram

It is a graphic presentation of two variables in the same person(s) or group(s) such as height and weight of student (male) aged 20 years. This indicates the nature of co-relation between two variables.

The observation of height and weight are plotted and each reading will give one scatter point. Varying frequencies of the characters give a number of such points or dots that show a scatter diagram (Fig. 10.6). A line can be drawn to indicate the nature of co-relation (positive or negative).

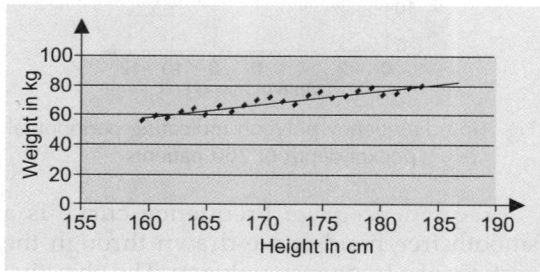

Fig. 10.6: Scatter diagram indicating positive co-relation between height and weight of students (male)

Presentation of Qualitative Data

1. **Bar Diagram:** Length of the bars, drawn vertical or horizontal, indicates the frequency of a variable. Bar chart or diagram is being adopted for visual comparison of the magnitude of different frequencies in discrete data, such as mortality, immunization status of population in different ages, sexes or places.

There are three types of bar diagrams: Simple, multiple and percentage bar diagram for visual comparison of data.

2. **Simple bar diagram:** Some simple bar diagrams are shown in Figs 10.7 to 10.9.

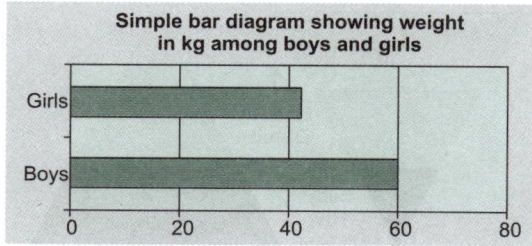

Source: indicative

Fig. 10.7: Simple bar diagram indicating weight in kg among boys and girls

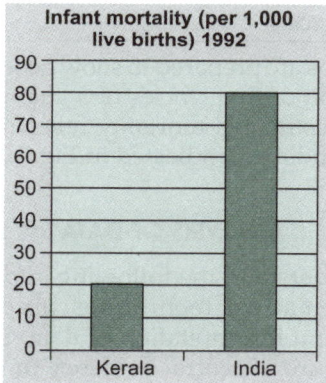

Source: Indicative

Fig. 10.8: Simple bar diagram indicating infant mortality

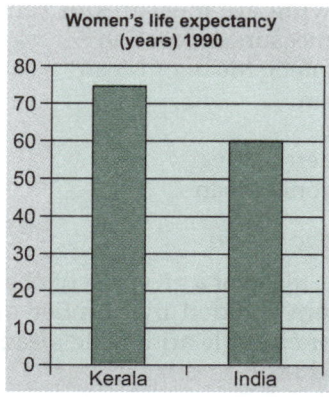

Source: Indicative

Fig. 10.9: Simple bar diagram indicating women's life expectancy

3. Multiple Bar diagram: This is being used to present two or more set of inter related variables (Fig. 10.10).

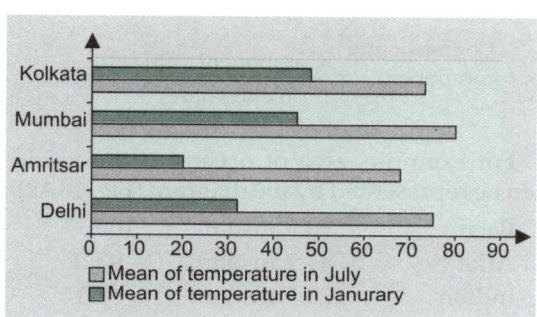

Fig. 10.10: Multiple bar diagram indicating mean of temperature for two months at four cities

4. Percentage Bar diagram: Components of a variable can be presented on percentage basis gives percentage bar diagram. Expenditure of a family (variable) on different items of consumption is indicated as percentage bar diagram (Fig. 10.11).

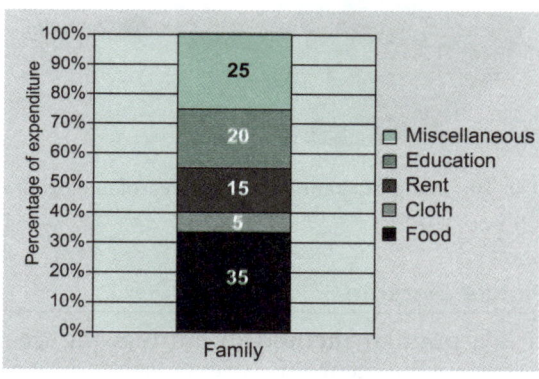

Fig. 10.11: Percentage bar diagram indicating expenditure of a family

Pie Diagram

This is another way of presenting the data such as blood groups, age groups, sex groups, causes of mortality in a population. The frequencies of the group are shown in a circle. Degrees of angle denote the frequency and area of the sector. It gives comparative difference at a glance.

$$\text{Degree of any component} = \frac{\text{Component value}}{\text{Total value}} \times 360°$$

For example, area of oceans of the world can be represented by pie diagram (Fig. 10.12).

Pacific	70.8 msq.m.	166.7°
Atlantic	41.2 msq.m.	97.0°
Indian	28.5 msq.m.	67.1°
Antarctic	7.6 msq.m.	17.9°
Arctic	4.8 msq.m.	11.3°

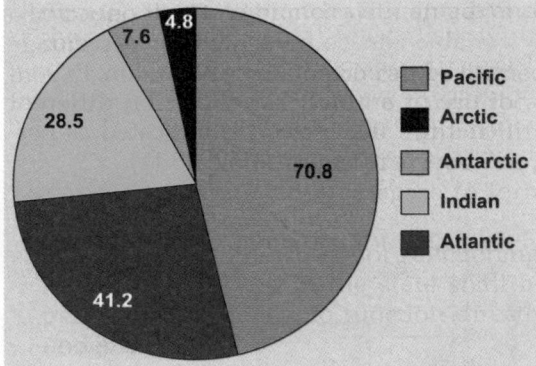

Fig. 10.12: Pie diagram indicating area of oceans of the world

Picture Diagram

It is a popular method to impress the frequency of the occurrence of events to common man such as attacks, deaths, number operated, admitted, discharged accidents in a population. For example, AIDS in developing and developed countries can be shown by picture diagram (Fig. 10.13).

The burden of disease caused by HIV infection is clear.

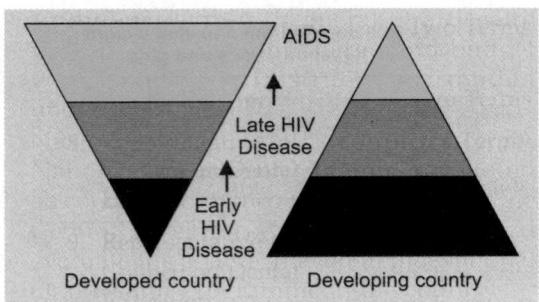

Fig. 10.13: Picture diagram indicating HIV infection and AIDS in developed and developing country

Map Diagram

These maps are prepared to show geographical distribution of frequencies of a character. For example, estimated mortality rates in various States of India are indicated in Fig. 10.14.

ANALYSIS OF DATA

Let us understand the following applications of mathematical techniques involved in analysis and interpretation of data.
    i. Measure of central tendency or measure of location
    ii. Measure of dispersion

Measure of Central Tendency

The following are measures of central tendency or measure of location :
    i. Arithmetic Mean or Mean
    ii. Median
    iii. Mode
    iv. Geometric Mean
    v. Harmonic Mean

i. Arithmetic Mean

Arithmetic mean of a given set of observation is their sum divided by number of observations. for example arithmetic mean of 5, 8 , 10, 15, 24, 28 is:

$$\frac{5+8+10+15+24+28}{6} = \frac{90}{6} = 15$$

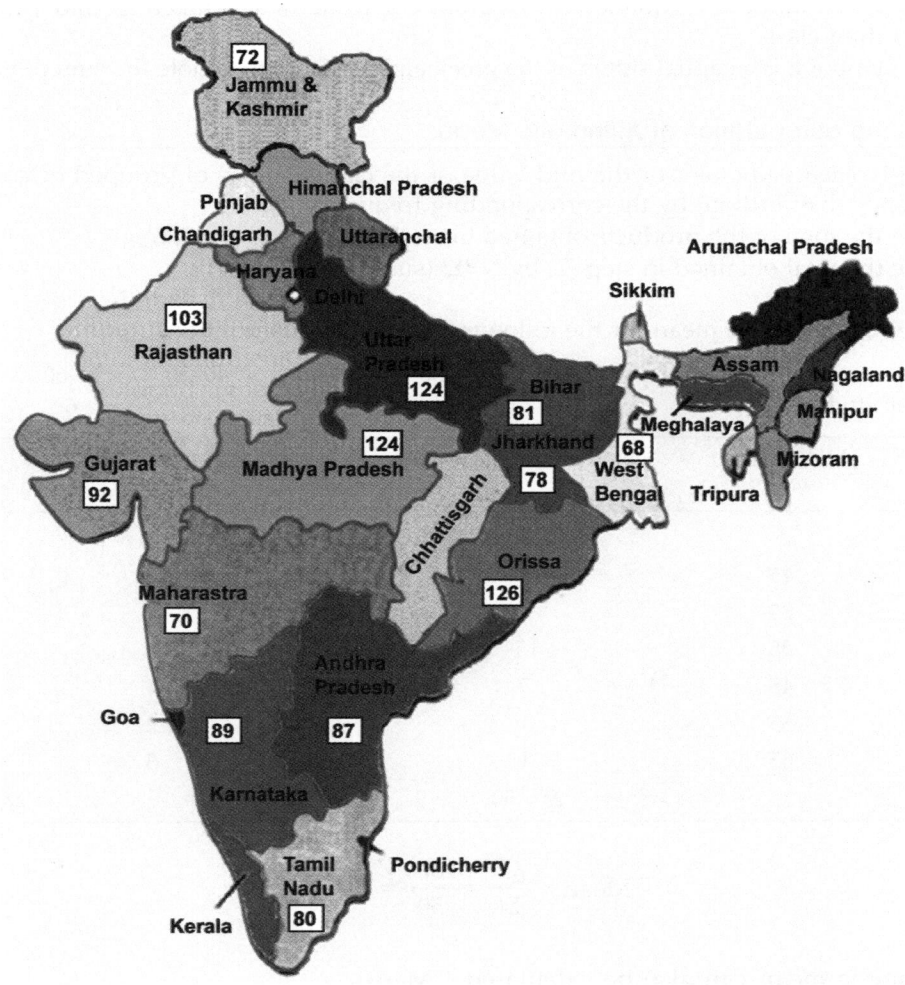

Source: Indicative

Fig. 10.14: Estimated infant mortality rates in various States of India

In general if $x_1, x_2, x_3\ldots\ldots x_n$ are values of 'n' observations then their arithmetic mean ($\bar{x}$) is given by:

$$\bar{x} = \frac{x_1 + x_2 + x_3 \ldots\ldots x_n}{n} = \frac{\Sigma x}{n}$$

Where 'Σx' is the sum of the observations and 'n' is the number of observations.

In case of frequency distribution, arithmetic mean is the sum of product of variable and their frequency divided by the sum of frequency, i.e.

$$\bar{x} = \frac{\Sigma fx}{N}$$

Where N is Σf i.e. sum of frequencies.

In case of continuous frequency distribution the value of x is taken as mid value of the corresponding class.

Note: Symbol Σ is a capital sigma of the greek alphabet and to denote the sum of values.

Steps for the computation of Arithmetic Mean

1. Multiply each value of x or the mid value of the class (in case of grouped or continuous frequency distribution) by the corresponding frequency (f).
2. Obtain the total of the products obtained in step (1) above to get Σfx.
3. Divide the total obtained in step (2) by $N = \Sigma f$ (sum of frequency).

Example: Calculate the mean for the following frequency distribution.

Marks:	0–10	10–20	20–30	30–40	40–50	50–60	60–70
Number of students:	6	5	8	15	7	6	3

Marks	Mid-value (x)	Number of students (f)	fx	$d = \dfrac{x-35}{10}$	f.d
0–10	5	6	30	–3	–18
10–20	15	5	75	–2	–10
20–30	25	8	200	–1	–8
30–40	35	15	525	0	0
40–50	45	7	315	1	7
50–60	55	6	330	2	12
60–70	65	3	195	3	9
		$\Sigma f = 50$	$\Sigma fx = 1670$		$\Sigma fd = 8$

$$\text{Mean} = \frac{\Sigma fx}{\Sigma f} = \frac{1670}{50} = 33.4 \text{ marks}$$

Arithmetic mean can also be calculated through step deviation method, which consists in taking the deviations (difference) of the given observation from any arbitrary value 'A'.

$$\text{Let, } d = \frac{x-A}{h}(A = 35 \text{ and } h = 10)$$

Where A is arbitrary number and h is magnitude or width of the class.

$$\bar{x} = A + \frac{h.\Sigma fd}{\Sigma f} = 35 + \frac{10 \times (-8)}{50} = 33.4 \text{ marks}$$

Merits
- It is rigidly defined.
- It is easy to calculate and understand.
- It is based on all the observations.

Demerits
- It is very much affected by the extreme observations i.e. two or three large values of variable may affect the value of mean.
- This cannot be used in the case of open end classes such as less than 10 or more than 20, etc.
- It cannot be located graphically.

ii. Median

The median is that value of the variable which divides the group in two equal parts, one part comprising all the values greater and the other, all values less than median.

Computation of Median

Ungrouped data: If number of observation is odd than the median is the middle value after the observations have been arranged in ascending or descending order. For example, median of five observations 3, 8, 7, 10, 5 is 7 **(middle value of series 3, 5, 7, 8, 10).**

In case number of observation is even than median is obtained as arithmetic mean of the two middle observations after they have arranged in descending or ascending order. For example if we consider one more observation say 15, than median of six observations 3, 5, **7, 8,** 10, 15 is the **mean of 7 and 8 that is 7.5.**

Frequency distribution: In case of frequency distribution, the following steps are involved for computation of median:

• Prepare 'less than' cumulative frequency distribution.

• Find $\frac{N}{2}$ and observed cumulative frequency just greater than $\frac{N}{2}$

• The corresponding value of the variable gives median.

Example 1: Eight coins were tossed together and the number of heads *(x)* obtained were observed. The operation was repeated 256 times and the frequency distribution of the number of heads is given below. Calculate median:

Number of : 0 1 2 3 4 5 6 7 8
heads (x)

Frequency (f) : 1 9 26 59 72 52 29 7 1

x	f	Less than c.f
0	1	1
1	9	1 + 9 = 10
2	26	10 + 26 = 36
3	59	36 + 59 = 95
4	72	95 + 72 = 167
5	52	167 + 52 = 219
6	29	219 + 29 = 248
7	7	248 + 7 = 255
8	1	255 + 1 = 256
N= Σf = 256		

Here N =256 and $\frac{N}{2}=128$

The cumulative frequency (c.f.) just greater than 128 is 167 and the value of *x* corresponding to 167 is 4. Hence median number of heads is 4.

Example 2: The following table shows the age distribution of persons in a particular region. Find median age:

Age (years)	Number of persons (in thousands)
Below 10	2
Below 20	5
Below 30	9
Below 40	12
Below 50	14
Below 60	15
Below 70	15.5
70 and over	15.6

Let us convert the above distribution into continuous frequency distribution as given below and then compute the median.

Age (years)	Number of persons (f)	Comulative frequeny (c.f.)
0–10	2	2
10–20	5–2 = 3	5
20–30	**9–5 = 4**	**9**
30–40	12–9 = 3	12
40–50	14–12 = 2	14
50–60	15–14 = 1	15
60–70	15.5–15 = 0.5	15.5
70 and over	15.6–15.5 = 0.1	15.6
	N = Σf = 15.6	

$$\text{Here } \frac{N}{2} = \frac{15.6}{2} = 7.8$$

Cumulative frequency (c.f.) greater than 7.8 is 9. Thus the corresponding class 20–30 is the median class. As this is continuous frequency distribution, the value of median can be obtained by using interpolation formula i.e.

$$\text{Median} = l + \frac{h}{f}\left(\frac{N}{2} - c\right)$$

Where

l is lower limit of median class,

f is frequency of median class,

h is width of median class,

c is cumulative frequency of class proceeding the median class.

$$\text{Median} = 20 + \frac{10}{4}(7.8 - 5)$$
$$= 20 + (2.5 \times 2.8)$$
$$= 20 + 7 = 27$$

Hence median age is 27 years.

Note: In this case, median is more suitable measure of central tendency than mean because the last class viz., 70 and over is open end class and as such arithmetic mean cannot be computed.

Merits

- It is rigidly defined.
- Median is easy to understand and easy to calculate.
- Since median is a positional average, it is not affected at all by extreme observations.
- Median can be computed while dealing with a distribution with open end classes.
- Median can sometimes be located by simple inspection and can also be computed graphically.
- Median is the only average to be used while dealing with qualitative characteristics which cannot be measured quantitatively but can still be arranged in ascending or descending order of magnitude. For example, to find the average intelligence, average beauty, average honesty, etc. among a group of people.

Demerits

- In case of even number of observations for an ungrouped data, median cannot be determined exactly between the two middle terms. In fact any value lying between the two middle observations can serve the purpose of median.
- Median, being a positional average, is no based on each and every item of the distribution. It depends on all the observations only to the extent whether they are smaller than or greater than it; the exact magnitude of the observations being immaterial. let us consider a simple example: The median value of 35, 12, 8, 40 and 60, i.e. 8, 12, 35, 40, 60 is 35. Now if we replace the values 8 and 12 by any two values which are less than 35 and the values 40 and 60 by any two values greater than 35 the median is unaffected.
- Median is relatively less stable than mean, particularly for small samples since it is affected more by fluctuations of sampling as compared with arithmetic mean.

iii. Mode

The mode of distribution is a value at the point around which the items tend to be most heavily concentrated. For example, if average size of shoe sold in Amritsar is 7, then this average is neither mean nor median but it is mode (most frequent value in distribution). Therefore, it means that there is a maximum demand for the shoe of size 7 in Amritsar.

Computation of Mode

In case of a frequency distribution, mode is the value of the variable corresponding to the maximum frequency. For example, in the following distribution, the maximum frequency is 40 and therefore, the corresponding value of x viz., 5 gives the value of mode.

Variable (x) : 1 2 3 4 5 6 7 8 9
Frequency (f) : 3 1 18 25 40 30 22 10 6

In case of continuous frequency distribution, the class corresponding to the maximum frequency is called the "modal class" and the value of mode is obtained by the interpolation formula:

$$\text{Mode} = l + \frac{h(f_1 - f_0)}{(f_1 - f_0) - (f_2 - f_1)}$$

$$= l + \frac{h(f_1 - f_0)}{2f_1 - f_0 - f_2}$$

Where

l is the lower limit of the modal class

h is the magnitude of the modal class

f_0 is the frequency of proceeding class

f_1 is the maximum frequency (frequency of modal class)

f_2 is the frequency of succeeding class

Example: Find the value of mean and mode from the following data:

Weight (in kg)	No. of students
93–97	2
98–102	5
103–107	12
108–112	17
113–117	14
118–122	6
123–127	3
128–132	1

Since the formula for mode requires the distribution to be continuous; therefore, let us first convert the classes into class boundaries as given in the Table 10.2.

Table 10.2: Computation of mean and mode

Weight (in kg)	Class boundaries	Mid-value(x)	Number of students (f)	$d = \dfrac{x - 110}{5}$	f.d
93–97	92.5–97.5	95	3	–3	–9
98–102	97.5–102.5	100	5	–2	–10
103–107	102.5–107.5	105	12	–1	–12
108–112	**107.5–112.5**	**110**	A **17**	**0**	**0**
113–117	112.5–117.5	115	14	1	14
118–122	117.5–122.5	120	6	2	12
123–127	122.5–127.5	125	3	3	9
128–132	127.5–132.5	130	1	4	4
			N = Σf = 61		**Σfd = 8**

Assume A = 110 and h = 5

$$\text{Mean} = A + \frac{h.\Sigma fd}{N} = 110 + \frac{5 \times 8}{61} = 110.66 \text{ kg}$$

Here maximum frequency is 17. The corresponding class 107.5–112.5 is the modal class. Using the mode formula, we get:

$$\text{Mode} = l + \frac{h(f_1 - f_0)}{2f_1 - f_0 - f_2}$$

$$= 107.5 + \frac{5 \times (17 - 12)}{2 \times 17 - 12 - 14}$$

$$= 107.5 + \frac{25}{8} = 107.5 + 3.125$$

$$= 110.625 \text{ kg.}$$

Merits

- Mode is easy to calculate and understand. In some cases, it can be located merely by inspection. It can also be estimated graphically from a histogram.
- Mode is not at all affected by extreme observations and as such is preferred to arithmetic mean while dealing with extreme observations.
- It can be conveniently obtained in the case of open end classes.

Demerits

- Mode is not rigidly defined. It is ill-defined if the maximum frequency is repeated or if the maximum frequency occurs either, in the very beginning or at the end of the distribution; or if the distribution is irregular.
- Since mode is the value of (x) corresponding to the maximum frequency, it is not based on all the observations of the series. Even in the case of the continuous frequency distribution, mode depends on the frequencies of modal class and the classes preceding or succeeding it.

- Mode is not suitable for further mathematical treatment. For example, from the modal values and the sizes of two or more series, we cannot find the mode of the combined series.

Relationship between mean (m), mode (mo) and median (md)

The *empirical* relationship between mean, mode and median is as follows:

Mode = Mean – 3 (Mean – Median)

Mean- Mode = 3 (Mean – Median)

iv. Geometric Mean (GM)

The geometric mean of a 'n' observations is the nth root of their product. Thus if $x_1, x_2 \ldots \ldots x_n$ are variable of 'n' observation then:

$$\text{GM} = [\, x_1 \times x_2 \times x_3 \ldots \ldots \ldots x_n]^{1/n}$$

For example, if there are two observation, i.e. 4 and 16 then G.M = $(4 \times 16)^{1/2} = (64)^{1/2} = 8$. if there are three observations, i.e. 1, 4, and 16 then GM = $(1 \times 4 \times 16)^{1/3} = (64)^{1/3} = 4$.

Merits

- Geometric mean is rigidly defined.
- It is based on all the observations.
- It is suitable for further mathematical treatment.
- Unlike arithmetic mean which has a bias for higher values, geometric mean has bias for smaller observations.
- It is not affected much by fluctuations of sampling.

Demerits

- Because of its abstract mathematical character, geometric mean is not easy to understand and to calculate for a nonmathematical observation.
- If any one of the observations is zero, geometric mean becomes zero and if any one

of the observations is negative, geometric mean becomes imaginary regardless of the magnitude of the other items.

v. Harmonic Mean (HM)

Harmonic mean is the reciprocal of the arithmetic mean of the reciprocals of given observations:

$$HM = \frac{\Sigma f}{\Sigma (f/x)} = \frac{N}{\Sigma f/x}$$

f = corresponding frequency of variable.

x = variable or mid-value class

Merits

- Harmonic mean is rigidly defined.
- It is based on all the observations.

- It is suitable for mathematical treatment.
- Since the reciprocals of the values of the variable are involved, it gives greater weightage to smaller observations and as such is not very much affected by one or two big observations.
- It is not affected very much by fluctuations of sampling.

Demerits

- It is not easy to understand and calculate.
- Its value cannot be obtained if any one of the observations is zero.
- It is not a representative figure of the distribution unless the phenomenon requires greater weightage to be given to smaller items. As such, it is hardly used in business problems.

Example: The following table depicts the weights of 31 students in a class. Calculate the mean weight using harmonic mean method.

Weight in kg (x)	:	130	135	140	145	146	148	149	150	157
Number of students (f)	:	3	4	6	6	3	5	2	1	1

Computation of Harmonic Mean (HM)

Weight in kg (x)	No. of students (f)	(f/x)
130	3	0.02307
135	4	0.02964
140	6	0.04284
145	6	0.04140
146	3	0.02055
148	5	0.03380
149	2	0.01342
150	1	0.00667
157	1	0.00637
	$\Sigma f = N = 31$	$\Sigma f/x = 0.21776$

$$HM = \frac{N}{\Sigma (f/x)} = \frac{31}{0.21776} = 142.36 \text{ kg}$$

Hence the mean weight of 31 students using harmonic mean is 142.36 kg.

Relationship between Arithmetic mean, Geometric mean, and Harmonic mean

The arithmetic mean (AM), geometric mean (GM), and harmonic mean (HM) of a series of 'n' observations are connected by a relation.

$$A.M \geq G.M \geq H.M$$

b. Measure of Dispersion

In order to explain the dispersion, let us consider the following three series A, B, and C of 9 items each.

Series										Total	Arithmetic Mean
A	15	15	15	15	15	15	15	15	15	135	15
B	11	12	13	14	15	16	17	18	19	135	15
C	3	6	9	12	15	18	21	24	27	135	15

All the three series A, B and C have the same size (n=9) and the same mean (15). Thus the mean of 9 observations is 15, therefore, series A or B or C cannot be determined. In fact any series of 9 items with total 135 will always indicate mean 15. Thus a large number of series with entirely different structures and compositions will have the same mean.

From the above example it is obvious that the measures of central tendency, i.e. arithmetic mean are inadequate to describe the distribution completely, thus the measures of central tendency must be supported and supplemented by some other measures. One such measure is *Dispersion.*

According to Spiegel *The degree to which numerical data tend to spread about an average value is called the variation or dispersion of the data.* In simple terms, *Dispersion is the measure of the variation of the items.*

There are three ways for measures of dispersion:
  i. Range
  ii. Mean deviation
  iii. Standard deviation

i. Range

The range is the simplest of all the measures of dispersion. It is defined as 'the difference between the two extreme observations of the distribution'. In other words, range is the difference between the greatest (maximum) and the smallest (minimum) observation of the distribution. Thus

$$\text{Range} = X\text{max} - X\text{min}$$

Where Xmax is the greatest observation and Xmin is the smallest observation of the variable.

In case of the grouped frequency distribution or continuous frequency distribution, range is defined as 'the difference between the upper limit of the highest class and the lower limit of the smallest class'.

Merits
- Range is the simplest measure of dispersion.
- It is rigidly defined
- It is readily comprehensible and is perhaps the easiest to compute, requiring very little calculations.

Demerits
- Range is not based on the entire set of data. It is based only on two extreme observations; as such range cannot be regarded as a reliable measure of variability.
- Range is very much affected by fluctuations of sampling. Its value varies very widely from sample to sample.
- Range cannot be used if we are dealing with open end classes.
- Range is not suitable for mathematical treatment.

Example: Calculate the range and the coefficient of range of a doctor's monthly earnings in a year.

Months	Monthly earnings (Rupees in thousands.)
1	139
2	150
3	151
4	151
5	157
6	158
7	160
8	161
9	162
10	162
11	173
12	175

Solution: Largest earnings (Xmax) = Rs. 175,000 Smallest earnings (Xmin) = Rs. 139,000
Range = 175,000 – 139,000 = Rs. 36,000

$$\text{Coeficient of range} = \frac{175-139}{175+139} = \frac{36}{314} = 0.115$$

ii. Mean Deviation (MD)

"Mean deviation is the average amount of scatter of the items in a distribution from either the mean or the median, ignoring the signs of the deviations. The average that is taken of the scatter is an arithmetic mean, which accounts for the fact that this measure is often called the mean deviation".

Merits

- Mean deviation is rigidly defined and is easy to understand and calculate.
- Mean deviation is based on all the observations and is thus definitely a better measure of dispersion than the range.

- As compared with standard deviation, it is less affected by extreme observations.
- Since mean deviation is based on the deviations about an average, it provides a better measure for comparison about the formation of different distributions.

Demerits

- The strongest objection against mean deviation is that while computing its value we take the absolute value of the deviations about an average and ignore the signs of the deviations.
- The step of ignoring the signs of the deviations is mathematically unsound and illogical.
- It is rarely used in sociological studies.
- It cannot be computed for distribution with open end classes.

Computation of Mean Deviation (MD)

If $x_1, x_2, x_3 \ldots\ldots\ldots x_n$ are observations, then mean deviation (MD) about arithmetic mean (M), median (Md) and mode (Mo) is as follows:

MD about mean	$= \dfrac{1}{N}\Sigma f(x - M)$
MD about median	$= \dfrac{1}{N}\Sigma f(x - Md)$
MD about mode	$= \dfrac{1}{N}\Sigma f(x - Mo)$

Example: Calculate the mean deviation about mean for the following data:

Class Interval :	2–4	4–6	6–8	8–10
Frequency :	3	4	2	1

Solution: First let us calculate the mean from the above data and then compute mean deviation about mean.

Class	Mid-Value(x)	Frequency (f)	d = x-A(A = 5)	fd	$\lvert x-\bar{x}\rvert$	$f\lvert x-\bar{x}\rvert$
2–4	3	3	–2	–6	2.2	6.6
4–6	5	4	0	0	0.2	0.8
6–8	7	2	2	4	1.8	3.6
8–10	9	1	4	4	3.8	3.8
		N = Σf = 10		Σfd = 2		Σf$\lvert x-\bar{x}\rvert$ = 14.8

Mean $(\bar{x}) = A + \dfrac{\Sigma fd}{N}$ where A is assumed as 5

$$= 5 + \frac{2}{10} = 5.2$$

MD about mean $= \dfrac{1}{N}\Sigma f\lvert x - \bar{x}\rvert = \dfrac{14.8}{10} = 1.48$

where $\lvert x - \bar{x}\rvert$ is absolute value, i.e. ignoring the negative sign.

Steps
- Calculate the arithmetic mean ($\bar{x}$) or mean
- Compute $\lvert x - \bar{x}\rvert$ of each variable with absolute value, i.e. ignoring the negative sign.
- Multiply each absolute value with frequency of variable.
- Divide the total obtained by N= Σf, get mean deviation about mean.
- Similarly get mean deviation about median and mode.

Example: Calculate mean deviation about median from the following data:

Marks less than	:	80	70	60	50	40	30	20	10
Number of students	:	100	90	80	60	32	20	13	5

Solution: First of all convert the given cumulative frequency distribution table into ordinary frequency distribution as given in Table 10.3.

			Table 10.3			
Marks	c.f.	Frequency (f)	Mid-value of class (x)	$\lvert x - Md\rvert$	$f\lvert x - Md\rvert$
0–10	5	5	5	41.43	207.15
10–20	13	8	15	31.43	251.44
20–30	20	7	25	21.43	150.00
30–40	32	12	35	11.43	137.16
40–50	60	28	45	1.43	40.04
50–60	80	20	55	8.57	171.14
60–70	90	10	65	18.57	185.70
70–80	100	10	75	28.57	285.70
	N = Σf = 100				Σf$\lvert x - Md\rvert$ =1428.6

Here N/2 = 50. Since the c.f. just greater than 50 is 60, the corresponding class 40–50 is the median class and width of class (h) is 10.

$$\text{Median (Md)} = l + \frac{h}{f}\left(\frac{N}{2} - c\right)$$

$$= 40 + \frac{10}{28}(50 - 32) = 40 + 6.43 = 46.43$$

Mean deviation about median

$$= \frac{1}{N}\Sigma f \mid x - Md \mid = \frac{1428.6}{100} = 14.29$$

iii. Standard Deviation (SD)

It is defined as 'the positive square root of the arithmetic mean of the squares of the deviations of the given observations from their arithmetic mean'. Thus if $x_1, x_2 \ldots \ldots \ldots \ldots x_n$ are observations then its standard deviation is given by:

$$SD = \sqrt{\frac{1}{N}\Sigma(x - \bar{x})^2}$$

where

$\bar{x}$ is the arithmetic mean of given observations

x is the value of variable or mid-value of the class.

N = Σf = Sum of frequencies

Computation of Standard Deviation

- Compute the arithmetic mean ($\bar{x}$) by the usual method.
- Compute the deviation ($x-\bar{x}$) of each value of variable.
- Find the suqare of the deviation of each value, i.e. $(x-\bar{x})^2$.
- Mutliply each of the above observation by corresponding frequency to get $f(x-\bar{x})^2$.
- Divide the sum of above values by N (total frequencies).
- The positive square root of the above value gives standard deviation of the distribution.

In case of frequency distribution

$$SD = \sqrt{\frac{1}{N}\Sigma f(x - \bar{x})^2}$$

Merits

- Standard deviation is the most important and widely used measure of dispersion.
- It is rigidly defined and based on all the observations.
- It is suitable for further mathematical treatment.
- It is least affected by fluctuation of sampling.

Demerits

- It is observed that standard deviation gives greater weight to extreme values; and as such not in favour of economists or businessman, who are more interested in the results of the modal class.

Example: Calculate the mean and standard deviation from the following data:

Value :	90–99	80–89	70–79	60–69	50–59	40–49	30–39
Frequency :	2	12	22	20	14	4	1

Solution: Let us calculate the arithmetic mean of the data and prepare the following

Class	Mid- value (x)	Frequency (f)	$d = \dfrac{x-A}{10}$	f.d	$(x-\bar{x})$	$f(x-\bar{x})^2$
90–99	94.5	2	3	6	26.4	1393.92
80–89	84.5	12	2	24	16.4	3227.52
70–79	74.5	22	1	22	6.4	901.12
60–69	**64.5 "A"**	**20**	**0**	**0**	**–3.6**	**259.2**
50–59	54.5	14	–1	–14	–13.6	2589.44
40–49	44.5	4	–2	–8	–23.6	2227.84
30–39	34.5	1	–3	–3	–33.6	1128.96
		N = Σf = 75		**Σfd = 27**		**Σf (x– x̄)² = 11728**

$$\text{Mean } (\bar{x}) = A + \frac{h.\Sigma fd}{N}$$

$$= 64.5 + \frac{10 \times 27}{75} = 64.5 + 3.6 = 68.1$$

$$\text{Standard deviation} = \sqrt{\frac{1}{75}\Sigma f(x-\bar{x})^2}$$

$$= \sqrt{\frac{1}{75} \times 11728}$$

$$= 12.5$$

Sampling and Sampling Technique

The science of statistics may be broadly classified as 'descriptive' and 'inductive'. The descriptive statistics consists of numerical data whereas the inductive statistics is termed as logic of drawing conclusion about the totality of items (known as population) on the basis of examining a part of population (known as sample). In our daily life most of our decision depends upon the examination of only few item out of total lot. For example, few grains of rice from a cooking vessel gets an fair idea whether the entire lot of rice is fully cooked or it requires further cooking. The process of studying the sample data and then generalizing the result to population involves an element of risk (making wrong decision). Therefore, sampling techniques plays a vital role for minimizing the risk.

The group of individual or items under study is known as population. For example if we want to study the expenditure habit of families in a city then the population will consists of all the households in that city. A finite subset of the population, selected from it with the objective of studying expenditure habit of families, is called a sample and number of units in the sample is termed as sample size. The objective of sampling is:

- Estimation of population parameters.
- Testing of hypothesis about the population.

Samples are like medicines. They can be harmful when they are taken carelessly or without knowledge of their effects. Every good sample should have a proper label with instructions about its use.

Types of Sampling

The choice of an appropriate sampling is very important during the execution of sample survey. The sampling techniques are generally utilized keeping in view of objective and the scope of statistical study. This can be further classified as follows:

- Purposive or Subjective or Judgment Sampling.
- Probability Sampling
- Mixed Sampling.

Purposive or Subjective or Judgment Sampling: In this method, a desired number of sample units is selected deliberately depending upon the objective of the study so that only important items representing the true characteristics of the population are included in the sample. This sampling technique is highly subjective in nature since the selection

of the sample depends entirely on the personal convenience and belief.

Probability Sampling: Probability sampling provides a scientific technique of drawing samples from the population according to some laws of chance (probability). Different types of sampling are as follows:

- Each sample unit has an equal chance of being selected
- Sampling units have varying probability of being selected
- Probability of selection of a unit is proportional to the sample size

Mixed Sampling: In this technique, samples are selected partly according to laws of chance (probability) and partly according to a fixed (subjective) sampling method.

In statistics, 'random' is a well defined concept, i.e. random samples are characterized by the way in which they are selected. Randomness is not used in the sense of hit or miss. Probability and mixed sampling can be broadly classified as follows:

 i. Simple Random Sampling
 ii. Stratified Random Sampling
 iii. Systematic Sampling
 iv. Multistage Sampling
 v. Cluster Sampling

 i. **Simple Random Sampling:** This is a technique in which *sample is so drawn that each and every unit in the population has an equal and independent chance of being included in the sample.*

This method is applicable when the population is small, homogeneous and readily available such as patients coming to hospital or lying in the wards. It is used in clinical trials like testing the efficacy of a particular medicine.

The sample may be drawn unit by unit, either by numbering the units such as persons, families or households of a particular population or from the published tables of random numbers. To ensure randomness of selection, one may adopt either lottery method or refer to table of random numbers.

Lottery Method: Suppose, 10 patients are to be put on a trial out of the 100 available. Note the serial number of patients on 100 cards and shuffle them well. Draw out one and note the number. Replace the card drawn, reshuffle and draw the second card. Repeat the process till 10 numbers are drawn. Reject the cards that are drawn for second time. The 10 cards drawn thus will indicate the patient's number to be put on trial and thus this selection of sample is through lottery method.

Table of Random Number: The other common method of drawing the sample is by making use of the published tables of random numbers.

ii. **Stratified Random Sampling:** This method is applicable when population is not homogeneous. The population under study is first divided into homogeneous groups called 'strata' and the sample is drawn from each 'strata' at random in proportion to its size. It gives representation to all strata of population such as selecting sample from defined areas, classes, ages, sexes, etc. This technique gives more representative sample than simple random sampling in a given large population. Therefore it gives greater accuracy and thus proportionate representative sample from each strata is secured.

iii. Systematic Sampling: Systematic sampling is slight variation of the simple random sampling in which only the first sample unit is selected at random and the remaining units are automatically selected in a definite sequence at equal spacing from one another. This technique of drawing samples is usually recommended if the complete and up-to-date list of the sampling units is available and the units are arranged in some systematic order such as alphabetical, chronological, geographical order, etc.

It is more often applied to field studies when the population is large, scattered and not homogeneous. Systematic procedure is followed to choose a sample by taking every Kth patient where K refers to the sample interval, which is calculated by the formula:

$$\text{Sample interval (K)} = \frac{\text{Total population}}{\text{Sample size desired}}$$

iv. **Multistage Sampling:** This method refers to the sampling procedures carried out in several stages using random sampling techniques. This is employed in large country surveys. In the first stage, random numbers of districts are chosen from all the States, followed by random numbers of talukas, villages and units respectively, For example-if we have to survey for dental problem in a district then choose 10% villages in each talukas and then examine teeth of all persons in every 10th house. This technique is known as multistage sampling.

v. **Cluster Sampling:** This method is used when units of population are natural groups or clusters such as villages, wards, blocks, slums of a town, factories, workshops or children of a school, etc. The technique of cluster sampling allows small number of the target population to be sampled while the data provided is statistically valid at 95% confidence level. From the chosen clusters, 30 in number, the entire population is surveyed. Cluster sampling gives a higher standard error but the data collection in this method is simpler and involves less time and cost than in other sampling techniques.

ERRORS AND TRIALS

In statistics 'error' refers to the difference between the true value of a population parameter and its estimate provided by sampling techniques. These errors in statistics are due to the followings:

- Approximations in measurement
- Approximations in rounding of figures
- Biases due to faulty collection and analysis of data and further biases in presentation and interpretation of results.
- Personal biases of the investigator.

The error in any statistical study may be classified as under:

i. Sampling errors
ii. Non-sampling errors
iii. Biased errors
iv. Unbiased errors

i. **Sampling Errors:** In a sample survey, small portion of the population is studied therefore its results are bound to differ from the population's results and thus have a certain amount of error. This error would always be there no matter that the sample is drawn at random or it is highly representative. This error is attributed to fluctuations of sampling and is called *sampling error*. Sampling error is due to the fact that only a subset of the population (sample) has been used to estimate the population parameters and draw inferences about the population.

Sampling errors are primarily due to the following reasons:

- Faulty selection of the sample
- Faulty demarcation of sampling units
- Error due to bias in the estimation method

ii. **Non-Sampling Errors:** Non-sampling errors are not attributed to chance and are a consequence of certain factors which are within human control. In other words, they are due to certain causes which can be traced and may arise at any stage of the study. Non-sampling errors are thus present in all studies. The following important factors are responsible for non-sampling errors in any study.

- Faulty planning

- Imperfect questionnaire which might result in wrong or incomplete information.
- Defective methods of interviewing and asking questions
- Exaggerated or wrong answers to the questions which appeal to the pride or prestige of self-interests of the respondents.
- Lack of trained and qualified investigators and lack of supervisory staff.
- Failure of respondent's memory to recall the events or happenings in the past.
- Improper coverage
- Publication errors

iii. **Biased Errors:** In any statistical study, biased errors are present due to the following factors:

- Bias on the part of investigator whose personal beliefs and prejudices are likely to affect the results of the study.
- Bias in the measuring instrument used for recording the observations.
- Bias due to faulty collection of the data and in the statistical techniques and the formulae used for the analysis of the data.
- Respondent's bias: Respondents may furnish wrong information to safeguard their personal interests. For example, for income-tax purpose, a person may give an understatement of his salary or income.
- Bias due to non-response: Bias due to non-response results if in a house-to-house survey the respondent is not available in spite of repeated visits by the investigator or if the respondent refuses to furnish the information.
- Bias in the technique of approximations.

Owing to their nature, the biased errors have a tendency to grow in magnitude with an increase in the number of the observations and hence are also known as *Cumulative Errors.* Thus, the magnitude of the biased errors is directly proportional to the number of observations.

iv. Unbiased Errors: If the chances of making an over-estimate is almost the same as the chances of making an under-estimate then this is known as unbiased error. Since these errors move in both the directions, the errors in one direction are more or less neutralized by the errors in the opposite direction and consequently the ultimate result is not much affected. For example, if the individual values, say, 385, 415, 355, 445 are rounded to the nearest complete (hundred) unit then each of them would be recorded as 400. In this case the values 385 and 355 give overestimating errors of magnitudes 15 and 45 respectively while the values 415 and 445 give under-estimating errors of magnitudes 15 and 45 respectively and in the ultimate result (approximation) they get neutralized. Thus, if the number of observations is quite large, these unbiased errors will not affect the final result much. Since the errors in one direction compensate for the errors in the other direction, unbiased errors are also termed as *Compensatory Errors*. Thus we observed that the unbiased errors do not grow with the increase in the number of observations but they have a tendency to get neutralized and are minimum in the ultimate analysis and *the magnitude of the unbiased errors is inversely proportional to the number of items.*

Trials in Statistics

Trials in statistic may be classified as 'Open' and 'Blind' trials.

Open trials: In an open trial, the researcher knows the full details of the treatment and so does the patient. Open trial may be appropriate for comparing two very similar treatment to determine which is most effective.

Blind trial: This is a part of the scientific method used to prevent research outcomes from being influence by others. To blind a person involved in research is to prevent them from knowing certain information about the process. There may be varying degree of blind i.e. single, double and triple blind.

Single blind trial: In a single-blind trial, the researcher knows the details of the treatment but the patient does not. Because the patient does not know which treatment is being administered (the new treatment or another treatment) there might be no placebo effect. In practice, since the researcher knows, it is possible for the researcher to treat the patient differently, thus influencing the outcome of the study.

Double blind trial: A double-blind trial is a clinical trial design in which neither the participating individuals nor the study staff knows which participants are receiving the experimental drug and which are receiving a placebo. Therefore double-blind trials are preferred, as they tend to give the most accurate results.

Triple blind trial: Some randomized controlled trials are considered triple-blinded, although the meaning of this may vary according to the exact study design. The most common meaning is that the subject, researcher and person administering the treatment (often a pharmacist) are blinded to what is being given. Alternately, it may mean that the patient, researcher and statistician are blinded. The team monitoring the response may be unaware of the intervention being given in the control and study groups. These additional precautions are often in place with the more commonly accepted term "double blind trials", and thus the term "triple-blinded" is infrequently used. However, it connotes an additional layer of security to prevent undue influence of study results by anyone directly involved with the study.

Trials in healthcare: In the hierarchy of evidence that influences healthcare policy and practice, randomized controlled trial are considered by most to be the top individual unit of research. They are considered the most reliable form of scientific evidence because they eliminate spurious causality and bias.

Sellers of medicines throughout the ages have had to convince their consumers that the medicine works. As science has progressed, public expectations have risen, and government health budgets have become ever tighter, pressure has grown for a reliable system to do this. Moreover, the public's concern for the dangers of medical interventions has spurred both legislators and administrators to provide an evidential basis for licensing or paying for new procedures and medications. In most modern health-care systems all new medicines and surgical procedures, therefore, have to undergo trials before being approved. Trials are used to established average efficacy of a treatment as well as learn about its side effects. Finally it has been proven that act of administering the medicine (treatment) may have direct or psychological effect on the patient which is known as "placebo effect". The meaning of word placebo is "I shall please". The phenomenon of an inert substance resulting in a patient's medical improvement is called "placebo effect" and negative effect is called "nocebo effect".

TESTING OF HYPOTHESIS

The statistical inference is based on deciding about the characteristics of the population on the basis of sample study. Such decisions involve an element of risk, i.e. the risk of taking wrong decisions. For example, a dentist may be interested to find if a particular mouthwash is really effective in reducing the gigival bleeding or a doctor may be interested to find a given food stuff is effective in increasing the weight of person. In such decision making, the theory of probability plays an vital role; and the branch of statistics,

which helps in arriving at the criterion for such decisions is known as "testing of hypothesis".

The fundamental concepts associated with testing of hypothesis are:
• Probability
• Statistical hypothesis
• Null hypothesis
• Tests of significance
• Level of significance
• Types of errors

Probability: Let us understand the fundamental rule of counting in statistics. If there are five routes of journey from Amritsar to Delhi then the total number of ways of making a to and fro journey i.e. going from Amritsar to Delhi and coming back from Delhi to Amritsar are 25 (5×5), since one can go in five ways and come back in five ways. It is established that an element of uncertainity is always associated with every experiment or research because complete information on all happenings might not be available. This uncertainity is numerically expressed as "Probability". Therefore, probability may be defined as the relative frequency (probable chances of occurrence) of a particular event happening by chance in long run. Probability is usually expressed by a symbol 'p'. It ranges from zero (0) to one (1). If $p = 0$ then it means that there is no chance that the event can happen (possible); but on the other hand if $p = 1$, then it means that chances of an event happening is 100 %. For example, chances of getting head or tail in one toss are fifty- fifty or half- half.

Similarly if a uniform die is thrown at random then the probability of getting 5 is $\frac{1}{6}$.

Mathematically:

$$p = \frac{\text{favorable number of cases to the event}}{\text{total number of cases}}$$

In order to explain, die can fall on any of the faces (1, 2, 3, 4, 5 and 6) i.e. total number of cases is 6. Number of cases favorable to the event (getting 5) is only one (1); therefore, probability of getting 5 is 1/ 6. If the probability of an event happening in a sample is 'p', then that of not happening is denoted by 'q'. Therefore, p + q is always one (1).

Statistical hypothesis: A statistical hypothesis is some assumption, which may or may not be true, about a population, which is to be tested on the basis of the evidence from a random sample. If the hypothesis completely specifies the population, then it is known as simple hypothesis, otherwise it is known as composite hypothesis. A test of a statistical hypothesis is two action decisions (acceptance or rejection) after observing a random sample from a given population.

Null hypothesis: The random selection of the samples from the given population makes the tests of significance as valid. For applying any test of significance, let us set a hypothesis – a definite statement about the population parameter(s). Such a statistical hypothesis, which is under test, is usually a hypothesis of no difference and hence is called Null hypothesis. According to Prof. R.A.Fisher:

Null hypothesis is the hypothesis which is tested for possible rejection under the assumption that it is true.

Tests of significance: A procedure to access the significance of a statistic or difference between two independent statistics is known as test of significance. Therefore a test of significance is a process by which the evidence is gathered as to how far the sample value matches with the population value.

In these tests, first formulate a null hypothesis, than assume that the factor under study has no effect and the observed difference is entirely due to chance.

There are following main ways for tests of significance:

• Coefficient of variation
• Standard error of mean
• Karl-Pearson coefficient for correlation

Coefficient of Variation (CV)

The relative measure of dispersion based on standard deviation is called the coefficient of variation. This is pure number, independent of unit of measurement and thus suitable for comparing the variability, i.e homogeneity of two or more distribution, for example, height and weight of Punjabi's and Tamilian's. Mathematically it is denoted as:

$$\text{Coefficient of variation (CV)} = \frac{\text{Standard deviation}}{\text{Mean}} \times 100$$

A distribution with smaller coefficient of variance is said to be more homogeneous (uniform) than the other distribution of higher coefficient of variance.

Standard Error of Mean (SE $\bar{x}$)

Difference between the mean of observed values from a sample and mean value of population measured by statistics is known as standard error of mean. Thus standard error is a measure of chance variation between sample and population. It does not mean error or mistake. Then SE of mean is calculated by the following formula:

$$(\text{SE } \bar{x}) = \frac{\text{SD}}{\sqrt{n}}$$

$$= \frac{\text{Standard deviation}}{\sqrt{\text{Number of observation in sample}}}$$

Standard error of mean varies directly with standard deviation. Therefore, greater the standard deviation, greater will be standard error. This can be minimized by reducing the standard deviation, which can only be done through a large sample. The standard error about mean varies inversely with the square root of number of sample. If the sample is increased to 100 times then this standard error is reduced to almost one tenth.

Karl-Pearson Coefficient for Correlation

Two variables are said to be co-related if the change in one variable results in a corresponding change in the other variable. The effect of correlation is to reduce the range of uncertainity in our prediction. Karl Pearson's coefficient of correlation is a mathematical method for measuring the magnitude of linear relationship between two variables and most widely used in studies. This is also known as 'covariance method'.

Coefficient of correlation 'r' between two variables x and y can be calculated by the following formula:

$$r = \frac{\Sigma dx.dy}{\sqrt{\Sigma dx^2 . \Sigma dy^2}}$$

where $dx = x - \bar{x}$

$dy = y - \bar{y}$

Example: Let sales in units (x) and expenses in rupees (y) of ten (10) firms in Amritsar are as follows:

x	y	$dx = (x - \bar{x})$	$dy = (y-\bar{y})$	dx^2	dy^2	$dx.dy$
50	11	−8	−3	64	9	24
50	13	−8	−1	64	1	8
55	14	−3	0	9	0	0
60	16	2	2	4	4	4
65	16	7	2	49	4	14
65	15	7	1	49	1	7
65	15	7	1	49	1	7
60	14	2	0	4	0	0
60	13	2	−1	4	1	−2
50	13	−8	−1	64	1	8
$\Sigma x = 580$	$\Sigma y = 140$	$\Sigma dx = 0$	$\Sigma dy = 0$	$\Sigma dx^2 = 360$	$\Sigma dy^2 = 22$	$\Sigma dx.dy = 70$

$$\bar{x} = \frac{\Sigma x}{N} = \frac{580}{10} = 58$$

$$\bar{y} = \frac{\Sigma y}{N} = \frac{140}{10} = 14$$

$$r = \frac{\Sigma dx.dy}{\sqrt{\Sigma dx^2 . \Sigma dy^2}} = \frac{70}{\sqrt{360 \times 22}}$$

$$= \frac{70}{\sqrt{7920}} = \frac{70}{88.99}$$

$$= 0.7866$$

This indicates that there is a positive correlation between sales in units and expenses in rupees.

Interpretation of Coefficient of Correlation (r)

- If r = +1, then it implies that there is a perfect positive correlation between the variables.
- If r = −1, then it implies that there is a perfect negative correlation between the variables.
- If r = 0, then the variables are uncorrelated. In other words, r always lies between (−1) to (+1).

Level of Significance

In order to find the parameter of the entire population, large number of samples cannot be drawn; therefore, calculate the parameter from a statistic of sampling. Then set up certain limits on both sides of the population and sample. For example, 20–25 sample size is required for 2000–2500 population. On the basis of the fact that statistical 'mean' of sample size are normally distributed around the population 'mean', these limits are called 'confidence limits' and range between two is called 'confidence interval'.

We have found the parameter of the population from that of sample but we cannot be confident because we are dealing with part of the population only (howsoever big the sample may be). We would be wrong in 5% cases only if we place the population value say mean within 95% confidence limits and in 1% cases only if we say the population mean lies within 99% confidence limits. The limit of the region at which we no longer regard the chance to be operating is called the **level of significance**.

In most of the statistical studies, the levels of significance are set at 5% (P, 0.05), 1% (P, 0.01) and 0.5% (P, 0.005). They are the yardsticks against which the probability or relative frequency of our sample estimate is measured. Significant or insignificant indicates whether a value is likely to occur by chance or it is unlikely to occur by chance.

Types of Error

As a routine, the concept of acceptance and rejection is followed to interpret the estimated difference from the population parameter at 5% level of significance.

In certain circumstances, the null hypothesis of no difference is rejected even when the estimate falls in the zone of acceptance at 5% level. It means the level of significance from 5% to 6, 8 or 10% is being changed. This is committing Type I error by changing the level of significance. The extent to which this may be rejected depends on the investigator and the circumstances, such as trial of two mouthwashes, when the investigator may think that the difference at 10% level of significance is enough.

There are other situations when null hypothesis is accepted when it should have been rejected because the estimate falls in the zone of rejection. Here the level of acceptance from 5% to 4, 3, 2 or 1% level of significance is being changed. This is committing Type-II error by changing the level of significance.

Inference	Accept it	Reject it
Hypothesis is true	Correct decision	Type I error
Hypothesis is false	Type II error	Correct decision

Type I error is usually fixed in advance by choice of the level of significance employed in the studies, e.g. if it is fixed at 5% level, we know that we shall be rejecting on an average 5% of all the true hypothesis. It may be noted that Type I error can be made as small as desired by changing the level of significance. In dental studies, Type I error is more serious as compared to Type II error. To minimize the error of chance, random sample as large as possible should be taken and interpret the results.

BIBLIOGRAPHY

1. Armitage, P. : Statistical Methods in Medical Research. Blackwell Oxford, 2nd Ed., 1973.
2. Darby, M.L. and Bowen, D.M. : Research methods for Oral Health Professionals – an introduction. St. Louis, C.V. Mosby Co., 1980.
3. Gupta, S.C. : Fundamentals of Statistics. Sixth Ed., 1997 Himalaya Publishing House, New Delhi.

4. Harris, E.. and Fitzergerald, J.D. : The principles and practice of clinical trials. Edinburgh, 1970.

5. Hyatt, T.P. and Lotka, A.J. : How dental statistics are secured in the metropolitan life insurance co. J.D.R. : 9, 411, 1929.

6. Pelton, W.J. and Wisan, J.M. : Statistics in Public Health. W.B. Saunders, London, 1960.

7. Petrie, A., Bukan , J.S. and Osborn, J.F. : Further statistics in dentistry Part 8 : systemic reviews and meta-analysis. B.D.J. : 194, 73, 2003.

8. Saleruo, F.R. : Of what value are dental biostatistics to the general population. W.V. Dent. J. 40, 30, 1966.

9. Slack, G.L. : Dental Public Health. John Wright and Sons, Bristol, 1974.

11   *General Epidemiology*

The health and disease phenomenon is not new. The features related with distribution of a disease have always been a subject of interest for the medical profession. The geographical distribution of a disease, the variation in its frequency at different times and the special characteristics of people affected by it should be clearly defined to ensure its better management. In simple terms, epidemiology is the study of occurrence and distribution of disease. The 'pattern' and the 'dynamics' of any disease is also involved in epidemiology process. The pattern implies variables such as age, sex, occupation and social characteristics, etc. and dynamics implies trends and timing of the concerned disease. Measurement of the frequency and changing pattern of disease is essential to ensure that the resources needed for the community's health care are sufficient. Management of ill health in any community requires a community diagnosis, which rests on epidemiological information. The data on morbidity (the frequency of illness) is also important for any community to manage the epidemics in a better way.

Clark has defined epidemiology as, *the science concerned with the study of factors that influence occurrence and distribution of a disease, defect, disability or death in aggregate of individuals.*

It has also been defined as *the science dealing with the relationship of the various factors which determine the frequency and distribution of a disease.*

The objective of epidemiology is to increase the understanding of the disease process, subsequently leading to the development of methods for its control and prevention. In addition, epidemiology attempts to discover population at high and low risk. The design, conduct and interpretation of clinical trials of preventive and curative measures are also included.

COMPONENTS OF EPIDEMIOLOGY

Three basic components of epidemiology are:
  i. Frequency of disease
 ii. Distribution of disease
iii. Determinants of disease

i. Frequency of disease: The frequency implies rates and ratios (prevalence, incidence, etc.) of any disease process. The disease frequency in different populations or subgroups of same population is an important factor in the development of strategies for its prevention and control.

ii. Distribution of disease: Health and disease are never uniformly distributed in human population. An important function of epidemiology is to study these distribution patterns in the given community. The epidemiologist examines the concentration of a particular disease in one subgroup and also increase/decrease of the same disease over the years. The variations so obtained are helpful in deciding the preventive regimes. An important outcome of this study is formation of etiological hypothesis. This aspect of epidemiology is known as *Descriptive Epidemiology.*

iii. Determinants of disease: The etiological factors or the risk factors of the disease are also analyzed in epidemiology. This is known as *Analytical Epidemiology*. Analytical studies help in developing programs and policies for sound health.

Measurement Tools in Epidemiology

The epidemiology usually expresses disease magnitude as a rate, ratio or proportion. A clear understanding of these is required for proper interpretation of an epidemiological data. Their description is as follows:

1. Rate: Rate measures the occurrence of any particular event in a population during a given period of time. It also indicates change in events that takes place in a population over a period of time. For example, births, deaths, etc.

$$\text{Rate (say death rate)} = \frac{\text{No. of events (say deaths) in one year}}{\text{population examined}} \times 1000$$

The rates are usually expressed per thousands and rarely per ten-thousands. The rates are further categorized as:

a. *Crude rates:* These are the unstandardized, actually observed rates that refer to the whole population. For example, birth and death rates.

b. *Specific rates:* These are the actual observed rates due to specific causes or occurring in specific groups or during specific periods or in a specified sub population.

c. *Standardized rates:* These are obtained by direct or indirect methods of standardization or adjustments. For example, age/sex standardized rates.

2. Ratio: Ratio expresses a relation between two random quantities. It is calculated by dividing one quantity with another. For exmaple, sex ratio, dentist-population ratio, child-woman ratio, etc.

3. Proportion: A proportion is a ratio which indicates the relation in magnitude of a part to the whole. The numerator is always included in the denominator. This is expressed as percentage.

$$\text{Proportion} = \frac{\text{No. of children with caries of 1st molars at a certain time}}{\text{Total number of children population}} \times 100$$

The **numerator** refers to the number of times an event has occurred in a population during a specified time period. The numerator is a component of the denominator in calculating a rate, but not in ratio. Numerator has little meaning unless it is related to the denominator. The epidemiologist has to choose an appropriate **denominator** while calculating a rate. It may be related to:

a. population
b. total events.

a. *Related to population:* The denominator related to population comprises the following:

- *Mid year population:* The 1st of July in any year is considered as the mid year population. This is because the population keeps on changing on account of births, deaths, migrations, etc.

- *Population at risk:* It means the population which is capable of having or acquiring the disease in question. The term is applied to all those to whom the event has happened or may happen.

- *Person-time*: In some epidemiological studies, e.g. cohort studies, a person may enter the study at different times. They are under observation for varying time periods. The most frequently used person-time is person-years. Sometimes this may be person-months, person-weeks and so on. These denominators have the advantage of summarizing the experience of persons with different duration of exposures or observations.

- *Person-distance:* A variant of person-time is person-distance, e.g. passenger miles.
- *Subgroups of the population:* The denominator may be subgroups of a population, e.g. age, sex, occupation, social status, etc.

b. *Related to total events:* In some instances, the denominator may be related to total events instead of the total population, e.g. in case of accidents, 'per thousand vehicles' or 'per million vehicles' would be more useful denominator rather than the total population.

Measurements in Epidemiology

The principle measurements used in epidemiology are *incidence* and *prevalence*. Another commonly used term is *Morbidity*, which is used to describe the percentage of a population suffering from a disease at any particular time. The term morbidity merely indicates the presence/absence of the disease. It does not give information about the severity, intensity of spread, extent and consequences of the disease process.

1. **Incidence:** It measures the rate of appearance of new cases in a population.

The incidence of a disease annually is expressed as:

$$\frac{\text{Number of persons in a population at risk during a given year who newly manifest the disease}}{\text{Average number of population in that year}} \times 1000$$

Incidence, therefore gives the frequency of new events or the first attacks.

In clinically presenting disease, the incidence may be accepted as the first appearance of a defined symptom. In malignant disease, the date of diagnosis is often accepted as the date of onset.

In subclinical disease, the detection of signs of a disease is considered as the onset.

2. **Prevalence:** Prevalence is defined as the number of cases of a disease at a specific time within a community or population. The prevalence is further described as:

- *Instantaneous/spot prevalence:* The prevalence of a disease calculated at a particular moment of time.
- *Period prevalence:* The number of cases of a disease which occur during a specified period of time. For example, weekly, monthly or annual.
- *Point prevalence:* The assessment is made at a specific point of time rather than over a period.
- *Prevalence rate:* The number of patients who have the disease at a particular time, divided by the population at risk of having the disease at that time gives the prevalence rate.

The prevalence is usually calculated for one point or cross section in time. The more chronic the condition, the greater is the difference between incidence and prevalence. The **point prevalence rate** of a disease is:

$$\frac{\text{Number of persons who manifest the disease at a given time in a defined population}}{\text{Number of persons in that population at that time}} \times 1000$$

The period prevalence may be calculated for a year. This is the proportion of the population manifesting the disease over the course of year; those already showing it at the beginning (point prevalence) plus the new cases and the relapses which occur subsequently.

The denominator is the average number in the population that has been studied during the same year.

The *attack rate* refers to the number of persons in the population at risk having a first or later attack during a stated period.

ANALYTICAL EPIDEMIOLOGICAL STUDIES

The analytical studies deal with individuals within the population. Although individuals are evaluated in such studies, the inference is drawn for the total population from which they are selected.

Two distinct types of such studies are:
A. Case control study
B. Cohort study

Each of these studies determine:
   i. Whether or not a statistical association exists between a disease and a suspected factor.
   ii. The strength of the association, if present, between a disease and suspected factor.

A. Case Control Study

These studies are also known as 'retrospective studies'. These are used to test the hypothesis. The case control studies have the following features:
   i. Both exposure and outcome of the disease have occurred before the start of the study.
   ii. The study proceeds from effect to cause.
   iii. It uses a control group to support or refuse an inference.

Case control studies are basically comparison studies. Cases and controls must be comparable with known factors such as age, sex, occupation, social status, etc. One can use children with local fluoride application as cases and children who have not been given such applications as control. These studies have their major use in the chronic diseases when the causal pathway may extend up to decades. The basic framework of the case control study is depicted in Table 11.1.

There are four basic steps in conducting a case control study:
1. Selection of cases and controls
2. Matching
3. Measurement of exposure
4. Analysis and interpretation

1. Selection of cases and controls: The first step is the selection of suitable group of cases and controls.

Case selection: The cases are selected according to following two criteria:

i. Diagnostic criteria: The 'diagnostic criteria' of the disease must be specified before the study is undertaken. Once the diagnostic criteria are determined, they should not be altered till the study is over.

ii. Eligibility criteria: The newly diagnosed cases within a specified period of time are eligible to be a part of study. The old cases or cases in advanced stages of the disease are usually not taken. The selected cases should fairly represent all cases present in the community.

Control selection: The 'controls' must be free from the disease under study. Difficulty may arise in the selection of controls if the disease under investigation occurs in subclinical forms whose diagnosis is difficult. Selection of an appropriate control group is therefore an important prerequisite because all inferences are drawn and judged against this.

Table 11.1: Framework of a case control study

Risk factors or suspected cases	Cases (disease present)	Control (disease absent)
Present	a	b
Absent	c	d
	a + c	b + d

The controls can be taken from relatives or from neighbours living in the same locality, persons working in the same factory or children attending the same school.

The selection of cases and controls is crucial to the interpretation of the results. Failure to select comparable controls can introduce 'bias' into the results of these studies.

2. *Matching:* Matching is defined as the process by which one selects controls similar to cases with regard to certain selected variables; for example, age. These variables definitely influence the outcome of the disease and if not matched properly, can distort the results. The controls may differ from the cases in a number of factors such as age, sex, occupation, social status, etc.

Different kinds of matching procedures are:

i. *Group matching:* Group matching is carried out by assigning cases to sub-categories based on their characteristics; for example, age, occupation, social status, etc. The frequency distribution of the matched variables must be similar in a particular study and those of the comparison groups.

ii. *Matching by pairs:* Matching by pairs means for each case, a control is chosen which is matched closely to it. For example, a 40 year old male with a particular disease in a given occupation and a 40 year old male of the same occupation without that disease as a control. Pairs can be matched by age/sex or severity of illness, etc.

3. *Measurement of exposure:* Information about exposure is as important as defining cases and controls. The required information may be obtained by interviews, questionnaires or studying past records of cases.

4. *Analysis and interpretation:* The following two features are to be analyzed:

i. Exposure rates among cases and controls

ii. Estimation of disease risk associated with exposure

i. *Exposure rates:* A case control study provides a direct estimation of the exposure rates (frequency of exposure) to a suspected factor in disease and non disease groups. Table 11.2 shows how exposure rates may be calculated from a case control study.

The results show that the frequency of oral cancer is definitely higher among betel chewers than among non-betel chewers.

ii. *Estimation of disease risk:* The second step is the estimation of disease risk associated with exposure. It is obtained by an index known as *Relative Risk (RR)* or *risk ratio,* which is defined as the ratio between the incidence of disease among exposed persons and incidence among non-exposed.

$$\text{Relative risk (risk ratio)} = \frac{\text{Incidence among exposed}}{\text{Incidence among non-exposed}}$$

Table 11.2: A case control study of betel chewing and oral cancer

		Cases with Oral Cancer)	Control (without Oral Cancer)
Betel Chewers		21 (a)	48 (b)
Non Betel Chewers		4 (c)	30 (d)
Total		25 (a + c)	78 (b + d)
Exposure rates	a. Cases = a/(a+c)	= 21/25 = 84%	
	b. Controls = b/(b+d)	= 48/78 = 61.5%	

A typical case control study does not provide incidence rates from which the relative risk can be calculated directly, because there is no appropriate denominator or population at risk to calculate these rates. The relative risk however can be determined from a cohort study.

ODDS RATIO

Odds ratio is a measure of the strength of the association between risk factor and outcome. Odds ratio is closely related to risk ratio. The deviations of Odds ratio are based on following three assumptions:

- A disease being investigated must be relatively rare.
- The cases must be representatives of the individuals with the disease.
- The controls must be representatives of the individuals without the disease.

The Odds ratio is represented in Table 11.3.

Table 11.3: Odds ratio		
	Diseases	
	Yes	*No*
Exposed	a	b
Not exposed	c	d

Odds Ratio = ad/bc

Using the data in Table 11.2,

Odds Ratio = ad/bc = 21 × 30/48 × 4 = 6.5

This shows that betel nut chewers show a risk of oral cancer 6.5 times more than that of non betel nut chewers.

BIAS IN CASE CONTROL STUDIES

Bias is any systematic error in the association between the control and the case groups. The Relative Risk estimate may increase or decrease as a result of the bias. It reflects some type of non comparability between the study and the control.

Many varieties of bias may arise, which can be:

a. Bias due to confounding.
b. Memory or recall bias.
c. Selection bias.
d. Berkesonian bias.
e. Interviewer's bias.

a. Bias due to confounding: Certain features are deleterious to some diseases. This can affect independently and also in combination with other factors. Such factors form the basis of bias due to confounding.

A *confounding factor* is one which is associated both with exposure and disease. For example, in the study of role of alcohol in oral cancer, smoking is a confounding factor because (i) it is associated with alcoholism and (ii) it is also an independent risk factor for oral cancer.

In such cases, the effect of alcohol can be determined only when effect of smoking is neutralized by matching.

b. Memory or recall bias: The past history of cases and controls should be comparable. In case they differ in recall of their past events, that leads to bias known as memory or recall bias.

c. Selection bias: The cases and controls may not be representatives of the general population. There may be systematic differences in characteristics between cases and controls. Care should be taken during selection.

d. Berkesonian bias: It has been termed after Dr. Joseph Berkeson who recognized this problem. It is because of different rates of admission to hospitals for people with different diseases, i.e. hospital cases and controls.

e. Interviewer's bias: Bias may occur when the interviewer knows the hypothesis to be evaluated. The prior information may lead him to question the cases more thoroughly than controls regarding a positive history of the suspected causal factor.

In such cases, the trial should be so planned that neither the doctor nor the participant is aware of the group allocation and the treatment received.

Advantages (Case Control Study)

- Relatively easy to carry out.
- Rapid and inexpensive.
- Comparatively few subjects are required.
- Particularly suitable to investigate rare diseases.
- Risk to subjects is minimum.
- Allows the study of several different etiological factors.
- Risk factors can easily be identified.
- Does not require follow up of individuals in the future.
- Ethical problems are minimal.

Disadvantages (Case Control Study)

- Problems of bias.
- Selection of an appropriate control group may be difficult.
- Only the relative risk is estimated, the incidence cannot be measured.
- Does not distinguish between causes and associated factors.
- Not suited to the evaluation of therapy or prophylaxis of disease.
- The cases and controls may not be truly representative.

B. Cohort Study

Cohort studies are usually undertaken to obtain additional evidence to refute or support the existence of an association between suspected causes and the disease.

The term 'cohort' is defined as a group of people who share common characteristics or experience within a defined time period (e.g. age, occupation, exposure) to a drug or vaccine. Examples of cohort are:

Birth Cohort

A group of people born on the same day, or in the same year, forms a birth cohort. For example, all those born in 1997 form the birth cohort of 1997.

Exposure Cohort

Persons exposed to a common drug, vaccine or infection within a defined period, form an exposure cohort.

Marriage Cohort

A group of males and females married on the same day or in the same period of time constitute a marriage cohort.

Features of Cohort Studies

The distinguishing features of these studies are:

    i. The cohorts are identified prior to the appearance of the disease under investigation.

    ii. The study groups so defined are observed over a period of time to determine the frequency of disease among them.

    iii. The study proceeds forwards from cause to effect.

Indications

The indications of Cohort studies are:

- When there is good evidence of an association between the exposure and disease as derived from clinical observations.
- When exposure is rare, but the incidence of disease is high among the exposed, e.g. exposure to industries, exposure to x-rays, etc.
- When follow up is easy.

Framework of a Cohort Study

The cohort study proceeds from cause to effect, i.e. exposure has occurred but the disease has not. The basic design of a simple cohort study shown in Table 11.4 begins with a group or cohort (a+b) exposed to a particular factor thought to be related to disease occurrence, and a group (c+d) not exposed to that particular factor. The former is known as *study cohort* and the latter as *control cohort*.

Table 11.4: Framework of a cohort study

Cohort	Diseases		Total
	Yes	No	
Exposed to putative etiologic factor	A	b	a + b
Not Exposed to putative etiologic factor	C	d	c + d

The following features are important for assembling cohorts:

a. The cohort must be free from the disease. The members who have the evidence of the disease are excluded.
b. Both the groups, i.e. study and control cohorts should be equally susceptible to the disease (keeping in mind the present knowledge of the disease).
c. Both the groups should be comparable in respect to all the possible variables, which may influence the frequency of the disease.
d. The diagnostic and eligibility criteria must be defined.

The groups are then followed under the same identical conditions over a period of time to determine the outcome of the exposure (e.g. onset of disease, disability or death) in both the groups. In chronic disease, the follow up time should be prolonged.

Types of Cohort Studies

Three types of cohort studies have been distinguished on the basis of time of occurrence of disease and the time at which the investigation is initiated and continued.

- Prospective cohort studies
- Retrospective cohort studies
- A combination of retrospective and prospective cohort studies

Prospective Cohort Studies

A prospective cohort study is also called 'Current' cohort study in which the outcome or disease has not occurred at the time the investigation begins.

Retrospective Cohort Studies

A retrospective cohort study is also called Historical; cohort study in which the outcome or disease has occurred before the start of investigation.

Combination of Retrospective and Prospective Cohort Studies

In this type of study, both the retrospective and prospective elements are combined. The cohort is identified from past records and is assessed to date for the outcome. The same cohort is followed up prospectively into future for further assessment of outcome.

Elements of a Cohort Study

The elements of a cohort study are:
1. Selection of study subjects.
2. Obtaining data on exposure.
3. Selection of comparison groups.
4. Follow up.
5. Analysis.

1. Selection of Study Subjects

The selection is usually carried out:

a. Either from the general population, or
b. Special groups of population (persons with different degrees of exposure to the suspected causal factor).

a. *General population:* When exposure or cause of death is fairly frequent in population, cohort may be assembled from the general population residing in well-defined geographical, political and administrative areas. If the population is large, an appropriate sample of the population is taken. The exposed and unexposed segments of the population to be studied should be a representative of the corresponding segment of the general population.

b. *Special groups:* The special groups amongst the population can be assembled from either of the following:

i. *Select groups:* These may be professional groups (e.g. doctors, nurses, lawyers, teachers, civil servants), insured persons, obstetric population, college alumni, government employees, volunteers, etc. These refer to a homogenous population.

ii. *Exposure groups:* These may be groups exposed to physical, chemical and other disease agents, e.g. radiologists exposed to x-rays, workers in the industries, etc.

2. Obtaining Data on Exposure

The information about exposure may be obtained as follows:

i. *Information can be obtained directly from:*
   - Cohort members
   - Through personal interviews
   - Through mailed questionnaires.

ii. *Review of records:* The requisite information, for example dose of radiation, types of medication or details of treatment can be obtained from record books.

iii. *Medical examination/tests:* Some types of information can be obtained only by medical examination or special tests; for example, blood pressure, serum cholesterols, ECG, fasting glucose level in blood, etc.

iv. *Environmental surveys:* This is the best way of obtaining information on exposure levels of the suspected factors in the environment where cohort lived and worked.

3. Selection of Comparison Groups

There are many ways of assembling comparison groups:

a. *Internal comparisons:* In case of cohort studies, the comparison groups are inbuilt, i.e. there is no comparison group from outside. On the basis of information obtained, the members may be classified into several comparison groups according to the degrees or levels of exposure.

b. *External comparisons:* In some cohort studies, outside comparison groups are required. When the available information on the degree of exposure is not satisfactory, it is necessary to have an external control for comparison.

c. *Comparison with general population rates:* In rare instances, if internal and external comparison groups are not available, the mortality of the exposed group is compared with the mortality experience of the general population in the same geographic area.

4. Follow up

In cohort study, it is necessary to carry out the regular follow up of all the participants. The procedures comprise of the following:

a. Periodic medical examination of each member of the cohort.

b. Reviewing physician and hospital records.

c. Routine surveillance of death records.

d. Mailed questionnaires, telephone calls, periodic home visits, preferably all three on an annual basis.

However, despite the best efforts, certain percentage of losses to follow up are due to: death, change of residence, migration or withdrawal of occupation, etc. These losses may bias the results.

5. Analysis

The data is analyzed in terms of:

a. Incidence rates.

b. Estimation of risk.

a. *Incidence rates:* In cohort study, incidence rates are determined directly in exposed and unexposed subjects. For example, incidence rates in betel nut chewers and non betel nut chewers are given in the Table 11.5.

b. Estimation of risk: After calculating the incidence rate, estimate the risk of outcome, e.g. disease or death in exposed and unexposed cohorts. The risk is estimated in terms of two indices, i.e.

- Relative Risk
- Attributable Risk

Relative Risk (RR) is the ratio of the incidence of disease (or death) among exposed and the incidence among non exposed cohorts.

$$\text{Relative risk} = \frac{\text{Incidence of disease (or death) among exposed}}{\text{Incidence of disease (or death) among non exposed}}$$

Estimation of relative risk is important in etiological enquiries. It is a direct measure (or index) of the 'strength' of the association between suspected cause and affect. A Relative Risk of one (1) indicates 'No' association. Relative Risk greater than one, suggests 'Positive' association between the exposure and the disease under study.

Attributable Risk is the difference in incidence rates of disease (or death) between an exposed group and non exposed group. It can also be termed as the risk difference. It is expressed as percentage. The formula is:

$$\frac{\text{Incidence of disease rate among exposed} - \text{Incidence of disease rate among non-exposed}}{\text{Incidence rate among exposed}} \times 100$$

The attributable risk indicates the disease under study can we attributed to the exposure.

Advantages (Cohort Study)

- Incidence can be calculated.
- Several possible outcomes related to exposure can be studied simultaneously.
- Cohort studies provide a direct estimate of relative risk.
- Dose response ratios can also be calculated.
- Since comparison groups are formed before disease develops, certain forms of bias can be minimized like misclassification of individuals into exposed and unexposed groups.

Disadvantages (Cohort Study)

- Cohort studies involve a large number of people.
- It takes a long time to complete the study and obtain results.
- Certain administrative problems such as lack of experienced staff, lack of funding and extensive record keeping are inevitable.
- Loss of substantial proportion of the original cohort - they may migrate, lose interest in the study or simply refuse to provide any required information.
- Selection of comparison groups (exposed and unexposed) is a limiting factor.
- There may be changes in the standard method or diagnostic criteria of the disease over prolonged follow up.
- Cohort studies are expensive.

Table 11.5: Hypothetical betel nut chewing and oral cancer			
Betel nut chewers	*Developed oral cancer*	*Did not develop oral cancer*	*Total*
Yes	70 (a)	6930 (b)	7000 (a + b)
No	3 (c)	2997 (d)	3000 (c + d)

Incidence rates
a. Among betel nut chewers = 70/7000 = 10 per 1000
b. Among non betel nut chewers = 3/3000 = 1 per 1000

- The study itself may alter people's behaviour.
- With any cohort study, we are faced with ethical problems of varying importance.
- In a cohort study, practical considerations indicate that we must concentrate on a limited number of factors possibly related to disease outcome.

Main differences between case control and cohort studies are as follows:

Case control study	Cohort study
1. Proceeds from 'effect to cause'.	Proceeds from 'cause to effect'.
2. Starts with the disease.	Starts with people exposed to risk factor or suspected cause.
3. Tests whether the suspected cause occurs more frequently in those with the disease than those without the disease.	Tests whether the disease occurs more frequently in those exposed, than in those not exposed to particular risk factor.
4. Usually the first approach to the testing of a hypothesis, but also useful for exploratory studies.	Reserved for testing of precisely formulated hypothesis.
5. Involves fewer number of subjects	Involves larger number of subjects.
6. Yields relatively quick results.	Generally long follow up period required, leading to delayed results.
7. Suitable for the study of rare diseases.	Inappropriate when the disease or exposure under investigation is rare.
8. Generally yields only estimate of Odds Ratio.	Yields incidence rates, relative risk and attributable risk.

Contd...

Case control study	Cohort study
9. Cannot yield information about the disease other than that selected for study.	Can yield information about more than one disease outcome.
10. Relatively inexpensive.	Expensive.

EPIDEMIOLOGICAL SURVEYS

Health surveys are usually carried out to evaluate the state of the disease process in a community. The surveys bring out statistical information which provides rational basis for the improvement of health care. The resources should be related to knowledge of the needs of community. It is a function of epidemiology to supply the information, either from routine statistics or from special surveys. The principle is to start with the most readily available data and then to proceed on with special surveys. It is important to be aware of the limitations as well as the scope of each kind of survey. The routinely used surveys are as follows:

I. Simple Descriptive Surveys

The basic epidemiological description of any disease entity is derived from relating the characteristics of a group of cases such as age, sex, occupation to the related population. The common problem is defining the related population, which comprises those individuals who are rationally at risk. Related population may be defined by geographical location or time span. For example, all births occurring during one year or by taking one characteristic of individuals. For example, age, sex, race, etc. The starting point in identifying cases is to maintain the register after the diagnosis. All patients may not be receiving the same treatment or may not be able to go to hospitals, such situations complicate the epidemiological surveys.

II. Cross-sectional Population Surveys

These studies depend on a single examination of a cross-section of a population in contrast to longitudinal studies which trace changes in a population over a period of time. The aims of such studies are:

  i. Description and distribution of a disease in the community.
 ii. Study of cause of the disease.
iii. Screening of undiagnosed cases.

The essential difference between a simple descriptive survey and cross-sectional population survey is that in the latter, the study group is a sample of complete population including sick or unhealthy. Such surveys truly represent the disease entity in the whole community.

The measure of disease frequency which a cross-sectional survey yields is 'Prevalence'. The terms cross-sectional survey and the prevalence survey are interchangeable. The probability of detecting a case disease is related to the disease's main duration and therefore the cross-sectional method is generally inappropriate for the study of acute conditions. The uncommon disorders are usually overlooked in these studies.

The main stages in the design and conduct of cross-sectional survey may be summarized as follows:

a. *Specify a precise aim:* A precise aim is specified which should be relevant to the practical problems studying the disease process. The correct size of the population needed, time, cost and other resources should be estimated in advance, since it is wasteful to start a study unless it is reasonably sure to achieve the aim.

b. *Definition of the study population:* The purpose of epidemiological studies is to measure the disease in a population. The persons in a given population are defined by some natural characteristics such as the area of residence, occupation, age and sex, etc. The term population is used in wider sense in epidemiological studies it is not only the people living in a particular area. An epidemiologist will term the particular population as the 'population of smokers' or the 'population of pan chewers', etc. Usually, the information is obtained from a sample of population and from that the general information can be drawn.

c. *Sample size:* The sample size is very important for any epidemiological survey. It should be considered before planning the survey process. Unplanned sample size may lead to unfruitful results. The sample size may be unrepresented, the size of this uncertainty being measured by the standard error of the prevalence rate, i.e.

$$SE = \sqrt{\frac{P(100 - P)}{n}}$$

where P = %age of affected persons
        n = Number in sample

It is noted that the sampling error depends on the prevalence of the condition. It is necessary to study the large sample for uncommon conditions rather than for common ones to achieve precision. The sampling error is proportional to the square root of the sample size. Small studies may not be able to identify the true state of the affairs, which may lead to false/negative conclusions.

Standard Error of Mean (SEM) is calculated as:

$$SEM = \sqrt{\frac{S^2}{n}}$$

Where S = Standard deviation subject wise
          n = Number of subjects.

Standard Error of Mean (SEM) is important in deciding the sample size.

d. *Recruitment of sample:* Taking appropriate sample in any population is important in any epidemiological study. Use of volunteers is usually convenient however, **volunteer samples** have been proved to be seriously biased. The principle of random sampling is that every person in the present population has a predetermined chance to be included in a sample. This becomes easier where an accurate and up to date age/sex register is maintained in a given population.

When the population has been enumerated, each individual is assigned a number and a sample is selected by use of random numbers. This constitutes a **simple random sample**. **Systematic sampling,** e.g. by taking every 8th / 9th (nth) sample on a list, may be less troublesome.

In order to obtain a representative sample of school children in a large city, it would be more convenient to first draw a random sample of schools. The sample of children can be selected from the schools already selected. This process is known as **multistage sampling**.

Another refinement in it is to draw a **stratified sample**. In a simple random sample a few of the subjects might be young, another few can be elderly and another few can be very old. In order to achieve even distribution among these categories, equal sized random samples should be drawn from within each stratum.

It is clear that the subject of sampling is not easy. Correct procedures should be followed for the success of any survey. Response rate is always important, though participation is voluntary. A small random sample should be taken from the non respondents and efforts should be made to encourage their participation.

e. *Methods of examination:* The ordinary methods of history taking and physical examination are usually not used in surveys. A standardized, simple and direct questionnaire is given to the individuals and their answers are recorded. The examinations should be carried out by experienced and trained examiners and whenever possible, two examiners should check to avoid observer variations.

f. *Records:* Since the number of subjects in any epidemiological survey is large, proper maintenance of records is necessary. The record form should be designed with the aim to have standardization speed and accuracy with which the results can be retrieved later.

The record starts with the subjects' serial number in the study. The same should be processed in the office for subsequent coding and data extraction. The record designs should be discussed with the statistician who will later be concerned with the analysis.

g. *Analysis:* The recorded results can be analyzed in various ways. Prevalence can be estimated in the study population as a whole. The results can be used to describe the range of normal variation in the population. The choice of the technique employed depends upon the size of the population and the other parameters taken. The results can be analyzed normally or by using computers. Various computer programs are available for carrying out such analyses.

III. Longitudinal Population Surveys

The observation on the given population over a period of time measures:
- The rate of occurrence of new cases (incidence).
- The association between initial characteristics and the risk of future disease.

The follow-up in any longitudinal study may take one of the several forms. The records of participants can be marked with a code. School records may be used to evaluate long term affects of complications on child growth and development.

Two problems usually arise in longitudinal studies. These are:

1. Because of an increasingly mobile population, maintaining of contact with study subjects over a long period of time is difficult.
2. The difficulty in maintaining stability of clinical and laboratory standards over a long period of time, since the staff keep on changing.

Longitudinal studies, usually have an added problem of sample size. The surveys are often large, lengthy and complex.

IV. Pathfinder Surveys

The pathfinder survey is a sampling technique, which aims to include the most important population subgroups, which is likely to have different disease levels. It also proposes appropriate numbers of subjects in specific index age groups. In this way, reliable and clinically relevant information for planning is obtained at minimum expense. The method is suitable for obtaining the following information:

- The overall prevalence of common oral diseases and conditions affecting the population.
- Variations in disease level, severity and need for treatment in subgroups of the population.
- Age profiles of oral diseases in the population to enable care needs for different age groups.
- The information about severity and progression of disease and provide indication as to whether the levels are increasing or decreasing.

Pathfinder surveys can be either pilot or national, depending on the number and type of sampling sites and the age groups selected.

A *pilot survey* is one that includes only the most important subgroups in the population and only one or two index ages (usually

12 years and one other age group). Such a survey provides the minimum amount of data sufficient to commence planning. Additional data should be collected in order to provide a reliable baseline for the implementation and monitoring of services.

A *national survey* incorporates sufficient examination sites to cover all important subgroups of the population that may have different disease levels or treatment needs, and at least three index ages. This type of survey design is suitable for the collection of data for the planning and monitoring of services. In a large country with many geographical and population subdivisions and a complex service structure, a large number of sampling sites are needed. The basic principle of using index ages and standard samples in each site within a stratified approach, however, remains valid.

The following method is recommended as a general guideline for basic oral health surveys for planning, monitoring and evaluation of oral care services.

Sub-groups

Sampling sites are usually chosen so as to provide information on population groups likely to have different levels of oral diseases. The sampling is usually based on the administrative divisions of a country—the capital city, main urban centers, small towns and rural areas; usually at least one sampling site in each area is selected.

If there are several distinct ethnic groups in the population with known, or suspected, differences in levels of oral disease, it may be necessary to include separate samples of each of these groups. It is necessary to know about variations between the different groups in order to limit the number of additional subsamples.

The assistance of local health administrators can be useful when the final decision is made as to which population subgroups are significant for the study and should be represented in the final sample. For a national pathfinder survey, 10 to 15 sampling sites are usually sufficient. If, however, there are large urban centers in the country, it may be necessary to locate additional sampling sites.

Index Age and Age Groups

The following age groups are recommended for examination 5 years for primary teeth and 12, 15, 35-44 and 65-74 years for permanent teeth.

- **5 years:** The children should be examined between their 5th and 6th birthdays; usually the child start schooling at this age. This age is of interest in relation to levels of caries in the primary dentition which may exhibit changes over a shorter time span than the permanent dentition at other index ages.

    In case the age group selected is 6–7 years, then the missing primary incisor teeth should not be scored as missing because of the difficulty in differentiating between primary incisors lost due to exfoliation and those lost because of caries or trauma.

- **12 years:** This age is important as it is generally the age at which children leave primary school. Also, it is likely at this age that all permanent teeth, except third molars, will have erupted. For these reasons, 12 year has been the *global monitoring age* for caries for international comparisons and monitoring of disease trends.

    In some countries, however, many school-age children do not attend school. In these circumstances, an attempt should be made to survey two or three groups of non-attenders, from different areas, in order to compare their oral health status with that of children attending school.

- **15 years:** At this age the permanent teeth have been exposed to the oral environment for pretty long time. The assessment of caries prevalence is therefore often more meaningful than at 12 years of age. This age is also important for the assessment of periodontal diseases in adolescents. In countries, where it is difficult to obtain reliable samples of this age group, it is usual to examine 15-year-olds in two or three areas only, i.e. in the capital city or an other large town, and in one rural area.

- **35–44 years (mean = 40 years):** This age group is the standard monitoring group for health conditions of adults. The full effect of dental caries, the level of periodontal involvement, and the general effects of care provided can be monitored using data from this age group. Sampling adult subjects is often difficult. Samples can, however, be drawn from organized groups, such as office or factory workers. Care must be taken to avoid obvious bias, such as sampling patients at medical care facilities.

- **65–74 years (mean = 70 years):** This age group has become more important with the changes in age distribution and increases in life span. Data for this group is needed both for planning appropriate care for the elderly and for monitoring the overall effects of oral care services in a population. Examination of members of this age group is often not as difficult as elderly people are more likely to be found in or near their homes.

BIBLIOGRAPHY

1. Ben-Shlomo, Y. and Kuh, D.: A life course approach to chronic diseases epidemiology : conceptual models, empirical challenges and interdisciplinary perspectives. Int. J. Epidem. : 31, 285, 2002.

2. Daniel, C. and Richmond, S.: The development of the index of complexity outcome and need (ICON). J. Orthodont. : 27, 149, 2000.

3. Destavola, B.L., Nitsch, D., dos Santos Silva, I., McCormack, V., Hardy, R. and Mann, V. :

Statistical issues in life course epidemiology. Am. J. Epidem. : 163, 84, 2006.

4. Firestone, A.R., Beck, F.M., Beglin, F.M. and Vig, K.W. : Validity of index of complexity outcome and need (ICON) in determining orthodontic needs. Augle Ortho. : 72, 15, 2002.

5. Nicolau, B., Marcenes, W., Bartley, M. and Sheiham, A. : Association between socio-economic circumstances at two stages of life and adolescents oral health status. J. Public Health Dent. ; 65, 14, 2005.

6. Namal, N. and Sheiham, A. : Comparison of ranking dental status using the significant caries index and the significant filled and sound-teeth index. Community Dental Health : 25, 103, 2008.

7. Namal, N., Vahid, S. and Sheiham, A. : Ranking countries by dental status using the DMFT and FS-T indices. International Dental Journal : 55, 373, 2005.

8. Nicolau, B., Marcenes, W., Hardy, R. and Sheiham, A. : A life course approach to assess the relationship between social and psychological circumstances and gingival status in adolescents. J. Clin. Periodontol. : 30, 1038, 2003.

9. Nicolau, B., Thomson, W.M., Steele, J.G. and Allison, P.J. : Life course epidemiology : concepts and theoretical models and its relevance to chronic oral conditions. Comm. Dent. Oral Epidem. : 35, 241, 2007.

10. Pearce, M.S., Steele, J.G., Mason, J., Walls, A.W. and Parker, L. : Do circumstances in early life contribute to tooth retention in middle age ? J.D.R. : 83, 562, 2004.

11. Susser, M. and Susser, E. : Choosing a future for epidemiology : 1. Eras and paradigms. Am. J. Public Health : 86, 668, 1996.

12. Susser, E. : Eco-epidemiology : thinking outside the black box. Epidemiology : 15, 519, 2004.

Indices are attempts to quantitate clinical conditions on a graduated scale that facilitate comparisons among populations examined by the same criteria and methods. Unlike the absolute or definitive diagnosis of disease that can be made in a solitary patient, an epidemiological index estimates only the relative prevalence or occurrence of the clinical condition. In general, indices are actually underestimates of a true clinical condition.

Russell has *defined* an index as 'a numerical value describing the relative status of a population on a graduated scale with definite upper and lower limits, that is designed to permit and facilitate comparison with other populations classified by the same criteria and method'.

An index has also been *defined* as 'an expression of clinical observation in numerical values which is used to describe the status of the individual or group with respect to a condition being measured'.

Oral indices are essential sets of values, usually numerical, with maximum and minimum units used to describe variables as specific conditions on a graduated scale, which use the same criteria and methods to compare specific variables in individuals, samples or population with the same variables as found in other individuals, samples or populations.

Properties of an Ideal Index

The purpose of any index is two-fold. Firstly, an index should make an accurate assessment of the extent and severity of the diseased state and compare the diseased status among individuals, communities, etc. Secondly, it should assess the efficiency of preventive or curative measures undertaken to overcome the disease. An ideal index should have the following properties:

1. **Simplicity:** An ideal index should be simple, easy to perform and understand.
2. **Validity:** The validity of index relies on its ability to detect either the presence or absence of a disease. The two components that describe the validity of an index are sensitivity and specificity.
   a. **Sensitivity:** It is the ability to identify the 'true positive cases', i.e. the persons actually suffering from the disease. It is calculated as follows:

$$\text{Sensitivity} = \frac{\text{True positive}}{\text{True positive} + \text{false negative}}$$

   b. **Specificity:** It is the ability to identify the persons who are actually not suffering from disease. It, thus, identifies the 'true negative cases'.

$$\text{Specificity} = \frac{\text{True negative}}{\text{True negative} + \text{false positive}}$$

3. **Reliability:** An ideal index should give reliable results if it is performed by different examiners under the same conditions. The term reliability can be used as a synonym of *reproducibility*, which means the ability to record, interpret and use of a particular index in the similar way. Reliability is determined by:
   a. **Intra-examiner reliability:** If the *same examiner* records the same results every

time and performs the index under similar conditions then it is termed as intra-examiner reliability.

b. **Inter-examiner reliability:** If *different examiners* record the same result every time and perform the index under similar conditions, the term inter-examiner reliability is used.

4. **Precisibility:** An index should be small and precise in its measurement so that it becomes easy for an individual to understand the need and importance of recording it.

5. **Objectivity:** An index should be unambiguous and clearly demarcate the presence or absence of a condition without any confusion.

6. **Quantifiability:** An index should be quantifiable and amenable to statistical analysis if needed.

7. **Acceptability:** The index should not be painful or traumatic to an individual. He should understand that the procedure is to be performed for his benefit and he should accept it with his full consent.

In true sense, there is not even a single index that satisfies all the needs of an ideal index. It is the duty of an examiner to record the particular situation by using the best possible index for that situation.

Purpose and Uses of an Index

The purpose and uses of an index depend on the motive behind the performance of an index. If an index is performed for:

i. **An individual:** It has following uses:

a. **Assessment:** An index can be used for recognition and assessment of the oral conditions of an individual by the dentist.

b. **Motivation:** An individual can be motivated so as to modify the index score for his benefit.

c. **Effectiveness:** It can be used to judge the effectiveness of oral hygiene practices performed and to be performed by him.

d. **Personal assessment:** A simple index can even be used by the individual for his/her assessment after he/she takes appropriate measures to prevent any oral disease; like use of disclosing agent for oral hygiene assessment.

ii. **For research:** In the field of research, an index can be used for:

a. **Determination of baseline:** It can be used to determine the baseline data before the introduction of experimental factors.

b. **Effectiveness of specific agents:** An index can be used to measure the effectiveness of specific agents—chemical (mouthwashes, drugs, etc.) or mechanical (toothbrushes, water irrigators, etc.) in controlled clinical trials.

iii. **In community health programs:** In community health programs, index can be used:

a. To assess the treatment needs of a community.

b. To record the incidence and prevalence of a particular disease in a particular community.

c. To provide baseline data for the existing dental problems.

d. To compare the effects of community health programs.

e. To evaluate the results of previous and present health programs.

Classification of Dental Indices

Dental indices are classified in the following ways:

A. Based on the *nature of disease* to be assessed, indices are classified as follows:

i. *Irreversible indices:* These indices assess the permanent damage caused by an active disease process that cannot be reversed to zero even after the disease has be2en cured completely.

The most typical feature of an irreversible index is that it assesses the damage caused by the disease rather than the disease itself. The DMF index for dental caries is an excellent example of an irreversible index as it only takes into consideration open cavities (D), filled cavities (F) and missing teeth (M). A carious lesion can never heal itself in the similar way as common cold, leaving no signs of disease behind it. Though, a carious (D) lesion can be filled (F) but this change does not lead to the overall reversal of the DMF score.

ii. *Reversible indices:* The reversible indices, as the name implies, returns to zero when the measured disease for some reason or the other, disappears. These indices are unlike the irreversible indices, which assess the permanent damage caused by the active disease; for example, PMA index, OHI, etc.

iii. *Composite indices:* The composite indices are a combination of reversible and irreversible aspects of the disease; for example, Periodontal Index by *Russell*. One class of index is exclusively concerned with the clinical signs of active gingival inflammation (Gingival index); while another class takes into account the destruction of the tissues as indicated by pocket deepening and bone resorption (Periodontal index).

B. Depending upon the *areas of the oral cavity* to be assessed, the indices are classified as:

i. *Full mouth indices:* These indices measure the whole dentition or its supporting tissues, for example, DMF index, Russell's periodontal index

ii. *Simplified indices:* These indices measure only a part of the dentition or its supporting tissues; for example, OHI-S index.

C. The indices have also been categorized as follows:

i. **General category indices:** These are sub-categorized as:

a. *Disease index:* An index that assesses the disease process, for example, D-component of DMF, DMFS or def index.

b. *Sign or symptom index:* An index that assesses a particular sign or symptom of a disease; for example, indices used to assess gingival bleeding, SBI, PBI, GBI, etc.

c. *Treatment index:* An index that assesses the treatment needed or treatment done in an individual; for example, CPITN, F-component of DMF, DMFS, etc.

ii. **Special categories:** The special categories are sub-classified as:

a. *Simple index:* A simple index is the one that detects the presence or absence of a condition presentable at the time of examination without assessing its effect on an individual; for example, the OHI only detects the amount of debris present on the teeth at the time of examination.

b. *Cumulative index:* These indices measure all the past and present evidences of a condition; for example, PMA, DMF index, etc.

D. Depending upon the disease to be assessed, the dental indices are classified in a manner as depicted in Table 12.1.

INDICES FOR ASSESSMENT OF DENTAL CARIES

The indices used to assess dental caries are categorized into (a) for permanent teeth (b) for primary teeth and (c) for both permanent and primary teeth.

INDICES USED FOR EVALUATING CARIES IN PERMANENT DENTITION

The indices used for evaluating caries in permanent teeth are:

DMF or DMFT (Decayed, Missing, Filled, Teeth Index)

The index was developed to record the prevalence of coronal caries in permanent teeth.

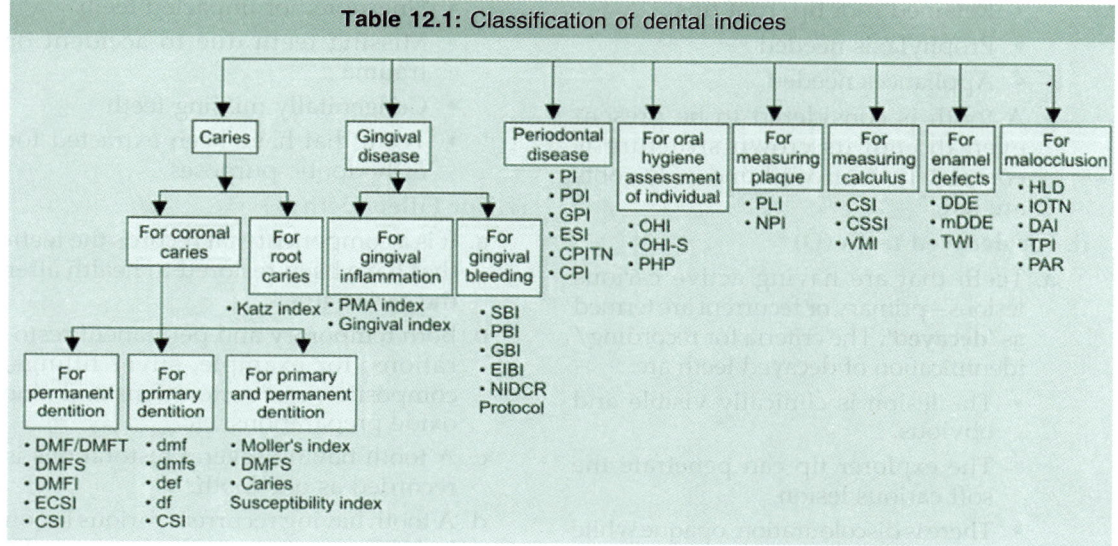

Table 12.1: Classification of dental indices

It is an *irreversible, cumulative index* and records the past and present caries experiences.

It expresses the sum of Decayed (D), Missing (M), Filled (F), Teeth (T), present per person.

Rules to be followed for recording DMF: There are certain rules that are to be followed while recording DMF index for an individual. These are as follows:

i. General

a. All the 28 permanent teeth are included.

b. No tooth should be recorded more than once. A single tooth can either be decayed, missing or filled - never all the three.

c. Deciduous teeth are not included in the DMF count.

d. A tooth is considered to be erupted when the occlusal or incisal angle is either totally exposed or can be exposed by gently reflecting the overlying gingival tissue with a mirror or explorer.

e. The teeth *not* included are:
  • Third molars (see WHO modifications)
  • Unerupted teeth

• Congenitally missing teeth
• Supernumerary and supplemental teeth
• Teeth removed for reasons other than dental caries; for example, orthodontic treatment, impacted or teeth lost during accidents.
• Teeth restored for reasons other than dental caries; for example, trauma, cosmetic purposes, bridge abutments, etc.
• Retained primary teeth regardless of whether the permanent successor has erupted or not. As DMF is a permanent teeth index, if the successor is erupted it is recorded in place of primary tooth.

f. The following criteria should be considered while determining the care needed:
  • Tooth decay
  • Gingival decay
  • Malocclusion
  • Abscess

- Retained root tip/root tips
- Prophylaxis needed
- Appliances needed

g. A tooth is considered to be present even though its crown structure is completely destroyed and only roots are left.

ii. For decayed teeth (D)

a. Teeth that are having active carious lesions – primary or recurrent are termed as **'decayed'**. The criteria for recording/identification of decayed teeth are:
- The lesion is clinically visible and obvious.
- The explorer tip can penetrate the soft carious lesion.
- There is discolouration, opaque white area showing the loss of translucency.
- There can be undermining or demineralization of enamel, marginal ridges, etc.
- There is a definite catch in the pit or fissure.

b. The tooth having recurrent caries under the restoration should be recorded as decayed and not filled.

c. Teeth that are grossly decayed to such an extent that they cannot be restored and must be extracted are not recorded as decayed – they are part of (M) component.

iii. For missing teeth (M)

a. The 'M' component includes those teeth that are lost due to caries. These are the teeth that have either been extracted or lost themselves due to caries. It is the component that is *most likely to give the false scores*.

b. It also includes the teeth that are grossly decayed and are beyond the limit of restoration.

c. The following teeth are not counted as missing:

- Unerupted or impacted teeth
- Missing teeth due to accident or trauma
- Congenitally missing teeth
- Teeth that have been extracted for orthodontic purposes.

iv. For Filled teeth (F)

a. It is a component that records the teeth that have been restored to health after the caries attack.

b. Both temporary and permanent restorations; for example, silver fillings, composites, cast restorations and zinc oxide preparations, etc.

c. A tooth having several restorations is recorded as one tooth.

d. A tooth having recurrent carious lesion is *NOT* counted as filled; it is a 'D' component.

Procedure

In DMFT index the permanent teeth are examined for three components: Decayed (D), Missing (M) and Filled (F) teeth.

Examination is carried out under adequate lighting conditions using No.3 plain mirror and a fine, pointed pig tail explorer.

Criteria for Coding

The examined teeth are coded as follows (Table 12.2).

Table 12.2: Coding criteria for DMFT

Code	Criteria
E	Excluded tooth or tooth space
O	Missing tooth – unerupted, impacted, congenitally missing
1	Sound permanent teeth
2	Filled permanent teeth
3	Decayed permanent teeth
X	Extracted permanent teeth

Calculation of index: The maximum number of an individual's DMFT score is 28 if 3rd molars are excluded or 32 if 3rd molars are included; for example, consider the following Fig. 12.1.

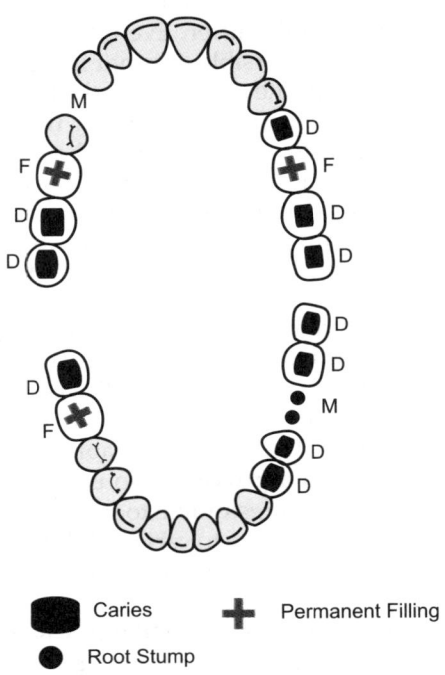

Caries   **+** Permanent Filling

Root Stump

Fig. 12.1: Example of DMFT

The above diagram depicts the oral cavity of a person from the occlusal aspect. Considering that no labial or lingual carious lesions are present and there are no recurrent carious lesions, the DMF score is calculated as follows:

- D (Decayed): These are

$$\frac{8\,7\ \big|\ 5\,7\,8}{7\ \big|\ 4\,5\,7\,8}$$

Thus, score for D is equal to 10.

- M (Missing):

$$\frac{4\ \big|}{\big|\ 6}$$

$\dfrac{4\ \big|}{\ }$ has been extracted due to caries; but

for $\dfrac{\big|}{\big|\ 6}$ as the tooth is grossly decayed (only root stumps remaining), so according to the rules it should be considered as 'M' component and not 'D'. Thus 'M' score is 2.

$\dfrac{\big|}{8\ \big|}$ is un-erupted in oral cavity (may be impacted), but as it is not missing due to caries it is not considered for scoring.

- F (Filled): As silver fillings are present in
$$\frac{6\ \big|\ 6}{\big|\ 6}$$
Thus, F score is 3. The **results** of scores obtained are compiled as follows:

- *Individual DMFT:* Here each component of D, M, F are recorded separately and then D + M + F is calculated, e.g. in above example. The DMFT score will be 10 + 2 + 3 = 15.

- *Group average:* Total DMF for each individual is calculated and then total is divided by total number of individuals in that group, i.e.

$$\text{Average DMF} = \frac{\text{Total DMF}}{\text{Total number of subjects examined}}$$

- *Percentage of care needed:* It is calculated by the calculation of 'D' component as follows:

$$\text{Percent of teeth lost} = \frac{\text{Total number of decayed teeth}}{\text{Total number of teeth examined}} \times 100$$

In the above example, percentage of care needed is 10/31 × 100 = 32.25%

- *Percent of teeth lost:* It is calculated by the calculation of 'M' component.

$$\text{Percent of teeth lost} = \frac{\text{Total number of missing teeth}}{\text{Total number of teeth examined}} \times 100$$

In the above case, percentage of teeth lost is $2/31 \times 100 = 6.45\%$

- *Percent of filled teeth:* It is calculated from 'F' component as follows:

$$\text{Percent of filled teeth} = \frac{\text{Total number of filled teeth}}{\text{Total number of teeth examined}} \times 100$$

In above example, percentage of filled teeth is $3/31 \times 100 = 9.68\%$

- *Missing permanent teeth per 100 children:* To calculate missing permanent teeth per 100 children, one has to divide the number of missing teeth by the total number of teeth examined and then multiply by 100, i.e.

$$\text{MPT}/100 = \frac{\text{Total number of missing teeth}}{\text{Total number of teeth examined}} \times 100$$

Shortcomings

Various shortcomings/limitations of DMF index score are:

a. The main and the most controversial drawback of DMF index is that **it tends to equate a desired state with a treated condition**. A carious tooth as well as the filled tooth is given equal score of one, thus making no differentiation in the treatment provided; for example, a person with 4 teeth which need filling, will be equated with the person who has already 4 teeth filled. The DMF index for both would be 4. Consequently the DMF index never changes even after the treatment. The four teeth of the same individual even after filling remain at DMF = 4. The investigators who are in favour of equating a carious tooth with a filled tooth, are of the view that

the carious disease is an irreversible one and the tooth cannot be taken as normal after the filling. These investigators may be right but practically there cannot be any disease process which does not leave a scar, whether minor or major. Any infectious disease can cause organic damage though the extent might differ. Even if the disease process is irreversible, it is not irreparable. With appropriate restorations, the tooth can be restored to functions. Even though a correctly restored tooth cannot be equated to a normal tooth, it should never be equated to an untreated carious tooth. Such teeth should be considered as 'treated' rather that 'diseased'. Even loss of tooth should be taken as treated if sufficient prosthetic rehabilitation has been done.

b. It does not determine the efficacy of treatment in controlling the disease.

c. It equates different stages of carious distribution. The easily restorable pit caries is equated to a grossly carious non-restorable tooth or a restorable tooth equated to a tooth missing due to caries. All the three are given a score of one, which is not justifiable.

d. Another drawback of DMF index is that it fails to compensate for the prosthetic replacement of lost teeth.

e. It does not include the criteria for arrested carious lesions.

f. DMF index is not an efficient tool for assessing long term effects of preventive techniques.

g. It does not depict the number of teeth at risk.

h. It can become invalid in old age where teeth are frequently lost due to periodontal reasons.

i. Preventive fillings can give false values.

j. It cannot be used for root caries.

Modifications of DMF

1. *WHO modifications:* The WHO has modified DMF index twice as follows:

a. **In 1986,** The WHO modified DMF index and included that:
  i. All the third molars should be included thus increasing the maximum score from 28 to 32.
  ii. Temporary restorations are considered as decayed teeth – 'D'.
  iii. Only frank carious defects are considered in 'D' component and not the initial lesions like chalky spots, stained fissures, etc.
b. **In 1997,** The WHO again modified DMF index as follows:

Originally only teeth lost due to caries were considered; but in 1997, the WHO included that for individuals aged 30 years or older, M-component should comprise teeth missing due to caries or for any other reason while for individuals less than 30 years, M-component should include teeth missing due to caries only.

2. *Procedural modifications* can be made to allow for the study of factors such as secondary caries, crown teeth, bridge pontics, and or any particular attribute for study.

DMC_sC_d index

It is equivalent to DMF index, but F component is broken down into C_sC_d as follows:

D – Decayed
M – Missing
C_s - Conserved (filled) and sound
C_d – Conserved but with cavities present on same or any other surface

CLR Index

Karthikeyan has suggested a new index simplifying the DMF index. The *Carious, Lost, Restored index* (Table 12.3).

Scoring in CLR Index is carried out as follows:
  C – is given as score 1
  L – is given as score 1
  R – is given as score ½
An arrested carious lesion without structural loss is given as score of ½ (It is treated as a restored tooth).

Modified DMFT Index

The *Modified DMFT Index* involves the division of 'D' component of DMFT into 4 parts that are as follows:

'D' splits as:

C: Unfilled teeth, that are carious.

CF: Filled teeth, that are carious: the caries can be recurrent or secondary around the margins of restorations or primary caries on tooth surfaces other than restored ones.

IX: Filled or unfilled carious teeth that are indicated for extraction, e.g. caries has destroyed the coronal architecture to such an extent that it cannot be restored – the whole coronal structure is destroyed and only root stumps remained.

IRC: Filled or unfilled carious teeth that are indicated for root canal treatment, i.e. during the debridement of tooth the pulp exposure is inevitable and ultimate treatment will be RCT only.

Table: 12.3: CLR Index		
C (Carious)	L (Lost)	R (Restored)
It can further be subdivided into:	Teeth lost due to caries	Restorations can be of any type like:·
C – Restorable carious		• Fillings
I – Non-restorable teeth indicated		• Crowns
for extraction		• Root canal treatment
		• Bridges, dentures, etc.

Shorthand Methods of Determining DMF

Several shorthand methods of DMF examination are devised for use in large surveys for determining the basic prevalence of caries. These are:

a. *WHO method (Half mouth method):* Half of the upper arch and the contralateral half of the lower arch is scored and results are doubled. Its objective is to obtain caries prevalence in a population which has not been previously scored.

b. *McLendon method*: He described a short-hand method where only first molars and upper central incisors are recorded. Its objective is to study caries prevalence in areas where DMF has a moderate to high value.

c. *Viegas Method*: In this method, only lower left molars and upper central incisors are examined in an individual.

d. *Graiger's Method*: A hierarchical pattern method, in which individuals are classified in hierarchial pattern according to which sites in the mouth have been attacked; for example, caries on proximal surfaces of mandibular incisors in an individual is graded in zone 5 (most severe zone); while caries on the labial surfaces of lower incisors is graded in zone 4 and so on.

DMFS Index

It was given along with the DMFT index to assess the prevalence of coronal caries. The DMFS index was originally a purely clinical index for field studies. DMFS index is simple, versatile, universally accepted and one of the best known indices. DMFS stands for:

D – total number of decayed surfaces of an individual tooth

M – total number of missing surfaces for an individual tooth

F – total number of filled surfaces for an individual tooth

Total score = D + M + F

D + F can also be calculated.

Surfaces examined: The following surfaces are to be examined for DMFS:

1. For anterior teeth – 4 surfaces (buccal, mesial, lingual, distal)
2. For posterior teeth – 5 surfaces (buccal, mesial, lingual, distal, occlusal)

Maximum score: The maximum score value that can be obtained for DMFS is:

a. 128, If third molars are excluded

Anterior teeth surfaces:		
Total number of anterior teeth present (6 + 6 = 12)	× Surfaces examined for an individual single anterior tooth (4)	= 48
Posterior teeth surfaces:		
No. of posterior teeth (8+8=16)	× Surfaces calculated for single posterior teeth (5)	= 80

Maximum total surfaces = Anterior teeth surfaces + Posterior teeth surfaces examined for an individual

$$= 48 + 80 = 128$$

b. 148, If third molars are included

Maximum score for anterior teeth = 48		
Maximum score for posterior teeth =		
No. of posterior teeth (10 + 10 = 20)	× Surfaces calculated for single posterior tooth (5)	= 100

Maximum total surfaces = 48 + 100 = 148

Procedure

The examiner records the index at a well illuminated place using No.3 plane mirror and fine pointed explorer. One must proceed systematically, beginning in the maxillary quadrant and then examining the mandibular segment on the right side following similarly on the left side. On each tooth, the following order of surfaces is examined: facial-occlusal-lingual/palatal-distal-mesial. Initially, the teeth are examined primarily by sight, and an explorer is used only in cases of doubt. It is convenient to use numbers rather than letters of the alphabet. Firstly, the clinical determination is made for all surfaces and subsequently the proximal surfaces are further evaluated radiographically.

The components are:

i. D (Decayed = 1,2,3,4)

In DMFS, initial lesions (chalky spots) as well as frank lesions (carious defects) are counted. Cervical portion of the tooth crown should be checked thoroughly for white spots.

- Grading of lesion severity *for pits and fissures*
  - Grade 0 : Healthy
  - Grade 1 : Thin light line, chalky margin.
  - Grade 2 : Thin, brown to black line
  - Grade 3 : Frank defect less than 2.0 mm.
  - Grade 4 : Frank defect greater than 2.0 mm.
- Grading of lesion severity for *smooth surfaces (proximal surfaces)*
  - Grade 0 : Healthy
  - Grade 1 : Chalky spot less than 2.0 mm.
  - Grade 2 : Chalky spot greater than 2.0 mm.
  - Grade 3 : Frank defect less than 2.0 mm.
  - Grade 4 : Frank defect greater than 2.0 mm.
- *Radiographic grade* of lesion severity on *proximal surfaces*.
  - Grade 1 : Radiolucency in the outermost half of the enamel, initial lesion.
  - Grade 2 : Radiolucency also in the inner half of the enamel, no dentinal alterations.
  - Grade 3 : Radiolucency extending completely through enamel with evident radiolucency in peripheral dentin substance.
  - Grade 4 : Obvious dentin radiolucency, close to the pulp.

When radiographically detectable radiolucencies exist on pits and fissures or on smooth surfaces, one is always dealing with clinical grade 4 carious defects, i.e. with a large cavity.

ii. F (Filled – grade 5)

If a filling with secondary caries is detected on a tooth surface, a separate category 'D+F' may be employed or taken as decayed 'D'.

If a gold crown or post-crown is present:
on molars   : count all '5' surfaces.
on bicuspids: count only '3' surfaces.
on anteriors : count all '4' surfaces.

iii. M (Missing – grade 6)

The same rules as given for crowned teeth are applicable here.

iv. Unerupted (grade 7)

Recording of DMFS Index: Practically, DMFS can be recorded by two methods:

I. Clinical DMFS

DMFS index recorded visually or with the aid of an explorer is called as clinical DMFS. The procedure given below is for clinical DMFS (Fig. 12.2).

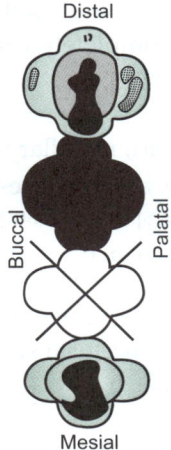

Fig.12.2: Example of DMFS calculation (clinical)

One should proceed systematically, beginning in the maxillary quadrant and then the mandibular segment on the right side following similarly on the left side. On each tooth, the following order of surfaces is examined. Facial-occlusal-lingual/palatal-distal-mesial. Initially, the teeth are examined primarily by sight, and an explorer is used only in case of doubt. It is convenient to use numbers rather than letters of the alphabet; for example,

0	= Means healthy
1,2,3,4	= Signify decay
5	= Means filled
6	= Means missing or extracted
7	= Means unerupted

Second molar, maxillary right (17)

Palatal : 5.0 mm chalky spot and carious defect < 2.0 mm score = 3.

Occlusal : Filling, score = 5.

Buccal : Chalky spot, score = 1

Distal : Healthy, score = 1

Mesial : Filling, score = 5

Write as : 3, 5, 1, 0, 5

First molar, maxillary right (16).
This tooth is completely restored.
Write as : 5, 5, 5, 5, 5

Second bicuspid, maxillary right (15)
This tooth, i.e. all 5 surfaces had to be removed. The space subsequently closed.
Write as : 6, 6, 6, 6, 6

First bicuspid, maxillary right (14)
The mesial and occlusal surfaces are filled.
Write as : 0, 5, 0, 0, 5

The findings can be entered in the form of rows and columns as:

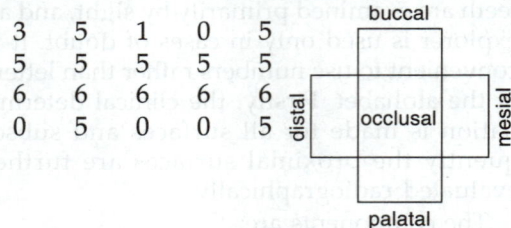

Fig. 12.3: Chart for recording clinical DMFS

II. Radiographic DMFS

The radiographic view in comparison to the clinical eye is better at diagnosing proximal caries, but is not very reliable in regard to occlusal and orofacial lesions. Sometimes, the proximal surfaces cannot be adequately examined because of the overlapping caused by X-ray projection or mal-alignment of teeth. In such cases an "x" is entered. Hence, *the final DMFS index is derived only from the clinical examination* (Fig. 12.4).

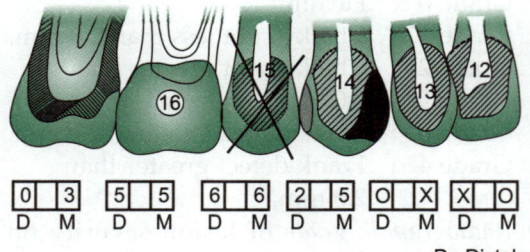

D : Distal
M : Mesial

Fig. 12.4: Example of DMFS calculation (radiographic)

Tooth No. 17 : For the mesial surface a "3" is entered instead of "5" because secondary caries of "grade 3" is noted beneath the filling.

Tooth No. 16 : Crowned distal and mesial surfaces, Hence enter 5,5

Tooth No. 15 : Missing , Hence enter 6,6

Tooth No. 14 : Proximal caries distally of Grade 2.

Tooth No. 13 & 12 : Due to overlapping, two proximal surfaces cannot be examined adequately. Hence enter "X" for these surfaces.

Merits

- It is a more sensitive index as compared to DMFT.
- It is the index of choice in clinical trials of caries preventive agent (because relative index is more likely to be detected over limited time period of clinical trial)

Demerits

- It takes a longer time to be scored.
- There are increased chances of an inconsistent diagnosis.
- To be fully accurate, for the detection of proximal carious surfaces, it requires the use of radiographs.

Relationship of DMFS and DMFT

Knutson found a high correlation between the mean DMFT (x) and the mean DMFS (y) prevalence in different populations and expressed this association as a straight line. According to *Knutson,* the straight line was selected to represent the association because it was simple to interpret. However, it is to be expected that the parameters of the equation may not be constant in different and variable circumstances.

DMFI Index

The DMF index was modified by the WHO to the DMFI index by subdividing decayed teeth into unfilled carious teeth (D), secondarily decayed filled teeth (DF) and decayed but indicated for extraction (I).

D - Unfilled teeth, that are carious.

DF - Filled teeth that are secondarily carious.

M - Teeth that are missing as a result of caries at the time of examination.

F - Filled teeth that show no signs of secondary caries.

I - Teeth either filled or unfilled which are in the examiner's opinion indicated for extraction.

Extrapolated Carious Surface Incremental Index *(ECSI Index)*

It is an index for evaluating caries progression *(Wagg et al 1974).* It is intended *to supplement rather than to replace existing indices.* It takes into account the enlargement of existing lesions as well as initiation of new ones. Distinct degrees of caries are defined as follows:

0 = a surface on which no carious attack can be demonstrated.

1 = a surface on which carious attack is confined to enamel.

2 = a surface on which carious attack involves tooth enamel and dentin, but has not involved the pulp.

3 = a surface on which the carious attack has involved the pulp.

The ECSI index is logically similar to the DMFS index but contains in addition a component representing the extension of existing lesions.

Caries Severity Index

It was given by the *WHO* and is known as **D1-D3** scale. It acts as an aid for diagnosing coronal dental caries. The scale assesses the earliest detectable non carious lesion to the pulpal involvement (Table 12.4).

It was developed to study the depth and extent of carious lesions along with the extent of pulpal involvement. It is used for assessing the carious progression.

Scoring Criteria

The scoring is carried out using both clinical and radiographic methods (Table 12.5).

Table 12.4: Caries severity index

0	Sound surface	a. No caries – either treated or untreated b. No caries - slightly stained sound fissure
D_1	Initial caries (Re-mineralizable)	Lesions show no clinically detectable loss of tooth substance with following features: a. Pits and fissures: those having staining, discolouration, rough spots in enamel that do not catch the explorer b. Smooth surfaces: showing white, opaque areas with loss of luster.
D_2	Enamel caries(may/may not be re-mineralizable)	Lesions show loss of tooth substance in pits and fissures or on smooth surfaces without the presence of softened floor or wall; or undermining of enamel. Enamel has chalky or crumbly appearance.
D_3	Caries of dentin(Never be Re-mineralized)	Lesions in category D_3 having the following features: a. Softened floor or wall b. Undermined enamel c. Explorer enters the lesions easily D_3 also includes temporary fillings. These lesions can never be re-mineralized and have to be restored.
D_4	Pulpal involvement	This categorizes lesions with deep cavities having probable pulpal involvement. This lesion should not be probed due to fear of iatrogenic pulpal exposure. D_4 is usually included with D_3 in surveys.

Table 12.5: Scoring criteria for caries severity index

Score	Criteria	Extent of caries
1	Superficial caries	In enamel only
2	Moderate caries	In enamel and superficial dentin
3	Moderately severe carious lesions	Enamel is undermined
4	Severe carious lesions	Caries approaching pulp, enamel collapsed
5	Pulpitis	Caused either by deep seated caries or by trauma without caries
6	Pulpal death	Caused either by deep seated caries or by trauma without caries
7	Periapical infection	Caused either by deep seated caries or by trauma without caries

INDICES USED FOR EVALUATION OF CARIES IN PRIMARY TEETH

The indices used for evaluating caries in deciduous dentition are as follows:

def Index

It is an age specific index and is equivalent to the DMFT index used for permanent teeth.

d – decayed primary teeth indicated for filling

e – decayed primary teeth indicated for extraction or already extracted due to caries.

f – filled primary teeth

Basic rules: The basic rules to be followed for recording def index are the same as for DMFT index.

The coding criteria (Table 12.6) is as follows:

Table 12.6: Scoring criteria for def index

Code	Criteria
E	Excluded tooth or tooth space
P_1	Sound deciduous tooth
P_2	Filled deciduous tooth
P_3	Decayed deciduous tooth

When a tooth is absent,

O – Missing tooth – un-erupted, congenitally missing or missing for any other reason.

X – Extracted deciduous tooth

For example, a child has a permanent molar and three deciduous molars are filled with amalgam, two other deciduous teeth that are carious, two deciduous upper incisors are extracted due to caries, then def score for that child is:

d = 2 (permanent molar is not included as def is a deciduous teeth index)

e = 2

f = 3

Then, def can be **calculated** as follows:

- *Individual def score:* It is calculated by recording d, e, f individually and adding them for total score.

d + e + f = def

The def score for above case = 2 + 2 + 3 = 7

- *Group average:* It is calculated by dividing the total def determined for all children by the number of children examined.

$$\text{Average def} = \frac{\text{Total def determined for all children}}{\text{Total number of children examined}}$$

- *Percent needing care:* It is calculated by dividing total 'd' component by total number of teeth examined. It determines the need of treatment to be provided to the children.

$$\text{Percent needing care} = \frac{\text{Total number of decayed teeth}}{\text{Total number of teeth examined}} \times 100$$

- *Percent affected:* It is determined as:

$$\text{Percent of teeth affected} = \frac{\text{Total number of teeth affected}}{\text{Total number of teeth examined}} \times 100$$

- *Percent of teeth filled:* It is calculated by dividing the total number of filled teeth by total def recorded for that individual.

$$\text{Percent filled} = \frac{\text{Total number of teeth filled}}{\text{Total def recorded by an exmainer}} \times 100$$

- *Extracted deciduous teeth per 100 children:* It is the number of deciduous teeth extracted per 100 children. It is calculated as:

$$\text{EDT}/100 = \frac{\text{Total number of extracted teeth}}{\text{Total number examined}} \times 100$$

df Index

It scores the decayed and filled deciduous teeth.

dmfs Index

It is similar to the DMFS index used for permanent dentition and scores the decayed, missing and filled deciduous teeth surfaces.

Dental caries Severity Index for Primary Teeth

While the caries severity index for permanent teeth is based on both clinical and radiographic findings, the CSI *for primary teeth is purely based on clinical findings only.* Scoring is carried out for different lesions as described in Table 12.7.

Table 12.7: Scoring criteria for Caries Severity Index (Primary teeth)

Lesion	1	2	3
Pit and fissure caries	a. Early pit and fissure caries b. Explorer catches or resists removal with moderate to firm pressure c. Softness at the base of pit or fissure d. Opacity adjacent to pit or fissure as an evidence of under-mined decalcification e. Softened enamel adjacent to pit or fissure which may be scrapped away with explorer	Cavitation of at least 1.0 mm across the smallest diameter at the tooth surface	Cavitation with break-down or undermining (as seen as obvious discolouration) of at least half of the cusp
Smooth surface caries (Buccal, Lingual and Palatal surfaces)	A white, soft and sticky lesion which is not extending to the embrasure areas	a. Cavitation of at least 1.0 mm but less than 2.0 mm across the smallest diameter or, b. Soft and sticky white lesion extending into one of the embrasure area	a. Cavitation of 2.0 mm or more than 2.0 mm in its smallest diameter or, b. Soft and sticky white lesion extending into both the embrasures
Proximal surfaces of i. Molars ii. Incisors and Canines	A discontinuity in enamel with catch and softness at base A discontinuity in enamel with catch and softness at base	Cavitation with early breakdown of marginal ridge or obvious dis-colouration indicating undermining of ridge cavitation with break-down or obvious dis-colouration, indicating undermining for at least 1.0 mm on buccal or lingual surfaces	Breakdown of marginal ridge with cavitation extending into mesial or distal extensions of occlusal fissures Cavitation with break-down or undermining of incisal edge

INDICES USED FOR EVALUATING CARIES IN BOTH PRIMARY AND PERMANENT TEETH

The indices that can be used to assess both primary and permanent dentitions are as follows:

Moller's Index for Both Primary and Permanent Teeth

It is a *standardized index* for diagnosing, recording and analyzing dental caries data. It is very sensitive index, both qualitatively and quantitatively, as it records all lesions ranging from incipient ones to frank carious lesions. It has:

i. A standardized criteria for diagnosis
ii. A standardized equipment for examination
iii. A standardized procedure for examination
iv. Standardized field records

Procedure

The patient is seated in a dental chair, under a high quality operating lamp light. Teeth are cleaned, isolated with cotton rolls and saliva ejectors, and dried with the use of compressed air.

Examination is carried out with plane mouth mirror and standardized dental probe- known as **Holst probe**. It is a simple probe and that is to be standardized after every use. Arrested caries should be recorded as decay because one cannot distinguish with certainty between acute and arrested caries, at least not on radiographs or clinically in pits or fissures.

a. **In the clinical procedure**, all teeth except third molars are examined. For posteriors, 5 surfaces are examined while for anteriors four surfaces are examined. Examination is started from the maxillary right to maxillary left side of the arch and then from mandibular left to mandibular right side of arch.

Each tooth is recorded on a field record form in **following sequence**:

1. Occlusal surface — O
2. Mesial surface — M
3. Vestibular or buccal surface — B
4. Distal surface — D
5. Lingual surface — L

The coding is carried out as described in Table 12.8.

Characteristics of Moller's scoring criteria (Tables 12.9 and 12.10) are:

Criteria for Primary Teeth

The criteria for indexing primary teeth using Moller's index are the same as that of permanent teeth.

DMFS Percentage Index

This is an age specific index and determines the caries activity as the percentage of surfaces involved with caries. Both the dentitions are recorded in the same manner and mixed dentition does not pose any problem.

Calculation of DMFS Percentage Index

Calculation of this index requires:

I. **Surface values:** These are the numerical values that determine the extent of carious involvement of tooth. The surface values (SV) are given to all the teeth of dentition.

Table 12.8: Coding criteria (Moller's Index)

Code	Criteria	Alphabetical code
0	Sound tooth	S
1	Type 1 caries	D_1
2	Type 2 caries	D_2
3	Type 3 caries	D_3
4	Type 4 caries	D_4
5	Filled tooth	F
6	Missing tooth due to caries	M
7	Un-erupted tooth or tooth surfaces	–
8	Tooth missing due to reason other than caries	–
9	Congenitally missing tooth, and not recordable	–

For (a) Clinical procedure:

Type	S	D₁	D₂	D₃	D₄

Table 12.9: Coding criteria (Moller's Index)-Clinical

Type	S	D_1	D_2	D_3	D_4
Score	0	1	2	3	4
Pit and fissure	Sound/Normal	Discolouration both with incident and transmitted light, confined to a small narrow line. No definite sticking of the probe	Slight discontinuity in enamel with sticky fissure, with or without discolouration, the probe requires a definite pull for removal	Definite cavity with dentin involvement	Probable pulp involvement
Smooth surface	Sound/Normal	White opaque area with loss of luster	Slight discontinuity in enamel	Definite dentin involvement	Probable pulpal involvement
Inference	No caries	Initial caries	Enamel caries	Dentinal caries	Probable pulpal involvement

For (b) Radiographic procedure:

Table 12.10: Coding criteria (Moller's Index)-Radiological

	S	D_1	D_2	D_3	D_4
Score	0	1	2	3	4
Proximal surfaces	Normal/Sound with distinct enamel surface contour and unbroken enamel surface	Broken enamel surface contour, shadow between enamel surface and a border not more than 1/4ᵗʰ through the enamel	Radiolucent shadow involves whole of enamel and has reached till DEJ	Radiolucent shadow involves dentin and extends to one half of the dentin	Radiolucent shadow extending more than half of dentin
Inference	No caries	Initial caries	Definite Enamel caries	Definite Dentinal caries	Probable pulpal involvement

They are as follows:

a. Incisors and canines have SV of 4 – M, D, B, L

b. Premolars and molars have SV of 5 – M, D, B, L, O

Scoring for:

i. **Carious tooth:** For every surface attacked by caries, *One*, caries surface value is given.

ii. **Missing teeth:** are allotted surface value equal only to their total surface, i.e. 4 for anteriors and 5 for posteriors. Teeth missing due to other reasons except caries are not included.

iii. **Restored teeth:** These are recorded as carious teeth.

iv. **Inter-proximal caries:**

    a. For incisors/canines: 'Three' caries surface values are given.

    b. For premolars/molars: 'Two' caries surface values are given.

II. **Age Factor:** To record the variation among the individuals of different ages the 'age factor', is applied while calculating the DMFS percentage index. The persons of different ages, have different number of erupted teeth and thus different number of surfaces are present in their oral cavities. The simplified age factors for different age groups (Table 12.11) are:

Table 12.11: Simplified age factor	
Age	*Age Factor*
6 to 7½ months	6
7-9 months	3
12-14 months	2
16-18 months	1.5
20 months-5 years	1
6-11 years	0.9
12-16 years	0.8
17 years	0.7

The age factor (for the particular individual's age group) multiplied by total number of surface values provides with the DMFS percentage index, i.e.

DMFS% = Total carious surface value × Age factor

Caries Susceptibility Index

This index assesses the susceptibility of an individual's teeth to caries attack.

For **calculation**, it requires the measurement of two factors:

I. Tooth surfaces of an individual at risk of caries attack.

II. Tooth surfaces of an individual developing caries during the period of observation.

I. **Tooth surfaces at risk:** All the tooth surfaces in the oral cavity of an individual that are free of carious lesions and had not been restored are at risk of developing caries, i.e. these are *susceptible tooth surfaces*.

    For anteriors (Incisors and Canines) - 4 surfaces (Mesial, Distal, Buccal, Lingual)

    For posteriors (Premolars and Molars) – 5 surfaces (Mesial, Distal, Buccal, Lingual, Occlusal)

    Thus, in full primary dentition, we have maximum of 88 tooth surfaces at risk while for permanent dentition the number is 148 (as in the DMFS index).

II. **Tooth surfaces developing caries during the period of observation:** This is the number of tooth surfaces developing caries lesions after the period of observation is completed.

Procedure and Calculations

a. During the initial examination of an individual the number of susceptible tooth surfaces to carious attack for that particular individual is calculated.

b. A gap period of six months or twelve months is given as an observation period.

c. Then, final examination of an individual is carried out to record the development of new carious lesions which were not present during the initial examination. This is called as **Caries Score**.

    From these two values, Susceptibility Ratio is calculated as:

$$\text{Susceptibility ratio (SR)} = \frac{\text{Caries score}}{\text{Total susceptibility tooth surfaces}}$$

Finally, susceptibility index is calculated as:

Susceptibility Index (SI) = SR × 100

The susceptibility Index (SI) is, thus, a percentage value that makes the result more simple by *eliminating the fractions*.

Murray and Shaw's Criteria for Dental Caries

Murray and Shaw developed clinical and radiographic criteria for the dental caries.

I. **Clinical criteria:** This criteria (Table 12.12) is based on the clinical findings.

Table12.12: Murray and Shaw's (clinical criteria)

Score	Criteria
C-1	Minute discontinuity of enamel surface without definite sticking of probe
C-2	A cavity in a pit, fissure or on a smooth surface with definite sticking of probe that requires a pull force for its removal
C-3	A large open cavity with probable involvement of pulp

II. **Radiographic criteria:** This criteria (Table 12.13) is based on the radiographic findings.

INDICES FOR ROOT SURFACE CARIES

Root surface caries, cemental or senile caries is defined as soft progressive lesion of root surfaces exposed to oral environment. These are observed within a 2.0 mm area of the cemento-enamel junction (CEJ). A root surface is always taken at risk if CEJ is involved.

Root surface caries is a common lesion of geriatric age group and is gaining importance in the modern times especially where the target is to reduce tooth loss due to caries among the elderly. With the increasing population of the elderly in developed

Table 12.13: Murray and Shaw's (radiographic criteria)

Score	Criteria
R-1	Radiolucent area present within the DEJ
R-2	Radiolucent area that has crossed DEJ and extends into the dentin without pulpal involvement
R-3	Gross caries with definite pulpal involvement
R-4	Absent (X) – No R-4 term exists in Murray's criteria
R-5	Filled tooth
R-6	Missing, un-erupted, extracted or congenitally absent tooth
R-7	Unreadable x-ray; overlapped image
R-8	Presumed carious lesion is not clear in radiograph
R-9	Presumed sound tooth is not clear in radiograph

countries, along with decreased tooth loss, root caries is certainly going to attract more attention in the future years.

Root Caries Index

Root caries index was proposed by *Ralph Katz* in 1984 to study the prevalence of root caries in an epidemiological survey. In this index, *risk as well as casualty, i.e. gingival recession as well as carious root surface,* are recorded.

Procedure

The patient is seated comfortably in the dental chair with adequate lighting facility. Mesial, distal, buccal and lingual surfaces of roots of the whole dentition are examined for recession, soft lesions or caries. The data is recorded for each tooth examined in a tabular form (Table 12.14) using the following codes:

Table 12.14: Root Caries Index			
M	*D*	*B*	*L*
R-N			
R-D			
R-F			
No-R			

The surfaces of roots are represented in vertical columns and lesions on these surfaces are recorded in horizontal rows.

These lesions are recorded (Table 12.15) as:

Table 12.15: Recording lesions of root surfaces	
Lesion	Surface (Mesial, Distal, Buccal, Lingual)
R-N	Root surface having recession but no decay, i.e. it is normal
R-D	Root surface having recession as well as decay
R-F	Root surface having recession and filled carious lesion
No-R	Root surfaces having no gingival recession, i.e. CEJ cannot be visualized
M	Missing root surfaces (this is, for whole tooth and not a single root surface; as tooth is missing completely)

Calculation of Index

Then, root caries index (RCI) is calculated as follows:

$$RCI = \frac{RD + RF}{RD + RF + RN} \times 100$$

RCI, is thus, recorded as a percentage and is considered as an important milestone in descriptive and analytical surveys. It takes the peculiar nature of root surface caries into account, i.e. it appears only on teeth with exposed cementum and they are lost when a particular tooth is extracted.

Katz's Diagnostic Convention for Root Caries Index (RCI)

Ralph Katz proposed following conventions (Table 12.16) for recording RCI.

INDICES USED FOR ORAL HYGIENE ASSESSMENT

These are indices that are used for assessing the oral hygiene status of an individual or population. These indices can be used simply to assess the oral hygiene status of an individual or to compare the oral hygiene status before and after treatment. The various indices used to assess oral hygiene are:

Oral Hygiene Index (OHI)

Oral Hygiene Index (OHI) was developed to study variations in gingival inflammation. It was regarded as a simple but sensitive and rapid method for assessing the oral hygiene status of an individual or group, quantitatively.

The Oral Hygiene Index (OHI) is composed of two parts: (a) Debris Index (DI) (b) Calculus Index (I)

Debris Index (DI)

Debris is defined as a foreign deposit on tooth surface that is soft in consistency and consists of mucin, bacteria and food particles, which provide it grayish white to green or orange colour.

Scoring of DI: For scoring, the exposed labial tooth surface is divided horizontally into three parts: Gingival 1/3rd, Middle 1/3rd and Incisal 1/3rd (Fig. 12.5).

The scoring is carried out as described in Table 12.17.

Debris index component of OHI records the amount of debris covering the tooth surface. It is estimated by running the side of No.5 explorer, i.e. shepherd's hook along the buccal/labial and lingual surfaces of tooth and noting the occlusal/incisal extent of debris as

Table 12.16: Katz's diagnostic convention

Convention No.	Convention
1	If diagnosis of root caries as carious lesion or filled lesion is uncertain – score surface as normal *(R-N)*
2	All caries detected on root surfaces near the CEJ are scored as decayed *(R-D)*; regardless of adjacent enamel condition
3	For coronal filling extending on root surface, the material must extend more than 3 mm to record that root surface as filled one; except cast crowns extending onto root surface (these root surfaces are never recorded as filled)
4	For recording filling as a multiple surface restoration, the particular restoration must extends across at least 1/3rd of each additional surface
5a	Recurrent decay associated with a root surface filling should be recorded as an independent disease category – *Recurrent Root Decay*
5b	Recurrent decay associated with coronal restoration or crown should be recorded as *Root Decay Contagious with Coronal Filling*
6	*Additional Root Caries Lesion* – used for any root surface that is already decayed and also has another separate additional lesion
7	Any root surface that appears to be about more than 20% of its surface area but is inaccessible to clinical examination due to plaque, calculus, etc. should be recorded as unreadable

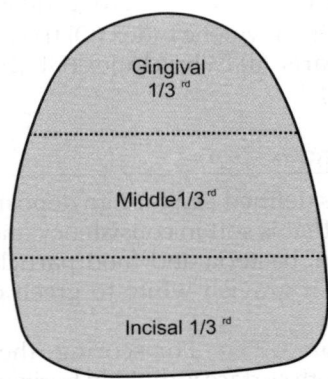

Fig. 12.5: Division of tooth surface for scoring Oral Hygiene Index (OHI)

it is removed from tooth surface. DI component is always recorded prior to the recording of CI component.

Calculus Index (CI)

The mineralized dental plaque or calculus is scored in this component. Examination is done

Table 12.17: Scoring of Debris Index

Score	Criteria	Diagrammatic
0	No debris or stain present	
1	Soft debris covering not more than one third of tooth surface and/or presence of extrinsic stains without debris regardless of tooth's surface area covered	
2	Soft debris covering more than one third, but not more than two thirds of exposed tooth surfaces	
3	Soft debris covering more than more than 2/3rds of exposed tooth surfaces.	

for both supra and sub-gingival calculus. The scoring is carried out (Table 12.18) as follows:

Table 12.18: Scoring of Calculus Index		
Score	Criteria	Diagrammatic
0	No calculus present	
1	Supra-gingival calculus covering not more than 1/3rd of exposed tooth surface	
2	Supra-gingival calculus covering more than 1/3rd but not more than 2/3rd of exposed tooth surfaces; and/or the presence of individual flecks of sub-gingival calculus around the cervical portion of tooth; or both.	
3	Supra-gingival calculus covering more than 2/3rd of exposed tooth surface; and/or continuous heavy band of sub-gingival calculus around the cervical one third of tooth; or both.	

Rules for assessing OHI: The rules followed for assessing OHI are:
- In this index only completely erupted permanent teeth are scored, i.e. teeth whose occlusal and incisal surfaces have reached the occlusal plane.
- Third molars and incompletely erupted teeth are not scored.
- The buccal and lingual scores in a segment, for both debris and calculus index, are taken on the tooth having the greatest surface area covered by debris and calculus.

Procedure

The patient is seated comfortably and examination is carried out under bright natural or artificial light. For the purpose of examination each dental arch is divided into three segments (Fig. 12.6), i.e. six segments for whole of the dentition (Table 12.19), which are:

Table 12.19: Segments of Oral Hygiene Index		
Segment 1	Upper right posterior	It extends from distal of right maxillary 7 to distal of right maxillary 3, i.e. it comprises upper right posteriors
Segment 2	Upper anterior	It comprises six anterior teeth, i.e. distal of right canine to distal of left canine
Segment 3	Upper left posterior	It includes upper left maxillary canine to distal of maxillary left second molar, i.e. distal to left canine
Segment 4	Lower left posterior	It includes lower left posteriors, i.e. teeth distal to lower left canine
Segment 5	Lower anterior	It comprises lower anteriors, i.e. distal of left mandibular 3 to distal of right mandibular 3
Segment 6	Lower right posterior	It comprises the posteriors of lower left arch, i.e. distal to right cuspid of mandibular arch

Each segment is examined for debris or calculus while one tooth from each segment is used for calculating the particular index. The examination is done in a sequence from segment No. 1 to segment No.6; with buccal or labial surfaces examined first followed by

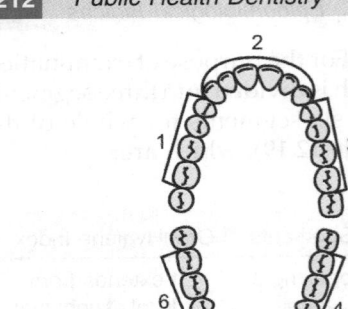

Fig. 12.6: Segmental division of Oral Hygiene Index (OHI)

lingual surfaces. Then, the indices are **calculated separately** as follows:

$$DI = \frac{\text{Total buccal/labial score} + \text{Total lingual score}}{\text{No. of segments scored}} \text{(for debris)}$$

$$CI = \frac{\text{Total buccal/labial score} + \text{Total lingual score}}{\text{No. of segments used}} \text{(for calculus)}$$

$$OHI = DI + CI$$

Results of OHI

- The minimum recordable value for either DI or CI is 0 while maximum value for them is 6.
- The minimum score for OHI is 0 while maximum score value is 12 (DI + CI, i.e. 6).
- The individual score for either debris or calculus ranges from minimum value of 0 to maximum value of 36 (as maximum scoring can be 3; if each segment gives a score of 3, then for 3 segments of either arch:

Maxillary buccal/labial score = 3 + 3 + 3 = 9
Maxillary lingual score = 3 + 3 + 3 = 9
(since we have to score only single tooth of the segment with maximum amount of debris/calculus – Rule 3).

Similarly,
Mandibular buccal/labial score = 3 + 3 + 3 = 9
Mandibular lingual score = 3 + 3 + 3 = 9
Thus, maximum score will be equal to 9 + 9 + 9 + 9 = 36

The higher the score, poorer is the oral hygiene status of the patient.

Limitations

Although this index is sensitive it requires more decision making and thus more time is to be spent in order to record it completely, which is not feasible in large surveys. It is quite lengthy an index and demands an extensive procedure for scoring.

Simplified Oral Hygiene Index (OHI-S)

This index was developed to overcome the limitations of the original OHI. The Simplified Oral Hygiene Index (OHI-S) differs from OHI in following ways:

i. The number of tooth surfaces to be scored is less for the Simplified Oral Hygiene Index (OHI-S) (6) than OHI (12).
ii. The maximum and minimum scores that can be obtained for a particular individual are less for the Simplified Oral Hygiene Index (OHI-S).

The Simplified Oral Hygiene Index (OHI-S) like the OHI is also composed of two parts:
a. Debris Index – Simplified (DI-S)
b. Calculus Index – Simplified (CI-S)
a. **Debris index:** Simplified (DI-S)
   DI-S is considered and scored in a manner similar to OHI giving a score of 0, 1, 2, 3 using a shepherd's crook.
b. **Calculus index:** Simplified (CI-S)
This component is also scored in a similar manner using exactly the same criteria as for CI component of OH-I. Basically the whole method of scoring the criteria is same for OHI and OHI-S except the number of tooth surfaces to be examined in OHI-S are decreased.

Procedure

The patient is seated comfortably and examination is carried out in bright sunlight or artificial light according to the available conditions. In OHI-S, only 6 teeth are examined with their following respective surfaces (Fig. 12.7) (Table 12.20).

Table 12.20: Simplified Oral Hygiene Index examination

Tooth	Surface
16 – Maxillary right first molar	Buccal
11 – Maxillary right central incisor	Labial
26 – Maxillary left first molar	Buccal
36 – Mandibular left first molar	Lingual
31 – Mandibular left central incisor	Labial
46 – Mandibular right first molar	Lingual

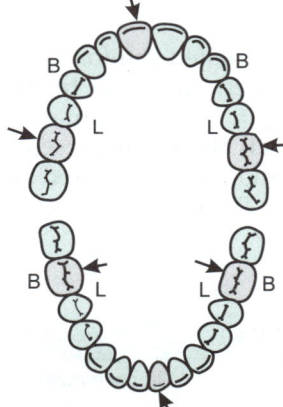

Fig. 12.7: Surfaces and teeth to be examined for Simplified Oral Hygiene Index

The teeth are examined and scores for debris and calculus are tabulated separately for particular tooth surface. Then, DI-S/CI-S is calculated as:

$$DI-S = \frac{\text{Total debris score for all surfaces examined}}{\text{Number of tooth surfaces scored}}$$

$$CI-S = \frac{\text{Total calculus score for all surfaces examined}}{\text{Number of tooth surfaces scored}}$$

The clinical level of oral cleanliness for debris/calculus that can be associated with DI-S or CI-S is as follows:

Good : 0.0 – 0.6
Fair : 0.7 – 1.8
Poor : 1.9 – 3.0

Then OHI-S is calculated by adding the DI-S and CI-S score, i.e.

OHI-S = DI-S score + CI-S score

The clinical levels of oral hygiene that can be associated with OHI-S are as follows:

Good : 0.0 – 1.2
Fair : 1.3 – 3.0
Poor : 3.1 – 6.0

Rules for Calculating OHI-S

- For OHI-S, each surface buccal/labial or lingual is considered as half the tooth circumference.
- Only fully erupted permanent teeth are considered for scoring, i.e. teeth whose occlusal or incisal surfaces have reached occlusal plane.
- Natural teeth with full crowns or surfaces/teeth reduced in height due to occlusal wear, trauma or caries are not scored.
- If the designated tooth is not available due to any reason then substitution tooth is measured. These substitutions are enumerated in Table 12.21.

Table 12.21: Substitution of teeth for Simplified Oral Health Index

Original tooth	Substitutions
16	17 or 18
11	21
26	27 or 28
36	37 or 38
31	41
46	47 or 48

- For an individual score, at least two of the six tooth surfaces possible, must have been examined and the scoring is done to one decimal place.
- A group score is calculated by calculating the average of the individual scores of the individuals in that particular group. The scoring can be done till one or two decimal places.

Uses of Simplified Oral Hygiene Index (OHI-S)

- It has been used extensively throughout the world to assess the oral hygiene status of an individual or a group and has contributed greatly to the understanding of periodontal diseases.
- It is easy to use because the scoring criteria are objective.
- A high level of reproducibility is possible with a minimum of training sessions.
- It is also used in National Health Surveys.
- It is used in epidemiological surveys, longitudinal studies and dental health education programs.
- It can be used for clinical trials.
- It is the standard companion of Periodontal Index in the epidemiological studies of the Interdepartmental Committee on Nutrition for National Defence (ICNND).
- It is used for evaluation of oral hygiene of school children in dental health education programs.
- It is also used to evaluate the cleansing efficiency of toothbrushes.

Glass Index

This index was developed to assess the presence and extent of debris accumulated on the surfaces of teeth in the oral cavity. This index put more emphasis on the debris accumulations on the **gingival thirds** of teeth than OHI and OHI-S.

This index scores the debris present on the surfaces of teeth and not the calculus.

The scoring is carried out (Table 12.22) as follows:

Procedure

The patient is seated comfortably and examination is carried out under bright natural or artificial light. Buccal/Labial and Lingual surfaces of **all the teeth** present in the oral cavity are examined and scored as per criteria described in Table 12.22. Glass Index (GI) is calculated by:

Table 12.22: Scoring for Glass Index

Score	Criteria	Diagrammatic
0	No visible debris	
1	Debris present at gingival margin but • is discontinuous and • is less than 1.0 mm in height	
2	Debris present at gingival margin and is continuous and greater than 1.0 mm in height	
3	Debris involving the whole gingival 1/3rd of tooth	
4	Debris scattered over the whole tooth surface	

$$GI = \frac{\text{Total debris score for all the teeth examined}}{\text{Tooth number of teeth examined for that person}}$$

More the score, poorer is the oral hygiene status of an individual.

Uses

- Assessing presence and extent of accumulated debris on tooth surface.
- Evaluating the efficacy of tooth brushing.
- Clinical trials of preventive or therapeutic agents.

Patient Hygiene Performance Index (PHP Index)

This index was introduced to assess the performance of an individual in maintenance of his oral hygiene. This index is usually performed twice; once at the first visit and secondly, after giving oral hygiene maintenance instructions to individual.

In this index, only debris is scored. Tooth is divided into five imaginary parts as follows (Fig. 12.8) (Table 12.23):

3 divisions vertically – mesial 1/3rd, middle 1/3rd, distal 1/3rd.

2 divisions horizontally – These are actually the divisions of middle 1/3rd, i.e. gingival, middle and occlusal/incisal third.

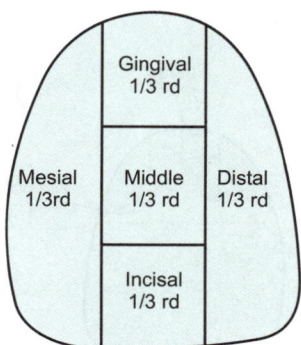

Fig. 12.8: Division of labial surface for Patient Hygiene Performance (PHP) scoring

Table 12.23: Scoring for Patient Hygiene Performance Index

Score	Criteria
0	No debris present
1	Debris definitely present

Procedure

The patient is seated comfortably and a disclosing agent is applied on his/her teeth for 30 seconds. He/she is asked to expectorate but not to rinse. Each tooth surface of the following teeth is then examined for debris (Fig. 12.9) by dividing it in five parts (Table 12.24):

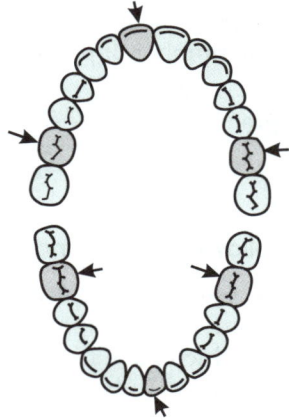

Fig. 12.9: Surfaces and teeth to be examined for Patient Hygiene Performance (PHP)

Table 12.24: Tooth surfaces for Patient Hygiene Performance index

Tooth	Surface
16 – Upper right first molar	Buccal
11 – Upper right central incisor	Labial
26 – Upper left first molar	Buccal
36 – Lower left first molar	Lingual
31 – Lower left central incisor	Labial
46 – Lower left first molar	Lingual

After scoring the five parts individually, all values are added to calculate the total debris score for an individual tooth.

Then, the scores for individual teeth are totaled to record the value of PHP-Index.

$$PHP\ index = \frac{Total\ scores\ for\ the\ individual\ teeth}{Number\ of\ teeth\ examined}$$

The rating is carried out as follows:

1. Excellent   -   0
2. Good   -   0.1 – 1.7
3. Fair   -   1.8 – 3.4
4. Poor   -   3.5 – 5.0

If PHP score for a group is to be calculated then the individual scores are totaled and divided by total number of people examined.

$$PHP\ for\ group = \frac{Total\ individual\ scores}{Total\ number\ of\ people\ examined}$$

Rules to be followed for PHP Index

- The six index teeth, that are used for scoring should be completely erupted.
- Index teeth, which have less than 3/4th of the crowns erupted, full crown restorations, are traumatized or broken are not scored. Instead the substitutions for these are used (these are the same as OHI-S substitutions).
- 'S' is marked with the tooth score if substituted tooth is used for scoring.
- 'M' is used for missing index tooth.

Uses of PHP Index

- Since disclosing agent is used in this index, it serves as a motivational factor for patient to encourage him to follow proper debris removal habits.
- As it is simple and rapid to perform so it becomes easy for the patient to understand it, so it also acts as an educational aid.

- It is used to score patient before and after oral hygiene instructions, thus, helping dentist to evaluate and analyze the effectiveness of home care methods performed by the patient.

INDICES USED FOR PLAQUE ASSESSMENT

Plaque is defined as *a soft deposit that forms the biofilm adhering to the tooth surface or other hard surfaces in the oral cavity, including removable and fixed restorations.*

The various indices used to measure plaque on the teeth are as:

Plaque Index (PLI)

This index was given by Silness and Löe to score the plaque thickness on the gingival one third of teeth without considering the coronal extent of plaque. It is one of the most reliable and widely used indices to assess the plaque score.

In this index, *only thickness of plaque at gingival one third* is considered and no significance is given to the extension of plaque on middle or incisal one thirds. The *gingival surfaces* of teeth are further divided into four parts as:

a. **Buccal/Labial** (Fig. 12.10): This is divided into:
   i. Distal-facial
   ii. Facial
   iii. Mesial-facial
b. **Lingual** (Fig. 12.11): This is scored as one unit.

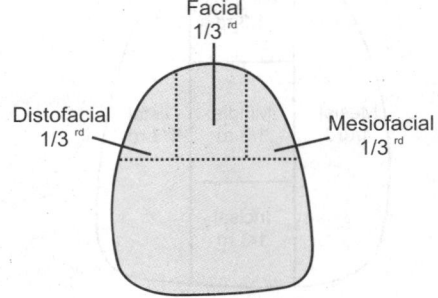

Fig. 12.10: Divisions of the labial surface for Plaque Index scoring

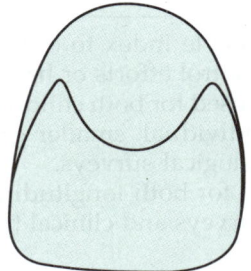

Fig. 12.11: Lingual surface for Plaque Index scoring

The plaque is scored on surfaces of teeth by the following criteria (Table 12.25).

Table 12.25: Scoring of Plaque Index	
Score	Criteria
0	No plaque
1	A film of plaque adhering to free gingival margin and adjacent area of tooth surface is seen in situ only after application of disclosing agent or by using probe on tooth surface
2	Moderate accumulation of soft deposits within the gingival pocket, on the tooth or on gingival margin which can be seen with naked eye
3	Abundance of soft matter within the gingival pocket and/or on the tooth/ gingival margin

Procedure

The patient is seated comfortably. The teeth and gingiva are properly air dried. The mouth mirror is used to examine the teeth visually. Visible plaque is given a score of 2 or 3 accordingly. If no plaque is visible then the explorer is passed across the cervical one third of tooth and entrance of gingival sulcus. If no plaque adheres to explorer, area is scored as 'O' and if plaque adheres, area is scored as '1'. Plaque on the dental restorations, calculus deposits, full crowns, etc. is also included in the scoring. There are two methods that can be followed for scoring:

i. **Full mouth index:** In this method whole of the present dentition is examined to assess the plaque status.

ii. **Index teeth method:** In this method six index teeth are examined for plaque score (Fig. 12.12). These teeth are:

16 – Maxillary right first molar
12 – Maxillary right lateral incisor
24 – Maxillary left first bicuspid
36 – Mandibular left first molar
32 – Mandibular left lateral incisor
44 – Mandibular right first bicuspid

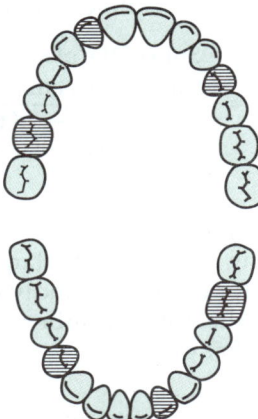

Fig. 12.12: Teeth to be examined for Plaque Index

If any of these six teeth are missing, full mouth index is to be recorded as there are **no substitutions** for the unavailable teeth.

After proper scoring for each area, the index is **calculated** as follows:

• *PLI for Area:* It is the score assigned to a particular area. Its value is 0–3 (as in Table 12.25).

• *PLI for an individual tooth:* The scores for four areas of tooth are totaled and the sum is divided by four. This gives average score for the individual tooth.

$$\text{PLI for individual tooth} = \frac{\text{Total score of four surfaces of that tooth}}{4}$$

- *PLI for group of teeth:* It is calculated by dividing the total score of the teeth present in a group by the number of teeth present in that group.

$$\text{PLI for group of teeth} = \frac{\text{Total score of individual teeth present in that group}}{\text{Total number of teeth present in that group}}$$

- *PLI for an individual person:* the plaque index values of all teeth are calculated and totaled. This sum is divided by the total number of teeth examined in that person.

$$\text{PLI for an individual} = \frac{\text{Sum of the plaque index values of all teeth examined}}{\text{Total number of teeth examined for that person}}$$

- *PLI for a group of persons:* The plaque index for a group of persons is calculated by dividing the sum of plaque indices calculated for each of the individual of the group by the total number of persons present in that group.

$$\text{PLI for a group of persons} = \frac{\text{Sum of plaque index values of each individual of that group}}{\text{Total number of persons present in that group}}$$

Evaluation of the patient based on this index is carried out as follows (Table 12.26):

Table 12.26: Evaluation for Plaque Index

Scores	Rating
0	Excellent
0.1 – 0.9	Good
1 – 1.9	Fair
2 – 3	Poor

Uses

- It is a reliable index to evaluate patient's plaque control efforts or habits.
- It can be used for both children and adults; for an individual, smaller group or large epidemiological surveys.
- It is used for both longitudinal epidemiological surveys and clinical trials.

Limitations

The major limitation of PI is that its scoring is completely subjective and can vary from the one investigator to another. In order to limit this bias, it is generally recommended that for a particular group or trial, a single investigator should be involved.

Modified Plaque Index

Plaque index was modified by Löe in the following ways:

1. *Sequence of examination:* Löe gave a particular sequence for the examination while recording plaque index for full dentition (Fig. 12.13). The sequence is as follows:

   a. **For maxillary arch:** The examination is started from the right maxillary second molar and is concluded at the left maxillary second molar. First buccal surfaces are scored in the sequence for teeth at right side of midline as Distal-Buccal, Buccal, Mesial-Buccal whereas for the teeth present on the left side as Mesial-buccal, Buccal and Distal. After buccal scoring, the lingual surfaces are scored for maxillary arch.

   b. **For mandibular arch:** The examination commences from the left mandibular second molar and concludes at the right mandibular second molar. Facial surfaces are examined first in the sequence of distal-buccal, buccal and mesial-buccal for left side and mesial-buccal, buccal and distal-buccal for right side. Thereafter, lingual surfaces of mandibular arch are scored.

2. Third molars are not scored in modified plaque index.

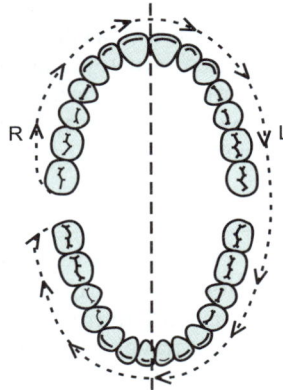

Fig. 12.13: Sequence of examination of teeth for Modified Plaque Index

3. If both plaque index and gingival index are to be scored for a particular individual then first plaque index should be scored.
4. According to Löe, the ideal method to score plaque index is for full mouth dentition.

Scoring criteria for modified plaque index: Löe also modified the scoring criteria slightly as follows (Table 12.27):

Table 12.27: Scoring for modified Plaque Index

Score	Criteria
0	No plaque
1	A film of plaque adhering to free gingival margin and adjacent area of tooth. The plaque can be recognized only by running a probe across a tooth surface
2	Moderate accumulation of soft deposits within the gingival pocket, on the gingival margin and/or adjacent tooth surface which can be seen with naked eye
3	Abundance of soft matter within the gingival pocket and/or on the tooth and gingival margin

The rest of the index, calculations, uses, rating, etc. are the same as that of original plaque index.

Modified Quigley-Hein Plaque Index

Quigley-Hein had developed a plaque index, which measures plaque on the facial surfaces of anterior teeth after using *basic fuschin as a disclosing agent*. The index was later modified by Gilmore and Glickman. The modified index is recognizable, reliable and valid index.

The index measures plaque at gingival one third of tooth surfaces but all the labial/buccal and lingual surfaces of dentition are scored in it. Thus, this is *a full mouth index* (unlike the original one) and scores the plaque from 0 to 5 as follows (Table 12.28).

Table 12.28: Scoring for Modified Quigley-Hein Plaque Index

Score	Criteria	Diagrammatic
0	No plaque	
1	Separate flecks of plaque at the cervical margin of tooth	
2	A continuous band of plaque, up to 1.0 mm in width at cervical margin of tooth	
3	A band of plaque, wider than 1.0 mm but covering less than whole gingival 1/3rd of tooth	
4	A band of plaque covering at least one third of tooth surface but less than two thirds of tooth surface	
5	Plaque covering 2/3rd or more than 2/3rd of crown of tooth	

Procedure

The patient is seated comfortably and *basic fuschin (a disclosing agent)* is applied on his teeth. After 30 seconds the patient is asked to expectorate. Then, the scoring of the plaque is carried out using the above criteria. There is no hard and fast rule for the sequence of examination but it is easy to start from the buccal surfaces of maxillary posterior teeth and finish at the mandibular arch, thus completing the circle formed by the maxillary and mandibular arches. After buccal surfaces are scored the lingual surfaces are scored in a similar manner (Fig. 12.14).

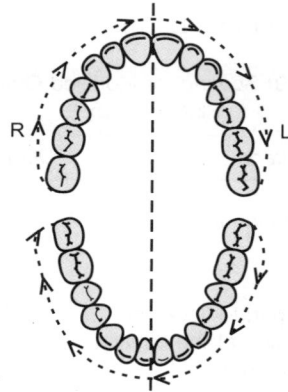

Fig. 12.14: Sequence of examination for Modified Quigley-Hein Plaque Index

Index value is **calculated** by dividing the sum of the scores of individual surfaces by the total number of surfaces examined, i.e.

Modified Quigley- Hein Plaque Index =	Sum of plaque scores of all the tooth surfaces examined
	Total number of surfaces examined

Advantages

The biggest advantage of this index is that the *scoring of this index is objective and not subjective*

(as it is used with a disclosing agent). Thus, investigator to investigator variations are minimum in its score.

Moreover, it is easy to *score stained plaque than the unstained one*. This index can be easily used for epidemiological surveys, as well as for evaluating the antiplaque procedures – both mechanical as well as chemical, accomplished either by clinician or patient.

Navy Plaque Index (NPI)

This index is called Navy Plaque Index because it was developed originally, to assess the plaque status and maintenance of oral hygiene among the naval personnel.

This index scores the facial and lingual surfaces of the six index teeth (Fig. 12.15) that are:

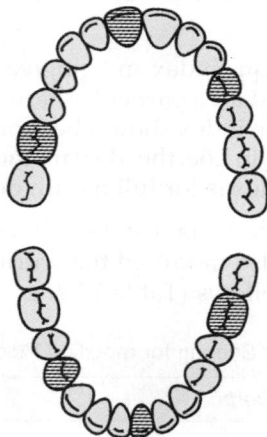

Fig. 12.15: Teeth to be examined for Navy Plaque Index (NPI)

16 - Maxillary right first molar
21 - Maxillary left central incisor
24 - Maxillary left first premolar
36 - Mandibular left first molar
41 - Mandibular right central incisor
44 - Mandibular right first premolar

Each facial/lingual surface is divided into three parts (Fig. 12.16).

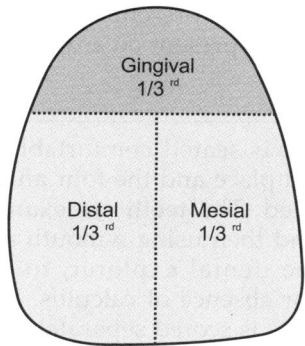

Fig. 12.16: Division of the labial surface for Navy Plaque Index (NPI) scoring

Gingival area (G): The area above the height of contour or contact are depending upon the absence or presence of adjacent tooth.

Mesial Proximal area (M): The area of tooth present mesially below the height of contour or contact area.

Distal Proximal area (D): The area of tooth present distally below the height of contour/contact area.

The scoring is carried out as follows (Table 12.29).

Table 12.29: Scoring for criteria Navy Plaque Index	
Plaque area	*Score*
M	3
G	2
D	3

When plaque is not found in contact with gingival tissue but is found on any of tooth surface, one point is added to facial/lingual score.

Procedure

The patient is seated comfortably and disclosing agent is applied on his teeth. The scoring of plaque is done using the above criteria for six index teeth. Then, finally NPI is **calculated** by adding the individual score for all the teeth surfaces, i.e.

NPI = Sum of the scores of the six index teeth for both facial and lingual surfaces

Advantages

- The index is easy to use because its criteria are dichotomous.
- It can be performed quickly.
- It can be used for educating the patient.

INDICES USED FOR ASSESSMENT OF CALCULUS

Calculus is **defined** as *the mineralized bacterial plaque that forms on the surface of natural teeth and dental prosthesis.*

According to its relation with gingival margin it is defined as:

Supra-gingival calculus: Calculus located coronal to gingival margin and therefore visible in the oral cavity is called supra-gingival calculus.

Sub-gingival calculus: Calculus located below the crest of marginal gingiva and therefore not visible on routine clinical examination is called sub-gingival calculus.

The indices used for calculus assessment are divided into three types, according to the trials with calculus inhibitory agents:

- Those used for **short term clinical studies,** i.e. maximum for six months duration, e.g. CSI, CSSI.
- Those used for **longitudinal studies**, generally for three to six months duration.
- Those used for **epidemiological surveys**.

The various indices used for rating of calculus are discussed below:

Calculus Surface Index (CSI)

Calculus Surface Index (CSI) is used for short term clinical trials of calculus inhibitory agents as it easily determines the effect of the agent on the calculus formation or initiation. It is simple, rapid, easy and reliable index for calculus assessment.

This index assesses both supra and/or sub-gingival calculus on the *four mandibular incisors*. Each incisor is divided into four scoring surfaces (Figs 12.17 and 12.18).

- *Labial/facial:* Scored as single unit.
- *Lingual surface:* It is divided into three sub-surfaces:

a. Disto-lingual one third
b. Lingual one third
c. Mesio-lingual one third

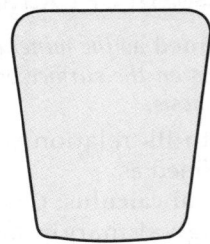

Fig. 12.17: Labial tooth surface for Calculus Surface Index (CSI) scoring

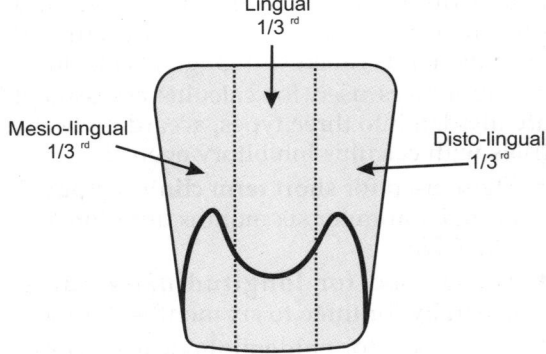

Fig. 12.18: Divisions of the lingual tooth surface for Calculus Surface Index (CSI) scoring

Scoring Criteria

The criteria for scoring for CSI is very simple and as follows:

0 – No calculus present
1 – Calculus present on any surface

Procedure

The patient is seated comfortably at a well illuminated place and the four anterior teeth are air dried. The teeth are examined first visually and then using a mouth mirror and sickle type dental explorer, to detect the presence or absence of calculus. Each of the four surfaces is scored separately as '0' or '1' accordingly.

The value of CSI is **calculated** by adding the individual scores of the four surfaces of four mandibular incisors, i.e.

CSI : Total score or surfaces having calculus present on them.

The maximum score that CSI can have is 16, i.e. 4 teeth each having maximum four surfaces which can have maximum score of 1. Thus, maximum score will be $4 \times 4 = 16$.

Calculus Surface Severity Index (CSSI)

This index is similar as CSI except the scoring criteria, that is given below:

0 – No calculus present
1 – Calculus present, but less than 0.5 mm in width and/or thickness.
2 – Calculus present, but not more than 1.0 mm in width and/or thickness.
3 – Calculus present, more than 1.0 mm in width and/or thickness.

Marginal Line Calculus Index (MLCI)

It is used to assess the development of only *supra-gingival calculus along the marginal gingiva* (thus MLCI). This index is also used *in short term* clinical trials of anti-tartar agents.

The index assesses the supra-gingival calculus present on the cervical margin of *lingual surfaces of four mandibular incisors. The cervical third* of each lingual surface of mandibular teeth is divided into two parts (Fig. 12.19).

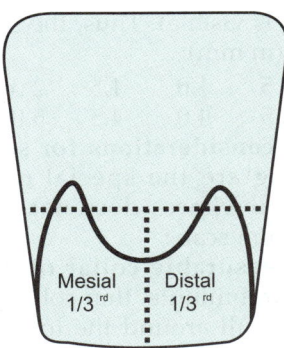

Fig. 12.19: Divisions of the lingual tooth surface for Marginal Line Calculus Index (MLCI) scoring

• Mesial half
• Distal half

The scoring of each half is carried out as a percentage value, depending upon the amount of tooth surface covered by calculus (Table 12.30).

Table 12.30: Scoring for Marginal Line Calculus Index

Score % age	Tooth surface covered by calculus
0	No calculus present
12.5	1/8th of the surface covered by calculus
25	1/4th of the surface covered by calculus
50	1/2 of the surface covered by calculus
75	3/4th of the surface covered by calculus
100	Total surface covered by calculus

Procedure

The patient is seated comfortably at a well illuminated place and the teeth are air dried. The examination of lingual surfaces of mandibular incisors is carried out using mouth mirror and specific score is assigned to each one of them. The score for each tooth is calculated by totaling the scores for each half of the individual tooth. The sum of scores of individual teeth divided by the number of teeth examined will give the value of marginal line calculus index, i.e.

$$MLCI = \frac{\text{Sum of scores for individual teeth for a person}}{\text{Total number of teeth examined in that person}}$$

Uses

• For motivating patient to maintain oral hygiene.
• Assessing the patient's progress after treatment procedure.
• For short term clinical trials (less than 6 months) of anti calculus agents.

Volpe Manhold Index (VMI)

Volpe Manhold Index (VMI) was developed to assess the *appearance of new deposits of supra-gingival calculus* after oral prophylaxis procedure.

In this index, the lingual surfaces of all the *six mandibular anterior* teeth are examined after dividing them into three parts/planes (Fig. 12.20).

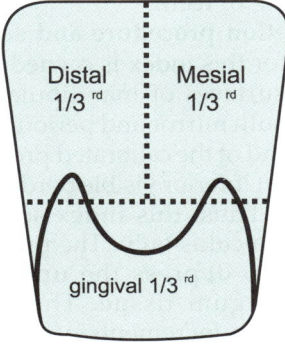

Fig. 12.20: Divisions of lingual tooth surface for Volpe Manhold Index (VMI) scoring

a. Mesial
b. Distal
c. Gingival

The scoring for the index is carried out on the basis of the amount the increments of calculus on the teeth.

Procedure

The procedure is precise and a complex one. It is carried out as follows:

1. **Preparation of instruments:** The periodontal probes to be used for examination should be recalibrated accurately with references to a millimeter gauge such as Boley gauge. The flat end of the probe should be incremented up to 5.0 mm using a green mounted stone or a triple edge orthodontic file (which accentuates the markings). Then, the rough edges are smoothened by rubber discs. Coloured tapes should also be applied to accentuate millimeter increments.

2. **Preparation of patient:** The patient is asked to brush his teeth thoroughly before the start of examination procedure. He is seated comfortably in a dental chair and his teeth are dried completely using compressed air. Adequate isolation is achieved by using saliva ejectors. For best results, assistant should provide the responsibility of isolation and clinician should be responsible for scoring of teeth.

3. **Examination procedure and scoring:** The scoring for this index is carried out for the lingual surfaces of mandibular anteriors using mouth mirror and periodontal probe. The flat end of the calibrated probe is placed at the most inferior visible border of formed calculus. Thus, this index scores supragingival calculus only. The probe can also be used to depress the unhealthy and displaced gum tissue. The calculus is measured in increments of 0.5 mm, from the minimum value of 0.0 mm, i.e. no visible calculus to 5.0 mm (i.e. 5.0 mm ring of

calculus is visible). Thus, the scoring is as follows (in mm):

| 0.0 | 0.5 | 1.0 | 1.5 | 2.0 | 2.5 |
| 3.0 | 3.5 | 4.0 | 4.5 | 5.0 |

4. **Special considerations for scoring:** The following are the special cases where calculus thickness does not lie between 0.5 – 5.0mm scale:
   a. **Un-measurable collar of calculus:** If there is a minute, thin collar of calculus present all around the tooth, less than 0.5 mm, then the entire tooth as a whole is assigned the value of 0.5 mm (i.e. for all the three surfaces one score is given).
   b. **Heavy calculus at inter-proximal areas:** If a large amount or heavy chunk of calculus is present between the anterior teeth, such that, even their inter-proximal surfaces are completely filled with calculus, then an imaginary vertical line is drawn through the total amount of inter-proximal calculus present, thus assigning first half of calculus to one tooth and second half to the adjacent tooth present.
   c. **Heavy calculus at lingual area:** If heavy calculus is present only at the lingual area of an individual tooth and is having thickness more than 5.0 mm, then it is assigned that particular value (i.e. 6.0 mm, 6.5 mm, 7.0 mm, etc.).

5. **Calculation of index**
   a. After scoring the tooth for its three planes, all the scores of that individual tooth are summed up. This is the VMI score for individual tooth.
   b. Then, score of each individual tooth is summed up to get total VMI score for that person.
   c. Finally, the index is calculated by dividing the total VMI score for a person by total number of lower anterior teeth examined, i.e.

$$VMI = \frac{\text{Total VMI score for that person}}{\text{Total number of lower anterior teeth examined}}$$

INDICES USED FOR ASSESSMENT OF GINGIVITIS

The tissues involving gingivitis are described as follows:

- **Gingiva:** Gingiva is the part of oral mucosa that covers the alveolar processes of the jaws and surrounds the necks of the teeth. It is anatomically divided into three types:

  i. **Marginal gingiva** or **unattached gingiva** is the terminal edge or border of gingiva that surrounds a tooth in collar like fashion.

  ii. **Attached gingiva** is the firm and resistant part of gingiva that is tightly bound to underlying periosteum of alveolar bone and is continuous with marginal gingiva. It is the distance between the muco-gingival junction and the projection of the external surface of the bottom of gingival sulcus or periodontal pocket.

  iii. **Inter-dental/papillary gingiva** is gingiva occupying the gingival embrasure, i.e. the inter-proximal space beneath the area of tooth contact is inter-dental gingiva. It can be of different shapes.

     a. *Pyramidal:* Tip of papilla is located immediately beneath contact point, as seen in anterior teeth.

     b. *Col:* It presents as a valley like depression that connects the facial and lingual papilla, as seen in posterior teeth.

- **Gingival sulcus:** The shallow crevice or space around the tooth bounded by surface of tooth on one side and the epithelium lining the free margin of gingiva on the other. It is V-shaped and barely permits the entrance of the periodontal probe.

- **Free gingival groove:** It is a shallow linear depression that separates marginal gingiva from the attached gingiva.

Gingivitis is defined as *the inflammation of gingiva in which junctional epithelium remains attached to the tooth at its original level.*

Although, the clinical signs of gingivitis are easy to detect, the amount of inflammation an individual must have to be considered as a case of gingivitis can never be accurately ascertained. Various indices have been used to study gingivitis. Depending on the study, the gingival unit may be an anatomic structure of gingiva (e.g. PMA index) or it may be a gingival site defined in relation to tooth, such as facial, lingual, mesial or distal gingiva (e.g. GI).

The indices for assessment of gingivitis are as follows:

Indices for Assessment of Gingival Inflammation

Papillary Marginal Attachment Index (PMA Index)

It was *probably the first reliable attempt to classify gingival inflammation* quantitatively using a numerical system. In the past, gingivitis was classified as mild, moderate and severe. It is also a *cumulative index*, like DMF, and is recorded as a sum total of the gingival units having gingival inflammation, regardless of the severity of inflammation.

This index scores the facial surface of gingiva after dividing it into anatomical units (Fig.12.21).

a. Papillary (P)

b. Marginal (M)

c. Attached (A)

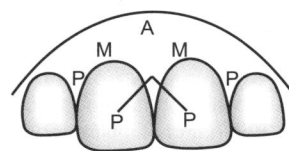

Fig. 12.21: Scoring units for Papillary Marginal Attachment Index (PMA)
P- Paillary gingiva
M - Marginal gingiva
A - Attached gingiva

Scoring: The scoring is carried out as follows for the above three anatomical units respectively (Table 12.31a, b, and c):

P – for papillary gingiva: The score ranges from 0 to 5.

Table 12.31a: Scoring for Papillary gingiva

Score	Criteria
0	Normal papilla showing no signs inflammation
1+	Mild papillary engorement with slight increase in size of papilla
2+	Obvious increase in size of papilla, with bleeding on probing
3+	Excessive increase in size of papillary gingiva with spontaneous bleeding
4+	Necrotic papilla
5+	Inflammation leading to atrophy and loss of papilla

Inflammation confined to papilla is the mildest form of inflammation.

M – for marginal gingiva: Its scoring range is also from 0 to 5.

Table 12.31b: Scoring for Marginal gingiva

Score	Criteria
0	Normal marginal gingiva without inflammatory signs
1+	Engorgement of marginal gingiva with slight increase in size
2+	Obvious engorgement of marginal gingiva with bleeding on pressure
3+	Swollen collar of marginal gingiva having spontaneous bleeding or/and beginning of infiltration into attached gingival
4+	Necrotic marginal gingival
5+	Recession of free marginal gingiva below the CEJ due to inflammatory changes

A – for attached gingiva: It is scored in range of 0-3.

Table 12.31c: Scoring for Attached gingiva

Score	Criteria
0	Normal attached gingiva showing stippling
1+	Slightly engorged attached gingiva with loss of stippling. Colour change may or may not be there.
2+	Obvious engorgement of attached gingiva showing marked redness with pocket formation
3+	Advanced periodontitis with deep pockets

Procedure

The patient is seated comfortably at a well illuminated place and examination is started from the left second molar to right second molar for maxillary arch and continued from right second molar to left second molar for mandibular arch. Scoring is carried out on the basis of presence or absence of inflammation for the facial gingiva. The three gingival units, i.e. P, M, A of facial gingiva are scored separately using the above criteria. *Third molars are not included in the PMA index score.* Separate numerical values of P, M, A are summed up first for each tooth and then for each arch and finally expressed as the total PMA score.

Thus, **PMA value of tooth** = Score of P + Score of M + Score of A for that tooth.

PMA value of each arch (maxillary/mandibular) = Sum of the scores of PMA for all the teeth present in the arch.

PMA value of an individual = Sum of PMA score for maxillary arch + Sum of PMA score for mandibular arch.

Uses of PMA Index

PMA index is used for assessing the gingival disease for:

- An individual patient
- Clinical trials
- Epidemiological surveys

Modifications of PMA Index

i. For large surveys, the examination of patient of PMA index can be carried out from premolar to premolar in order to save time.

ii. Papillary Marginal Index (PMI): This is simplified form of PMA index to be used in the school surveys. The basis behind this modification is that 'A' unit, i.e. attached gingiva is rarely inflamed/diseased in school going children (mostly the inflammation is limited to papillary or marginal units).

The examination procedure is similar to PMA index while scoring criteria is as follows (Table 12.32).

Table 12.32: Scoring criteria for Papillary Marginal Index	
Score	Criteria
0	No inflammation, healthy gingiva
1	Gingiva appearing normal visually (i.e. colour, contour), but bleeding on gentle probing present
2	Bleeding on probing with change of colour; contour normal (no oedema)
3	Bleeding on probing, change of colour, edematous swelling altering gingival contour present
4	Ulceration or additional symptoms

The index is calculated by:

$$PMI = \frac{\text{Sum of all the scores for an individual}}{\text{Number of areas scored}}$$

Gingival Index (GI)

This index was developed by *Löe and Silness* for assessing the severity of gingivitis by examining the qualitative changes of gingival soft tissue without considering the quantitative changes of periodontium (like pocket depth, alveolar bone loss, etc.). It rates the gingivitis into mild, moderate and severe gingivitis according to the GI scores obtained.

Gingival Index (GI) scores the gingival inflammation after dividing the gingival tissues into four scoring units (Fig. 12.22).

a. Distal-facial papilla
b. Facial marginal gingiva
c. Mesial-facial papilla
d. Lingual-gingival margin

Lingual-gingival margin is scored as a single unit because it is most likely to be viewed indirectly using mouth mirror and thus has maximum chances of being scored inadequately (Fig.12.23).

The scoring can be carried out for:

- **Full mouth dentition:** It is not routinely followed but is the ideal method.

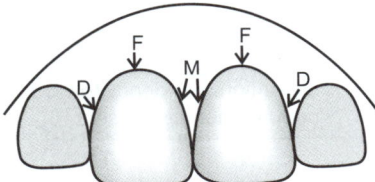

Fig.12.22: Papillae to be examined for Gingival Index (GI)
M - Mesial facial papilla
D - Distal facial papilla
F - Facial marginal gingiva

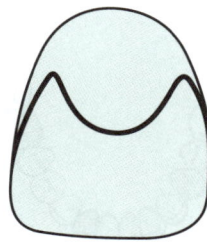

Fig. 12.23: Lingual marginal gingiva for Gingival Index scoring

- **Selected teeth:** The selected index teeth that are scored are (Fig.12.24) as follows:

16 – Maxillary right first molar
12 – Maxillary left lateral incisor
24 – Maxillary left first premolar
36 – Mandibular left first molar
32 – Mandibular left lateral incisor
44 – Mandibular right first premolar

The *scoring criteria* for Gingival Index (GI) are as follows (Table 12.33):

Table 12.33: Scoring criteria for Gingival Index

Score	Criteria
0	**Normal gingiva**, without any signs of inflammation
1	**Mild inflammation**, gingiva showing slight color change and edema; no bleeding on probing
2	**Moderate inflammation**, gingiva showing moderate glazing redness, hypertrophy and edema. Bleeding on probing present
3	**Severe inflammation** of gingiva with marked redness, hypertrophy and ulceration. Tendency towards spontaneous bleeding present

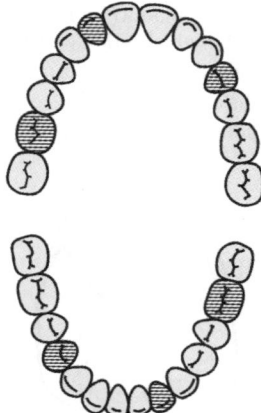

Fig. 12.24: Teeth to be examined for Gingival Index (GI)

Procedure

The patient is seated at a well illuminated place and the teeth and gingiva that are to be examined are dried with cotton rolls. The use of blast of air to dry teeth should be avoided as it can start bleeding in an inflamed gingiva. Each of the four units of a tooth is examined and scored according to the scoring criteria. Examination for each tooth is carried out using a blunt instrument such as periodontal probe to assess the bleeding potential of the inflamed tissues.

The GI score for a single tooth is obtained by dividing the sum of the scores of all the four units examined for that tooth by four, i.e.

$$\text{GI of tooth} = \frac{\text{Total score of all the four units of that tooth}}{4}$$

And, the GI for an individual is obtained by dividing the sum of all the obtained scores per tooth by the number of teeth examined, i.e.

$$\text{GI of a person} = \frac{\text{Sum of scores obtained for all teeth examined for that person}}{\text{Number of teeth examined for that person}}$$

The numerical scores of GI are correlated clinically with disease as follows (Table 12.34).

Table 12.34: Gingival index score and disease

GI scores	Clinical disease
0.1 – 1.0	Mild gingivitis
1.1 – 2.0	Moderate gingivitis
2.1 – 3.0	Severe gingivitis

Uses of Gingival Index

The gingival index is used.

a. **In epidemiological surveys:** To determine the prevalence and severity of gingivitis.

b. **For controlled clinical trials:** To assess the clinical efficacy of the preventive or therapeutic agents

c. **In individual dentition:** To assess the severity of gingivitis in an individual

d. **In deciduous dentition:** To assess the gingival inflammation of children

Limitations of Gingival Index

The major limitation of Gingival Index is that, it takes only **qualitative changes of gingiva** into account and does not consider the quantity of disease. Disease can be classified only as mild, moderate and severe; the middle range in between any two of them cannot be accomplished.

Gingival Index is a widely accepted index. Its validity, reliability and easy procedure make it one of the most widely used indices for assessing gingival inflammation.

Modifications of Gingival Index

The modifications are:

a. **Löe's modification of Gingival Index:** Like plaque index, Löe also modified Gingival Index by giving a detailed sequence for the examination of individual's full dentition instead of six index teeth. The examination procedure should be as follows:

 i. **For maxillary arch:** The procedure should commence at the maxillary arch, from the buccal aspect of the right second molar and continue over the midline to end at buccal aspect of the left second molar. For the right side, the buccal surface of gingiva of each tooth is scored in sequence of distal facial papilla, facial margin, mesial-facial papilla while for left side the sequence will become mesial-facial papilla, facial margin and distal-facial papilla. After that lingual surfaces of maxillary teeth are scored; starting from the upper left second molar.

 ii. **For mandibular arch:** The examination is started with the buccal-gingiva of the lower left second molar and is continued over the midline to end at the buccal-gingiva of the lower right second molar. For left side, the sequence is distal-facial papilla, facial margin and mesial-facial papilla while on right side it is mesial-facial papilla, facial papilla, distal-facial papilla. Afterwards all the lingual surfaces are scored, starting from the right mandibular second molar.

The GI is calculated by dividing the total score obtained for an individual (for all the four areas) by the total number of teeth examined (i.e. 28 if whole dentition is present; *third molars are not included*).

$$GI = \frac{\text{Total score for an individual}}{\text{Total number of teeth examined}}$$

b. **Modified Gingival Index (MGI)**

 This index is a modification of Löe and Silness Gingival Index. The motive behind its development was to increase the sensitivity of assessment in the low region of the scoring scale. Since its development, the MGI has been *widely used in the clinical trials of therapeutic agents.*

 The index is same as Gingival Index except that scoring criteria have been changed (Table 12.35).

Table 12.35: Scoring criteria for Modified Gingival Index	
Score	*Criteria*
0	**Normal gingiva** (without signs of inflammation)
1	**Mild inflammation** (slight change in color and texture without any edema) of any portion of gingival unit
2	**Mild inflammation** of entire gingival unit
3	**Moderate inflammation** (moderate glazing, redness, edema and/or hypertrophy) of entire gingival unit

Contd...

Score	Criteria
4	**Severe inflammation** (marked redness, edema/hypertrophy or ulceration) of gingival unit – spontaneous bleeding present

Procedure

The examination procedure for Modified Gingival Index (MGI) is almost the same as Gingival Index except that the MGI is a noninvasive index in which the periodontal probe is not used for examination (see scoring also, criteria of bleeding on probing is eliminated). The scoring is typically based on visual observation, which has maintained high visual sensitivity, especially for incipient gingivitis.

Examination can be carried out for six index teeth (same as GI) or full dentition. The labial/buccal and lingual surfaces of gingival margins and inter-dental papillae of teeth are examined and scored using above criteria. Here, the gingiva is not divided into four parts for scoring and papillary, facial and lingual marginal gingiva is scored. *Third molars are not included in examination.*

Maximum gingival units for full dentition to be scored are (Table 12.36):

Table 12.36: Scoring for Gingival Units

	Maxillary	Mandibular	Total
Facial Margins	14	14	28
Lingual Margins	14	14	28
Facial Papilla	13	13	26
Lingual Papilla	13	13	26

Total gingival units scored are 52 marginal and 52 papillary, i.e. 108 gingival units.

The MGI is **calculated** as:

$$MGI = \frac{\text{Sum of papillary and marginal scores obtained for an individual}}{\text{Total number of sites (i.e. gingival units) examined}}$$

INDICES USED FOR ASSESSMENT OF GINGIVAL BLEEDING

This is the category of indices that assess the gingival inflammation by considering the amount and extent of bleeding from gingival tissue. The *earliest sign of gingival disease that can be detected clinically is bleeding on probing.* This is the basic criterion behind the development of these indices. The various indices used are as follows:

Sulcus Bleeding Index (SBI)

Sulcus Bleeding Index (SBI) was developed to detect and assess the early gingival disease. This index is basically a modification of Papillary Marginal index.

Sulcus Bleeding Index (SBI) locates the areas of gingival sulcus that bleed after gentle probing. It is a full mouth index in which four gingival units of teeth are scored (Fig. 12.25a, b). The units are:

(P) – Papillary units – 2 papillary units – Mesial and distal papilla.

(M) – Marginal units – 2 marginal units – Facial and Lingual.

The scoring criteria for each gingival unit are as follows (Table 12.37):

Table 12.37: Scoring criteria for each gingival unit

Score	Criteria
0	Normal, healthy gingival
1	Apparently healthy P and M units, showing normal color and contour, but bleeding on probing present
2	Bleeding on probing present, reddening of gingiva, without swelling; macroscopic edema or changed contour
3	Bleeding on probing, redness with slight edematous swelling present

Contd...

Score	Criteria
4	Bleeding on probing and redness with obvious swelling
5	Spontaneous bleeding with color change; marked swelling with or without ulceration of gingival unit

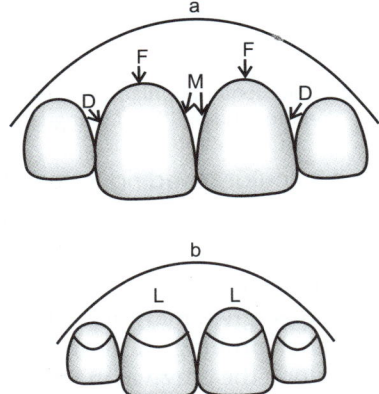

Fig. 12.25a, b: Units to be examined for Sulcus Bleeding Index (SBI)

(P) Unit	M: Mesial papilla
	D: Distal papilla
(M) Unit	F: Facial Marginal gingiva
	L: Lingual Marginal gingiva

Procedure

The patient is seated comfortably at a well-illuminated place and the gingiva is dried and cleaned gently. Teeth present in the dentition are examined in a systematic manner. Scoring each of the four gingival units (2M and 2P) is carried out for each tooth after using the above criteria. First, visual examination is carried out for the evaluation of change in color and contour of gingival unit followed by the probing using blunt periodontal instrument. The probe should be held parallel to the long axis of tooth to be examined for the M units

and should be directed towards 'col' area for P units. One must wait for 30 seconds after probing to detect any delayed bleeding. Each unit is assigned its score from 0–5.

Calculation of Index

The index can be calculated for:

a. **Single tooth:** The index is obtained by dividing the sum of scores for the four units of that tooth by 4, i.e.

$$\text{SBI single tooth} = \frac{\text{Sum of scores of four gingival units of that tooth}}{4}$$

b. **An Individual:** It is obtained by dividing the sum of scores of all the individual teeth recorded by the total number of teeth examined.

$$\text{SBI for individual} = \frac{\text{Sum of tooth scores of individual teeth for that person}}{\text{Total number of teeth examined in that person}}$$

Modifications of SBI

Sulcus Bleeding Index (SBI) being time consuming and a little complex for large surveys, several modifications of SBI were introduced to simplify it. These are:

Papillary Bleeding Index (PBI)

Papillary Bleeding Index (PBI) is a modified version of SBI. In this index only inter-dental papilla (mesial and distal) is scored (Fig. 12.26).

This is a full mouth index but the scoring of teeth is carried out after dividing the mouth into four quadrants as follows:

a. *Maxillary right quadrant:* In this, lingual inter-dental papillae of teeth are scored.

b. *Maxillary left quadrant*: In this, buccal inter-dental papillae of teeth are scored.

c. *Mandibular right quadrant:* In this, buccal inter-dental papillae of teeth are scored.

d. *Mandibular left quadrant*: In this, lingual inter-dental papillae of teeth are scored.

The intensity of bleeding is scored on scale of 0–4 (Table 12.38).

Table 12.38: Scoring criteria for intensity of bleeding	
Score	Criteria
0	No bleeding after probing
1	A single discrete bleeding point that appears after probing
2	Several isolated bleeding points or single fine line of blood appears
3	The inter-dental triangle fills shortly after probing
4	Profuse bleeding occurs after probing and blood flows immediately into marginal sulcus

Procedure

The patient is seated comfortably at a well illuminated place and the teeth are cleaned gently. Papillary Bleeding Index (PBI) is scored on mesial and distal aspects of inter-dental papilla on the assigned surfaces of teeth in particular quadrants according to above criteria. The blunt periodontal instrument is introduced into the gingival sulcus on the mesial aspect and moved coronally to papilla's tip. The same procedure is repeated for the distal side of same papilla and bleeding intensity is recorded. Examiner must wait for 30 seconds after probing to give an adequate score to the papilla.

Papillary Bleeding Index (PBI) is finally **calculated** by dividing the sum of scores for all teeth by the total number of teeth examined, i.e.

$$PBI = \frac{\text{Sum of scores for all the papillae examined for a person}}{\text{Total number of teeth examined for that person}}$$

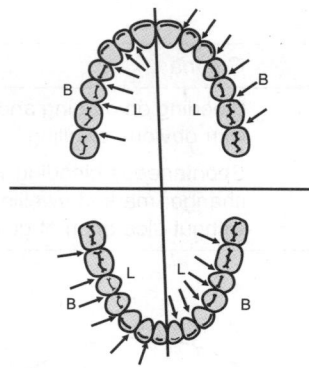

Fig. 12.26: Interdental papillae to be examined for Papillary Bleeding Index (PBI), L: Lingual, B: Buccal

Modified Sulcular Bleeding Index (mSBI)

This index is modification of the Papillary Bleeding Index (PBI) that assesses the severity of gingival bleeding.

Here, the gingival margin is scored for the bleeding after probing. A periodontal probe is passed along the gingival margin and scoring is carried out using following criteria (Table 12.39):

Table 12.39: Scoring criteria for modified Sulcular Bleeding Index	
Score	Criteria
0	No bleeding on probing, when probe is passed along the gingival margin
1	Isolated visible bleeding spots emerge after probing on gingival margin
2	Blood forms a confluent line on gingival margin
3	Profuse bleeding from gingival margin
5	Inflammation leading to atrophy and loss of papilla

The mSBI is **calculated** by dividing the total score obtained for teeth by total number of teeth examined, i.e.

$$\text{mSBI} = \frac{\text{Sum of scores obtained for all the teeth examined for that individual}}{\text{Total number of teeth examined for that individual}}$$

Gingival Bleeding Index (GBI)

Gingival Bleeding Index (GBI) was developed to detect gingival inflammation by presence or absence of bleeding from the inter-proximal gingival sulci.

For Gingival Bleeding Index (GBI) there are **no particular scoring criteria** as this index does not make any attempt to quantify the gingival disease. Bleeding indicates the presence of disease, while its absence means healthy gingiva. Each of the inter-proximal area has two sulci; mesial and distal, which are scored separately or together as an inter-dental unit.

Procedure

The patient is seated comfortably at a well-illuminated place and examination procedure is started with unwaxed dental floss. The floss is first passed inter-proximally on one side of the papilla and then on the other. The floss is then curved around the adjacent tooth, brought below the gingival margin and moved up and down for one stroke gently to prevent the laceration of gingiva. The used floss is then discarded. A new floss of adequate length should be used for each of the remaining areas. Occurrence of bleeding is noted. One must wait for at least 30 seconds so as to ensure that there is no delayed bleeding from the gingiva. Gingiva can be slightly retracted to improve visibility from facial and lingual aspects. All inter-proximal areas are examined one by one and these areas are recorded as areas of risk. Certain areas can be excluded from scoring because of inaccessibility, mal-positioning (rotations, supernumerary teeth) diastema, etc. Third molars are excluded from this index. Thus, a full complement of teeth will have 26 inter-dental scoring units for this index.

The total of all the bleeding areas is Gingival Bleeding Index (GBI) for that person, i.e.

Gingival Bleeding Index (GBI) = Sum of the bleeding points in individual's dentition

Advantages

- The index is simple and easy to perform.
- The procedure basically requires the use of dental floss, so it is easy for the individual to understand.
- Patient participation in observing and recording over series of appointments helps to enhance the motivation.

Eastman Inter-dental Bleeding Index (EIBI)

Eastman Inter-dental Bleeding Index (EIBI) detects the gingival inflammation in inter-dental area (like GBI) by considering presence or absence of bleeding.

In this index also, quantification of severity of gingival bleeding is not recorded. Simply, number of bleeding sites are recorded and totaled to get Eastman Inter-dental Bleeding Index (EIBI) score.

Procedure

Eastman Inter-dental Bleeding Index is also a full mouth index and examination is carried out on each inter-dental area of the entire dentition. However, instead of floss, wooden inter-dental cleanser with a triangular tip is used for performing it. An inter-dental cleanser is inserted into each inter-dental area, depressing it by 1 to 2.0 mm and is removed gently. The insertion and removal should be carried out consecutively for four times and then examiner should proceed towards next inter-dental area. The path of insertion of cleanser should be parallel to the occlusal surface and it should not point apically. One must wait for **15 seconds** to record the bleeding.

The number of bleeding sites are recorded and sum of this EIBI score divided by total number of areas examined for an individual multiplied by 100 will give EIBI. Thus, EIBI is expressed as a percentage value.

$$EIBI = \frac{\text{Total number of bleeding areas in an individual}}{\text{Total number of areas examined in that individual}} \times 100$$

NIDCR Protocol for Assessment of Gingival Bleeding

National Institute of Dental and Craniofacial Research (NIDCR) has used the presence or absence of gingival bleeding as an indication of gingival disease. It is just a component of one of the several components of NIDCR protocol for the assessment of periodontal disease.

This index assesses the facial and mesio-facial sites of teeth in two randomly selected quadrants- one maxillary and one mandibular. This index, also, calculates the total number of bleeding units without quantifying the disease.

Procedure

Two quadrants are selected randomly (one maxillary and one mandibular) and each tooth present in them is assessed for the gingival bleeding using a special NIDR probe. This is a color coded probe graduated at 2, 4, 6, 8, 10 and 12.0 mm. To begin with assessment, the selected quadrant is air dried. Starting with the most posterior tooth of the first quadrant (excluding third molars), the probing is begun on the facial side and the probe is carefully swept into the mesial inter-proximal area. Each probed site is assessed for the presence or absence of bleeding. The same procedure is repeated for the remaining teeth in the quadrant. The sum of the total bleeding sites or percentage of the total sites examined can be used to assess the gingival disease.

INDICES FOR PERIODONTAL DISEASES

The study of epidemiology of periodontal diseases requires precise rules, which can be applied while determining and recording the periodontal status of the individuals being studied. Indices are used to express clinical observations in terms of numeric values. These values may further be used for quantitating and evaluating the factors being studied.

Like dental caries, periodontal disease is also a pathologic process. It begins as a microscopic lesion which cannot be positively diagnosed with confidence and develops into a clinically obvious lesion. Gingivitis and pocket formation are steps in the development of periodontal disease and the ability to recognize the signs of these conditions depends on a number of factors. However, all the factors cannot be controlled and accurately determined by the examiner. A simple present/absent type of classification for recording clinical signs of periodontal diseases should be used to provide valid indications of disease status and estimation of treatment requirements. To assess the periodontal status of individuals, the various indices used are:

Periodontal Index (PI)

The increasing popularity of gingival indices motivated *Russell* to develop an index that can be used to measure the advanced stages of periodontitis in the population, popularly known as *Russell's Periodontal Index*. It is a **composite index** as it records both reversible as well as irreversible changes of periodontal tissues.

Russell's Index can be based solely upon the clinical examination, or it can make use of dental radiographs, if available. Each tooth can be scored separately according to following criteria (Table 12.40).

Procedure

Periodontal Index is quite fast and easy to use. It requires minimum equipment: a light

	Table 12.40: Scoring criteria for Russell's Index		
Score		*Criteria for field studies*	*Additional radiographic criteria for clinical studies*
0	Negative	There is neither overt inflammation in the investing tissues nor loss of function due to destruction of supporting tissues	
1	Mild-gingivtis	An overt area of gingival inflammation in free gingiva that does not completely circumscribe the tooth.	
2	Gingivitis	Inflammation completely circumscribes the tooth, but there is no apparent break in epithelial attachment.	
4		Used only if radiographs are available as there is no clinical basis of this criteria.	There is an early notch like resorption of alveolar crest (First radiographic criteria)
6	Gingivitis with pocket formation	Epithelial attachment has been broken and there is pocket formation (not merely a deepened gingival crevice due to swelling) without any interference with normal masticatory functions; tooth is firm in its socket and has not been drifted.	X-ray shows horizontal bone loss involving entire alveolar crest, up to half of the root length
8	Advanced destruction with loss of masticatory function	The tooth may be: • Mobile • Sound dull on percussion with mouth mirror • Or may be depressible in the socket	X-ray shows advanced bone loss involving more than half of root length and/or a definite infrabony pocket with widened periodontal ligament and/or root resorption or rarefaction at root apex.

source, a mouth mirror and an explorer. The supporting tissues for **each tooth in the mouth** are scored according to the progressive scale which gives less weightage to gingivitis and relatively more weightage to advanced periodontal disease. Probing is avoided, as according to Russell – *probing adds little and has been proved to be a troublesome focus of* examiner disagreement. If an examiner is in doubt about the scoring, **Russell's rule**, i.e. *whenever in doubt, always assign the lower score*

may be applied. Ultimately the index can be **calculated** in the following ways:

a. PI for an Individual: It is calculated by dividing the sum of scores obtained for an individual by total number of teeth examined.

$$\text{PI for an individual} = \frac{\text{Total score obtained for an individual}}{\text{Total number of teeth examined for that individual}}$$

b *PI for a population:* It is the average of the individual scores in population examined.

$$PI \text{ for population} = \frac{\begin{array}{c}\text{Total PI score of}\\\text{all the individuals in}\\\text{population examined}\end{array}}{\begin{array}{c}\text{Total number of individuals}\\\text{examined in that population}\end{array}}$$

Interpretation

The minimum score value is 0 while the maximum score value is 8. The score can be correlated with the index values as follows (Table 12.41 a, b):

Table 12.41a: Periodontal Index score (Individual)

PI score	Clinical condition
0 – 0.2	Clinically normal periodontal tissues
0.3 – 0.9	Simple gingivitis (Reversible)
1 – 1.9	Initiating destructive periodontal disease (Reversible)
2 – 4.9	Established destructive periodontal disease (Irreversible)
5 – 8	Terminal disease (Irreversible)

Table 12.41b: Periodontal Index score (Population)

PI score	Clinical condition
0 – 0.2	Clinically normal periodontal tissues
0.3 – 0.9	Simple gingivitis (Reversible)
0.7 – 1.9	Initiating destructive periodontal disease
1.6 – 5	Established destructive periodontal disease (Irreversible)
3.8 – 8	Terminal disease (Irreversible)

Limitations

• Due to its method of examination and scoring criteria, this index has been found to be of limited use for individual or small groups.
• It tends to underestimate the true level of periodontal disease, especially the changes due to early bone loss.
• The number of periodontal pockets with supra-gingival calculus is also under-estimated in PI.

Uses

It is used for:
• Epidemiological surveys
• National Health Surveys (NHS)
• Judging individual's periodontal status (but not much reliable)

Periodontal Disease Index (PDI)

Taking the positive features of existing indices and adding new criteria to compensate for their shortcomings, *Sigurd Ramfjord*, developed Periodontal Disease Index. It is basically a clinician's modification of the Russell's Periodontal Index that can be used for a large population as well as for small groups or individuals with equal accuracy.

This index basically consists of three components of scoring that are:
A. The gingival and periodontal component
B. The plaque component
C. The calculus component

Each of the above is scored by an independent criteria.

Ramfjord Teeth

The specific teeth (Fig. 12.27) selected by Ramfjord for recording the index are known as *Ramfjord teeth*. These are:

16	-	Maxillary right first molar
21	-	Maxillary left central incisor
24	-	Maxillary left first premolar
36	-	Mandibular left first molar
41	-	Mandibular right central incisor
44	-	Mandibular right first premolar

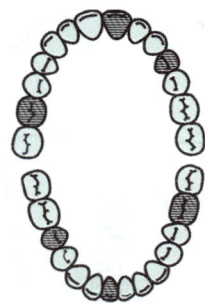

Fig. 12.27: Teeth to be examined for the Peridonal Disease Index (PDI)

A. The gingival and periodontal component:
To begin the assessment, the examiner dries the areas around six teeth to assess the severity of gingival inflammation. Scores from G-0 to G-3 are provided after assesing the gingiva around the tooth for:

a. Color change: The color changes from coral pink to red, blue or purple in gingivitis.

b. Contour: The blunting or rounding of gingival margin; thickening of papilla or swelling due to edematous fluid can change the contour during gingivitis

c. Consistency: The gentle probing pressure can detect the change from normal firm and resilient consistency of gingiva to soft/spongy one.

d. Stippling: The presence/absence of stippling can be considered, but is never the deciding factor due to marked individual variation.

e. Gingival ulceration: It indicates severe gingivitis.

f. Gingival crevice depth: The depth is recorded in millimeters with respect to the cemento-enamel junction. University of Michigan Number 'O' probe is used for recording the crevicular depth. A deepened gingival sulcus is called pocket. This pocket can be:

   i. Gingival pocket/Pseudo pocket: This pocket is formed by gingival enlargement with the destruction of underlying periodontal tissues. Increased bulk of gingiva causes deepening of gingival sulcus.

  ii. Periodontal pocket: This type of pocket occurs due to destruction of supporting periodontal tissues leading to loosening and exfoliation of teeth.

    Thus, by measuring the crevicular depth, examiner can detect loss of the periodontal attachment apparatus.

Ramfjord's Method

One of the unique aspects of *Ramfjord Index* was the use of cemento-enamel junction (CEJ) as a fixed landmark for measuring the periodontal attachment loss (Fig. 12.28)

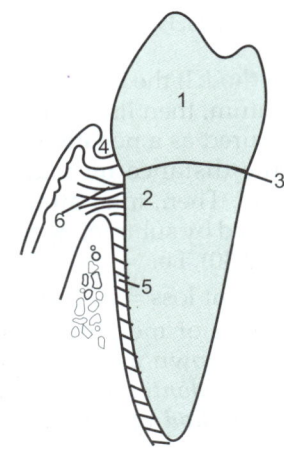

Fig. 12.28: Normal attachment appratus

1. Crown	4. Gingival crevice
2. Root	5. Periodontal ligament
3. CEJ (Fixed landmark)	6. Gingival fibres

   The following criteria are used for measurement of attachment loss in PDI considering according to the position of gingival margin:

a. Direct Method: *If free gingival margin is on enamel* then the distance of gingival margin from the CEJ measured first (x) and then the distance from the margin to bottom of gingival sulcus is measured (y). The later value (y) is the depth of gingival sulcus. By the subtraction of former from latter the attachment loss can be calculated (shaded portion).

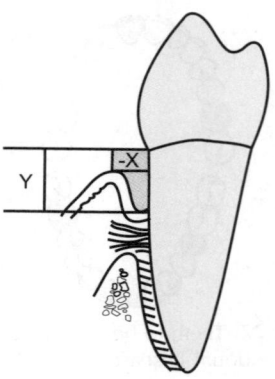

Fig. 12.30: Loss of attachment-indirect method (Y + X)

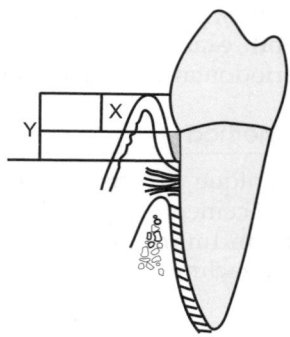

Fig. 12.29: Loss of attachment-direct method (Y–X)

b. Indirect method: If the free gingival margin is on cementum, then its distance from the CEJ is measured as a negative value (say -x). Also, the distance measured (sulcus depth, say y). Then, total attachment loss can be obtained by subtracting former from later (Fig. 12.30), i.e.

Attachment loss = y - (-x) = y + x

This method of measuring the attachment loss is known as *indirect method of measuring periodontal attachment loss or* **Ramfjord's method of measuring attachment loss.**

Examination Technique

The University of Michigan Number 'O' probe, graduated at 3.0, 6.0, 8.0 mm from end, is used for examination. The probe end is placed against the enamel surface coronally to the margin of gingiva such that the working end of probe is at an angle of 45° to the long axis of crown. The probe is passed towards apical direction maintaining the contact with tooth, pointing towards apex of single rooted tooth or the central axis of multi-rooted teeth. The distance of free gingival margin to CEJ is measured moving the probe along the cemental surface of tooth. It can be achieved only if there has been loss of periodontal attachment.

The examination is performed for mesial, facial, distal and lingual sides of six index teeth. Buccal measurements should be made at middle of buccal surface, while mesial measurement is made at buccal aspect of inter-proximal contact area with probe touching both teeth if adjacent tooth is present in the arch. Probe should point towards the long axis of tooth that is to be scored.

Scoring Criteria

The scoring criteria for Periodontal Disease Index are as follows (Table 12.42).

Table 12.42: Scoring criteria for Periodontal Disease Index	
Score	Criteria
0	Absence of inflammation – Healthy tooth
1	Mild to moderate gingival changes not extending all around the tooth

Contd...

Score	Criteria
2	Mild to moderately severe gingival changes that extend all around the tooth
3	Severe gingivitis, characterized by marked redness, tendency to bleed and ulceration
4	Gingival crevice in any of the four measured areas extending apically to the CEJ but not more than 3.0 mm.
5	Gingival crevice in any of the four measured areas extending 3.0-6.0 mm apically to CEJ.
6	Gingival crevice in any of the four measured areas extending apically more than 6 mm from CEJ.

In surveys:

a. If gingival sulcus in none of the measured areas extends apical to the CEJ, the recorded score for gingivitis is the PDI score for that tooth (i.e. 0–3).
b. However, if the gingival sulcus in any of the two measured areas extends apical to the CEJ but its extension is not more than 3.0 mm the PDI score is '4'. The gingivitis score is disregarded for that tooth.
c. If the gingival sulcus extends 3.0–6.0 mm apical to the CEJ in either of the recorded areas of tooth, PDI score is 5 (disregard the gingivitis score for that tooth).
d. If the gingival sulcus extends more than 6.0 mm apical to the CEJ in any of the measured areas of the tooth, then PDI value for it is 6 (again disregarding gingivitis score).

The index is **calculated** as follows:

For an individual:

The average of PDI score obtained in a group is the score for an individual, i.e.

$$\text{PDI for an individual} = \frac{\text{Sum of PDI scores of each tooth examined}}{\text{Total number of teeth examined for that individual}}$$

For a population (group):

It is the average score of the individual of that group, i.e.

$$\text{PDI for population (group)} = \frac{\text{Sum of PDI scores of each individual present in group}}{\text{Total number of individual examined}}$$

B. The plaque component: The plaque component scores the plaque present on the surfaces of the teeth. It was the first index that attempted the use of numerical scale to assess the biofilm present on teeth.

The following scoring criteria are used for the plaque assessment (Table 12.43).

Score	Criteria
\multicolumn{2}{c}{**Table 12.43:** Scoring criteria for Plaque Assessment}
0	No plaque present
1	Plaque present on some but not all inter-proximal, buccal and lingual surfaces of the tooth
2	Plaque present on all inter-proximal, buccal and lingual surfaces, but covering less than one half of these tooth surfaces
3	Plaque extending over all the inter-proximal, buccal and lingual surfaces, covering more than half of these tooth surfaces

Procedure

The patient is seated at a well illuminated place and a disclosing solution is applied on the teeth. Bismark brown (the disclosing solution) is poured in a dappen dish. Get two Richmond cotton pellets completely saturated in solution. One pellet is picked up using cotton plier (don't use hands) and is touched gently on the buccal, lingual and occlusal surfaces of mandibular teeth while the second one is used for maxillary teeth in similar manner. The patient is then instructed to spit and rinse thoroughly. Then, the scoring is carried out for the facial, lingual, mesial and distal surfaces of the Ramfjord teeth using above mentioned criteria. Only fully erupted teeth are scored without making any substitutions for missing teeth.

The plaque score for an individual is calculated as the average value of the scores of individual's teeth, i.e.

$$\text{Plaque score of an individual} = \frac{\text{Sum of the scores for the Ramfjord teeth examined in an individual}}{\text{Total number of Ramfjord teeth examined for him}}$$

Shick and Ash Modification of Plaque Component of PDI

Simplifying the plaque component of PDI, *Schick and Ash* modified the scoring criteria of the plaque component of PDI. The modified criteria consists of scoring the plaque present on the gingival half of facial and lingual surfaces of six Ramfjord teeth, without scoring the inter-proximal surfaces.

The new scoring criteria are as follows (Table 12.44):

Table 12.44: Scoring criteria for Plaque Component of PDI

Score	Criteria
0	Absence of dental plaque
1	Dental plaque present at the gingival margin covering less than 1/3rd of gingival half of facial or lingual surfaces of tooth
2	Dental plaque covering more than 1/3rd but less than 2/3rd of the gingival half of the facial or lingual surfaces of the tooth
3	Dental plaque covering 2/3rd or more of the gingival half of facial or lingual surfaces of the tooth

The procedure of examination and calculation methods is similar to that of the PDI-plaque component.

C. **The calculus component:** The calculus component assesses the hard mineralized deposits present on the surfaces of teeth.

The six Ramfjord teeth are examined on the facial and lingual surfaces only (not inter-proximal) for the presence/absence of calculus using following scoring criteria (Table 12.45):

Table 12.45: Scoring criteria for Calculus component of PDI

Score	Criteria
0	No calculus present
1	Supra-gingival calculus extending only slightly below the free gingival margin (less than 1.0 mm)
2	Moderate amount of supra-gingival and sub-gingival calculus or only moderate sub-gingival calculus present without the presence of supra-gingival calculus
3	An abundance of supra-gingival and sub-gingival calculus.

Procedure

The patient is seated comfortably and the teeth are cleaned gently with a cotton swab. The presence and extent of calculus on the facial and lingual surfaces of six index teeth is evaluated using a mouth mirror and dental explorer; or a periodontal probe sequentially. An adequate scoring is provided to them using above mentioned criteria.

The average value for the individual's calculated score is the PDI-calculus value.

Advantages

- It is the first index that assesses the periodontal status of an individual completely.

- It has a high degree of examiner reproducibility.
- It can be performed easily and the scores are quite reliable.

Uses

It is used for:
- Longitudinal studies of periodontal disease.
- Epidemiological surveys.
- Clinical trials of preventive or therapeutic agents.
- Individual's as well as group's periodontal status assessment.

Gingival Periodontal Index (GPI)

Gingival Periodontal Index (GPI) was developed as a modification of Ramfjord's PDI for screening of individuals so as to determine the need of treatment for those suffering from periodontal diseases. The GPI assess following three components of PDI.
a. Gingival status
b. Periodontal status or crevice depth
c. Irritational factors; like material alba, calculus and overhanging restorations.

Six Segments of GPI

While PDI used six Ramfjord's teeth for assessment, GPI divides the whole maxillary and mandibular arch into six segments for scoring. The primary objective of this segmentation is to determine the tooth or its surrounding tissues, having the severest condition within each segment. The six segments are (Fig. 12.31):

1. Maxillary right third molar to right first premolar
2. Maxillary anterior area, i.e. right canine to left canine
3. Maxillary left first premolar to left third molar
4. Mandibular left third molar to left first premolar
5. Mandibular anterior area – right canine to left canine
6. Mandibular right first premolar to right third molar.

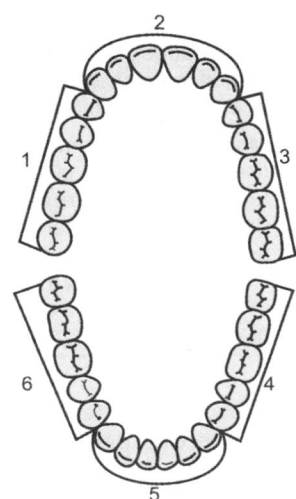

Fig. 12.31: Segments of teeth to be examined for Gingival Periodontal Index (GPI)

Each tooth of the segment is examined and scored accordingly. The components are scored separately using different criteria for each one.

To record gingival status: The scoring criteria used to record gingival inflammation are (Table 12.46):

Table 12.46: Scoring criteria for Gingival Inflammation	
Score	Criteria
0	*Absence of inflammation* – Tissue tightly adapted to the tooth, has firm consistency and shows normal physiological architecture
1	*Slight to moderate gingival inflammation* – gingiva shows colour changes, becomes edematous with blunting or slight enlargement of

Contd...

Score	Criteria
	marginal or papillary gingiva; involving one or more teeth in the same segment, but not completely surrounding any one tooth
2	The changes of score 1 criteria, if extend to *encircle* one or more teeth in a segment completely
3	*Marked inflammation* – loss of surface continuity, ulceration, spontaneous haemorrhage, marked deviation from normal contour [such as gross thickening or enlargement covering more than one third of anatomic crown]; recession, and gingival clefts are present.

To record periodontal status: The scoring criteria used to record periodontal inflammation are (Table 12.47):

Table 12.47: Scoring criteria for Periodontal Inflammation	
Score	Criteria
0	The probe does not extend 1.0 mm apical to CEJ of any tooth in the segment and there is no exposure of CEJ.
4	The probe can extend up to 3.0 mm apical to CEJ of any tooth in any segment
5	The probe extends 3.0 mm to 6.0 mm apical to CEJ of any tooth in the segment
6	The probe extends 6.0 mm or more apical to CEJ of any tooth in the segment

Procedure

The patient is seated comfortably and the gingival status of each tooth present in the arch is assessed segment-wise starting from segment No.1 to No.6. The area with the highest score is the gingival score for entire segment, and gingival status of mouth is obtained by dividing the sum of gingival score by the number of segments examined, i.e.

$$\text{GPI (gingival component score)} = \frac{\text{Sum of gingival scores obtained for each segment}}{\text{Total number of segments examined}}$$

Secondly, each segment from 1 to 6 is examined for the periodontal disease. The recording is made at the mesio-facial or buccal line angle of every erupted tooth of each segment with a probe placed parallel to the long axis of tooth and directing it towards the CEJ at 45° angle. The distance of the free gingival margin to the CEJ is located first and then the probe is advanced to the base of pocket so as to record the depth of pocket. Subtracting the latter from the former gives the attachment loss on that tooth.

Extent and Severity Index (ESI)

Extent and Severity Index (ESI) was developed to assess the extent and severity of the loss of periodontal attachment. The PI and PDI scores depict the severity of periodontal disease in an individual or populations, but these scores do not provide any information on the extent of the disease. Unlike, PI and PDI, ESI does not assess the gingival inflammation, rather it estimates the attachment loss for the teeth examined.

Extent and Severity Index (ESI) assesses the extent (E) and severity (S) of the periodontal disease. Loss of periodontal attachment (LPA) is determined by using Ramjford's indirect method (as prescribed for PDI). In ESI the tooth site is considered diseased only if LPA exceeds 1.0 mm. The components of ESI are discussed below:

Extent (E)

This component describes the number of sites affected with periodontal disease. E, is expressed as the percentage of sites among examined sites with LPA greater than 1.0 mm, i.e.

$$E = \frac{\text{Total number of sites having LPA more than 1.0 mm}}{\text{Total number of sites examined}} \times 100$$

If a decimal value, ESI is rounded off to the nearest whole number value.

Severity (S)

This component describes the mean loss of attachment, more than 1.0 mm, for the affected or diseased sites. The loss of attachment for all the sites examined is totaled and divided by the total number of sites examined, i.e.

$$S = \frac{\text{Total LPA for all the sites examined}}{\text{Total number of sites examined}}$$

'S' value can be decimal or a whole number.

The ESI is expressed as bivariate number statistics, i.e. ESI = (E, S), e.g. ESI for an individual = (50, 2.5 mm) means, 50% of the examined sites show evidence of disease (E), with an average severity of 2.5 mm LPA per diseased site.

The ESI for population would be the average ESI for the individuals examined in that population.

Procedure

The examination is carried out for two quadrants—one maxillary and another mandibular. One maxillary quadrant is selected randomly and the opposite contralateral quadrant in the mandibular arch is selected. The two designated quadrants are examined for LPA of each tooth present in them, *except the third molar*, using Ramfjord's indirect method. Thus, a maximum of 28 measurements (7×2, i.e. 14 for each quadrant) are recordable for ESI. Larger values of E accompanied by smaller values of S imply a generalized milder form of disease; while smaller E but larger S values signify a severe localized form of periodontal disease.

Advantages

- It is a simple and reproducible index that can be performed relatively easily.
- It is equally reliable for partial as well as full mouth examination.

Limitations

It is not considered a true index as it summarizes data, thereby describing it rather than analyzing it. Thus it is a descriptive index, that is intended not for diagnosis of an individual's disease but for contrasting the patterns of disease among different populations.

Uses

It is used for population prevalence surveys and longitudinal surveys.

Community Periodontal Index of Treatment Needs (CPITN)

The Community Periodontal Index of Treatment Needs (CPITN) was developed by the World Health Organization (WHO) and the Federation Dentaire Internationale (FDI), collectively to survey and evaluate treatment needs rather than determining past and present periodontal disease.

As the name suggests, CPITN is an index that assesses the treatment needed for a population. 'Treatment Needs' includes those conditions that are reversible and potentially responsive to treatment; for example, plaque retaining factors, dental calculus, gingivitis, periodontitis, etc.; but not the non-treatable or irreversible conditions like alveolar bone loss. Primarily, it is a screening procedure for identifying actual and potential problems posed by an individual or community and is not a comprehensive assessment of total past and present periodontal disease experience.

For assessment of an index, the mouth is divided into six sextants. In each of the sextant, we examine only index teeth of CPITN. Index teeth are:

For young adults (less than 19 years of age): The six index teeth examined are (Fig. 12.32).

16 – Maxillary right first molar

11 – Maxillary right central incisor

26 – Maxillary left first molar

46 – Mandibular right first molar

31 – Mandibular left central incisor

36 – Mandibualr left first molar

For adults (more than 20 years): Second molars are also examined for each patient in addition to the above teeth – thus, ten index teeth are examined (Fig. 12.32).

17 – Maxillary right second molar

27 – Maxillary left second molar

37 – Mandibular left second molar

47 – Mandibular right second molar

Third molars, if functioning in place of second molars are included in the index; but if not functioning, they are not included.

Molars are examined in pairs and only highest single score is recorded. Each sextant is given one highest score.

CPITN Probe: This probe was designed by WHO (for TRS 621-1978). It measures pocket depth and detects sub-gingival calculus. This is a thin, light weight probe (5 gms) that is designed for gentle manipulation even of sensitive soft tissues around the teeth.

The probe has a ball tip of 0.5 mm diameter that allows the easy detection of sub-gingival calculus; and color coding with a black marking from 3.5 mm to 5.5 mm.

For recording deep pockets, two additional black lines at 8.5 mm and 11.5 mm from the working tip are present on it. Nowadays, two variants of CPITN probes are present there:

CPITN-E: CPITN-epidemiological probe (Fig.12.33) has a ball tip of 0.5 mm diameter and black coding from 3.5 mm to 5.5 mm.

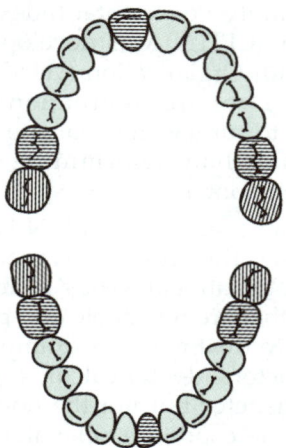

▨ Teeth to be examined for young individuals

▨ Additional teeth to be examined for adults

Fig. 12.32: Teeth examined in CPITN

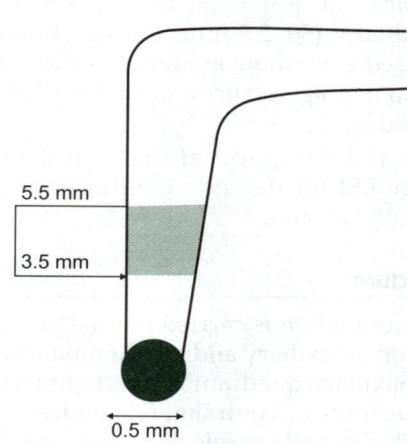

Fig. 12.33: CPITN-E Probe

CPITN-C: CPITN-clinical probe (Fig.12.34) has additional marking from 8.5 to 11.5 mm. This is used for clinical surveys.

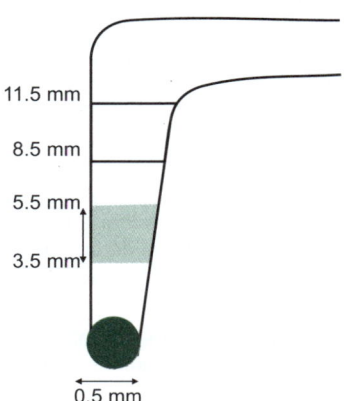

11.5 mm

8.5 mm

5.5 mm

3.5 mm

0.5 mm

Fig. 12.34: CPITN-C Probe

Rules for Selecting Teeth for Coding for CPITN

The following substitutions are made for the missing or extracted index teeth at the time of examination:

a. For a sextant to be scored, at least two index teeth should be present in it for quality score.

b. But in case of posterior sextant, if only one index tooth is present, then the recording is based on the examination of that tooth.

c. If both index teeth in the posterior segment are absent or excluded, then all the remaining teeth in the sextant are examined and the highest score recorded.

d. For anterior maxillary sextant if tooth 11 is excluded, substitute 21 for it; if 21 is also missing then one has to identify the worst score for remaining teeth.

e. For subjects less than 20 years of age, if first molar is not present or has been excluded, then adjacent premolar is examined.

f. If all teeth, in the sextant are missing or only single tooth is present (which is not an index tooth, see pt. 8) in whole sextant, then sextant is coded as missing X.

g. A single tooth in the sextant is considered as a tooth in the adjacent sextant and is subjected to the rules for that sextant.

h. If the single standing tooth is an index tooth, then worst index tooth score recorded for that tooth is the score of sextant.

The codes and criteria to be determined for a sextant are listed in the descending order of treatment complexity as follows (Table 12.48).

The treatment needed for a person is determined by the code and criteria obtained after examination. Population groups or individuals are allocated to the appropriate 'Treatment Need (TN)' category on following basis (Table 12.49):

Procedure

The patient is seated comfortably at a well illuminated place and the teeth are cleaned gently with a cotton swab. The dentition is divided into six sextants and each sextant is examined to determine its validity for scoring, i.e. for epidemiological purposes, the score is identified by examination of specified index teeth, whereas for clinical examination, highest score in each sextant is provided after examining all teeth. The CPITN probe is inserted gently with the force of 20 gms or even less, along the long axis of tooth. The 20 gm force is that force with which a probe can be inserted under a finger nail without causing any pain and discomfort. The ball end of the probe should always be kept in contact with root surface of the tooth to be examined. The six sites—mesio-buccal, mid buccal, disto-buccal, mesio-lingual, mid lingual and disto-lingual are examined for each tooth. The probing can be carried out by withdrawing the probe between each point or the probe can be moved around the tooth with probe tip remaining in the sulcus. The short upward and downward movements are sufficient.

After probing is completed, bleeding from the sulcus is also inspected. One should wait for at least 30 seconds before the completion of coding criteria.

The appropriate highest score is determined for each sextant and as the highest score

Table 12.48: Coding for CPITN

Code	Criteria	Explanation
X	When no index teeth are present or only one tooth present in the examined sextant	
4	Black area of CPITN probe is not visible, i.e. pathological depth of 6.0 mm or more is present	This is the highest score that any sextant can have. So if the score 4 is determined, there is no need to determine the lower score for that sextant (i.e. 0, 1, 2, 3).
3	Pathological pocket of 4.0 mm or 5.0 mm is present, gingival margin is on the black area of the probe.	We can examine the sextant for higher score but there is no need to examine for lower score (i.e. 0, 1, 2).
2	Calculus or plaque retaining factors are either felt or seen during probing	–
1	Bleeding observed during or after probing within 30 seconds	–
0	Healthy gingival tissues, no signs of disease are present.	This is the minimum score that can be provided to a sextant.

Coding for CPITN (diagrammatic)

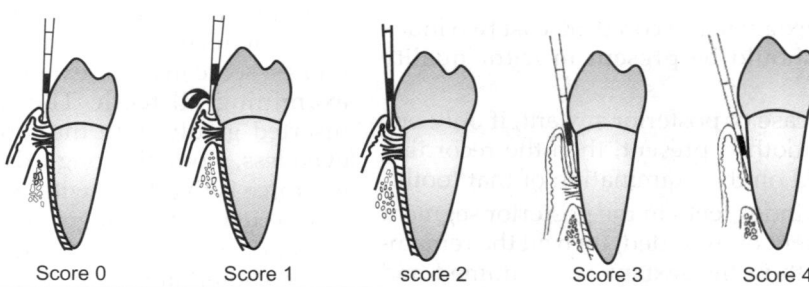

Score 0   Score 1   score 2   Score 3   Score 4

has been established there is no need to examine other teeth for the presence of lower score in that particular sextant.

Then, the CPITN is calculated as follows:

• The number of charts with different codes is counted and their coding score is summed up individually.

• The percentage of subjects with codes 0, 1, 2, 3, 4 as their score is calculated by dividing the counts of codes respectively by the total number of dentate subjects examined, e.g. to calculate the percentage of subjects with code value '3';

$$\% \text{ of subjects} = \frac{\text{Total counts having the code value 3}}{\text{Total number of dentate subjects examined}} \times 100$$

The percentage value is the prevalence of that particular code value in the population examined.

• MNS – mean number of sextants for each condition per person can be calculated by dividing the total number of sextants with highest score for the person by the total number of dentate subjects examined.

TN group	Codes included in TN group	Treatment needed
Table 12.49: Categories based on Treatment need groups		
TN-O	Code-O, Code-X	No treatment is needed; proper oral hygiene instructions can be repeated
TN-1	Code-1	An individual has to improve his personal oral hygiene; provide him with the instructions and demonstrate them.
TN-2	Code-2, Code-3	Code 2 indicates the need for professional cleaning of teeth and removal of plaque retentive factors along with oral hygiene instructions. Code 3 also indicates the need for professional cleaning of teeth. Scaling will reduce inflammation and will reduce pocket depth from 4.0–5.0 mm to 3.0 mm or even less than 3.0 mm. Thus, both code 2 and 3 are placed in same TN category, i.e. TN-2
TN-3	Code-4	These individuals or population needs complex treatment like deep curettage, root planning and more complex surgical procedures.

Modifications of CPITN

The following indices have been evolved as the modifications of CPITN:
- Simplified Periodontal Examination (SPE) that was afterwards termed as Basic Periodontal Examination (BPE)
- Periodontal Screening and Recording (PSR) Index

INDICES FOR ASSESSMENT OF MALOCCLUSION

Occlusion is the inter-cuspation of upper and lower teeth in different positions achieved by neuromuscular components of the masticatory system, i.e. teeth, periodontium, maxilla, mandible, temporomandibular joints and their associated muscles and ligaments.

In an epidemiological study, the terminology of occlusion includes all the occlusal variations from ideal occlusion to normal occlusion and malocclusion; that are discussed below:
- **Ideal Occlusion:** It is the hypothetical concept based on the anatomy of teeth and is rarely

found in nature. In an ideal occlusion, the skeleton basis of maxilla and mandible are of correct size relative to each other and the teeth are in correct relationship in all the three planes of space at rest. It can be precisely described and therefore is used as a standard by which other occlusions can be judged.
- **Normal occlusion:** The occlusion is said to be normal when the upper and lower molars are in a relationship whereby the mesiobuccal cusp of upper molar occludes in the buccal groove of lower molar and the teeth are arranged in a smooth curved line of occlusion.
- **Malocclusion:** The World Health Organization has included malocclusion under the handicapping dentofacial anomaly and defines it as an anomaly which causes disfigurement, impedes function, becomes an obstacle for patient's physical or emotional well being and often requires an adequate treatment.

Various indices of malocclusion have been developed for providing an objective method for the assessment of severity of malocclusion and for estimating priorities of orthodontic treatment. In all malocclusion indices, the presence of morphological traits is expressed numerically by using a proper scoring system. A common characteristic of all the indices is that the index scores are based on clinical estimation of the severity of various traits, i.e. the scores are assigned according to the adverse effect of the traits on the facial appearance, function and oral health. These indices have been employed in epidemiological surveys to determine the severity of malocclusion in different individuals or communities, for studying relationships between malocclusion severity and other dental diseases. The main purpose of these indices is to interpret malocclusion severity objectively in terms of the treatment priorities.

Malocclusion indices are categorized into following five categories according to the purpose they are used for:

- Diagnostic Indices
- Epidemiological Indices
- Treatment Priority Indices
- Treatment Outcome Indices
- Treatment Complexity Index (none at present)

The most commonly employed malocclusion indices are described as follows:

Handicapping Labio-Lingual Deviations Index (HLD)

Handicapping Labio-Lingual Deviations Index (HLD) was introduced to assess the degree of physical dento-facial handicaps. It only identifies the presence or absence of dental deformities without diagnosing the extent of malocclusion. The index can be used to determine the treatment needs of an individual.

This index assesses the seven components, according to which the degree of facial handicaps can be judged. These components are:

1. Cleft palate
2. Traumatic deviation
3. Over jet
4. Over bite (including reverse overbite)

5. Mandibular protrusion
6. Open bite
7. Labio-lingual flaring

1. *Cleft palate:* It is a congenital, developmental oro-facial deformity, that severely affects the routine procedures of an individual (eating, speaking, etc.) (Fig. 12.35)

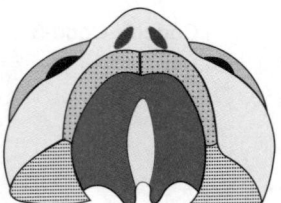

Fig.12.35: Cleft palate

2. *Traumatic deviation:* Any deviation from the normal patterns that is injurious for the hard and soft tissues of the oral cavity is called traumatic deviation (Fig. 12.36).

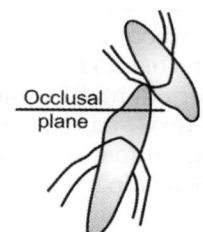

Fig.12.36: Traumatic deviation

3. *Over jet:* The horizontal distance between maxillary and mandibular teeth is called over jet (Fig. 12.37).

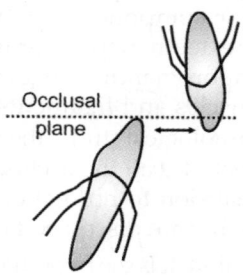

Fig.12.37: Over jet

4. *Over bite:* The vertical overlap of maxillary and mandibular teeth is called overbite (Fig. 12.38).

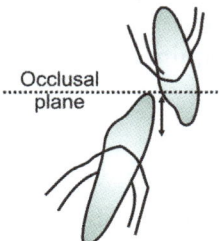

Fig.12.38: Over bite

5. *Mandibular protrusion:* If the mandibular anterior tooth or teeth are placed in front of maxillary teeth, then the condition is termed as mandibular protrusion (Fig. 12.39.).

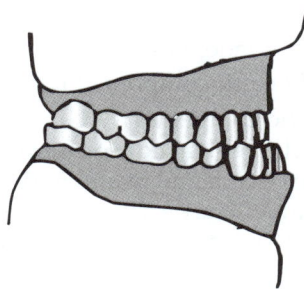

Fig.12.39: Mandibular protrusion

6. *Open bite:* It is the deviation in which there is an absence of occlusal contacts in the anterior dentition (Fig. 12.40).

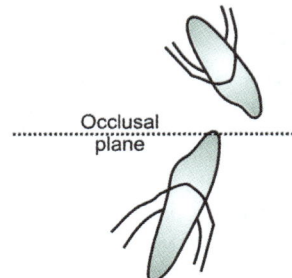

Fig.12.40: Open bite

7. *Labio-lingual flaring:* The flaring of mandibular teeth in labial and/or lingual direction from the normal dental arch pattern is termed as labio-lingual spread (Fig. 12.41).

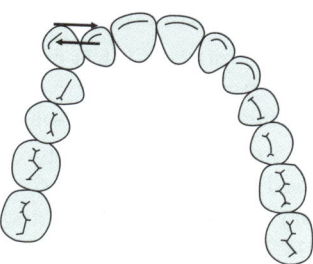

Fig.12.41: Labio-lingual flaring

Procedure

The patient is seated comfortably at a well illuminated place and examined for the above seven components of HLD. The teeth are positioned in centric occlusion and the numerical measurements (over jet, over bite/reverse over bite, open bite, mandibular protrusion and labio-lingual spread) are measured in millimeters using Boley's gauge. The data is recorded using following codes and criteria (Table 12.50):

Table 12.50: Codes for HLD index	
Code	*Used for*
O	If the condition is absent
X	If the condition is present
M	If mixed dentition is assessed
A	Clinically approved condition
D	Clinically disapproved condition

The conditions are detected using following criteria:

- *Cleft palate and traumatic deviations:* These can be judged as present or absent.
- *Over jet:* It is measured for a single tooth or for the whole arch (in mm).

- *Overbite:* The overlap of teeth can be marked with a pencil or a marker to assess the extent of overbite (in mm).
- *Open bite:* It is measured from incisal edges of maxillary incisors to incisal edges of mandibular incisors (in mm).
- *Mandibular protrusion:* It is measured from the labial surface of lower incisor to the labial surface of upper incisor (in mm).
- *Labio-lingual spread:* If labially or lingually displaced anterior teeth are present in maxillary or the mandibular arch; then the measurement from the incisal edge of displaced tooth to that of the tooth placed at normal position of dental arch should be taken.

If any of *multiple measurements* (as in a crowded dental arch where multiple teeth are out of alignment), the most severe measurement should be recorded. However, the condition is simply considered present or absent; the extent of condition is not relevant in HLD.

The scoring is carried out (Table 12.51) as follows:

Table 12.51: Scoring for HLD index

	Code	Score
Cleft Palate	X	13
Severe traumatic deviations	X	13
Over jet (in mm)	X	Measured score
Over bite (in mm)	X	Measured score
Mandibular protrusion	X	Measured score
Open bite	X	Measured score
Labio-Lingual spread	X	Measured score

Total HLD score = Sum of the scores of the components assessed

If HLD score is > 13 – Individual is considered as dental handicap

If HLD score is <13 – Individual is not considered as dental handicap.

Advantages

- It is simple, objective, valid and reliable index.
- Is can be performed easily on patients and on study models.
- It does not require any special equipment for scoring.

Limitations

- It is unduly sensitive to the developing symptoms of the malocclusion.
- It is meant only for identification of handicapping malocclusions and not for assessing the degree or severity of malocclusion.

Index of Orthodontic Treatment Needs (IOTN)

Index of orthodontic treatment needs (IOTN) was developed to assess the orthodontic treatment needed for an individual.

Index: The index is scored in two components:
a. Dental health component (DHC)
b. Aesthetic component (AC)
a. **Dental Health component (DHC):** It assesses the dental health and functions of the individual's dentition using five different grades using the following five occlusal traits:
   i. Missing teeth (Fig. 12.42)

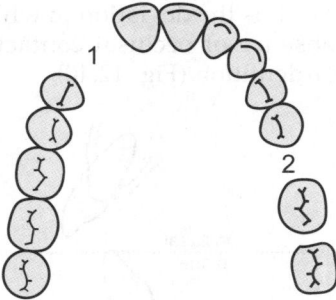

Fig.12.42: 1. Missing anterior tooth
2. Missing tooth resulting in mesial migration of posterior tooth

ii. Over jet (Fig. 12.37)
iii. Cross bite (Fig. 12.43)
iv. Contact point displacement (Fig. 12.44)
v. Over bite (Fig. 12.38)

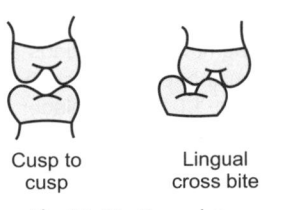

Cusp to   Lingual
cusp   cross bite

Fig.12.43: Cross bite

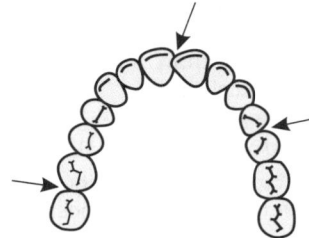

Fig.12.44: Contact point displacement

Dental health component (DHC) scores the dentition into five grades using the following criteria (Table 12.52).

b. **Aesthetic Component (AC):** A Standardized Continuum of Aesthetic Need (SCAN) scale was used for the development of aesthetic component of Index of orthodontic treatment needs. It is a visual 10 point scale, illustrated by series of 10 photographs, scored from 0.5 to 5. Patient's score is based on matching his or her dental appearance with a series of 10 photographs showing the labial aspect of different Cl-I or Cl-II malocclusions ranked according to their attractiveness.

These scores are used for:
– Patient's counseling
– Priorities of cosmetic treatment needed
– Studies and research regarding the effectiveness of the treatment
– Determining the urgency of the treatment

The SCAN can also be useful for estimation of treatment needed at the community level.

Grade	Treatment needs	Criteria
Table 12.52: Dental Health component of IOTN		
1	No treatment needed	• Occlusal variations including displacements equal to or less than 1.0 mm
2	Little treatment needed	• Over jet more than 3.0-5.0 mm but less or equal to 6.0 mm with competent lips • Reverse over jet more than 0.0 mm but less than or equal to 1.0 mm • Increased overbite greater than 3.5 mm with absence of gingival contacts· • Anterior or posterior cross bites with less than or equal to 1 mm displacement between retruded contact position and inter-cuspal position • Lateral or anterior open bite more than 1.0 mm but less than or equal to 2.0 mm • Cl-II or Cl-III occlusions without any anomalies • Displacement of teeth greater than 1.0 mm but less than/equal to 2.0 mm
3	Moderate treatment needed	• Over jet more than 3.5 mm but less than or equal to 6 mm with incompetent lips at rest

Contd...

Grade	Treatment needs	Criteria
		• Reverse over jet greater than 1.0 mm but less than or equal to 3.5 mm
		• Increased and complete overbite with gingival contacts, without any signs of trauma or indentations
		• Anterior or posterior cross bites with less than or equal to 2.0 mm but greater than 1.0 mm displacement between retruded contact position and inter-cuspal position
		• Lateral or anterior open bite greater than 2.0 mm but less than or equal to 4.0 mm
		• Displacement of teeth greater than 2.0 mm but less than or equal to 4.0 mm
4	Great treatment needed	• Increased overjet greater than 6.0 mm but less than or equal to 9.0 mm
		• Reverse overjet greater than 3.5 mm without any masticatory or speech difficulties
		• Reverse overjet more than 1.0 mm but less than or equal to 3.5 mm with reported speech and masticatory difficulties
		• Anterior or posterior cross bites with more than 2.0 mm displacement between retruded contact position and inter-cuspal position
		• Posterior lingual cross bites without contacts in one or both buccal segments
		• Lateral or anterior open bites greater than 4.0 mm
		• Increased or complete overbites with indentations on the palatal or labial gingiva
		• Patients referred by qualified, registered dentists for orthodontic treatment, for example, by periodontists, oral surgeons, endodontists, etc.
5	Very great treatment needed	• Cleft lip or cleft palate or both
		• Over jet more than 9.0 mm
		• Reverse over jet, more than 3.5 mm with masticatory and speech difficulties
		• Impeded eruption of teeth (with the exception of third molars) due to crowding, displacement, supernumerary teeth, or any other pathological cause
		• Extensive hypodontia with restorative implications (more than one missing tooth in any quadrant)

Advantages

The advantages of SCAN scale used for recording aesthetic component are:

• It is simple and can be easily conceptualized.

• It can be used in day to day practice and in epidemiological studies.

- Taken together with dental health appraisal, estimate of the relative treatment needed is possible with this index.
- It can be used for individual patient's counseling.

Limitations

- It has poor ability to represent dentofacial imbalance in antero-posterior plane.

1. Over jet of upper anterior segment (Fig. 12.45)
2. Reversed over jet of lower anterior segment (Fig. 12.46)
3. Over bite of upper anteriors over the lower anteriors (Fig. 12.38)
4. Anterior open bite (Fig. 12.40.)
5. Congenital absence of incisors
6. Disto-occlusal molar relation (Fig. 12.47a, b)

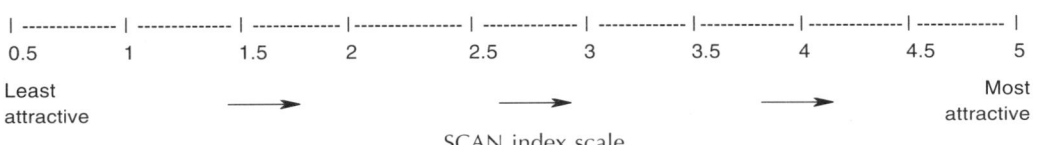

| -------------- | -------------- | ------------- | ---------------- | -------------- | ------------- | -------------- | -------------- | ------------- |
| 0.5 | 1 | 1.5 | 2 | 2.5 | 3 | 3.5 | 4 | 4.5 | 5 |

Least attractive   Most attractive

SCAN index scale

- For SCAN index, Photographs from an older sample may be required; (some of the 12 year old samples having transitional dentition).

Procedure

The patient is seated at a well illuminated place, and examined using a mouth mirror and retractors for the criteria discussed before (in DHC and AC). The order of examination of these occlusal traits is not significant; however, each trait should be assessed independently and the most severe grade to the individual's treatment needs to be assigned. The treatment needed for the patient is planned according to the assigned grade. Larger the grade, more is the severity of malocclusion and greater treatment is needed for the patient.

Orthodontic Treatment Priority Index (TPI)

Orthodontic treatment priority index (TPI) or simply treatment priority index was developed as a modification of the Malocclusion Severity Estimate (MSE) to determine the orthodontic treatment needed in an individual after assessing the severity of malocclusion and degree of handicap present in him.

Orthodontic treatment priority index (TPI) assesses the dentition for following parameters:

7. Mesio-occlusal molar relation (Fig. 12.48)
8. Posterior cross bite with maxillary teeth buccal to normal position (Fig. 12.49 a, b)
9. Posterior cross bite with maxillary teeth lingual to normal position (Fig. 12.50)
10. Displacement of individual teeth

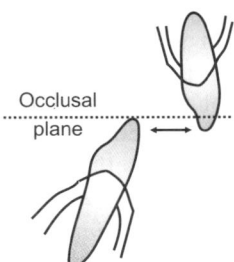

Occlusal plane

Fig.12.45: Over jet

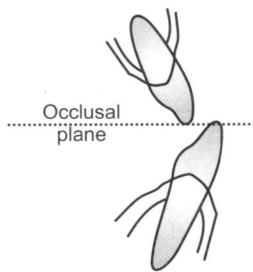

Occlusal plane

Fig.12.46: Reverse over jet

Procedure

Index can be performed in the individual or on the study models. TPI is used for the assessment of permanent dentition by considering all the above ten factors.

The measurements are recorded using a steel millimeter ruler.

1. *Maxillary over jet:* Horizontal distance between the labial surface of lower central incisor and labial surface of most prominent maxillary central incisor is recorded in millimeters as follows:

   0 1 2 3 4 5 6 7 8 9 9+

2. *Reversed over jet:* Horizontal distance between the labial surface of maxillary central incisor and labial surface most prominent lower central incisor is recorded in millimeters as follows:

   0 1 2 3 4 5 6 7 8 9 9+

3. *Overbite:* Overbite is recorded after dividing the palatal surface of maxillary central incisor into three parts.

   0 1   2   3   4   5

4. *Open bite:* It is the greatest distance, in millimeters, present between the incisal surfaces of upper and lower central incisors while teeth are in their centric occlusion position. It is recorded as:

   (in mm) 0 1 2 3 4 5

5. *Congenitally absent incisors:* Suspicious absence of incisors is clinically confirmed with the use of radiographs and scoring is carried out for individual/multiple quadrants, i.e.

   0   1   2   2+

6. *Disto-occlusion:* Disto-occlusion present is recorded for each quadrant and scoring can be given as follows:

   0   1   2   3   4

7. *Mesio-occlusion:* Similarly mesio-occlusion will be scored for each quadrant as follows:

   0   1   2   3   4

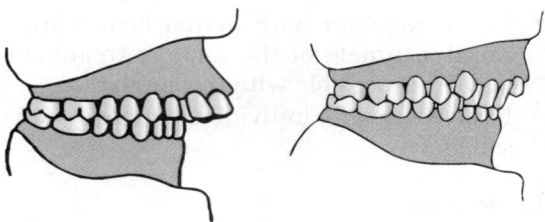

Fig.12.47a, b: Disto-occlusion of molars

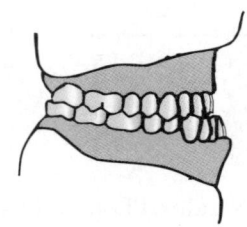

Fig.12.48: Mesio-occlusion of molars

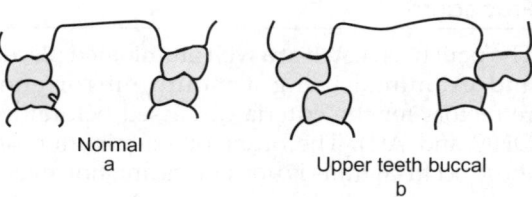

Normal
a

Upper teeth buccal
b

Fig.12.49a, b: Posterior cross bite

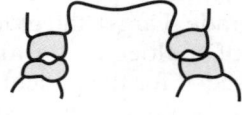

Upper teeth Palatal

Fig.12.50: Posterior cross bite

8. *Buccal cross bites:* The cross bites in which maxillary posteriors are present buccally with respect to the lower posteriors are scored in both quadrants as follows:

   0 1   2   3   4   5   6   7

9. *Lingual cross bites:* The cross bites in which maxillary posteriors are present lingually

with respect to the mandibular posteriors are scored as follows:

0   1   2   3   4   5   6   6+

10. *Displacement of individual teeth:* After dividing the maxillary and mandibualr arches into three quadrants, the score is assigned to the displaced/rotated teeth, using two criteria:

i. Number of rotations less than 2.0 mm; or degree of rotation less than 45 in the segment examined as follows:

Upper left (UL)	Upper Anterior (UA)	Upper right (UR)
Lower left (LL)	Lower Anterior (LA)	Lower right (LR)

ii. Number of rotations more than 2.0 mm or degree of rotation more than 45 in the segment examined as follows:

Upper left (UL)	Upper Anterior (UA)	Upper right (UR)
Lower left (LL)	Lower Anterior (LA)	Lower right (LR)

If the displacement or rotation is absent then score 0 is provided; and if these are present score 1 is provided to them.

After each of the above components is measured/assessed and scored, the sub-score weights are summed up to compute TPI (Fig. 12.51).

TPI = Sum of the sub-scores obtained for the above criteria

Higher the score, more severe is the malocclusion.

The interpretation of the score is carried out (Table 12.53) as follows:

Table 12.53: Interpretation of score

0	-	near ideal occlusion
1-3	-	mild malocclusion, low requirement for treatment
4-6	-	moderate malocclusion, moderate requirement for treatment
7-9	-	severe handicap, high requirement for treatment
10 or greater	-	Very severe, handicap, treatment mandatory.

Advantages

- It is a versatile index with epidemiological applicability.
- It can be 'Screening' method to determine treatment need in public health programs.
- It provides a rough description of case type (scores only occlusal characteristics, excluding skeletal and facial components).
- It helps to estimate malocclusion severity in population groups.

Peer Assessment Rating Index (PAR)

Peer Assessment Rating Index (PAR), also known as *Index of Treatment Standards*, was developed to measure malocclusion and to assess the outcome of orthodontic treatment during or after the treatment procedure.

This index consists of 11 components, which are assessed and scored for normal and abnormal parameters that are given below:

1. Upper right segment
2. Upper anterior segment
3. Upper left segment
4. Lower right segment
5. Lower anterior segment
6. Lower left segment
7. Right buccal occlusion
8. Over jet
9. Over bite
10. Center line
11. Left buccal occlusion

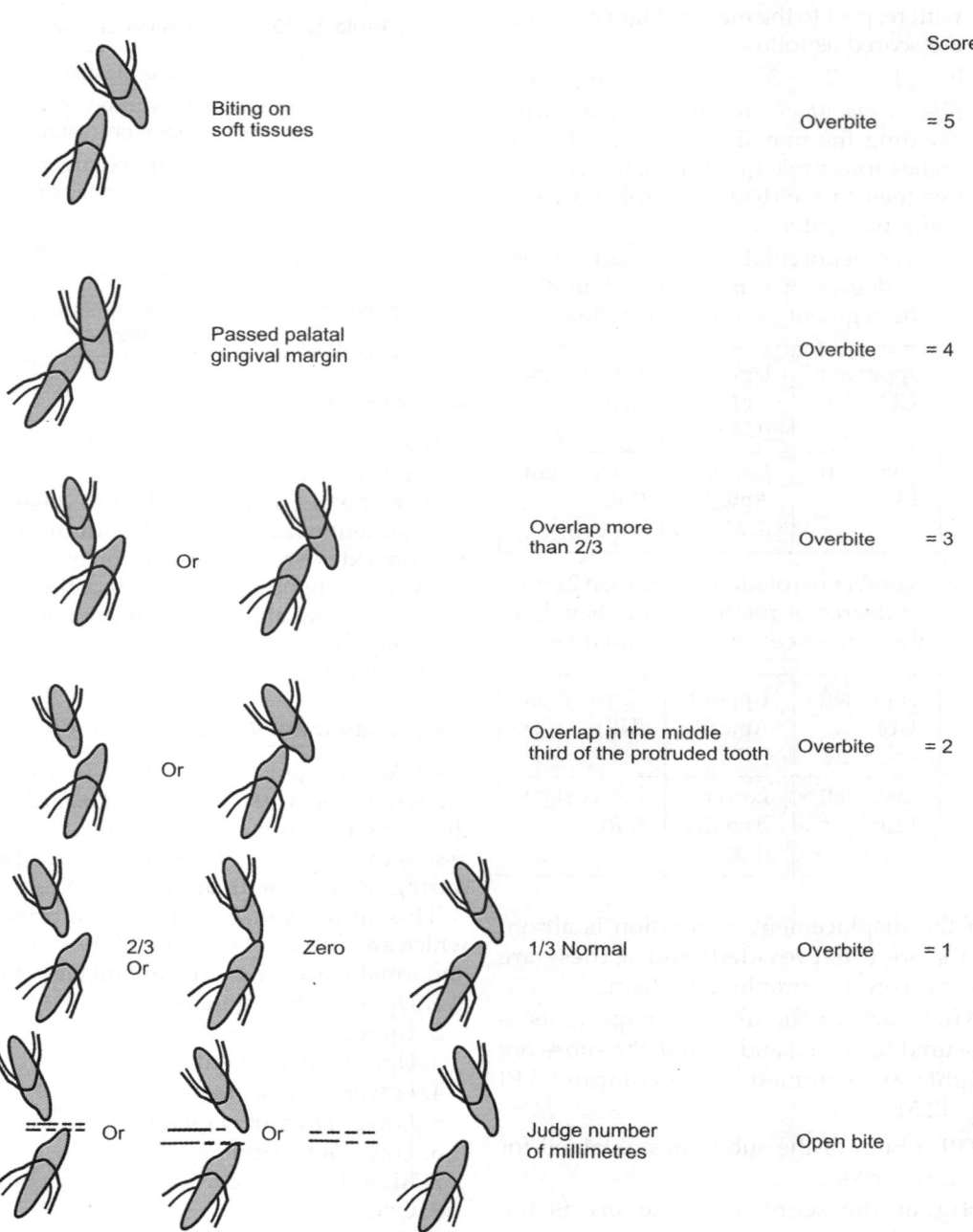

Fig.12.51: Scoring pattern for Orthodontic Treatment Priority Index

Guidelines for Recording PAR Index

The guidelines for recording PAR index are as follows:

I. General

a. All the scores are summed up.
b. There is no maximal, cutoff value.
c. The occlusion is scored irrespective of functional displacements.
d. The contact points between first, second and third molars are not recorded.
e. Contact point displacements because of poor restorations are not recorded.
f. Contact points of deciduous teeth are not recorded.
g. Extraction spaces are not recorded if the prosthesis is to be given. However, if space closure is intended, the distance between adjacent teeth should be noted.

II. Specific

A. For incisors
a. If maxillary incisor is absent or is lost due to trauma or caries, then:
  • If the space is to be maintained (for a prosthesis); the distance between adjacent teeth is not recorded.
  • If the space is to be closed then the distance between adjacent teeth should be recorded.
b. If mandibular incisor is extracted or missing then there is no need to record centre line.

B. For canines
a. Cross bite due to canines should be recorded in over jet section.
b. If canines are missing, then the displacements created by their spaces (i.e. between lateral incisors and premolars) are recorded in anterior segment.
c. The distal contact point of canine and the midpoint on the mesial surface of adjacent premolar is the most acceptable relationship between canine and premolar.

C. **For molars:** If the first molars are extracted, then the contact point of second molar is to be recorded.

D. **For impaction:** An un-erupted and displaced tooth from line of arch; either bucally or palataly, due to insufficient space is considered as an 'impaction'. If the tooth is erupted and displaced, then only the displacement score is given and not impaction.

Procedure

It is performed on the dental casts mounted at centric occlusion position using a specially designed, translucent, PAR ruler (Fig. 12.52) which has the PAR components along with their scoring codes and criteria listed on it.

PAR index divides maxillary and mandibular arches into six segments for scoring. These are:

1. *Maxillary right segment:* From mesial contact point of right first permanent molar to distal contact point of right maxillary cuspid.
2. *Maxillary anterior segment:* From mesial contact point of right maxillary cuspid to mesial contact point of left maxillary cuspid.
3. *Maxillary left segment:* From distal contact point of left maxillary cuspid to mesial contact point of left maxillary permanent first molar.
4. *Mandibular right segment:* From mesial contact point of right first permanent molar to distal contact point of right mandibular cuspid.
5. *Mandibular anterior segment:* From mesial contact point of right mandibular cuspid to mesial contact point of left mandibular cuspid.
6. *Mandibular left segment:* From distal contact point of left maxillary cuspid to mesial contact point of left maxillary permanent first molar.

ANT-POST
0 None 1< 1/2 unit distance 2= 1/2 unit distance

TRANSVERSE
0 None bite 1 cross bite tend > = 11 2 1 tooth in cross bite 3 >1 tooth in cross bite 4 > 1 tooth in open bite

VERTICAL
0 None 1open bite 2 teeth > 2mm

CENTRE LINE
0 < = 1/4 1 1/4 -1/2 2 > 1/2

OVER BITE	
0 0-1/3	Open bite
1 1/3-2/3	—
2 > 2/3	—
3 > = FTC	—
4	→

CONTACT POINT
0 — 1 — 2 — 3 — 4 → 5 impacted tooth

THE PAR INDEX

OVERJET
4 > 21x b 3 21 x b 2 11 x b 1 10 0

Fig.12.52: The PAR ruler

I. Segments

Each of the above listed segments is assessed for:

a. Crowding of teeth (Fig. 12.53)

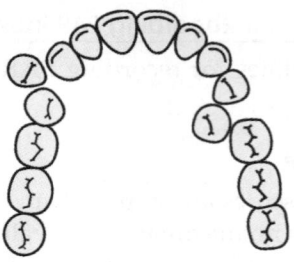

Fig.12.53: Crowding of posterior teeth

b. Spacing in teeth

c. Impacted teeth: If the space for a tooth is less than 4.0 mm then it is considered as impacted.

d. Displacements: The shortest distance between the contact points of adjacent teeth which is parallel to the occlusal plane is measured and displacement is scored according to the following discrepancy criteria (Fig.12.54) (Table 12.54):

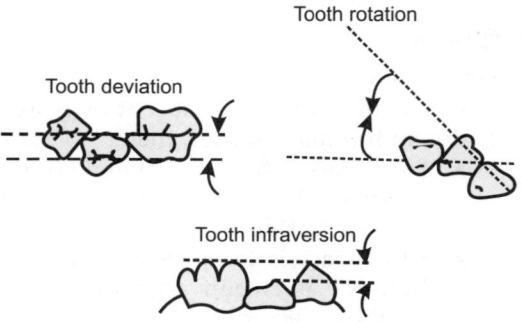

Fig.12.54: Displacements

Table 12.54: Displacement in PAR Index	
Displacement	
Score	*Discrepancy (in mm)*
0	0 – 1.0
1	1.1 – 2.0
3	4.1 – 8.0
4	> 8.0
5	Impacted teeth*

* Impacted teeth are mostly canines in the anterior segment and third molars in posterior segments.

However, as the contact areas in mixed dentitions are not well defined, so assessment of future potential of crowding in permanent dentition is done using the average mesio-distal width measurements of teeth in mixed dentition that are as follows (Table 12.55a, b):

Table 12.55a: Mixed dentition period (Maxillary arch)

Tooth	Width (mm)
Canine	8.0
Ist premolar	7.0
2nd premolar	7.0
Total	**22.0**

If the total width is less than 18 mm then the impaction of permanent tooth in arch is expected.

Table 12.55b: Mixed dentition period (Mandibular arch)

Tooth	Width (mm)
Canine	7.0
Ist premolar	7.0
2nd premolar	7.0
Total	**21.0**

If their total width is less than 17 mm, then the impaction of permanent tooth is expected.

II. Buccal Occlusion

The second component of PAR index, buccal occlusion is assessed with respect to three planes, i.e. antero-posterior (sagittal), vertical and transverse (Horizontal) for both right and left side as follows (Table 12.56).

Table 12.56: PAR Index (Buccal Occlusion)

Antero-posterior (Sagittal) plane	
Score	Discrepancy
0	Good inter-digitation, CI-I, C-II, C-III
1	Less than half unit discrepancy
2	Half unit discrepancy (cusp to cusp)
Vertical plane	
Score	Discrepancy
0	No discrepancy in inter-cuspation
1	Lateral open bite on at least two teeth greater than 2.0 mm
Transverse (Horizontal) plane	
Score	Discrepancy
0	No cross bite
1	Cross bite tendency
2	Single tooth in cross bite
3	More than one tooth in cross bite
4	More than one tooth in scissor bite

III. Over Jet

It includes over jet and cross-bites from left lateral incisor to right lateral incisor (most prominent incisor is scored). PAR ruler is held parallel to the occlusal plane and radial to line of arch. The sum of over jet and cross bite scores is considered as 'Total Over jet Score' (Table 12.57a, b):

Table 12.57a: Over jet measurement

Score	Discrepancy (mm)
0	0 – 3.0
1	3.1 – 5.0
2	5.1 – 7.0
3	7.1 – 9.0
4	> 9.0 mm

Table 12.57b: Anterior cross bite measurement

Score	Discrepancy (mm)
0	No discrepancy
1	One or more teeth present in edge to edge relation
2	Single tooth in cross bite
3	Two teeth in cross bite
4	More than two teeth in cross bite

IV. Over Bite

It assesses the vertical overlap or open bite of maxillary anterior teeth in relation to coverage of lower incisors or degree of open bite using following criteria (Table 12.58a, b):

Table 12.58a: Open bite

Score	Discrepancy
0	No open bite
1	Open bite less than and equal to 1.0 mm
2	Open bite 1.1 to 2.0 mm
3	Open bite 2.1 to 3.0 mm
4	Open bite greater than or equal to 4.0 mm

Table 12.58b: Over bite

Score	Discrepancy
0	No discrepancy
1	One or more teeth present in edge to edge relationship
2	One single tooth in cross bite
3	Two teeth in cross bite
4	More than two teeth in cross bite

V. Center Line

The center line is assessed with respect to lower central incisors (Fig.12.55). If lower incisor has been extracted, then center line assessments need not be assessed. The scoring criteria are as follows (Table 12.59):

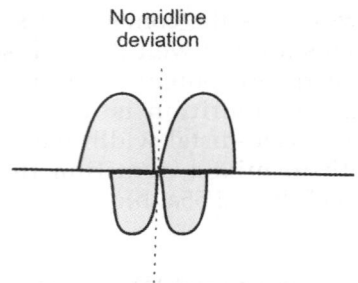

No midline deviation

Fig. 12.55: Center line (without discrepancy)

Table 12.59: Discrepancy with center line

Score	Discrepancy
0	Center line is coincident and is up to 1/4th of lower incisor width
1	Center line one quarter to one half of lower incisor width
2	Center line width greater than one half of lower incisor

Once the total 11 components are scored, then the scores are summed up for PAR index score.

PAR Index = Sum of scores obtained for each component

Uses

- It measures malocclusion
- It assess the outcome of orthodontic treatment at any stage
- It assess the pre and post treatment changes obtained in an individual

Advantages

- It is a quick, valid and highly reliable index.
- It provides a single summary score for all occlusal anomalies found in a malocclusion.
- It provides an estimate of how far a case deviates from normal alignment and occlusion.

Differences in pre and post treatment scores reflect the degree of improvement, and therefore, the success of treatment.

INDEX FOR DEVELOPMENT DEFECTS OF ENAMEL (DDE)

Developmental defects of enamel are defined as disturbances in hard tissue matrices and their mineralization during odontogenesis. Disturbances may be genetic, localized when affecting single or multiple teeth or systemic when affecting groups of teeth. Defects may affect primary teeth, permanent teeth or both and may also involve dentin, cementum or both.

The defects can be single (only one lesion is visible on the tooth surface) or multiple (more than one defect, with margins well demarcated from the adjacent normal enamel). It can also be diffuse with fine white lines or diffuse with a patchy appearance.

The types of defects can be:

a. **Hypoplasia:** It is defined as a quantitative defect of enamel, identified visually and morphologically as involving the surface of the enamel, which is associated with a reduced enamel thickness. The defective enamel may occur as (a) shallow or deep pits or rows of pits arranged horizontally in a linear fashion across the tooth surface (b) it may occur as small or large, wide or narrow grooves, (c) there may be partial or complete absence of enamel over small or considerable areas of dentin.

b. **Opacity:** It is defined as a qualitative defect of enamel identified visually as an abnormality in the translucency of enamel. It is characterized by a white or discolored (cream, yellow, brown) area. The enamel surface is smooth and the thickness is normal, except in some instances when associated with hypoplasia.

Combinations of hypoplasia and opacities can occur on the same tooth surface.

c. **Discolored enamel:** It is defined as an obvious abnormal appearance of the enamel because of its color and it cannot be considered within the normal range of variation in color and shade of tooth enamel. This category excludes colored opacities.

Coding of Enamel Defects

The coding of enamel defects is carried out as follows:

Clinical Examination

The tooth surfaces should be inspected visually and explored with a probe to determine abnormalities of surface contour. Natural or artificial light is used depending on field conditions. When using artificial light, the intensity and incidence of the source should be altered to overcome 'burning out' of the defects.

Ideally, the teeth should receive a prophylaxis and be dried at the time of examination. Teeth cleaned of stains and soft deposits show more defects than uncleaned and stained surfaces. This is also true for dried teeth as compared to wet teeth.

In certain instances when it is difficult to decide the abnormality, the tooth surface should be scored normal. Where an abnormality is obviously present but cannot readily be classified into one of the listed categories of defects, it should be scored 'other'. After completion of the examination and recording of dental, medical and other relevant details, a tentative diagnosis of etiology should be attempted.

A recording chart is designed which permits the identification of the various types, number and location of defects on the lingual and buccal surfaces of 28 teeth. In addition, basic demographic data, treatment needs, dental and medical history are also recorded.

- Un-erupted, missing, restored, decayed, fractured teeth and teeth which for any reason cannot be classified under defects must be coded as X. This implies that it will be disregarded from statistical evaluation.
- Type of defect: Permanent teeth are coded with numbers and primary teeth are coded with letters. Tooth surfaces with no defects are coded 'O' for permanent teeth and 'A' for primary teeth. When a defect is observed

it is classified with respect to the type of defect it resembles most closely.

Treatment Needs

This is intended to provide information on the significance of defects as a clinical problem. It is not expected that all defects have a treatment need. For example, defects not having a functional or esthetic problem need not be treated. An opacity on the buccal surface of an upper anterior tooth may require cosmetic treatment, whereas the same defect on a posterior tooth would best remain untreated.

The classification and coding of enamel defects are given in Table 12.60.

Modifications of the DDE Index

The Modified DDE index is simple, flexible and can be used extensively. This index is used for screening surveys and for general epidemiological studies. The three primary defects which have emerged as being central to this index are:

a. Demarcated opacity
b. Diffuse opacity
c. Hypoplasia

For general screening purposes, only the three above mentioned basic types of defects are recorded. If defects do not fall in these categories they are scored as 'other defects'. Hence with this screening index, a single

Table 12.60: Coding and recording of Enamel defects for DDE

	Code permanent teeth	Code deciduous teeth
1. Types of Defects		
a. Normal	0	A
b. Opacity (white/cream)	1	B
c. Opacity (yellow/brown)	2	C
d. Hypoplasia (pits)	3	D
e. Hypoplasia (horizontal grooves)	4	E
f. Hypoplasia (vertical grooves)	5	F
g. Hypoplasia (missing enamel)	6	G
h. Discolored enamel (not associated with opacity)	7	H
i. Other defects	8	J
j. Combination of defects (both the codes are given)		
2. Number and Demarcation of Defects		
a. Single	1	A
b. Multiple	2	B
c. Diffuse, white lines	3	C
d. Diffuse, patchy	4	D
3. Location of Defect		
a. Gingival one half	1	A
b. Incisal one half	2	B
c. Occlusal	3	C
d. Cuspal	4	D

scoring system applies with the scores ranging from 0 to 4 (Table 12.61).

Table 12.61: Modified DDE Index for use in screening surveys

Normal	0
Demarcated opacity	1
Diffuse opacity	2
Hypoplasia	3
Other defects	4
Combinations Code	
Demarcated and diffuse	5
Demarcated and hypoplasia	6
Diffuse and hypoplasia	7
All three defects	8

Developmental defects of enamel are defined as *deviations from the normal appearance of tooth enamel resulting from enamel organ dysfunction.* Almost all enamel defects in human teeth can be classified into one of the three types, based on their microscopic appearance. These are:

a. **Demarcated opacity:** It is an alteration in the translucency of enamel, which varies in degree. The defective enamel is of normal thickness and with a smooth surface. It has a distinct and clear boundary with the adjacent normal enamel. The lesions vary in extent, position on the tooth surface, and distribution.

b. **Diffuse opacity:** It is also a defect involving an alteration in the translucency of enamel to varying degrees. The defective enamel is white in colour, has normal thickness and is relatively smooth at eruption. There is no clear boundary with the adjacent normal enamel.

   i. **Lines:** Distinctive white lines of opacity, which follow the lines of development of the teeth. Confluence of adjacent lines may occur.

   ii. **Patchy:** Irregular, cloudy areas of opacity lacking well defined margins.

   iii. **Confluent:** Diffuse patches merged into a chalky white area extending from mesial to distal margins which can cover the entire surface or be confined to a localized area of the tooth surface.

   iv. **Confluent/patchy plus both staining and loss of enamel:** Post-eruptive change of colour and or loss of enamel related only to the hypomineralized zone, i.e. punched-out appearance of pits or large areas of missing enamel surrounded by chalky white or stained enamel.

c. **Hypoplasia:** A defect involving the surface of the enamel associated with a reduced localized thickness of enamel. It can occur in the form of pits [single or multiple, shallow or deep, scattered or in horizontal rows] or grooves [Single or multiple, narrow or wide (maximum 2.0 mm); or partial or complete absence of enamel over a considerable area of dentin].

Photographic Interpretations

Color reproductions are typical examples of demarcated opacities, diffuse opacities and hypoplastic defects.

Even with more precise definitions and more extensive photographs, investigators may continue to have difficulty in differentiating between the different types of defects. Training and calibration by experienced users of the index on individual subjects with a variety of defects is therefore strongly recommended.

Clinical Examination

Tooth surfaces are inspected visually for defects under the guidelines of the Table 12.62.

Table 12.62: Modified DDE index

Normal	0
Demarcated opacities	
white/cream	1
yellow/brown	2

Contd...

Diffuse opacities	
lines	3
patchy	4
confluent	5
Confluent/Patchy, staining and loss of enamel	6
Hypoplasia	
Pits	7
Missing enamel	8
Any other defects	9
Combinations	
Demarcated and diffuse	A
Demarcated and hypoplasia	B
Diffuse and hypoplasia	C
All three defects	D

TOOTH WEAR INDEX

With the increase in awareness of communities regarding dental health, more and more people are likely to have more number of teeth at an older age. One of the many dental health problems which these senior citizens are likely to face will be that of tooth wear. Presently, very less number of studies have been conducted on tooth wear as a whole and little is known about the epidemiology of tooth wear among adult population.

Tooth wear may be defined as the gradual loss of tooth substance due to repetitive physical contacts or the chemical dissolution. Physical contacts may be with opposing or adjacent teeth or with a foreign objects such as food or tooth brush. Chemical attack of bacterial origin, i.e. from plaque is usually not included in tooth wear. Tooth wear is usually recognized by attrition, abrasion or erosion.

Attrition refers to the loss of tooth substance caused by contact between opposing and adjacent teeth occurring during function and parafunction. **Abrasion** involves the progressive loss of mineralized tissue caused by mechanical factors other than tooth to tooth contact. **Erosion** describes the chemical dissolution of hard tooth substance as a result of action of acids other than bacterial plaque.

Tooth wear can be physiological or pathological. The process occurs during normal function and consequently, a degree of tooth wear is normal at any given period. It is pathological, if the teeth involved are judged as unable to survive to their expected life span if wear continues at a given rate.

The proposed Tooth Wear Index *(Smith and Knight)* has the following features:

• Each tooth is assessed by visual examination.
• Separate records are made of cervical, buccal, occlusal and incisal surfaces. The affect of tooth wear on occlusal and incisal surfaces is not the same hence different criteria are used.
• The total number of surfaces possible to be recorded are 4 per tooth. Hence, for 32 teeth in a patient 128 surfaces are to be recorded.
• Heavily restored teeth and missing teeth are not recorded.
• The index is recorded on a specially designed chart and can be entered from this into a computer record.
• The index can be recorded clinically as well as from photographs.
• Acceptable tooth wear scores at each age group is proposed. Comparison with patients score, extent and distribution of pathological tooth wear can be recorded.

The diagnostic criteria for Tooth Wear Index are given in Table 12.63. In case of doubts lower score is taken.

There is very little data on the prevalence of tooth wear. **Pollman et al (1987)** surveyed a population using an index which grades loss of tooth substance from incisal and occlusal surfaces as 0-4. The surface which showed no wear was given a score of 0 and 5 was given in case of pulp exposure. They observed that

Table 12.63: Tooth Wear Index scoring criteria

Score	Buccal, lingual and occlusal	Incisal	Cervical
		Surface	
0	No loss of enamel surface characteristics	No loss of enamel surface characteristics	No change in contour
1	Loss of enamel surface characteristics	Loss of enamel surface characteristics	Minimal loss of contour
2	Loss of enamel exposing dentin for less than 1/3 the surface	Loss of enamel just exposing dentin	Defect less than 1.0 mm deep
3	Loss of enamel exposing dentin for more than 1/3 of the surface	Loss of enamel and substantial loss of dentin, but not exposing pulp or or secondary dentin	Defect 1.0–2.0 mm deep
4	Complete loss of enamel, exposure of secondary dentin	Loss of enamel and substantial loss of dentin with exposure of secondary dentin	Defect 2.0–3.0 mm deep with exposure of secondary dentin
5	Complete loss of enamel and pulp exposure	Loss of enamel and substantial loss of dentin with pulp exposure	Defect more than 3.0 mm deep or pulp exposure

men displayed more tooth wear than women. They also noted that tooth wear increased with age.

In a study conducted by **Sikri and Sikri (1992)** on 460 patients between the age group of 30–70 years; the total patients were divided into four groups for convenience; from 31–40 years, 41–50 years, 51–60 years and 61–70 years. 11,040 teeth were examined in all 460 patients and out of all 2760 were cervically abraded. The incidence of cervical abrasion was maximum in the age group of 51–60 years. Males showed more cervical abrasions while the total number of teeth present was more in females. A reasonable explanation for this may be the higher utilization of dental services by females and also the females are more conscious towards their dental problems. The lesions were classified by shape as well as depth. The observations are recorded in the Table 12.64. The shape could be:

a. Notch (N) - Where the occlusal and cervical walls intersect at a certain depth. Definite axial walls may not be present.

b. Undercut concave (UC) - Where occlusal and cervical walls intersect with definite axial walls present.

c. Divergent box (DB) - Where the width of the axial wall increases with cervical and occlusal walls diverging.

The depth could be;

   i. Shallow (S) - Shallow lesions were 0.1–0.5 mm in depth

   ii. Deep (D) - more than 0.5 mm without pulp exposure

   iii. Pulp exposure (E) - where pulp was exposed

Smith and Knight (1984) suggested that the threshold level of Tooth Wear Index could be established for individual tooth surface, beyond which the level of wear should be

Table 12.64: Percentage of shape and depth of cervical lesions

Shape (%age)	No. of teeth Shallow (%age)	Deep (%age)	Depth Exposure (%age)	
Notch (N) (34.78)	960 (26.08)	720 (8.69)	240 (0)	0
Undercut Concave (UC)	1088 (39.42)	277 (10.03)	783 (28.36)	28 (1.01)
Divergent Box (DB)	712 (25.79)	185 (6.70)	450 (16.60)	67 (2.42)
All 2760	1182 (42.12)	1483 (53.73)	95 (3.44)	

considered 'pathological'. The tooth can be termed to have pathological wear if it cannot function effectively or its appearance is seriously marred. Many authors are of the view that the term 'pathological' is misleading and should be avoided. The principle of establishing the extent and severity of wear which might be regarded as acceptable for a given age, however, allows comparison between population groups. It would be more useful from an epidemiological standpoint to report wear score in relation to the number of individuals in any given group who have one or more teeth above a specific threshold value. In this way, both the prevalence of given levels of wear and its severity should be assessed and comparison can be made more readily.

The acceptable level of wear, however, varies with the individuals at different ages. The sensitivity of Tooth Wear Index should be increased to take into account the capacity of elderly to have adequate oral function even after significant tooth wear has occurred. Older people especially are concerned more with function rather than the appearance.

Tooth wear can be regarded as pathological if the teeth become so worn that they do not function effectively or are lost through other causes. Examples of conditions which may produce rapid but short term tooth wear are erosion from crushed diets like excessive amount of citrus fruits, bruxism, the use of abrasive tooth cleaning techniques, gastric disturbances producing regurgitation and dentists adjusting occlusions.

Certain clinical features which are regarded as diagnostic of pathologic wear are as follows:
1. Pulp exposure
2. Loss of vitality attributing to wear
3. Exposure of secondary dentin
4. Exposure of dentin on buccal and lingual surfaces
5. Notched cervical surfaces
6. Cupped occlusal and incisal surfaces
7. Wear in one arch more than the other
8. Restoration projecting above the tooth surface
9. Wear producing persistent sensitivity
10. The cervico-incisal length is out of proportion with the width

THE EXACT TOOTH WEAR INDEX

A modified tooth wear index, the exact tooth wear index was developed following the basic principles of Smith and Knight index.

The wear on teeth was graded separately for enamel and dentin using 5 and 6 point scales (Table 12.65). Changes in the enamel surface texture were graded according to the criteria listed in Table 12.65. The area around the cemento-enamel junction or the zone just above the gingival margin (if not visible), was considered as the cervical area. The part of tooth coronal to this area was considered to be on the facial/buccal surface. In case of doubt the lower score is given.

Table 12.65: Recording of exact tooth wear index

The Exact Tooth Wear Index for Enamel

0 No tooth wear : no loss of enamel characteristics or change in contour

1 Loss of enamel affecting less than 10% of the scored surface

2 Enamel loss affecting between 10% and one third of the scored surfaced

3 Enamel loss affecting at least one third but less than two thirds of the scored surface

4 Enamel loss affecting two thirds or more of the second surface

The Exact Tooth Wear Index for Dentin

0 No dentinal tooth wear : no loss of dentin

1 Loss of dentin affecting less than 10% of the scored surface

2 Dentin loss affecting between 10% and one third of the scored surface

3 Dentin loss affecting at least one third but less than two thirds of the scored surface

4 Dentin loss affecting two thirds or more of the scored surface, without pulpal exposure

5 Exposure of secondary dentin or pulpal exposure.

BIBLIOGRAPHY

1. Adam, R.A. and Nystrom, G.P. : A periodontitis severity index. J. P. : 57, 176, 1986.
2. Aherne, C.A., Mullene, D.O. and Barrett, B.E. : Indices of root surface caries. J.D.R. : 69, 1222, 1990.
3. Ainamo, J. and Cutress, T.W. : An epidemiological index of developmental defects of dental enamel (DDE Index). Int. Dent. J. : 32, 159, 1982.
4. Ainano, J., Barmes, D. and Beagrie, G. : Development of WHO Community Periodontal Index of treatment needs. Int. Dent. J. : 32, 281, 1982.
5. Atchison, K.A. and Dolan, T.A. : Development of Geriatric Oral health assessment index. J. Dent. Educ. : 54, 680, 1990.
6. Barnett, M., Ciancio, S. and Mather, M. : The modified papillary bleeding index : comparison with gingival index during the resolution of gingivitis. J. Prevent. Dent. : 6, 135, 1980.
7. Benn, D.K. : A review of the reliability of radiographic measurements in estimating alveolar bone changes. J.C.P. : 17, 14, 1990
8. Ben-Shlomo, Y. and Kuh, D. : A life course approach to chronic diseases epidemiology : conceptual models, empirical challenges and interdisciplinary perspectives. Int. J. Epidem.: 31, 285, 2002.
9. Burke, F.J.T., Worthington, H.V. and Wilson, N.H.F. : Oral Health Index. B.D.J. : 178, 168, 1995.
10. Burke, T.J.F. and Wilson, F.H.F. : Measuring oral health : an historical view and details of a contemporary oral health index (OHX). Int. Dent. J. : 45, 358, 1995.
11. Carter, H.G. and Barnes, G.P. : The gingival bleeding index. J. Periodontol. : 45, 801, 1974.
12. Ciancio, S.G. : Current status of indices of gingivitis. J. Clin. Periodontol. : 13, 375, 1986.
13. Clarkson, J. : A review of the developmental defects of enamel index (DDE Index). I.D.J. : 42, 411, 1992.
14. Daniel, C. and Richmond, S. : The development of the index of complexity outcome and need (ICON). J. Orthodont. : 27, 149, 2000.
15. Demers, M., Brodeur, J., Simard, P.L., Mouton, C., Vcilleun, G. and Frechette, S. : Caries predictors suitable for mass screenings in children : a literature review. Comm. Dent. Health: 7, 11, 1990.
16. Destavola, B.L., Nitsch, D., dos Santos Silva, I., McCormack, V., Hardy, R. and Mann, V. : Statistical issues in life course epidemiology. Am. J. Epidem. : 163, 84, 2006.
17. Fares, J., Shirodaria, S., Chiu, K., Ahmad, N., Sherriff, M. and Bartlett, D. : A New Index of Tooth Wear. Caries Res. : 43, 119, 2009.
18. Firestone, A.R., Beck, F.M., Beglin, F.M. and Vig, K.W. : Validity of index of complexity outcome and need (ICON) in determining orthodontic needs. Augle Ortho. : 72, 15, 2002.
19. Grewe, J.M., Godin, R.J. and Meskin, L.H. : Human tooth mortality : A clinical statistical study. J. Am. Dent. Assoc. : 72, 106, 1996.

20. Heather Beckett and Graeme Zaki : An index of implant treatment need (II TN). B.D.J. : 182, 160, 1997.

21. Karthikeyan, K.S. : DMF Index : Its shortcomings and suggested rectification. J.I.D.A.: 68, 19, 1997.

22. Katz, R.V. : Development of an index for the prevalence of root caries. J.D.R. : 63 (Spl. Issue), 814, 1984.

23. Namal, N. and Sheiham, A. : Comparison of ranking dental status using the significant caries index and the significant filled and sound-teeth index. Community Dental Health : 25, 103, 2008.

24. Namal, N., Vahid, S. and Sheiham, A. : Ranking countries by dental status using the DMFT and FS-T indices. International Dental Journal: 55, 373, 2005.

25. Nicolau, B., Marcenes, W., Bartley, M. and Sheiham, A. : Association between socio-economic circumstances at two stages of life and adolescents oral health status. J. Public Health Dent. : 65, 14, 2005.

26. Nicolau, B., Marcenes, W., Hardy, R. and Sheiham, A. : A life course approach to assess the relationship between social and psychological circumstances and gingival status in adolescents. J. Clin. Periodontol. : 30, 1038, 2003.

27. Nicolau, B., Thomson, W.M., Steele, J.G. and Allison, P.J. : Life course epidemiology : concepts and theoretical models and its relevance to chronic oral conditions. Comm. Dent. Oral Epidem. : 35, 241, 2007.

28. Pearce, M.S., Steele, J.G., Mason, J., Walls, A.W. and Parker, L. : Do circumstances in early life contribute to tooth retention in middle age ? J.D.R. : 83, 562, 2004.

29. Ripa, L.W. : Nursing caries : a comprehensive review. Pediat. Dent. : 10, 268, 1988.

30. Sikri, Poonam and Sikri, V.K. : Prevalence, classification and management of cervical lesions. I.S.P. Bull. : 17, 1992.

31. Sikri, V. and Sikri, P. : Clinical and Radiological Examination of root surface caries: An in-vitro study. I.J.D.R. : 2, 1, 1991.

32. Smith, B.G.N. and Knight, J.K. : An index for measuring the wear of tooth. B.D.J. : 156, 435, 1984.

33. Susser, E. : Eco-epidemiology: thinking outside the black box. Epidemiology : 15, 519, 2004.

34. Susser, M. and Susser, E. : Choosing a future for epidemiology : 1. Eras and paradigms. Am. J. Public Health: 86, 668, 1996.

35. Wagg, B.J. : ECSI : caries progression data. Comm. Dent. Oral Epidem. : 2, 219, 1974.

Epidemiology of Oral Diseases

Epidemiological studies of oral diseases mainly aim to describe the prevalence and distribution of a disease in a community so as to contribute to the solutions for public health problems concerned with the identification, detection, treatment planning and treatment of that oral condition. The epidemiological studies of main oral conditions are described below.

EPIDEMIOLOGY OF PERIODONTAL DISEASES

Periodontal disease, an ancient disease of mankind, is usually referred by layman as 'Pyorrhea'. The World Health Organization has stated that it is one of the most widespread diseases affecting more than ninety percent of the population. Research and clinical evidences indicate that the damage caused to the supporting structure of the teeth in early adult life is irreparable while in middle adult life it destroys a large part of the natural dentition. Since periodontal disease and caries are large scale public health problems, so the epidemiological surveys of these diseases become mandatory. The developing countries need more attention in order that preventive programs can be used efficiently despite of limited resources of finances and manpower.

The factors affecting the prevalence and distribution of periodontal disease are:

1. Age

  a. *Primary dentition:* Gingivitis is present in almost all the children (almost 100% prevalence); however, it rarely proceeds into periodontitis except in the cases of aggressive periodontitis.

  b. *Mixed dentition:* Due to fluctuating and unfavourable local conditions during the mixed dentition period, it is difficult to evaluate prevalence during this period.

  c. *In younger adults:* The prevalence of gingivitis and periodontitis increases in this period. Periodontal pockets may be observed in some children in their teens, but periodontitis does not often lead to tooth mortality before the age of 20 years.

  d. *In older adults:* The prevalence of periodontitis and bone resorption increase by 40 to 50 years of age.

2. Sex: The periodontal conditions are significantly better in females than in males. However, during puberty, pregnancy and lactation periods the prevalence of periodontal diseases is more in females as compared to males.

3. Oral hygiene: Oral hygiene has strong association with the oral diseases and the prevalence of periodontal disease is more in the population with poor oral hygiene.

4. Socio-economic status: The prevalence of periodontal disease is more in the persons of low socio-economic status.

5. Tobacco/Betel nut consumption: The prevalence of periodontal diseases increases in the individual having regular consumption of tobacco and betel nut.

6. Systemic diseases: Diabetics have high prevalence of periodontal diseases; however, other diseases like AIDS, cardiac

and renal disorders have been associated with the increased rate of periodontal diseases.

7. **Nutritional factors:** The nutritional factors are more significant in the developing countries as compared to developed countries and the prevalence of periodontal diseases is more in the malnourished communities.

8. **Dental caries:** Prevalence of periodontal disease is more in the persons having more prevalence of dental caries. It may be because of the similar etiological factor.

9. **Malocclusion:** Gingivitis is more prevalent in the crowded, malaligned or rotated teeth as they are not completely accessible to the oral hygiene measures.

10. **Traumatic occlusion:** The prevalence of periodontal diseases increases in individuals having traumatic occlusion.

11. **Race:** It may be a secondary factor in determining the prevalence of periodontal diseases.

Epidemiological Studies

Many studies have been carried out in the past to assess the prevalence of various forms of periodontal diseases in Global and Indian populations. These studies have a remarkable impact on our understanding of periodontal diseases.

An epidemiologic survey of the Indian population was carried out by **Marshall-Day et al in 1955.** They assessed alveolar bone height to distinguish between gingivitis and destructive periodontal disease in 1187 dentate subjects. They observed a decrease in the percentage of subjects with 'gingival disease without any bone involvement' with increasing age. Concomitant with this observation was an increase in the percentage of subjects with 'chronic, destructive periodontal disease'. Further, the authors reported 100% destructive periodontitis after the age of 40 years.

An epidemiological study of periodontal disease in and around Bombay, India, and in Atlanta, Georgia (U.S.A.), was conducted by **Greene in 1957.** The study involved 1,613 males, aged eleven, thirteen, fifteen, and seventeen in India and 577 males of the same age groups in Atlanta. In addition, 63 Indian males, eighteen to thirty years of age, were examined in a rural area near Bombay. Periodontal disease was found to be highly prevalent in both groups, but was significantly more severe in India than in Atlanta. Oral calculus was also abundant in the Indian group. The rural persons studied in India were reported to have severe periodontal disease, more calculus, and more debris than those in urban India.

Dutta (1965) studied the prevalence of periodontal disease in a group of school going children in Calcutta. The author examined 1424 children in the age group of 6–12 years. A prevalence of periodontal disease of 73.4% in 6 year-olds and 96.5% in 12 year-olds was reported. In addition 91.6% of boys were affected by periodontal disease in comparison with 87.6% of girls.

A study was conducted in rural areas of Delhi by **Pandit et al (1986)** to determine the prevalence of periodontal disease and dental caries amongst children of both sexes, aged 5 to 14 years. 458 primary school children from lower socio-economic group families were examined. Prevalence of periodontal disease and dental caries was found to be low despite a perfunctory oral health care system with no fluoridation of water supply. The authors attributed their findings to the consumption of coarse and fibrous food by the children.

Vyas and Damle (1991) conducted a prevalence study on dental caries and periodontal disease in 94 mentally subnormal, 92 physically handicapped, 74 juvenile delinquents and 206 normal children (11–14-year-old). They found a high prevalence of periodontal disease in handicapped (95 to 100%) and a low prevalence in normal children (54.37%).

Dixit et al (1980) studied the occurrence and severity of gingivitis in 80 pregnant and 40 non-pregnant women in Lucknow, Uttar Pradesh. They found a significantly higher severity of gingivitis in pregnant subjects as compared to non-pregnant ones. They also observed an increase in the severity of gingivitis in the second trimester of pregnancy.

Singh (1982) surveyed a Semi-urban community of Pune and found that 95.8% of the subjects had calculus, 62.2% had gingivitis and 34.3% showed advanced periodontal involvement (pocket depths more than 3.0 mm and visible signs of periodontal disease).

Venkatesh (1987) reviewed earlier studies conducted in North India and Amritsar. He quoted the prevalence of periodontal diseases to be 60.0% and 86.6% respectively. He further quoted studies carried out in Trivandrum and Madras, which showed that 90.3% and 95.0% subjects suffered from periodontal disease.

Anil et al (1990) assessed the periodontal condition of 2756 subjects aged 15–44 years from urban and rural areas of Trivandrum, Kerala using the CPITN index. They reported that calculus and bleeding were more frequent (86%) in the age group of 15–19 years; shallow pockets were observed in the age group of 25–29 years, and deep pockets more than 6.0 mm were seen in 33% of the subjects, aged 35–44 years.

Rao and Bharambe (1993) compared the periodontal status among urban, rural and tribal school children in Sewagram, Maharashtra. Bleeding, calculus and abscesses were taken as prevalence criteria. It was observed that periodontal diseases tended to be limited to children using ash, coal, and manjan. Rural children (22.6%) were more likely to suffer from periodontal diseases than urban (10.5%) and tribal children (15%).

Maity et al (1994) examined 5960 subjects aged 15–65 years in a rural population in West Bengal. A surprisingly low prevalence of deep periodontal pockets was found. However, dental calculus was found to be a widespread finding in this study.

In a population of rural women in Pondicherry, **Jagadeesan et al (2000)** found that only 0.8% had bleeding gums, 20.1% had calculus and 20.6% showed shallow periodontal pockets.

Singh et al (2005) studied the prevalence of periodontal diseases in rural and urban areas of Ludhiana, Punjab. 96.8% urban and 97.2% rural subjects showed presence of calculus while gingival bleeding was seen in 68.6% urban and 69.2% rural subjects. 42.3% of urban subjects aged above 15 years showed presence of shallow periodontal pockets as compared to 31.7% of rural subjects. 22.9% subjects in urban areas had deep periodontal pockets as compared to 11.0% in rural areas. 22.9% subjects belonging to urban areas showed loss of tooth attachment as compared to 13.2% subjects belonging to rural areas. The authors were of the view that advanced stages of periodontal disease were significantly more prevalent in urban areas as compared to rural areas.

Dhar et al (2007) recorded the prevalence of gingivitis, fluorosis and malocclusion among 1,587 government school children of Udaipur district in the age group of 5–14 years. Gingivitis was found in 84.37% children, malocclusion in 36.42% and fluorosis in 36.36%.

The summary of the aforementioned studies are tabulated in Table 13.1.

EPIDEMIOLOGY OF DENTAL CARIES

Dental caries is a multi-factorial disease influenced by diet, socio-economic status, and fluoride exposure. Recent epidemiological studies in economically developing countries show that the prevalence and severity of dental caries has increased with the industrialization and exposure to a western type diet.

Factors Determining Epidemiology of Caries

1. **Sex:** Girls usually have a higher rate of caries in younger age, chiefly because of the earlier eruption of their teeth and the

Table 13.1

Year	Author	Place	Study population	Findings
1955	Marshall-Day et al.	India	1187 dentate subjects	- Increase in percentage of subjects with "chronic, destructive periodontal disease" with age - 100% occurrence of destructive periodontitis after 40 years
1957	Greene	Bombay and Atlanta (Georgia, U.S.A.)	1,613 Indian males, 577 American males, 63 males from rural areas	- Periodontal disease is more severe in India - Calculus more abundant in India - Rural subjects had more severe disease
1965	Dutta	Calcutta	1424 school going children aged 6-12 years	- Prevalence of 73.4% in 6 year-olds and 96.5% in 12 year-olds - 91.6% of boys and 87.6% of girls were affected
1980	Dixit et al.	Lucknow	80 pregnant and 40 non-pregnant women	- Higher severity of gingivitis in pregnant subjects - Increase in severity of gingivitis in the second trimester
1982	Singh	Pune	Semi-urban community	- 95.8% had calculus - 62.2% had gingivitis - 34.3% showed advanced periodontal involvement
1986	Pandit et al.	Rural areas of Delhi	458 primary school children aged 5 to 14 years from lower socio-economic groups	Low prevalence of periodontal disease and dental caries despite poor oral health care
1987	Venkatesh	Quoted earlier studies conducted in Northern India, Amritsar, Madras, Trivandrum	Review of earlier studies	Prevalence of Periodontal disease - Northern India - 60.0% - Amritsar: 86.6% - Madras: 95.0% - Trivandrum : 90.3%
1990	Anil et al.	Trivandrum	2756 subjects aged 15-44 years from urban and rural areas	- Calculus and bleeding more frequent (86%) in 15-19 age group

Contd...

Year	Author	Place	Study population	Findings
				- Shallow pocketing more frequent in 25-29 age group
				- Deep pockets seen in 33% of subjects aged 35-44 years
1991	**Vyas and Damle**	Bombay	94 mentally subnormal, 92 physically handicapped, 74 juvenile delinquents, 206 normal children (11-14 yrs)	High prevalence of periodontal disease in the handicapped (95 to 100%) and low in normal children (54.37%)
1993	**Rao and Bharambe**	Sewagram, Maharashtra	Urban, rural and tribal school children	Rural children more likely than urban and tribal children to suffer from periodontal diseases
1994	**Maity et al.**	Rural areas in West Bengal	5960 subjects aged 15-65 years	- Surprisingly low prevalence of deep periodontal pockets - Dental calculus widespread
2000	**Jagadeesan et al.**	Pondicherry	Rural women	- 0.8% had bleeding gums - 20.1% had calculus - 20.6% showed shallow periodontal pockets
2005	**Singh et al.**	Ludhiana, Punjab	Rural and urban populations	Advanced stages of periodontal disease more prevalent in urban areas as compared to rural areas
2007	**Dhar et al.**	Udaipur district, Rajasthan	1,587 government school children aged 5-14 years	84.37% of children had gingivitis

consequent longer exposure time. Boys have higher caries rate during teens and as they approach adult life.

2. **Race:** Racial characteristics influence caries not only by heredity, but also influencing cultural characteristics and individual habits. The Chinese and Black groups show lower caries than white group. The difference may be attributed to different general and family environment and genetics.

3. **Heredity:** In general, children of parents with low caries susceptibility have lesser carious lesions as compared to children whose parents have extensive carious involvement. An ongoing Minnesota study on twins living in different environments

has determined genetics to be of considerable importance.

4. **Genetic effects:** The Amelogenin (AMELX) gene is responsible for x-linked amelogenesis imperfecta. The decreased amount of Amelogenin protein leads to disruption of formation of enamel matrix and therefore increased caries susceptibility.

5. **Pregnancy:** Pregnancy may lead to hormonal fluctuations, salivary alternations, immune suppression and other physiological changes that would adversely affect the host resistance to caries.

6. **Diet:** Diet influences caries prevalence in different ways.
   - The *Vipeholm study* on adult inmates in a mental institution showed that the physical form of carbohydrates is more important than the total amount of sugar ingested.
   - The *Hopewood House study* on children between 3 and 14 years of age residing at Hopewood house on an institutional diet, showed that dental caries can be reduced by a particular diet, even in the presence of unfavourable oral hygiene.

7. **Systemic Disturbances:** There is no evidence that any particular systemic disease influences the initiation of dental caries. Diseases of nutritional deficiencies and dominant gene transfers may produce alteration in the calcification of enamel and dentin, but there are no convincing data that such alteration affects the initiation of dental caries. However, these disturbances may influence its progress.

Caries Susceptibility in Primary Dentition

The deciduous teeth are more susceptible to caries, may be because the brushing habits and other oral hygiene measures are not followed properly during this period. It has been shown that at the age of two, occlusal caries accounts for over 60% of carious lesions. However, the proximal caries of molars is insignificant. The difference may be associated with spacing which exists between erupted primary teeth and the short period of exposure of primary second molars at the age of 2 years. At the age of 6 years, the proximal caries is as prevalent as occlusal caries.

The distal surfaces of 'd' or mesial surfaces of 'e' are more susceptible. With eruption of first permanent molars, the susceptibility of distal surfaces of 'e' increases 10 times and the mesial surfaces of 'd' are less susceptible because of spacing that normally exists between primary cuspids and first molars. Also, the broader area of contact between 'd' and 'e' predisposes to development of caries.

The relative susceptibility of various surfaces of deciduous teeth is as follows:

Mesial surface of cuspid < distal surface of cuspid = mesial surfaces of 'd' < distal surface of 'd' = mesial surface of 'e' (until first permanent molar erupts)

Caries Susceptibility in Permanent Dentition

The first permanent molar is more susceptible to caries, mainly because of early eruption and considering it a part of deciduous dentition. It is observed that 20% of children at age 6 experience tooth decay in permanent dentition. By the age of 8 and 10 years, 60 to 85% children are affected and at the age of 12 years, 90% are affected.

DMFS approximates DMFT from age 6–8. Beyond this point, the DMFS increases at an accelerated rate and at the age of 12 years, 7.5 DMFS may be expected.

The maxillary permanent central and lateral incisors are involved only in case of rampant caries. During 10–12 years, the maxillary and mandibular cuspids and premolars erupt and approximately 5% of premolars may be affected.

The second permanent molars which erupt at 12 years are quite susceptible to caries.

20% mandibular and 10% maxillary second permanent molars are affected by the age of 19 years.

Occlusal surfaces are the most prevalent among the surfaces which develop carious lesion. At 12 years of age, caries involving occlusal surfaces are 50%; proximal surface 30%; buccal and lingual surface 20%; labial, incisal and cervical surface are less than one percent.

Global Decline in Caries

In any country, high caries prevalence was known from the excessive burden of restorative treatment and the frequent destruction of teeth beyond repair. Children 12 years of age, usually have more than 5 DMFT, and by the age of 15, the average DMFT was above 10.

Such situations initiated the search for preventive measures. The discovery of the cariostatic effects of fluoride rapidly inspired activities in both research and practical dentistry. Local use of fluorides was preferred in the Scandinavian studies while in couple of European countries daily intake of fluoride tablet was preferred.

The early **Scandinavian report** of caries decline was cited by **Von der Fehr and Haugejorden (1997)**. They observed that in 5 of the 14 Norwegian countries, the decline began around 1967. In Switzerland, Germany and Austria, decline of caries became obvious in the early sixties. It was concluded that the decline started when fluoride brushing or rinsing were introduced.

The decline in caries took various courses in Europe. The average DMFT of 12 year old children decreased steadily from 8 in 1965 to one in 1993 in Netherland.

The data on the decline up to 1993 were presented at the 'Second International Conference on Declining Caries'. The decline of the DMFT in several European countries was found to be continuing until late nineties. The earlier statistics showed that the fluoride level in the drinking water had been the main determinant of dental caries prevalence.

In recent years, it has been established that caries prevalence was highest in the lower socio-economic strata.

Reasons for the Decline

The reasons for the decline of caries have not been established. It is hypothesized that the daily use of fluoridated toothpastes, preferably twice a day, was considered to be the most important single factor. In controlled randomized studies comparing dentifrices with and without fluoride, the reductions were often between 20 and 40% and rarely exceeded 50%. However, in several countries, the DMFT averages have fallen to 60% or even below. It may be due to improved tooth brushing habits, since more frequent and more thorough toothbrushing would strengthen the fluoride effect, lower the 'aggressivity' of dental plaque and remove fermentable food remnants more thoroughly. However, other important factors are likely to be involved in the dramatic decline of dental caries prevalence at school age.

Among the factors considered unimportant by **Bratthall et al. (1996),** placement of sealants needs to be reconsidered. In case of DMFT averages above 3, there will be much caries apart from fissures and pits and the role of sealants will be limited. The fact is that the declines above 70% were obtained in several European countries before fissure sealants were commonly used. However, in the countries in which DMFT averages are below 2.0, most of the caries occur in fissures and pits of the first molars until the age of 12 years. Subsequently, it is assumed that sealants can be a very important, or even the main factor in lowering the DMFT.

The decline phase ended by the late nineties. The dmfs and DMFS of Dutch children between 1996 and 2002 are tabulated in Table 13.2.

Table 13.2: Average dmfs and DMFS counts of the Dutch children (1996–2002)

	Dutch nationals
Age 6, dmfs	
1996	0.8
1998	0.5
2002	0.7
Age 12, DMFS	
1996	.3
1998	0.1
2002	0.4

In statistical studies of any country, the number of migrants usually poses problems. For proper interpretation of epidemiological data, the immigration status, country of origin as well as the length of stay in the guest country needs to be recorded and reported.

The effect of immigrated children on overall caries experience is more obvious in Switzerland. 7 years old Swiss children in the city of Zurich had dmft averages between 1.5 and 1.8. It was showed that immigrant children had 6.0 dmft, more than thrice that of Swiss children in the nineties. When the Swiss children were counted along with migrants, the dmft average increased from 1.7 to 2.7 (1998).

It is established that once the average dmf or DMF counts are low, there will be instability. The 'White' fillings have also become a problem. It is inevitable that part of them are not identified by the examiner with the effect that the F component, which in Europe has long become much larger than the D and M component, is underestimated to some extent. At the low caries levels in highly industrialized countries, it is difficult to identify minor changes in caries prevalence. However, the conventional examination procedures are sufficient to detect substantial increase in caries prevalence.

New diagnostic methods, particularly for fissure caries, where the majority of carious lesions and fillings occur, may provide more reliable bases for determining whether decay levels decrease, remain constant or increase.

It is important to note that the decline is carried on into adult age. In Switzerland, the DMFT at age 20 was 16.0 in 1970 but by 1996 had decreased to 4.8 (including extracted premolars) or 4.4 (counting only extracted first molars). It is summarized that the average reductions ranged from 18 to 66% in recent years.

Global increase in Dental Caries

Recent studies have reported increase in caries incidence. The increase is in children and adults, primary and permanent teeth, which include both coronal and root caries.

The causes of this increase is not clear; however, it is possible that the benefits of prevention might not be reaching these people. The use of bottled water and dietary changes might be the cause. The influx of immigrants and the movement of rural people to urban areas, changing their life style might also be the reason for global increase in caries.

Epidemiological Studies

Ray E. Stewart (2003) conducted a study in California and made two significant observations. First, high caries index patterns run in families and are passed vertically from mother to child from generation to generation. The children of high caries index mothers are always at a higher risk. Secondly, the modification of the mother's dental flora at the time of inoculation of the child can significantly affect the child's caries index.

An estimated 90% of school children worldwide and most adults have experienced caries, with the disease most prevalent in Asian and Latin American countries and least prevalent in African countries. In the US, dental caries is the most common chronic childhood disease, being at least five times more common than asthma. It is the primary pathological cause of tooth loss in children. Between 29% and 59% of adults over the age of fifty, experience caries.

In the Northern Philippines, a study of 993 children aged 2 to 6 years using Decayed, Missing and Filled Teeth reported increase in caries (DMFT) index, prevalence from 59% (4.2 DMFT) to 92% (10.1 DMFT). Caries was diagnosed using the World Health Organization (WHO) criteria. Only obvious frank cavitation was recorded as caries. The authors stated that caries rates were similar to those of developing countries with untreated lesions dominating all age groups (Carino et al 2003).

A longitudinal study of the permanent dentition was reported on 6–9 year olds in Campeche, Mexico. Two examiners conducted dental examinations. Prevalence of caries in permanent teeth increased from year 1999 to 2000 by over 20%. The percentage of children with new dental caries increased from 14.2% to 34.7%. The authors concluded that the study demonstrated significant increments in dental caries in as short a time period as 18 months, stating that priorities need to be set to identify children who will likely develop new caries so that preventive methods can be provided (Vallejos et al 2006).

Hougejorden et al (2006) reported from Norway for the years 1985–2004 showing a reversal of caries decline and similar trends of increasing caries in permanent teeth of children aged 12 years. This study included samples of over 50,000 children using aggregated data reported from clinics to the national level. Results indicated a linear decline in caries in 12 year-old children from 1985 to 2000. This decline was followed by a rise in caries from 2000 to 2004. The increase was 3.3% per year, in contrast to a decline of 3.0% before 2000. More of 12 year-old Norwegian children were affected by caries in 2004 than in 2000 (59.8% versus 52.2%).

A WHO study conducted across 188 countries to get an estimate of global DMFT for 12 years old children, reported that 200, 335, 280 teeth were either decayed, filled or missing among just that age group (Brathall et al, 2006). This was based on the data available in 2004 from the WHO Oral Health Database, Country/Area Profile Program (CAPP).

Du, M. et al (2007) conducted a cross-sectional survey on a representative sample of Chinese preschool-children aged 3–5 years. The sample included 2,014 children and examinations were conducted using the World Health Organization (WHO) criteria. Results demonstrated a prevalence of 55% with regular dental caries and 14% with rampant dental caries. Caries prevalence and severity increased with age. A high proportion of young children had dental caries and most decayed teeth were untreated.

Pandit et al (1986) conducted a study in four primary schools of Mehrauli block of rural Delhi.

Four hundred and fifty eight primary school children of both sexes in the age group of 5–14 were examined. Regularity of teeth cleaning habits and associated caries prevalence was noted.

Dental caries prevalence was 33.19% and DMF index was 0.52.

The regular teeth cleaning group showed significantly less caries prevalence while 'not regular' and 'never cleaning' groups had higher caries prevalence.

Rao and Bharambe (1993) studied the oral health status in school children of Wardha to find out the geographical differences and to relate it with the teeth cleaning habit and nutritional status. A sample of 778 children studying in two urban, four rural and two tribal primary schools was selected.

The study indicated that dental caries and periodontal diseases were prevalent among primary school children. Periodontal diseases were prevalent among rural children who were using coarse teeth cleaning materials.

Dental decay was less prevalent among rural and tribal children than urban children. The relationship of nutritional status and dental caries was observed as controversial.

Grover and Evans conducted a study in industrialized areas of Haryana (India) to investigate the effect of diet, natural level of fluoride in drinking water, oral health habits and socio-economic status on dental caries.

They included a cross-sectional survey of 1403 school children aged 6 and 12 years in the study. The caries experience was severe among poor urban children.

DMFT = 0.53 (in 6 years aged children)

= 0.23 (in 12 years aged children)

Dash et al (2002) conducted the study on 1257 school children in the age group of 5, 8, 11 and 15 years respectively in the city of Cuttack, Orissa.

The examination was carried out under natural light and dental caries was diagnosed according to the WHO criteria 1983. The point prevalence of dental caries was recorded to be 64.3% with an average DMFT of 2.38.

The prevalence of caries showed a pattern of occurrence; prevalence consistently increased from 5 years to 8 years age group and subsequently decreased at 11 years and 15 years age. The reason could be that caries being a continuous and cumulative process increases within a span of 3 years. The fall in point prevalence at 11 years age is understandable, because most of the deciduous teeth have been exfoliated and succeedaneous premolars have not been in the oral cavity long enough for caries process to set in.

David and Wang (2005) conducted a study to describe the dental health status of 12 year old school children in Thiruvanthapuram, Kerala (India).

A cross-sectional survey of 838 children in urban primary schools was carried out and the prevalence of dental caries in the permanent dentition was found to be 27%.

The study indicated that caries were associated with urban living conditions. Since urbanization is rapid in India, timely oral health promotion would be beneficial to prevent caries.

Saravanan and Madivanan (2005) studied the pattern of prevalence of dental caries in the primary dentition among 5 year old school children, selected from the area of urban Pondicherry. A total of 1009 children of both sexes were included in the study. Dental caries was assessed by the dentition status and treatment needs (WHO, 1997).

The prevalence of caries was 44.4% among the study population, being higher in the boys.

Regarding prevalence pattern in arches, the mandibular arch was affected more than the maxillary arch. On comparing caries prevalence in relation to right and left side of the oral cavity, it was evident that dental caries occurs predominantly as a bilateral phenomenon. Caries prevalence was higher in posterior teeth as compared to anterior teeth in both the sexes, may be due to complex morphological nature of the posterior teeth.

It was also seen that, among posterior teeth, primary first molars in both the arches were less susceptible to caries than the primary second molars. The difference in individual tooth susceptibility was due to the fissure topography of molars. The pits and fissures in second primary molars were deeper and less completely coalesced.

The sequence of caries attack follows a specific pattern: Mandibular molars, maxillary molars and maxillary anterior teeth were predominantly affected by caries; however, mandibular anterior teeth were least affected

The prevalence of caries was higher in the maxillary arch than the mandibular arch among the anterior teeth whereas in the posterior teeth, the prevalence was higher in the mandibular arch as compared to the maxillary arch.

Goyal et al (2007) considered caries trends in Chandigarh school children over the last 25 years. The spurt in dental caries can be attributed to the limited use of fluoride-tooth paste, greater consumption of sugary food stuffs and neglect of oral hygiene.

Patro and Ravi Kumar (2008) estimated the prevalence of dental caries in the adult population (aged 35–44 years) and in the elderly (60 years and above) in an urban resettlement colony in New Delhi.

The prevalence of dental caries among adults was found out to be on higher side. The awareness about good and bad dental practices was found to be low among the participants. Also, a statistically significant association was found between tobacco consumption and dental caries.

Khan et al (2008) evaluated persons suffering from dental caries in relation to different factors. They reported high incidence of dental caries in females and amongst vegetarian population. Further, it was observed that the 21–30 years age group was more susceptible to caries.

Maru and Narendaran assessed dental caries using DMFT and DMFS indices.

The study population consisted of 189 volunteer subjects from the village of Kachchh, with the mean age of 34.9 ± 14.2 years.

More than 80% of the participants had untreated caries and the mean DMFT and DMFS scores were 5.1±3.9 and 13.8±17.8 which did not show any gender differences. The results indicated high levels of dental caries as well as dental treatment needs among a rural East Indian population.

Shenoy et al (2009) assessed the dental caries experience of 3–5 years old anganwadi and kindergarten children in Mangalore city. The assessment was carried out by dentition status and treatment need (WHO oral health assessment form, 1997). The prevalence of dental caries among anganwadi children was 81.4%; however, among the kindergarten children, the prevalence of dental caries was 62.3%.

The mean dmft among the anganwadi children was 4.62 (3.82) and among kindergarten children, the mean dmft score was 3.42 (3.77). It was found that the caries prevalence and mean dmft was higher among anganwadi children, and the prevalence of filled teeth was higher among kindergarten children.

Sunayana et al (2009) examined a total of 3,315 school children in Chennai city by multiphase cluster sampling technique. The 12 year olds consisted of 1,448 school children of which 706 were males and 723 were females. The 15 year olds consisted of 1,867 school children of which 959 were males and 908 were females. The data was collected and recorded.

They observed that the prevalence of dental caries was high in the 15 year old age group (48.9%) when compared to the 12 year old age group (46.5%). The 12 year old age group has the Significant Caries Index (SiC) value (2.8) which is in proportion with the WHO proposed value of 3; however the 15 year old age group has marginally higher SiC value (3.4). It was recommended that oral health education and prevention strategies should be implemented at all levels of school education for promoting oral health.

Sikri and Sikri (1993) determined the prevalence and distribution of root surface caries in a population of older adults residing in Amritsar city and adjoining villages.

Seven hundred and sixty patients were chosen on the criteria of patients' age (should be above fifty) and number of teeth (at least fifteen teeth present in both the arches).

The diagnosis of caries was based on the visual findings of darkened/discoloured lesions and tactile criteria of leathery feel upon probing. An area softer and darkened than the surrounding teeth surfaces, with or without a cavity was taken as carious.

When both the coronal and root surfaces were affected by a single carious lesion, only its most likely site of origin was scored as decayed. A root surface was considered at risk if the cemento-enamel junction was visible.

As the age advanced, the Root Caries Index (RCI) rate increased (maximum in the age group of 60–69 years; then declining after age of 70). The decline in the RCI after 70 years of age may be due to a small number of samples in these age groups.

The RCI rate was more for males than females (due to higher utilization of dental services by females). Mandibular molars showed the maximum RCI (12.72 ± 6.77) and the mandibular incisors the least (1.90 ± 6.42). Maxillary canines were the maximum affected in the maxillary arch and are comparable to mandibular molars.

As regards tooth surfaces the mesial was more susceptible than distal, then buccal and followed by lingual.

The RCI rates in mandibular molars were 16 times more than mandibular incisors, comparing the surfaces at risk of both the teeth. These findings should encourage further research to evaluate the controlling factors, which determine the preferential oral attack.

EPIDEMIOLOGY OF MALOCCLUSION

Malocclusion, being not a disease but a deviation from normal; the epidemiological studies for it cannot be assessed as easily as in case of other dental diseases like caries, periodontal diseases, etc.

Earlier, the epidemiological studies were based on the Angle's classification for assessing the malocclusion and treatment needs of a community, but later it was observed that the Angle's classification does not completely define all the individual morphogenetic traits. Now-a-days, most of the studies use different malocclusion indices for the assessment of occlusal status of an individual or community. The present epidemiological studies chose index according to goal of study, feasibility of examiner and accessibility to community. These indices assess different morphological traits and give more reliable results as compared to Angle's classification.

Criteria for Malocclusion Epidemiological Studies

Because of the complexity of malocclusion, the epidemiological studies are based on certain criteria, which are as follows:

I. **Criteria for sample selection**

a. *Sample size:* The size of the sample should always be calculated on the basis of population to be examined and earlier prevalence if reported. 45% of the target population should be included in sample.

b. *Sample age:* The age of the sample should minimally be more than 10 years and preferably more than 12 years to avoid the discrepancies during mixed dentition period.

II. **Criteria for sampling area:** A town, community, district, , village, etc. should be clearly specified in a survey to avoid any misunderstandings.

III. **Criteria for registration method:** The method of registration should be objective, reliable and easily quantifiable.

IV. **Criteria for examiners:** The study should be conducted by professional or trained persons, who can assess the malocclusion traits correctly.

Prevalence of Malocclusion

The prevalence of malocclusion varies greatly among different geographical areas, ethnic groups, races and communities. Some of the trends for the estimated prevalence of malocclusion areas are:

I. Class I Malocclusion or Crowding

a. *Maxillary incisors:* Incisor crowding tends to increase with the eruption of permanent incisors as permanent incisors require more space than their predecessors.

b. *Mandibular incisors:* Lower incisor crowding generally does not correct without interception (serial extractions, etc.) and continues to worsen in adulthood if left untreated.

c. Nearly 15% of adolescents and adults have been found to have severely crowded or rotated incisors requiring extractions for alignment.

d. Bi-maxillary protrusion is more common in Negroes.

II. Class II Malocclusion (Over jet more than 5.0 mm)

a. It is found in 23% of children, 15% of adolescents and 13% of adults.

b. It is more prevalent in whites of Europe.

III. Class III Malocclusion/Reverse Over jet:
These are more prevalent in Asian populations (2%–5%) than in American populations (less than 1%).

IV. The following prevalence of malocclusion is found in the US population:

Normal occlusion	- 30%
Cl I Malocclusion	- 50%
Cl II Malocclusion	- 15%
Cl III Malocclusion	- less than 1%

V. Racial factors:
It has been found that prevalence of malocclusion is more in whites as compared to blacks. It may be due to more refined eating habits of developed nations.

VI. Geographical area:
The presence of malocclusion is more in the urban areas than in rural areas due to more sophisticated eating styles of the rural population.

Epidemiological Studies

Esa-R, Razak (2001) evaluated malocclusion and orthodontic treatment needs in 12–13 years old school children, and also assessed the relationship between malocclusion and socio-demographic factors, perceptions of need of orthodontic treatment, aesthetic perfection and social functioning. They concluded that from 1,519 school children, 62.6% required no orthodontic treatment while 7% had handicapping malocclusion for whom orthodontic treatment was mandatory. The prevalence of malocclusion between different races and different genders was not significantly different.

Data from the third *National Health and Nutrition Examination Survey* (NHANES III) provide a clear picture of malocclusion in the US population which is as follows:

Noticeable incisor irregularity occured in the majority of all racial/ethnic groups, with only 35% of adults having well aligned mandibular incisors. In 15% of the population, severe mandibular incisor irregularity affecting esthetics and function was present, which required a definite arch expansion or extraction of some teeth with progressive orthodontic treatment for correction.

About 20% of the population had deviations from the ideal bite relationship; in 2%, these deviations were severe enough to be disfiguring. In Mexican-Americans, compared to the rest of the population, incisor irregularity and severe Class II and Class III malocclusions were more prevalent, but deep bite and open bite are less prevalent.

Application of the Index of Treatment Needs to the survey data revealed that 57% to 59% of each racial/ethnic group has at least some degree of orthodontic treatment needs.

Over 30% of white youths, 11% of Mexican-Americans, and 8% of blacks had received orthodontic treatment in one form or other. Severe malocclusion was observed more frequently among blacks, which might reflect their lower level of treatment.

Shourie in 1952 examined children of 13–16 years age in Punjab and found that 50% of them suffered from malocclusion.

Sven Helm (1968) examined 1,700 Danish children (742 boys and 958 girls) to determine the prevalence of malocclusion during adolescent dentition. He concluded that frequency of malocclusion was similar in boys and girls.

Kharbanda et al (1995) reported prevalence of malocclusion in Delhi based on survey of 4500 school children in the age group of 5–13 years. The sample size represented three subdivided locations, i.e. urban, peri-urban and rural. The sample data were essentially presented in two major groups: the mixed dentition group which comprised 2817 school children in the age group of 5–9 years and the late mixed/permanent dentition groups, in the age group 10–13 years, which comprised of 2737 children.

Jalili, Sidhu and Kharbanda (1995) surveyed 1085 children of 6–14 years of age living in remote villages of Mandu in Madhya Pradesh. The tribal children exhibited a low prevalence of malocclusion as compared to the urban children. The prevalence of malocclusion was only 14.4%. A majority of these (10.5%) were of mild malocclusion and a smaller number (3.7%) had moderate to severe malocclusion. The 'handicapping malocclusion' was observed in 0.2% only.

Guaba et al (1998) investigated 3164 rural children in Raipur Rani and Naraingarh blocks of district Ambala and found that 29.2% of the rural children had malocclusion. Among them, CI-I molar relation was found in 14.4% children, Cl-II molar relation in 13.5% and CIII in 1.3%. 3% of rural children also had abnormal oral habits, predominantly tongue thrusting and thumb sucking along with malocclusion.

Proffit and Plante published findings of prevalence of malocclusion and orthodontic treatment need in the United States; estimates from the NHANES III survey. About 25%

were found to have definite malocclusion for which 'treatment' was considered to be 'elective'. Treatment was found to be 'highly desirable' in 13% and 'mandatory' for an additional 16%. An estimated 10.2 million young/adults had specific occlusal defects, such as severe incisor overbites or open bites, which required 'evaluation by orthodontists to determine the need for treatment'.

According to Zhang et al, prevalence of malocclusion among Chinese children was 67.82%. A study by Lew et al on 1050 Chinese school children (aged 12–14 years) reported a high incidence of class III malocclusion in Chinese compared with Caucasians. However, the incidence of class II malocclusions was quite similar to those reported in Caucasians. Crowding occurred in about 50% of cases. Japanese are known to have higher prevalence of class III malocclusion compared to other races.

Dinesh (2003) examined 329 handicapped children among age group of 11–30 years, attending special schools in South India using Dental Aesthetic Index. He observed that prevalence of malocclusion was definitely higher in handicapped children with 53% requiring no treatment; 24% had definite malocclusion requiring elective treatment and 12% needed desirable treatment. 11% had handicapping malocclusion requiring mandatory treatment.

Shivkumar (2009) examined 1000 children (518 males and 482 females) among the age group of 12–15 years in Davangere (India). He observed that 80.1% of children had no or minor malocclusion requiring no or slight treatment while 19.9% had definite handicapping malocclusion requiring definite or mandatory treatment.

EPIDEMIOLOGY OF ORAL CANCER

Oral cancer is any cancerous tissue growth located in the oral cavity. It may arise as a primary lesion originating in any one of the oral tissues; by metastasis from a distant site of origin; or by extension from a neighbouring anatomic structure, such as the nasal cavity, maxillary sinus, etc. Oral cancers may originate in any of the tissues of the mouth, and may be of varied histologic types - teratoma, adenocarcinomica, lymphoma or melanoma. There are several types of oral cancers, but around 90% are squamous cell carcinomas, originating in the tissues that line the mouth and lips. Oral or mouth cancer most commonly involves the tissue of the lips or the tongue. It may also occur on the floor of the mouth, cheek lining, gingiva or palate. Most of oral cancers look very similar under the microscope and are called as squamous cell carcinomas. These are malignant and tend to spread rapidly.

Factors Affecting the Prevalence of Oral Cancer

1. **Betel quid:** The placement of betel quid on the oral mucous membrane, definitely increases the prevalence of oropharyngeal malignancies.
2. **Tobacco:** Use of tobacco in any form; smoking, chewing, sucking leads to increased incidence of malignancies.
3. **Alcohol:** The concurrent intake of alcohol increases the incidence of malignancies.
4. **Chronic irritation:** Chronic irritation due to an intrinsic cause (sharp tooth, ill fitting denture) or an extrinsic cause (U.V. rays, occupational hazards) has been associated with the increased incidence of oral malignancies.
5. **Others:** Poor oral hygiene, nutritional deficiencies may affect the incidence of oral malignancies.
6. **Age:** The average age of occurrence of malignancies is above 45; however, even younger patients may suffer from oral cancer.
7. **Sex:** Oral cancers are more common in males as compared to females.

8. **Race:** The role of genes in oral malignancies have been proved. Blacks have higher incidence of cancer with the exception of Basal cell carcinoma which most frequently occurs in whites as they are more sensitive to UV rays.

Epidemiological Studies

The epidemiological data on oral cancer can be obtained from two sources; the malignancies reported in the hospitals for treatment and the mortalities registered due to the malignancies. It has been found that cancers of oral cavity and pharynx accounted for 3% of all malignancies in US. The National Cancer Institute of US recorded the incidence of 10.4 per one lakh population and mortality rate of 2.9 per one lakh population in US people. The annual incidence of 15.7 per lakh in males and 6 per lakh in females has been reported. The incidence, prevalence and mortality is more in black males as compared to white ones. The maximum mortality rate was reported in persons above 60 years of age; however the mean age of the registered cases was 45.

In USA, about 34,000 individuals were diagnosed with oral cancer in 2008. Low public awareness of the disease is a significant factor, but these cancers could be diagnosed at early survivable stages through a simple, painless, five minute examination by a trained professional.

The average incidence of oral cancer in UK is 2 per one lakh population and 1.6 per one lakh population in Japan.

Despite the fact that there are limitations in the reporting of malignancies in a developing country like India, the incidence of oral cancer is the highest in the world and is preceded mostly by premalignant lesions. The most important of *all premalignant lesions is* oral submucous fibrosis. It is characteristically found in people of South-East Asian origin and is associated with the chewing of betel nut. Its prevalence has increased manifold in the past three decades due to increased consumption of paan masala and gutka by persons of all age groups, including children. The condition has a high malignant potential; 7.5% of the lesions become malignant over a 10 year period and more than one lesion may develop at different sites in the oral cavity.

R. Sankaranayan (1990) reviewed the epidemiological and clinical aspects of oral cancer in India and concluded that the disease ranked number one among all the cancers in male patients and number three among the female patients. Most of the patients used betel quid or tobacco. The malignancy was preceded by one or another kind of precancerous lesions; with oral submucous fibrosis being most common. They reported the prevalence ratio of 2:1 for males and females. Among the lesions only 10–15% were present at a localized site and 85–90% were having generalised spread in whole body.

National Cancer Registers in Mumbai and Chennai recorded the average incidence rate of 2165 per one lakh population (29 for males and 143 for females). The reported incidence rate is much higher in Indian population as compared to the rest of the world with double incidence in males as compared to females.

BIBLIOGRAPHY

1. Abdul Arif Khan, Sdhir K. J. and Archana, S.: Prevalence of dental caries and among the dental population of Gwalior in relation of different associated factors. Euro. J. Dent. : 2, 81, 2008.

2. Anil S, Hari S, Vijayakumar T. Periodontal conditions of a selected population in Trivandrum District, Kerala, India. Community Dentistry and Oral Epidemiology 18, 325, 1990.

3. Bagramian, R.A., Garcia-Godoy, F. and Volpe, A.R. : The global increase in dental caries. Am. J. Dent. : 22, 3, 2009.

4. Binod Kumar Patro and Ravi Kumar, B. : Prevalence of dental caries among adults and elderly in an urban resettlement colony of New Delhi. Indian J. Dent. Res.: 19, 95, 2008.

5. Brathall, D., Hansel, P.G. and Sundberg, H.: Reasons for the caries decline : What do the experts believe ? Eur. J. Oral Sci.: 104, 416, 1996.

6. Brathall, D. : Estimation of global DMFT for 12-year olds in 2004. Int. Dent. J. : 55, 14, 2004.

7. Carino, K.M., Shinada, K. and Kawaguchi, Y. : Early childhood caries in northern Philippines. Comm. Dent. Oral Epid. : 31, 81, 2003.

8. Dash, J.KI., Sahoo, P.K. and Bhuyan, S.K. : Prevalence of dental caries and treatment needs among children of Cuttack (Orissa). J. Indian Soc. Pedo. Prev. Dent. : 20, 139, 2000.

9. David, J. and Wang : Dental caries and associated factors in 12 years old school children in Thiruvananthapuram, Kerala, India. Int. J. Pediat. Dent. : 15, 420, 2005.

10. Dhar V, Jain A, Van Dyke TE, Kohli A. Prevalence of gingival diseases, malocclusion and fluorosis in school-going children of rural areas in Udaipur district. J Indian Soc. Pedod. Prevent. Dent. 25, 103, 2007

11. Dinesh, R.B. and Arnitho, H.M. : Malocclusion and orthodontic treatment need of handicapped individuals in South Canara; India. Int. Dent. J. : 53, 18, 2003.

12. Dixit J : Pregnancy Gingivitis and multiparity. J Ind. Dent Assoc.: *52, 303, 1980*

13. Downer, M. : Caries prevalence in the United Kingdom. Int. Dent. J.: 44, 365, 1994.

14. Du, M., Luo, Y., Zeng, X., Alkhatib, N. and Bedi, R. : Caries in preschool children and its risk factor in 2 provinces in China. Quint. Int. : 38, 143, 2007.

15. *Dutta, A.:* A study in the prevalence of periodontal disease and dental caries amongst school going children in Calcutta. J Ind. Dent Assoc: 37, 367, 1965.

16. Esa, R. and Razak, I.A : Epidermiology of malocclusion and orthodontic treatment need of 12-13 year old Malaysian school children. Comm. Dent. Health : 18, 31, 2001.

17. Goyal, A., Gauba, K. and Chawla, H.S. : Epidemiology of dental caries in Chandigarh school children and trends over the last 25 years. J. Indian Soc. Pedod. Prevent. Dent. : 115, 2007.

18. Grover. P. and Evans, R.W. : Dental Survey of children in Haryana, India. Google website.

19. Guaba, K. and Ashima, G. : Prevalence of malocclusion and abnormal oral habits in North

Indian rural children. J. Indian Soc. Of Pedodontics and Preventive Dentistry : 16, 26, 1998.

20. Haugejorden, O. and Magne Birkeland, J. : Ecological time trend analysis of caries experience in 12-18 year old children in Norway from 1985 to 2004. Acta Odontol Scand. : 64, 368, 2006.

21. Jacob, P.P. and Mathew, C.T. : Occlusal pattern study of school children (12-15 years) of Tiruvananthapura city. J. Indian Dent. Assoc.: 41, 271, 1969.

22. Jagadeesan M, Roti SB, Danabalan M.: Oral health status and risk factors for dental & periodontal diseases among rural women in Pondicherry. Indian Journal of Community Medicine 25, 31, 2000.

23. John C. Greene.: Periodontal Disease in India: Report of an Epidemiological Study. J Dent Res. 39, 302, 1960.

24. Johnson, M. and Harkness, M. : Prevalence of malocclusion and orthodontic treatment need in 10 year old New Zealand children. Aust. Orthodont. J. : 16, 1, 2000.

25. Kharbanda, O.P., Sidhu, S.S., Sundaram, K.R. and Shukla, D.K. : Prevalence of malocclusion and its traits in Delhi children. J. Indian Orthod. Soc. : 26, 98, 1995.

26. Lew, K.K., Foong, W.C. and Loh, E. : Malocclusion prevalence in an ethnic Chinese population. Aust. Dent. J. : 38, 442, 1993.

27. Lussi, A. and Francescut, P. : Performance of conventional and new methods for the detection of occlusal caries in deciduous teeth. Caries Res.: 37, 2, 2003.

28. Maity AK, Banerjee K, Pal TK.: Low levels of destructive periodontal disease in a rural population in West Bengal, India. Community Dentistry and Oral Epidemiology: 22, 60, 1994.

29. Marshall-Day CD, Stephens RG, Quigley L.F Jr. : Periodontal disease: prevalence and incidence. J Periodontol: 26, 185, 1955.

30. Marthaler, T., Menghini, G. and Steiner, M. : Use of the Significant Caries Index in quantifying the changes in caries in Switzerland from 1964 to 2000. Community Dent. Oral Epidemiol. : 33, 159, 2005.

31. Marthaler, T.M. : Changes in dental caries 1953-2003. Caries Res. : 38, 173, 2004.

32. Marthaler, T.M., Steiner, M., Menghini, G.D. and Bandi, A. : Caries prevalence in Switzerland. Int. Dent. J: 44, 393, 1994.

33. Pandit K., Kannan, A.T., Sarna, A. and Aggarwal, K.: Periodontal disease and dental caries in primary school children in rural areas of Delhi. Indian Journal of Pediatrics: 53, 525, 1986.

34. Pandit, K., Kannan, A.T., Sarna, A. and Aggarwal, K. : Prevalence of dental caries and associated teeth cleaning habits among children in four primary schools of Mehrauli block of rural Delhi. Int. J. Epidem.: 15, 581, 1986.

35. Pitts, N.B., Evans, D.J. and Nugent, Z.J. : The dental caries experience of 14-year-old children in the United Kingdom. Surveys coordinated by the British Association for the Study of Community Dentistry in 1998/99. Comm. Dent. Health: 17, 48, 2000.

36. Pitts, N.B., Evans, D.J., Nugent, Z.J. and Pine, C.M. : The dental caries experience of 12-year-old children in England and Whales. Surveys coordinated by the British Association for the Study of Community Dentistry in 2000/2001. Comm. Dent. Health: 19, 46, 2002.

37. Proffit, W.R., Fields, H,W. Jr. and Moray, L.J. : Prevalence of malocclusion and orthodontic treatment need in the United States : estimates from the NHANES III survey. Int. J. Adult Orthognath. Surg.: 13, 97-106, 1998.

38. Rao, S.P. and Bharambe, M.S. : Dental caries and periodontal disease among urban, rural and tribal school children. Department of Community Medicine, M.G. Institute of Medical Sciences, Sewagram. Indian Paediatrics. : 30, 759, 1993.

39. Saravanan, S. and Madivanan, I. : Prevalence pattern of dental caries in the primary dentition among school children. I. J. Dent. Res. : 16, 140, 2005.

40. Shankranarayan, R. : Oral cancer in India. An epidemiology and clinical review. Elsevier J. O. Surg., O. Med., O. Path. : 69, 325, 1990.

41. Shenoy, R., Sequeira, P.S. and Rao, A. : Denta caries experience of pre-school children in Manglore, India. J. Nepal Dent. Assoc. : 10, 25, 2009.

42. Shiv Kumar, V.M. and Chandu, G.N. : Prevalence of malocclusion and orthodontic treatment needs among middle and high school children of Davangere city; India by using Dental Aesthetic Index. J. of Indian Society of

Pedodontics and Preventive Dentistry : 27, 211, 2009.

43. Sikri, V. and Sikri, P. : Prevalence of root surface caries and intraoral distribution in older adults. J.I.D.A. : 64, 193, 1993.

44. Singh, A., Singh, B., Kharbanda, O.P., Shukla, D.K, Goswami, K. and Gupta, S. : Malocclusion and its traits in rural school children from Haryana. J. Indian Orthod. Soc.: 31, 76, 1998.

45. Singh GPI, Bindra J, Soni RK, Sood M. : Prevalence of Periodontal Diseases in Urban and Rural areas of Ludhiana, Punjab. Indian Journal of Community Medicine. 30, 128, 2005.

46. Sunayana, G., John, J., Sarvanam, S. and Meignana, A.I. : Prevalence of dental caries among 12 and 15 years old school children in Chennai city. J.I.A. Public Health Dentistry: 13, 54, 2009.

47. Sven Helm : Malocclusion in Danish children with adolescent dentition : An epidermiological study. Am. J. Orthodontics : 54, 352, 1968.

48. Vallejos-Sanchez, A.A., Edina-Solis, C.E., Casanova-Rosado, J.F., Maupome, G., Minaya-Sanchez, M. and Perez-Olivares, S. : Caries increment in the permanent dentition of Mexican children in relation to prior caries experience on permanent and primary dentitions. J. Den. : 34, 709, 2006.

49. Von der Fehr, F.R. and Haugejorden, O. : The start of caries decline and related fluoride use in Norway. Eur. J. Oral Sci. : 105, 21, 1997.

50. Vyas HA, Damle SG.: Comparative study of oral health status of mentally sub-normal, physically handicapped, juvenile delinquents and normal children of Bombay. J Indian Soc. Pedod. Prev. Dent. 9, 13, 1991.

14 Prevention of Oral Diseases: General Considerations

Man's fight with 'disease' is a continuous process. Since time immemorial, researchers remained active finding causes and cure of various diseases inflicting human beings. It took very long for the dental ailments to be recognized, since superstitions and ignorance have been engulfing the early population. The need to prevent a disease process or at least to slow down its effect on living tissues has always been a challenge for the medical professional. Preventive dentistry is that branch of dental practice, *which deals with establishment and maintenance of oral environment conducive for the preservation of sound and healthy stomatognathic system*. The rationale is to promote optimal health of the oral tissues and to prevent the future damages also.

Until recently, the preventive measures were based on the old theories of etiology of oral and dental disease; however, the knowledge of mechanism of inception and progress of oral/dental diseases has increased manifolds now.

It is essential that every effort should be made to translate our present knowledge of etiological factors in oral diseases to preventive dentistry. This knowledge should then be transmitted to practicing dentists so as to enable them to refresh themselves regarding preventive aspects which can be involved in oral diseases.

There are significant differences between the developed and the developing countries as regard the resources and development of professional oral care services are concerned. These differences may affect the choice of priorities in health care and their practical implementation.

Preventive regimens are broadly divided into four components Table 14.1.

- *Primordial prevention* is the prevention of risk factors, beginning with change in social and environmental conditions in which these factors are observed to develop and continue for high risk children, adolescent and young adults.

- *Primary prevention* refers to those procedures applied prior to the inception of a disease. This is also known as *pre-pathogenic prevention*, which is accomplished by avoidance of the factors responsible for inception of the disease.

- *Secondary prevention* is to diagnose and manage the disease in its early stages so that the subsequent damages are minimized. It is also called *pathogenic prevention*.

- *Tertiary prevention* refers to utilizing restorative procedures to prevent any further damage from the disease. It is also designated as *post-pathogenic prevention*.

Guidelines for Preventive Dentistry at Community Level

Since oral health is an integral part of overall well-being of any individual, its care should be a part of comprehensive preventive regimens carried out at community level. The following principles should apply:

- Basic oral health care information should be provided to each and every individual, if otherwise not possible.

- The oral hygiene is an essential part of the general body hygiene is to be emphasized.

Table 14.1: Components of preventive regimens

Primordial prevention (preventing risk factors)	Primary prevention (pre-pathogenic)	Secondary prevention (pathogenic)	Tertiary prevention (post-pathogenic)

1. Changing lifestyles	1. Fluoride therapy
	  a. Systemic
	  b. Topical
		1. Restorative dentistry	1. Fixed prosthesis

2. Policy to curb smoking	2. Diet control	2. Periodontics	2. Removable prosthesis
3. Program to promote physical activities	3. Plaque control	3. Endodontics	3. Implants
4. Modify food habits	4. Sealants	4. Orthodontics	
	5. Preventive Orthodontics	5. Oral surgery	
	6. Pulp protection	6. Tissue biopsy	
	7. Tissue protection		
	8. Mouth guards, etc.		

- Fluoride containing tooth pastes (wherever required) and an adequate non-cariogenic diet should be recommended.
- When resources are limited, the least costly and appropriate approach should be chosen.
- Even in the same community with same resources, less than ideal approach for some individuals can be accepted.
- Propose a program, which is compatible with existing activities in that particular community.

Community preventive services are:
- Organized to ensure that care is equitably distributed and accessible to as much of the population as possible.
- Aimed at improving the overall oral health of the population rather than providing specified care for the individuals.
- Organized to use appropriate material and personnel resources to maximum advantage.
- Oriented towards health promotion, health awareness, self-care and self-reliance.

Community Oral Health Care (A Model)

It may be difficult to include every possible aspect of oral care in a community program. However, it is possible to set priorities for the introduction of different types of oral care. These criteria can guide the progress of oral care service in a particular community. The community oral health care model has emergency and plus four care levels for organized preventive regimes (Fig. 14.1).

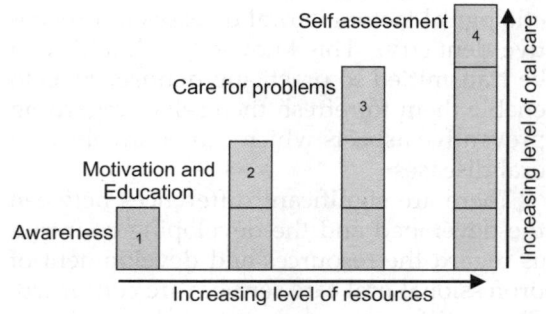

Fig. 14.1: A model for developing Oral Health Care in Communities

Emergency Care

All communities need an emergency service. However, emergency set-ups are rarely provided separately for oral diseases. In principle, general medical emergency care facilities will also provide oral emergency care.

Oral emergencies include gum shot injury traumatic teeth and bones, bleeding from extraction wounds or any other wound or even acute pulpits, etc.

Organized Preventive Care

The organized preventive regime is divided into four levels, which are as follows:

Care Level 1: Aims at increasing awareness of oral health, educating and motivating the public to adopt preventive measures and also to assess themselves.

Care Leve 2: Includes informing the community of available preventive aids and their clinical use.

Care Level 3: Cares for moderate problems, which include initial restorative procedures, physical removal of etiologic factors and also encouraging the individuals to visit dentists regularly.

Care Level 4: Deals with care of oral and other related complex problems along with tertiary preventive regimes.

Care level 1: Awareness, Education, Motivation and Self assessment

The individuals at community level should be provided information towards a better understanding of the role of healthy oral tissues in retaining a functional dentition for life. The information should emphasize upon the advantage of a clean and healthy mouth. The awareness is required not only for public but also for the health professionals. The awareness messages should be clear and non-conflicting. The medium used should cover majority of the population. For example, radio, television, posters, etc. in public places.

The program includes specific aims, goals and strategies. Evaluation of health and hygiene promoting campaigns are carefully coordinated. Different agencies and institutions can be involved in the implementation of such programs, e.g. government agencies, non-government organizations and educational institutions.

Promotion of self-assessment and self-care should be a part of general awareness campaigns. Self-care begins with regular self-assessment, i.e. evaluation of the condition of oral tissues by an individual to enable him to make a judgement on the need of extra self-care or professional assistance. Bleeding gums as a result of tooth brushing or other physical stimulus and black spots over the teeth are the common signs which indicate impending periodontal problems and caries. Any abnormal discolouration of the mucous membrane of cheeks, tongue, etc. should be consulted with professionals.

Care Level 2: Introduction of preventive aids and their clinical use

The community is informed about the available preventive aids in the market and their clinical use. The groups of people are motivated and educated to know the availability of home care devices which can help prevent the oral diseases. The most common preventive aid is tooth brush and other inter-dental cleaning devices. Protective guards for children during their playtimes should also be made known to parents.

The second step in care level 2 is *self-care*. This includes knowledge regarding preventive measures for caries and periodontal diseases which can be carried out at home.

Care Level 3: Monitoring, Screening and Initial Treatments

A system to monitor trends in health and disease is essential in planning any health service.

The primary aim of screening is to identify individuals within the community who may require further investigations and/or professional assistance. The community at large cannot be screened because of the resources and organization available to provide care for the identified disease. Specific population groups are targeted, which differ according to circumstances and needs.

Screening increases awareness and reinforces, self-assessment and self-care programs. It is an efficient way of categorizing individuals according to basic treatment needs.

Care Level 4: Care for complex problems

The practical difficulties in the professional management of complex problems are important to be analyzed. Furthermore, an extensive range of sophisticated treatment modalities fall into the category of complex oral care. Oral care personnel will need a scientific background and appropriate training to function at this level.

In situations where there are insufficient resources, complex treatment should be given a low priority in community services. Where there are reasonable resources and care level 1, 2 and 3 have already been instituted, complex treatment can be introduced but still be restricted to smaller and needy groups. Treatment of complex diseases in the elderly population should be considered only when preventive oral care of younger age groups has been established.

Motivation

Motivation is an art of stimulating people to take the course of action usually desired by others. If the goal is desired by the person himself, that is known as self-motivation. Motivation is derived from the word 'motive'. Motive means an idea, need, emotion or organic state that prompts a man to act. It is defined as *The process of attempting to influence others to do your will through the possibility of gain or reward.*

Self-motivation can be – *All those forces operating within the individual which impels him to act or not to act in certain ways.*

From the motivation cycle (Fig. 14.2), it is evident that a motive or need compels the person to obtain certain goals and when the person achieves them, he feels satisfied.

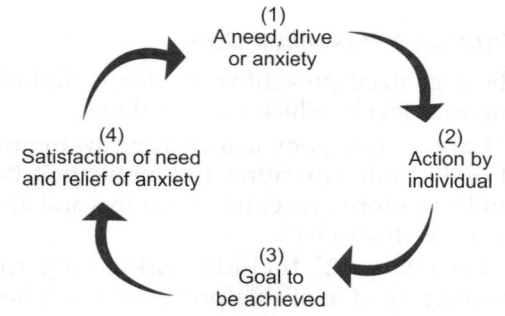

Fig. 14.2: Motivation cycle

The factors, which may influence motivation are:
• An individual's experience of life.
• Literacy level
• Family circumstances
• Culture and environment during growth
• Social standards
• Financial constraints
• Whether ambitions or not
• Emotional quotient
• Psychological complexes in personality

Education

It is a joint effort of the dentist as well as the patient for achieving success in any preventive regime. Visiting a dental office for dental and oral care will not eliminate the disease completely unless the patient is educated regarding the preventive and therapeutic procedures. There are many sources of information for educating the patient. Though dentist is an important source of information, but other sources also play an important role. These sources are:

- *Mass media:* television, radio and magazines, etc.
- Family and friends
- *Other authorities:* physician, school teachers, nurses, etc.
- Computers
- Pamphlets

Most of the patients are aware of dental, periodontal and oral lesions because they hear through media, magazines and advertisements. Lectures are delivered to small groups in a community on dental and oral health. More attention should be focused upon informing and convincing the opinion makers in the community. Physicians, nurses and other health professionals are powerful opinion makers in the community. School teachers should be informed and motivated for effective oral care means which would have long lasting impact on the students.

Patients should be informed about the importance of periodic checkups. Since most of the dental and oral lesions are painless in their initial stages and the patient is unaware of the disease in the oral cavity, it is the dentist who can guide the patient for proper treatment at an early stage.

BIBLIOGRAPHY

1. Ainamo, J. and Holmberg, S.M. : The oral health of children of dentists. Scand. J. Dent. Res. : 82, 547, 1974.
2. American Association of Dental Schools : Curriculum guidelines for predoctrol preventive dentistry. J. Dent. Educ. : 55, 746, 1991.
3. Bernick, S.M., Cohen, D.W., Baker, L. and Laser, L. : Dental disease in children with diabetes mellitus. J. Period. : 46, 241, 1975.
4. Bloom, M. : Towards a code of ethics for primary prevention. J. Primary Prev. : 13, 173, 1993.
5. Bergman, J.D., Wright, F.A. and Hammond, R.H.: The oral health of the elderly in Melbourne. Aust. Dent. J. : 36, 280, 1991.
6. Dawson, A.S. and Makinson. O.F. : Dental treatment and dental health. Review of studies in support of a philosophy of minimum intervention dentistry. Aust. Dent. J. : 37, 126, 1992.
7. Emalie, R.D. : A dental health survey in the republic of Sudan. Br. Dent. J. : 120, 167, 1966.
8. FDI working group : Nutrition, diet and oral health. Int. Dent. J. : 44, 599, 1994.
9. Goodson, J.M. : Pharmacokinetic principles controlling the efficacy of oral therapy. J. Dent. Res.: 68, 1025, 1989.
10. Horowitz, A.M. : The public's oral health : the gaps between what we know and what we practice. Adv. Dent. Res. : 9, 91, 1995.
11. Hyatt : Prophylactic odontotomy : The ideal procedure in dentistry for children. Dent. Cosmos. : 78, 353, 1936.
12. Wilson, T. : Compliance – a review of the literature with possible application to periodontics. J. Period. : 58, 706, 1987.

Prevention of Periodontal Diseases

It has been established that the periodontal disorders affect nearly the entire dentate population worldwide. The major dental public health problems are caries and periodontal diseases as documented by various prevalence studies. The etiological factors for these two diseases are many and varied, but one common agent, the aggregate of bacteria—the plaque, affects both. There exists a definite association between bacterial colonization on the tooth surface and inflammation of the gingiva.

Motivation of Patients with Periodontal Disease

For long term success of periodontal treatment, motivation plays a key role. Make the patient understand the pathogenesis, treatment and prevention of periodontal diseases. Patient should adopt a successful, self administered daily plaque control regimen and follow oral hygiene habits.

The patient must be aware of periodontal disease and its effect on the general health. Whether or not the patient is susceptible to this disease should also be analyzed. The patient must be aware of plaque control measures and adopt a manual technique for successful plaque control.

Patient should be shown areas of gingivitis and stained plaque after disclosing the same in their oral cavity. Additional plaque control measures must be advocated in those areas where they have missed cleaning. Mostly, the patient can self evaluate prevailing conditions. The dentist can also compare the previous records with the recent ones.

Oral Hygiene Instructions

The primary aim of oral hygiene is to control gingival bleeding by reducing the level of bacterial plaque. Periodontitis may also be reduced in prevalence and severity utilizing oral hygiene measures.

Oral hygiene advice and instruction should preferably be aimed at periodontal awareness including the effects on general health. The program should emphasize that oral care is a part of normal body hygiene procedures and should be included in one's daily routine. Written or visual instructions should convey two messages.

  i. Teeth should be cleaned regularly and effectively, at least once a day.
 ii. Effective cleaning is more important than frequency; thorough cleaning once a day is preferred rather partial cleaning many times a day.

The toothbrush is the most routinely used oral hygiene aid. However, improved cleanliness can also be achieved with traditional chew sticks. The sticks should be encouraged in the population where there is religious, cultural or economic relevance. Inter-dental aids should also be popularized amongst community groups. The use of anti-plaque and anti-gingivitis tooth pastes can be recommended.

Repeated instructions and encouragement must be given to the patient for effective self acquired oral hygiene. Instructions can be given in the dental office, community and schools. Videos and pamphlets can be used to augment personalized instructions. Sometimes the patient may have to be demonstrated repeatedly for the correction of mistakes.

Initially, individuals are instructed how to use tooth brushes and other inter-dental aids; further, control of diet and other chemical preventive regimens can be explained.

Subsequent instructions should be given to reinforce or modify previous instructions. The patients who have adopted favourable habits should be encouraged.

The relationship between plaque and the threshold of disease is dependent on the specific bacterial composition of the plaque and the resistance of the host. However, there is no clear relationship between the amount of plaque and the extent of the disease. Though site-to-site and patient-to-patient variables exist as far as plaque accumulation is concerned, its removal and control definitely prevent periodontal disease.

Periodontal disease has also been associated with smoking. Various authors have observed alveolar bone loss associated with cigarette smoking and other tobacco products. Smokers tend to have more extensive plaque, calculus, bleeding on probing, deep periodontal pockets and tooth mobility. Cigarette contains toxic materials that may influence plaque retention through a number of local and systemic mechanisms. Local effects on the periodontium are gingival mucosal irritation, altered salivary flow and microbial growth. Systemically, nicotine and other toxins absorbed into the blood stream suppress immunologic activity and increased epinephrine levels subsequently induce vasoconstriction. Gingivitis has been considered to be an early form of periodontitis. The progression from gingivitis to periodontitis is relatively common and it is recognized that a useful and logical approach to prevention of periodontitis is to control gingivitis through effective plaque removal and control.

Since microbial plaque is responsible for gingival inflammation and is one of the important etiological factors producing periodontal disease, the aim of any preventive regimen should be to control the accumulation of plaque. It has been established that the removal of microbial plaque leads to resolution of gingival inflammation; subsequently, periodontal diseases can be prevented. Every individual should be encouraged to adopt a plaque control program.

Plaque control will lead to:
- Preservation of a healthy periodontium
- Optimal healing following the treatment of periodontal disease
- Prevention of recurrence of the periodontal disease

The most dependable mode of plaque control is mechanical cleaning with a tooth brush and other oral hygiene aids. Chemical inhibitors are used as adjuncts to mechanical measures. In every periodontal treatment plan, the patients should be introduced with oral hygiene measures. The patient is taught how to clean all the surfaces of teeth. For the routine patient, a short headed brush with straight-cut, round-ended, soft to medium nylon bristles arranged in three or four rows of tufts is recommended. Dental floss should be used on smooth proximal surfaces only. Flossing around sharp edges and coarse surfaces causes the floss to shred and break, leading to ineffective plaque removal.

Various brushing techniques have been introduced for effective plaque control. The most common method of brushing is the scrub technique whereas for patients with periodontal disease, the sulcular technique is most frequently recommended. However, no one method can be considered as superior and most effective.

TOOTH BRUSHING METHODS

Various tooth brushing techniques introduced for the hygienic care of the oral cavity are given below. The types of brushes are exhibited in Fig. 15.1.

Leonard's Method

Leonard described a tooth brushing method in which maxillary and mandibular teeth are

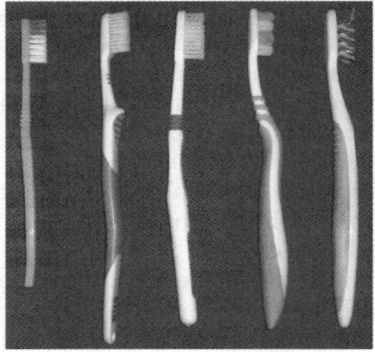

Fig. 15.1: Type of tooth brushes
(straight and angled shanks)

brushed separately using vertical strokes. The upper and lower teeth are placed edge to edge so that the brush does not slip incisally or occlusally (Figs 15.2a and b). The filaments of the brush are then placed at an angle of 90° to the long axis of the teeth. It was suggested that mostly up and down strokes should be used, with just a slight rotation of the brush head after striking the gingival margin with force. The pressure should be sufficient to force the filaments of the brush into embrasure areas.

This method of tooth brushing may encourage gingival trauma and abrasion of tooth substance. In addition, it is sometimes insufficient for plaque control in inter-dental areas.

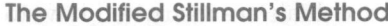

The Modified Stillman's Method

The tooth brush is placed with bristle ends resting partly on the cervical portion of the teeth and partly on the adjacent gingiva pointing in an apical direction at an oblique angle to the long axis of the teeth. Pressure is applied laterally against the gingival margin so as to produce a perceptible blanching. The brush is activated with 20 short back and forth strokes and is simultaneously moved in a coronal direction along the attached gingiva, the gingival margin and the tooth surface.

The process is repeated on all tooth surfaces. To reach the oral surfaces of maxillary and mandibular incisors, the handle of the brush is held in a vertical position, engaging the 'heel' of the brush. The occlusal surfaces of molars and premolars are cleaned with the bristles perpendicular to the occlusal plane and penetrating deeply into the sulci and grooves (Figs 15.3a and b).

With this technique, the sides rather than the ends of the bristles are used and penetration of the bristles into the gingival sulci is avoided.

The Charter's Method

The tooth brush is placed on the teeth with the bristles pointing towards the crown at a 45 degree angle to the long axis of the teeth.

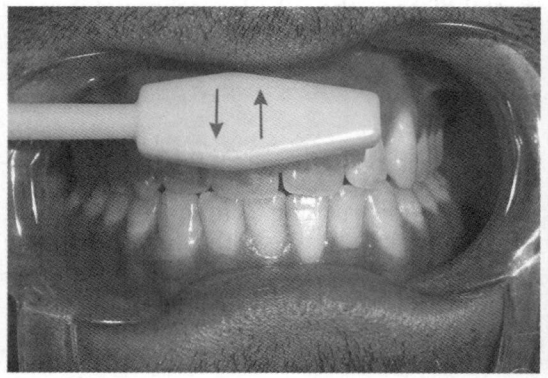

a

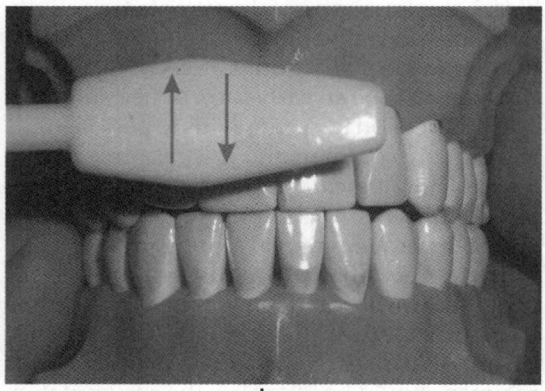

b

Figs 15.2a and b: Leonard's method a. Intra-oral; b. On model

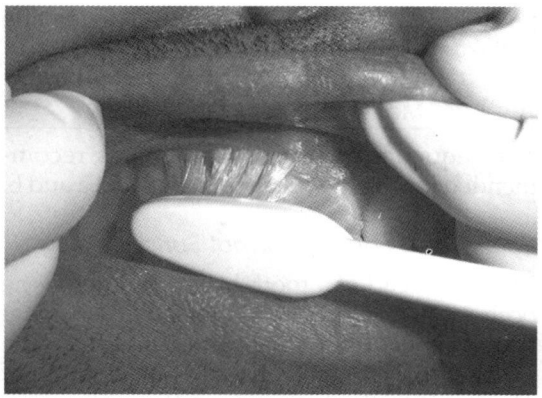

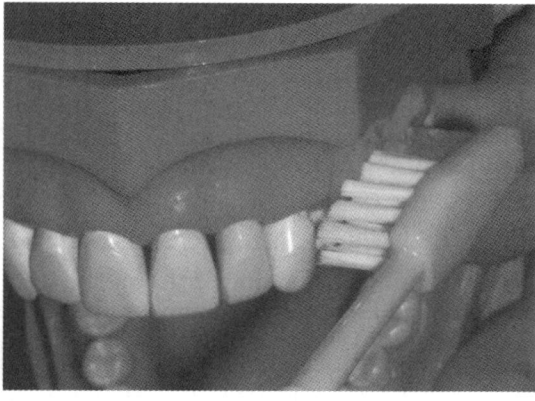

a

b

Figs 15.3a and b: Modified Stillman's method a. Intra-oral; b. On model

The brush is then moved along the tooth surface until the sides of the bristles engage the gingival margin preserving the 45 degree angle. Twist the brush lightly flexing the bristles so that the sides press on the gingival margin, the edges touch the tooth and some bristles extend inter-proximally. Without dislodging the bristles, rotate the head of the brush, maintaining the bent position of the bristles. Move the brush to the adjacent area and repeat the procedures, continuing area by area on the entire facial surface and then move to the lingual. Care should be taken to enter every embrasure (Figs 15.4a and b).

To cleanse the occlusal surfaces, gently force the bristle tips into the pits and fissures and activate the brush with a rotary motion (not sweeping or sliding). Without changing the position of the bristles repeat area by area until all chewing surfaces are cleansed.

The Fone's Method

In this technique, the brush is pressed firmly against the teeth and gingiva; with the handle

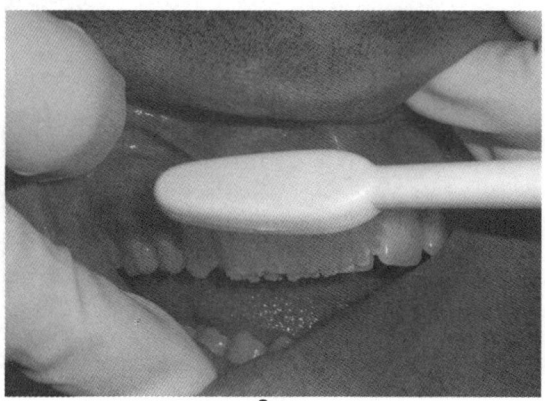

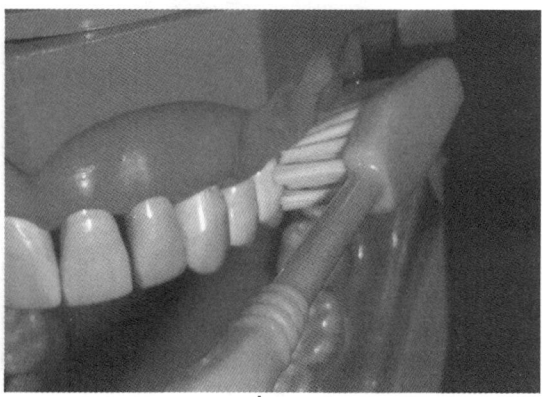

a

b

Figs 15.4a and b: Charter's tooth-brushing technique a. Intra-oral; b. On model

of the brush parallel to the line of occlusion and the bristles perpendicular to the facial tooth surfaces. The brush is then moved in a rotary motion with the jaws closed and the spherical pathway of the brush is confined by the limit of the muco-gingival fold.

The Scrub Method

With this technique of tooth brushing the teeth are scrubbed essentially as one would scrub a floor with a brush. The bristle ends are placed at right angles to the tooth surface. The brush is then moved with back and forth motion antero-posteriorly in the posterior teeth and side to side in the anterior teeth (Figs 15.5a and b).

The Bass Method (Sulcus Cleansing)

The sequence of brush positions as recommended by Bass is exhibited in Figs 15.6a and b.

Facial and Facio-proximal Surfaces

Place the head of a tooth brush parallel to the occlusal plane with the 'tip' of the brush distal to the last molar. Place the bristles at the gingival margin, establish an apical angle of 45 degree to the long axis of the teeth, exert

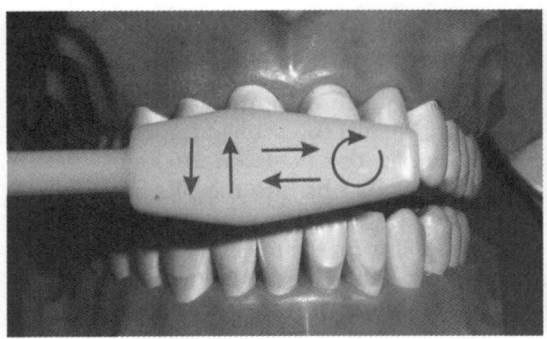

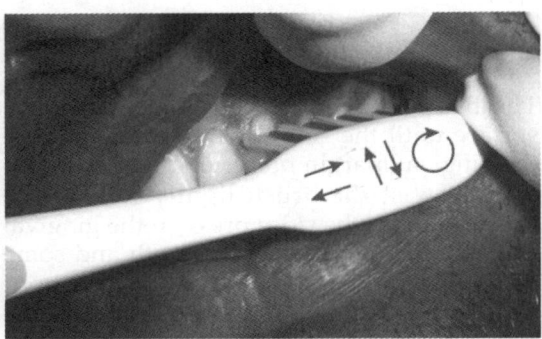

a   b

Figs 15.5a and b: The Scrub method a. Intra-oral; b. On model

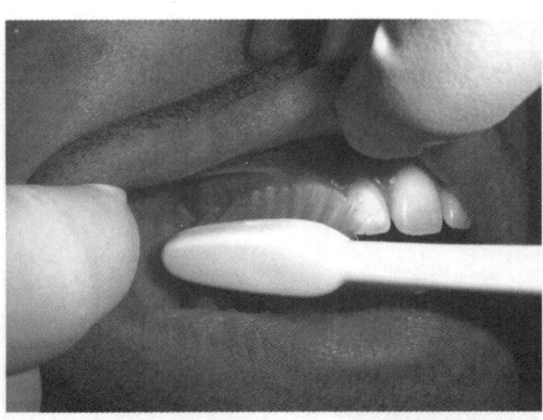

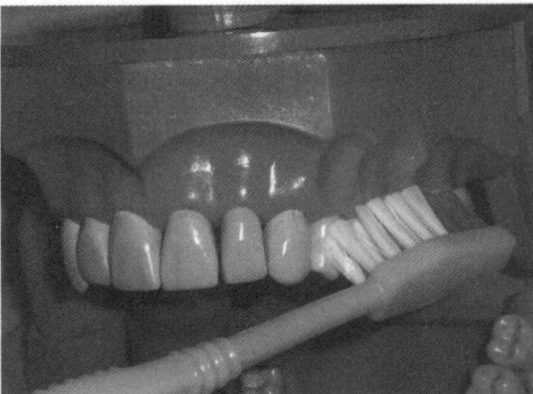

a   b

Figs 15.6a and b: The Bass method a. Intra-oral; b. On model

gentle vibratory pressure along the long axis of the bristles, and force the bristle ends into the facial gingival sulci, as well as into the inter-proximal embrasures. This should produce perceptible blanching of the gingiva. Activate the brush with a short back and forth motion without dislodging the tip of the bristles. Complete 20 such strokes in the same position. Lift the brush, move it anteriorly.

Occlusal Surfaces

Press the bristles firmly on the occlusal surfaces with the ends as deeply as possible into the pits and fissures. Activate the brush with 20 short back and forth strokes, advancing section by section until all posterior teeth in all four quadrants are cleaned.

Palatal and Palate-proximal Surfaces

Engage the brush at a 45 degree apical angle in the molar and premolar areas, covering three teeth at a time. Clean each segment with 20 short back and forth strokes. To reach the palatal surface of the anterior teeth, insert the brush vertically at 45 degree angle to the long axis of the teeth. Activate the brush with 20 short up and down strokes.

Sequences of Positions

The Bass technique requires approximately 40 different tooth brush positions to cover a full dentition. Therefore, the oral cavity should be divided into sections and a systematic cleaning sequence is followed.

Advantages

The Bass method has the following advantages over other techniques:

- The short back and forth motion is easy to master because it requires the same simple movement familiar to most patients; who are used to the scrubbing technique. Except for the 45 degree sulcus position of the bristles and a considerably shorter stroke, there is no difference between the two methods.

- It concentrates the cleaning action on the cervical and inter-proximal portions of the teeth, where microbial plaque accumulates and is injurious to gingiva.

- This technique can be recommended for the routine patient with or without periodontal involvement.

Contraindications for Tooth Brushing

Open lesions are formed during the acute phase of periodontal diseases or diseases of oral mucous membrane. The involvements can be irritated if the bristles are drawn over the lesion. Once the lesion is epithelized, the patient should be encouraged for brushing with a soft tooth brush.

Powered Brushes

The powdered brushes (Figs 15.7a and b) have been established as an alternative to manual method of tooth brushing. Their mode of action resembles that of manual tooth brushes.

Methods of Cleaning

The electrical brushes do not require special techniques as various mechanical motions are in-built in these brushes.

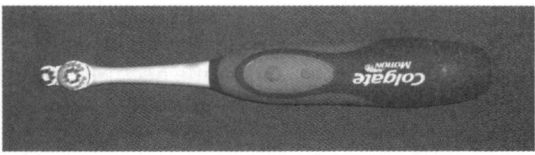 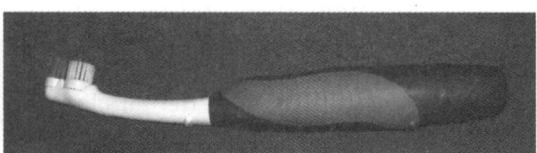

a   b

Figs 15.7a and b: Powered brush

Powered brushes resemble the dental prophylaxis hand piece. Patients must be taught to place the brush head next to the teeth and proceed systematically around the dentition. Additional hand movements can also be used. The three methods used for manual brushing, viz. Bass method, Modified Stillman's method and Charter's method, are also suitable for powered tooth cleaning.

Several researchers have different opinions regarding the efficacy of electric tooth brushes and manual brushes. *Walmsley (1997)* has exhaustively reviewed the effectiveness of electric tooth brushes. The electric brushes are very effective in removing plaque and improving gingival health. They produce less abrasion of the tooth substance and restorative materials than manual brushes, unless the manual brush is used in a vertical rather than a horizontal direction.

Electrical brushes are recommended in the following cases:
• Individuals lacking fine motor skills for any reason.
• Young children or handicapped or hospitalized patients who need someone else to clean their teeth.
• Patients with orthodontic appliance.
• Personal preference.

Inter-dental Cleansing Aids

A variety of inter-dental cleansers are available for removing soft accumulated materials in between the teeth and other inaccessible axial surfaces.

The inter-dental cleansers are effective even to the irregular tooth surfaces, concave root surfaces, furcation areas and large or open inter-dental spaces in normal and periodontally treated dentitions.

The routinely used inter-dental cleansers (Fig. 15.8) are:
• Dental floss
• Dental tape

• Wood sticks
• Inter-dental stimulators
• Inter-dental brushes

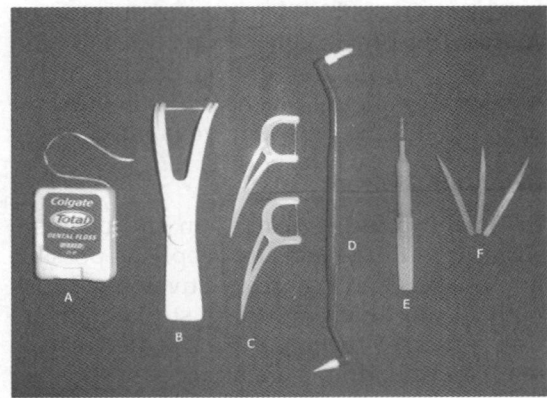

Figs 15.8a to f: Inter dental cleansers
a, b, c. dental floss; d. Rubber tip and unitufted brush; e. Inter-dental brush; f. Wooden tips

Dental Floss

Periodontal diseases originate in the inter-dental areas where routine mechanical plaque removal is difficult. Flossing is recommended as an accepted method of cleaning the proximal surfaces, especially in individuals with tight tooth contacts.

Floss is available as a multifilament nylon yarn or a thin strand of silk thread with or without wax coating, twisted or non twisted, thin or thick and bonded or non-bonded (Figs 15.8a to c). There is no significant difference in the ability of various types of floss in terms of plaque removal. The choice of floss is based upon individual factors like: tightness of the tooth contacts, roughness of the tooth surfaces and the patient's manual dexterity. Earlier it was thought that thin waxy film may be left on proximal surfaces after flossing contributing to plaque accumulation; however, later, waxed dental floss was found to be equally effective.

Dental floss can be used by several methods. It must contact the proximal surface from line angle to line angle for effective cleaning (Fig. 15.9). A piece of floss about one foot long is taken. The ends are tied together in a loop or may be wrapped around the fingers. The floss is stretched tightly between the thumb and the forefingers and passed gently through each contact area with a firm sideward swing motion. The floss should not be pushed downward from the contact areas; otherwise it may injure the inter-dental gingiva.

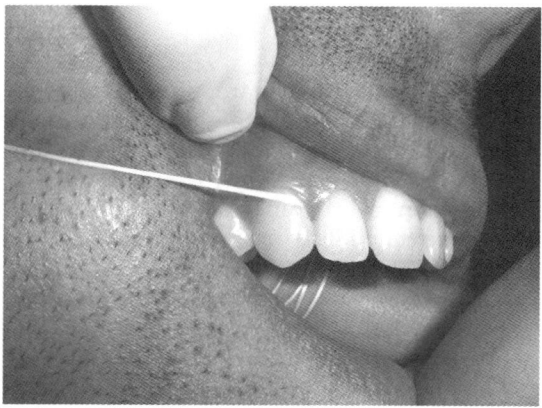

Fig. 15.9: Use of dental floss

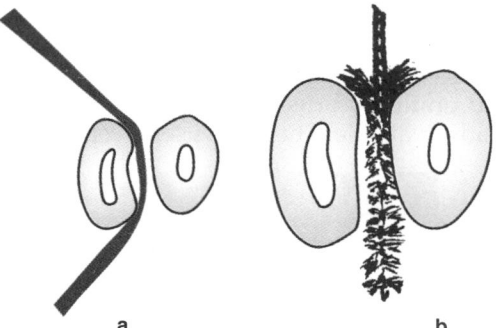

a   b

Figs 15.10a and b: Cleaning of concave surfaces. Dental floss a. is less effective than an; b. inter-dental brush

The floss is wrapped around the proximal surface of one tooth, and slipped to the base

of the gingival sulcus. It is then moved across the inter-dental gingiva and the procedure is repeated on the proximal surface of the adjacent tooth. This method is continued throughout the dentition, including the distal surface of the last tooth in each quadrant. When the working portion of the floss becomes soiled or begins to shred, a fresh portion of the floss is used.

Flossing can be made easier by using a floss holder. Though it is more time consuming, it is helpful for the patients lacking manual dexterity and also for nursing personnel assisting handicapped and hospitalized patients.

Dental Tape

Dental tape is thicker than dental floss and is flattened, like a ribbon. Strands of tape can be used to loosen retained debris over the proximal surfaces and gingival surfaces. Since it is flattened it presents a greater working surface than floss. Tape should be carefully adapted to the curved surfaces of teeth because its edges are narrower and sharper than floss and can hurt the soft tissue.

Wood Sticks

Wood sticks are used as an adjunct to other inter-dental cleansing aids (Fig. 15.11).

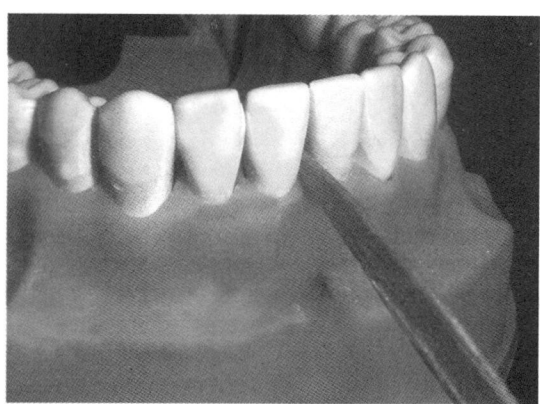

Fig. 15.11: Use of wooden tips

Functions of the wood stick are:
- Cleaning the embrasure areas
- Reshaping the soft tissues to functional form
- Increases keratinization of the inter-dental col

The sticks are not used as tooth picks. They are available with or without a handle. These are triangular in shape and should be placed at an oblique angle to the tooth so that the point passes through the embrasure without touching or hurting the lingual papillae. The sides of the triangular stick are functional parts of the stick, which remove the plaque from the proximal surfaces of the teeth in the depth of the embrasure. The base of the triangle rests on the gingiva.

Wood sticks are usually used on the facial surfaces of anterior teeth. Wood sticks should be discouraged in the presence of sub-gingival calculus, otherwise it will tear the junctional epithelium and may increase existing inflammation.

Inter-dental Stimulators

Inter-dental stimulators are used to massage inter-dental gingiva and to remove debris from exposed proximal surfaces of teeth (Fig. 15.8d). This device is made of rubber, wood or plastic, which is attached to a handle. The stimulator is inserted from the facial or lingual aspect into an open inter-dental embrasure with the tip of the cone pointing slightly towards the occlusal plane. The tip is inserted until the cone fills the space. Light pressure is exerted against the soft tissue and the handle is rotated gently. Sides of the cone bump against the soft tissue for massaging and against the teeth to loosen the debris. There should be sufficient space in the inter-dental embrasure to insert stimulators without injuring the soft tissue. The stimulator should never be "pushed" uncomfortably otherwise it would cause further recession and break down of the epithelial attachment (Figs 15.12a and b).

Inter-dental Brushes

The inter-dental brushes are recommended for proximal cleaning of teeth with large or open inter-dental spaces, concave root surfaces and furcations (Figs 15.8e and 15.13).

Inter-dental brushing has been proved to be very effective. The brush is made up of tufts of bristles, two rows wide and six tufts long, placed apart with tapering ends. Such a small brush readily passes between the teeth when gentle pressure is exerted on the handle.

Place the brush at right angle to the long axis of the teeth. Force the bristles between the teeth. Rotate and vibrate the brush with wrist motion. This will remove the accumulated soft materials in between the teeth and do gingival massage as well.

Recently, cone shaped inter-dental brushes and unitufted brushes (Fig. 15.8d) have been made available. These are useful especially in

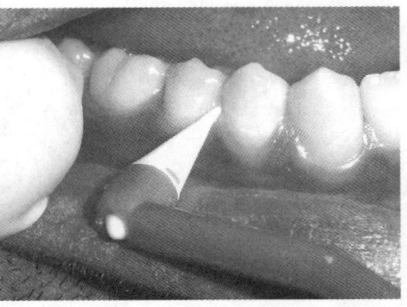

a

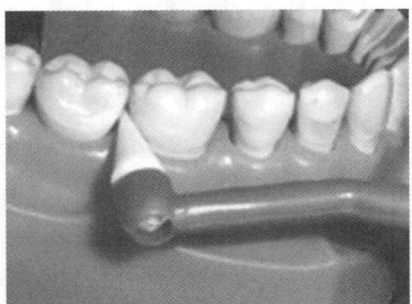

b

Figs 15.12a and b: Use of rubber tips a. Intra-oral; b. On model

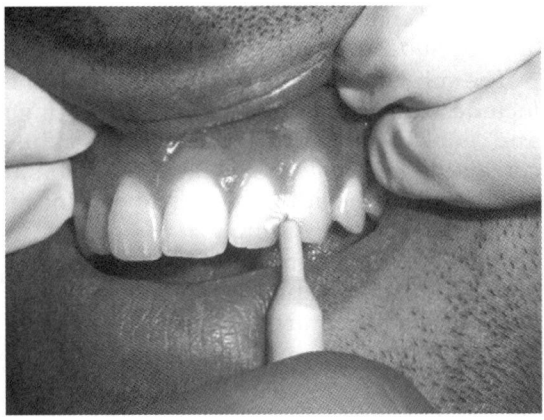
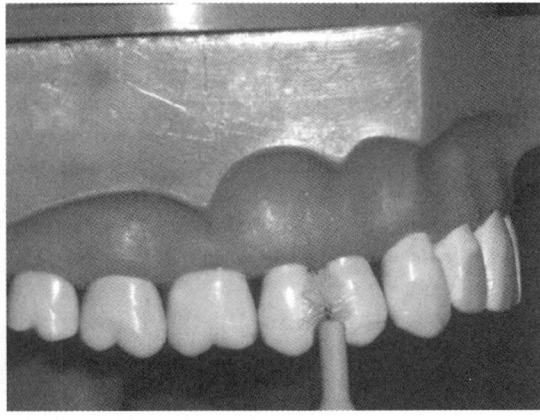

a   b

Figs 15.13a and b: Use of proxa brush a. Intra-oral; b. On model

areas with large gingival embrasures. These are also used to clean crowns and the region distal to the last molars.They are inserted inter-proximally and are activated with short back and forth strokes in between the teeth. For best cleaning efficiency, the diameter of the brush should be slightly larger than the gingival embrasure so that the bristles can exert gentle pressure on the proximal surfaces and concavities of the root. On the lingual surfaces of mandibular premolars and molars, where the tongue often interferes in brushing and for isolated areas of deep recession, unitufted brushes are highly effective.

Oral Irrigation Devices

Oral irrigator is an effective aid for removing non adherent bacteria and debris from the inaccessible areas like periodontal pocket, inter-dental areas, furcations, orthodontic appliances and fixed prosthesis.

It not only increases gingival keratinization but also has beneficial effects on periodontal health by minimizing plaque accumulation. It can deliver high concentration of a drug to the desired site. Various antimicrobial agents viz. normal saline, stannous fluoride, iodine, sanguinarine, essential oils, chlorhexidine and antibiotics have been tested. Even though oral irrigation devices can deliver the drug to the base of the pocket, the drug level declines rapidly. However, water irrigation may lead to transient bacteremia.

The oral irrigator along with a pulsating stream of water is pushed through a nozzle on to the tooth surfaces. It is relatively easy to use.

Gingival Massage

Gingival massage can be carried out with tooth brush, inter-dental cleaners and gum massager. The effects of tooth brushing and inter-dental stimulators on the gingiva are as follows:

- It produces epithelial thickening.
- It increases keratinization.
- Blood circulation is improved, which provides substantial protection against microorganisms and other local irritants.

There is, however, no direct evidence that the above changes are much beneficial. However, massage may remove plaque, thus improving periodontal status.

Chemical Plaque Control

Mechanical plaque control measures are the primary methods for the prevention of dental and periodontal diseases. Since these diseases are infectious in nature, the chemical plaque inhibitors have also been tried as anti-plaque agents. However, chemical inhibitors cannot replace the mechanical measures completely. These are used as adjuncts to mechanical techniques and should be prescribed according to the needs of the individual.

The following are the requisites of the anti-plaque agents:

• They should eliminate the pathogenic bacteria.
• These agents should not develop resistance.
• Substantivity (these should remain in contact with the surface for a considerable period).
• Safety to the oral tissues at the recommended concentration and dosages.
• They should not stain the teeth or alter the taste.
• Easy to use.
• Preferably cost effective.

The following three agents have been accepted as chemical agents minimizing plaque.

I. Chlorhexidine

II. Listerine.

III. Delmopinol (Decapinol)

I. Chlorhexidine

Chlorhexidine gluconate has a broad antimicrobial spectrum including yeasts. It was used as wound and general skin cleanser for pre-surgical preparation of the patient and surgical scrub and hand wash for health care personnel. It is established that 0.2% chlorhexidine inhibits development of dental plaque, subsequently gingivitis and other periodontal diseases.

The local antibacterial effect of chlorhexidine is a result of its ability to interact with organic and inorganic components of the tooth surface. It gets adsorbed on to these surfaces and remains potent for long periods and is gradually released. This quality of prolonged contact time between the substance and the substrate is known as substantivity.

The sub-gingival delivery of chlorhexidine includes sub-gingival irrigation with syringe and packing of cellulose dialysis tubes containing 0.2% chlorhexidine in periodontal pockets. Chlorhexidine has also been incorporated in chewing gum.

Chlorhexidine substantially reduces gingival bleeding in geriatric patients as well as patients wearing orthodontic appliances. Plaque reduction and gingivitis has been reported in medically compromised patients and patients lacking manual dexterity.

However, chlorhexidine produces some undesirable side effects. They include brown staining of teeth, resin restorations and even the tongue. Some persons have complained of alteration of taste, burning sensation, feeling of soreness, dryness of mouth, desquamation and increased supra-gingival deposits.

Chlorhexidine does not have significant toxic effects in humans, nor any appreciable resistance of oral microorganisms and teratogenic alterations.

II. Listerine

The essential oil mouth washes or phenol mouth washes having germicidal properties have been used since long. Listerine is one of the phenols, commonly used as mouth rinse and is the only non-prescription mouthwash.

The composition of Listerine is as follows:

• Menthol   0.04%
• Thymol   0.06
• Eucalyptol   0.09%
• Benzoic acid   0.15%
• Ethyl alcohol   21.6 to 26%
  Colour   Fast green to Caramel

Listerine has been seen to substantially reduce plaque scores when tested in human beings. When listerine and chlorhexidine were compared, it was found that both mouth rinses improved the oral hygiene status but listerine was less effective in reducing the plaque and gingival scores than chlorhexidine. *Yoshihika et al (1997)* have observed that most of the plaque bacteria were killed completely by a 10 second exposure to listerine. They further reported that in dental plaque, bacteria and *candida albicans* were reduced by a 30 second exposure to listerine.

The adverse effects of listerine are bitter taste, burning sensation and occasional staining of teeth.

Listerine contains alcohol so it should not be used along with metronidazole/ tinidazole. The antiviral effect of Listerine has also been established.

III. Delmopinol (Decapinol)

Delmopinol is an ethanol derivative, which has been shown to be effective in the inhibition of dental plaque and gingivitis. It is available as a delmopinol hydrochloride mouthwash and toothpaste. Mouth rinsing with delmopinol, particulary at a concentration of 0.2%, is seen to provide adjunctive benefits to plaque control by mechanical methods. The reduction in both plaque and gingivitis suggest that it may be used as an anti-plaque agent.

Mechanism of action: Delmopinol hydrochloride is a surface active agent. Its chemical nature permits it to access plaque structures effectively. It is established that delmopinol interferes with plaque matrix formation and reduction of bacterial adherence. Subsequently plaque adheres loosely to the tooth so that it can be easily removed by mechanical cleaning procedures. Delmopinol is suitable as a pre-brush mouthrinse. A number of studies have shown its effectiveness against development of gingivitis. This may imply that delmopinol has an anti-inflammatory effect as well.

However, delmopinol, unlike chlorhexidine, has a low antimicrobial effect. In addition, it has much lower substantivity than chlorhexidine. But inspite of this difference, the effectiveness of delmopinol against plaque

and gingivitis is by virtue of its effect against the maturation of plaque matrix.

Adverse effects: The most frequently observed adverse effect is a transient numbness of the dorsal aspect of the tongue. Alteration of taste perception has also been reported. Other less frequently reported local adverse events include tooth and tongue discolouration (much less than chlorhexidine), and rarely mucosal soreness and erosion.

Other products: Several other products have shown plaque reduction; however, they are less potent than chlorhexidine and listerine. These products are:

1. Fluorides
2. Iodine
3. Iodophores
4. Chloroxylenol
5. Sanguinarine
6. Enzymes
7. Triclosan
8. Oxygenating agents
9. Quaternary ammonium compounds
10. Sodium benzoate
11. Antibiotics

1. *Fluorides:* Fluorides have a significant role in the prevention of dental caries and show potential therapeutic, adjunctive and preventive use in the treatment of periodontal disease as well. Stannous fluoride is the most effective amongst commonly available fluorides. A significant reduction in plaque and gingivitis in subjects brushing with 0.4% stannous fluoride has been observed. Stannous fluoride is usually applied in an aqueous gel with a tooth brush. When used as a rinse, it can reduce organisms responsible for caries and periodontal disease. Subgingival irrigation with 1.64% stannous fluoride was found to be effective in those sites which were inaccessible to mechanical plaque control. However, the use of

stannous fluoride as oral rinse is limited due to its instability in aqueous solution.

2. *Iodine:* Iodine is a powerful antiseptic with a wide spectrum of activity. The tubercle bacilli, leptospira, entamoeba, fungi, yeasts and viruses are all susceptible to iodines. 2.0% solution of iodine in 70% alcohol virtually sterilizes the skin in 30 seconds. However, it cannot be used satisfactorily on mucous surfaces and may produce skin sensitivity. It can also produce deep brown colour in the skin.

3. *Iodophores:* Newer iodine compounds were tried in an attempt to overcome the shortcomings of iodine. One such compound is an Iodophore. Iodophores are complexes of iodine with surface active agents such as nonionic detergents, quaternary compounds and macromolecules. 70–80% of iodine may be released as available iodine when a concentrated solution is diluted. They are generally non-toxic, non-irritating, non-staining and miscible in all proportions with water. They do not produce sensitivity when applied to mucous or skin surfaces. Use of 0.5% povidone iodine before prophylaxis significantly reduces gingival surface bacteria.

4. *Chloroxylenol:* Chloroxylenol is a widely used and relatively nonirritant antiseptic with occasional skin sensitivity. It is active against streptococci and less active against staphylococci and almost inactive against pseudomonas and proteus. Though its activity is reduced in the presence of blood or serum, it retains significant bactericidal activity in these circumstances. The commercial preparation, Dettolin, which contains 1.02% chloroxylenol and menthol is a satisfactory mouth wash.

5. *Sanguinarine:* Sanguinarine, a herbal extract obtained from the roots of the plant *Sanguinaria canadensis*, is a potent anti-plaque agent. Sanguinarine when used as mouth wash is retained by plaque rather than saliva.

The antimicrobial and anti-inflammatory properties of sanguinarine have been confirmed. The inhibitory concentration of sanguinarine for a wide spectrum of oral microorganisms is less than or equal to 16 mg/ml. This concentration is readily detected in plaque several hours after use of an oral rinse containing 0.03% sanguinaria extract.

The antiplaque action of sanguinaria may be related to its bacterio-static and bactericidal actions; i.e. it interferes with the adherence of certain bacteria to the tooth surface by blocking specific receptors either on the bacteria or on the tooth pellicle.

The antiplaque efficacy of sanguinarine was found to be less when compared with chlorhexidine. Various authors after combining sanguinarine tooth paste and mouth wash have observed significant reduction in plaque and gingivitis. However, *Cullinan et al (1997)* have observed no significant improvement in periodontal status with the use of sanguinarine. The combined use of sanguinaria tooth paste and oral rinse is particularly useful to orthodontic patients, because the presence of fixed orthodontic appliances poses difficulty in maintaining good oral hygiene by mechanical means alone.

Sanguinarine contains 11.5% alcohol; so it may produce burning sensation in the oral tissues. It should not be used in combination with metronidazole/tinidazole preparations.

6. *Enzyme:* Enzyme preparations have been used to inhibit formation of dental plaque by interfering with the mechanism of bacterial attachment and also breaking apart the existing plaque. The enzymes commonly used are:

a. Mucinase
b. Viokase

- Trypsin
- Chymotrypsin
- Carboxypeptidase
- Amylase
- Lipase
- Nucleases

Substantial reduction in plaque accumulation and subsequently, gingival inflammation was observed with the use of enzymes. The pancreatic enzyme preparation has also been incorporated into chewing gum. Although calculus formation was reduced, the chewing gum was found to be unpleasent. It is necessary that enzymes should be slow acting and have prolonged contact with plaque deposits. A combination of enzymes such as Mytolysin, Lysozyme and Dextranase might prove better. However, the enzymes damage the oral mucosa. So appropriate and effective formulation is required that may interfere with bacterial attachment. The formulation should not develop the resistance or produce adverse changes in the oral mucous membrane.

7. *Triclosan:* Triclosan as an antibacterial agent has been added to several dentifrice formulations to inhibit plaque and gingivitis. Triclosan is effective against both gram-positive and gram-negative organisms.

Even at sub-minimal concentration levels, triclosan can interfere with bacterial metabolism and acid production. No adverse effects are associated with its use; however, it has poor substantivity. To increase its retention and to boost its antiplaque activity, triclosan is combined with zinc citrate or with a copolymer, polyvinyl methyl ether maleic acid.

Significant improvement in gingival health is reported with the use of 0.5% triclosan and 1.0% zinc citrate. The commercially available tooth pastes usually contain 0.2% triclosan with or without zinc citrate. Zinc citrate is more effective on existing plaque and triclosan inhibits plaque formation on clean surfaces.

The addition of a co-polymer, polyvinyl methyl ether maleic acid to triclosan enhances retention of triclosan to tooth and mucous membrane. Long-term clinical trials of 6 weeks to 6 months duration have demonstrated that dentifrices containing triclosan and co-polymer significantly inhibit both supragingival plaque and gingivitis.

8. *Oxygenating agents:* The oxygenating agents are commonly used disinfectants. They release oxygen with effervescence which is bacteriostatic. Hydrogen peroxide combined with baking soda was popularized as a chemotherapeutic adjunct to non surgical treatment of periodontal disease. Chlorine dioxide gas was developed as a bleaching agent having better taste and odour. Chlorine dioxide (purogene) when added in tooth pastes and mouth rinses showed insignificant antiplaque and antigingivitis effects.

9. *Quaternary Ammonium Compounds:* Quaternary ammonium compounds are cationic antiseptics and surface active agents.

The commonly available Quaternary Ammonium Compounds are:

- Benzethonium chloride
- Benzalkonium chloride
- Cetylpyridinium chloride
- Domiphen bromide

These compounds react with cell membranes of microorganisms and disrupt the cell wall, thereby increasing its permeability leading to cell death. Quaternary amines are also used, which are more effective against gram-positive than gram-negative organisms. These antiseptics are beneficial antiseptics against early developing plaque.

However, if compared to chlorhexidine, their effectiveness is limited. The oral retention is twice that of chlorhexidine but desorption of Quaternary Ammonium Compounds in saliva is much more rapid. This may be because the doubly charged chlorhexidine may bond more effectively to oral sites than the monovalent Quaternary Ammonium Compound molecules.

Some undesirable side effects of Quaternary Ammonium Compound mouth rinses are burning sensation yellowish brown discolouration of tongue and aphthous ulceration of the oral mucosa.

10. *Sodium benzoate:* Sodium benzoate is used as a pre-brushing cleaning agent. This agent is meant for loosening plaque before brushing. A few authors, however, are of the view that the pre-brushing use is not much effective. No side effects have been reported with its use.

11. *Antibiotics:* The bacterial nature of dental plaque and its primary role in the etiology of both caries and periodontal diseases has led to a considerable research in the use of antibiotics in prevention and control of these diseases. The various antibiotics used are:

a. **Penicillin:** Penicillin has the potential to reduce caries and inflammation, especially in children suffering from rheumatic fever. However, certain authors have revealed conflicting results with the use of penicillin dentifrice.

It is established that daily use of penicillin for plaque control is not preferred because of development of resistant strains and hypersensitivity reactions.

b. **Vancomycin:** Vancomycin is primarily active against gram-positive micro-organisms. The topical application of vancomycin in an adhesive paste reduces incidence of periodontal diseases. However, it is reported that anti-plaque effect of vancomycin is temporary and do not prevent plaque formation in persons who do not mechanically remove plaque. These limitations as well as its narrow spectrum and emergence of resistant strains do not justify its use.

c. **Kanamycin:** Kanamycin has a broader spectrum of activity than vancomycin. It is observed that 5.0% topical application of kanamycin when used in place of mechanical removal of plaque, produced improvement in moderate to severe gingivitis. However, it did not eliminate gingivitis as it was not effective against anaerobic bacteria. The studies have shown that the reduction in plaque mass was primarily due to the inhibitory action upon streptococcal organisms.

d. **Macrolide antibiotics:** Several antibiotics like erythromycin, niddamycin and spiramycin belong to this group. These are moderately effective in reducing gingivitis and plaque scores.

   i. *Niddamycin:* Niddamycin when used twice daily in a concentration of 0.01% produced significant reduction in plaque and gingivitis. However, bacterial resistance to niddamycin is very common.

   ii. *Erythromycin:* Erythromycin has a spectrum similar to that of penicillin. Significant reduction of plaque has been reported with its use. Patients sensitive to penicillin can be given erythromycin as a substitute.

   iii. *Spiramycin:* Spiramycin has a similar spectrum to that of niddamycin and erythromycin.

The use of antibiotic preparations to inhibit plaque growth has reduced considerably. Bacterial resistance and hypersensitivity reactions are greater than potential benefits of using antibiotics for longer periods. These limitations discourage their use for prevention of periodontal diseases.

BIBLIOGRAPHY

1. Addy, M. : Chlorhexidine compared with other locally delivered antimicrobials. A short review. J. Clin. Period. : 13, 957, 1986.

2. Aguirre-Zero, O., Zero, D.T. and Proskin, H.M. : Effect of chewing xylitol chewing gum on salivary flow rate and the acidogenic potential of dental plaque. Caries Res. : 27, 55, 1993.

3. Ainamo, J. and Etemadzadeh, H. : Prevention of plaque growth with chewing gum containing chlorhexidine acetate. J. Clin. Periodontol. : 14, 524, 1987.

4. Ainamo, J., Nordblad, A. and Kallio, P. : the use of the CPITN in populations under 20 years of age. Int. Dent. J. : 34, 285, 1984.

5. Ash, M.M : A review of the problem and results of studies on manual and power tooth brushes. J. Periodontol. : 35, 202, 1964.

6. Axelsson, P. and Lindhe, J. : Effect of controlled oral hygiene on caries and periodontal disease in adults. J. Clin. Periodontol. : 5, 133, 1978.

7. Axelsson P. and Linde P. : Efficacy of mouth rinses in inhibiting dental plaque and gingivitis in man. J. Clin. Periodontal : 14, 205, 1987.

8. Bellini, H.T., Arneberg, P. and Vonder, F.R. : Oral hygiene and caries : A review. Acta. Odont. Scand. : 39, 257, 1981.

9. Bergstrom, J., Eliasson, S and Preber, H. : Cigarette smoking and periodontal bone loss. J. Periodontol. : 62, 242, 1991.

10. Bhambani, P.K. and Nayak, R.P. : The effect of different tooth brushes on plaque removal. J. Ind. Dent. Assoc. : 50, 149, 1978.

11. Bouwsma, D.J., Yost, K.G. and Baron, H.J. : Comparison of a chlorhexidine rinse and a wooden interdental cleaner in reducing inter-dental gingivitis. Am. J. Dent. : 5, 143, 1992.

12. Ciancio, S.G. : Medications as risk factors for periodontal diseases. J. Periodontol. : 67, 1055, 1996.

13. Ciancio, S.G. : Agents for the management of plaque and gingivitis. J. Dent. Res. : 71, 1450, 1992.

14. Ciancio, S.G. : Chemotherapeutic agents and periodontal therapy : Their impact on clinical practice. J. Periodontol. : 57, 108, 1986.

15. Ciancio, S.G., Shibley, O. and Mather, B.S. : Clinical effects of a stannous fluoride mouthrinse on plaque. Clin. Prev. Dent. : 14, 27, 1992.

16. Cullinan, P. Mary, Powell, N. Robin, Faddy, J. Malcolm and Seymour, J. Gregory : Efficacy of a dentifrice and oral rinse containing sanguinaria extract in conjunction with initial periodontal therapy : Aust. Dent. J.: 42, 7, 1997.

17. Dennison, D.K., Meredith, G.M., Shillitoe, E.J. and Caffase, R.G. : The antiviral spectrum of Listerine antiseptic. O. Surg., O. Med., O. Path. : 79, 442, 1995.

18. Engel, D., Nessly, M. and Morton, T. : Safety testing of a new electronic tooth brush. J. Periodontol. : 69, 941, 1993.

19. Fardal, O. and Turnbull, R.S.: A review of literature on use of chlorhexidine in dentistry. J. Am. Dent. Assoc. : 112, 863, 1986.

20. Katayama, T., Nagagawa, E., Honda, O., Tani, H., Okado, S and Suzuki, S. : Incidence and distribution of Streptococcus mutans in plaque from confectionary workers. J. Dent. Res. : 58, Abstr. 11, 1979. pp. 2251.

21. Gibson, W.A. : Antibiotics and periodontal disease : A selective review of the literature. J. Am. Dent. Assoc. : 104, 213, 1982.

22. Gjermo, P. an Flotra, L. : The effect of different methods of interdental cleaning. J. Periodontol. Res. : 5, 230, 1970.

23. Glass, R.L. : A clinical study of hand and electric tooth brushing. J. Periodontol. : 36, 322, 1965.

24. Jenkins, S., Addy, M. and Newcombe, R. : Toothpastes containing 0.3% and 0.5% triclosan I. Effects on 4 day plaque regrowth. Am. J. Dent. : 2, 211, 1989.

25. Johnson, B.D. and Melnnes, C. : Clinical evaluation of the efficacy and safety of a new sonic tooth brush. J. Periodontol. : 65, 692, 1994.

26. Kalio, P. : Self-assesed bleeding in monitoring gingival health among adolescents. Comm. Dent. Oral Epidem. : 24, 128, 1996.

27. Kawanabe, J., Hirasawa, M., Tatceuchi, T., Oda, T. and Ekede, T. : Non cariogenicity of Erythritol as a substrate. Caries. Res. : 26, 358, 1992.

28. Khambay, B.S. and Walmsley, A.D. : An in-vitro evaluation of electric tooth brushes. Quint. Int. : 26, 841, 1995.

29. Mandinier, I.M., Fesse, T.M. and Montell, R.A. : Oral carriage of Helicobacter plylori. A review. J. Periodontol. : 68, 1, 1997.

30. Parson, J.C. : Chemotherpay of dental plaque : a review. J. Periodontol. : 45, 117, 1974.

31. Shilosh, J. and Hovious, L.A. : The role of subgingival irrigation in the treatment of periodontitis. J. Periodontol. : 64, 835, 1993.

32. Silverstone, L.M. and Featherstone, M.J. : A scanning electron microscopic study of the end rounding of bristles in eight toothbrush types. Quint. Int. : 19, 3, 1988.

33. Spolsky, V.A., Perry, D.A. and Meng, Z. : Evaluating the efficacy of a new flossing aid. J. Clin. Periodontol. : 20, 490, 1993.

34. Stolze, K. and Bay, L. : Comparison of a manual and a new electric toothbrush for controlling plaque and gingivitis. J. Clin. Periodontol. : 21, 86, 1994.

35. Tellesen, G., Larsen, G., Kaligithi, R., Zimmerman, J.G. and Wikesjo, M.E. : Use of chlorhexidine chewing gum significantly reduces dental plaque formation compared to use of similar xylitol and sorbitol products. J. Periodontol. : 67, 181, 1996.

36. Terezhalmy, G.T., Iffland, H., Jelepis, C. and Waskowski, J. : Clinical evaluation of the effect of an ultrasonic tooth brush on plaque, gingivitis and gingival bleeding. J. Prosth. Dent. : 73, 97, 1995.

37. Tenovuo, J. an Soderling, E. : Chemical aids in the prevention of dental disease in the elderly. Int. Dent. J. : 42, 355, 1992.

38. Trahn, L. : Xylitol : a review of its action on mutans streptococci and dental plaque and its chemical significance. Int. Dent. J. : 45 (suppl.), 77, 1995.

39. Walmsley, A.D. : The electric toothbrush : a review. B.D.J. : 182, 209, 1997.

40. Yoshihiko, K., Hajime, I. and Okuda, K. : Bactericidal effects of mouth rinses on oral bacteria. Bull. Tokyo Dent. Coll. : 38, 297, 1997.

16   *Prevention of Caries*

Dental caries is a multi-factorial disease. To understand its preventive protocol, it is important to get familiarize with the etiology and progress of the disease process. For initiation and progress of dental caries, three factors are essential: presence of an adequate number of cariogenic bacteria, susceptible tooth surface and available foodstuffs to support the growth of cariogenic bacteria (Fig. 16.1). The caries process can be prevented or interrupted if any one of these conditions can be modified. Therefore, therapies effective on these three directions should be recommended to patients for reducing dental caries.

Dental caries is considered as the disease of 'have nots', though it exists in developed as well as underdeveloped regions of the world. Taking into consideration the harsh realities of mal-distribution of resources and individual's susceptibility, the total eradication of caries may remain a dream in near future.

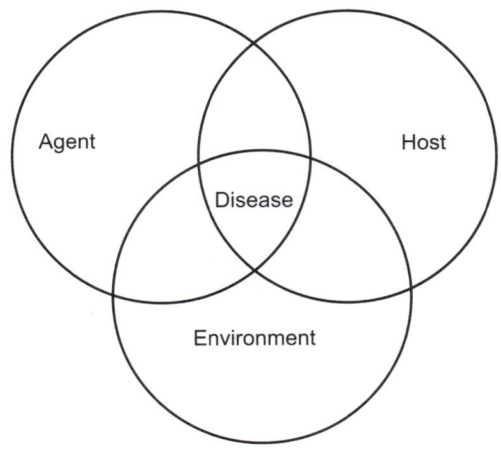

Disease	Agent	Host	Environment
Dental caries	Cariogenic Bacteria	Tooth	Foods
i. Crowns	i. Streptococcus mutans	i. Enamel	i. Fermentable carbohydrates
ii. Root	ii. Lactobacillus	ii. Dentin	
		iii. Cementum	

Fig. 16.1: Essential factors for the development of disease

There is a marked increase in tooth retention across the world. In older adults, recession is an accompanying problem leading to root caries. When secondary caries and root caries are considered, the aggregate caries increment may come to be higher, especially in older adults. The caries and its sequel, rather than periodontal disease, are the primary cause of tooth loss in our aging population.

According to the World Health Organization Global Oral Data Bank, caries is on the increase in many countries in South and Central America, Asia and the Middle East countries. There is a need for improvement in our existing preventive techniques and materials.

The following three point strategy was evolved at National Caries Preventive Programs along with creating awareness among masses through motivation and education.
A. Control of caries inducing microorganisms
B. Modification of caries promoting diet
C. Increasing the resistance of the teeth to decay

A. Control of Caries Inducing Microorganisms

The most accepted method of controlling the microorganisms is the personal oral hygiene. The emphasis should be laid on the mechanical removal of the plaque and the substrate with proper brushing and flossing. Whether these methods lead to reduction in caries or not, remains controversial. A few authors were of the view that supervised brushing and flossing led to a decrease in plaque and gingivitis but not caries. However, others were of the view that tooth brushing and flossing have definite impact on caries reduction.

The commonly used agents which help reducing or eliminating the plaque are as follows:

a. Chlorhexidine and Allied Agents

Since caries is an infectious disease, the chemotherapeutic approach for caries pre-vention is gaining importance. Chlorhexidine is the accepted antiseptic and effective anti-plaque agent. The potential efficacy of chlorhexidine against Streptococcus mutans vis-à-vis human dental caries has been established. Currently, 0.2% chlorhexidine is recommended for short duration as a mouth wash. However, the most effective mode of use of chlorhexidine is application of chlorhexidine gel or varnish in a concentration of 40%. Since Streptococcus mutans has been recognized as more than one bacterial species, this group of bacteria has been functionally labelled as mutans streptococci. The mutans streptococci titre in saliva and caries risk is directly proportional. Use of chlorhexidine mouthwash for 30 seconds, prior to sleep is beneficial. The salivary flow decreases at night and the concentration of the drug remains high till morning. This increases the amount of time the drug remains in contact with microorganisms and prolongs its effectiveness.

The effectiveness of chlorhexidine lies in its chemical charge. Chlorhexidine is a biguanide and strongly cationic. Since almost all oral surfaces are negatively charged, the positive charge of this cationic drug causes it to adhere to almost everything giving the drug the best substantivity (*substantivity is the ability to keep an agent in contact with an organism, long enough to kill or disable the organism*). The drug maintains the bactericidal activity even during sleep and by continuous use of chlorhexidine, the caries risk is lowered.

Chlorhexidine is accepted as a safe and effective way of preventing caries. The teratogenic safety has been established. Chlorhexidine is poorly absorbed from the gastrointestinal tract. The lethal dose for this drug is estimated to be 2000 mg per kg body weight which means that a 50 kg child must drink 83 liters of chlorhexidine to be at risk of dying which is certainly impossible.

It is established that the bacterial count in the oral cavity changes in a characteristic way, being highest in the morning, 50% after meals and again high in between meals. Each brushing and rinsing can reduce bacterial count up to 50% which again reaches peak value within half an hour.

Various antiseptics have been tried from time to time. Earlier, quarternary ammonium salts were used, which were efficient against gram-positive organisms. It was observed that by rinsing with chloramines (quarternary ammonium salt), the plaque flora was reduced to about 10–30%.

Many studies have documented the benefits of xylitol as a sugar substitute in one form or the other in reducing dental caries. The beneficial effects of xylitol chewing gum in reducing caries have been established. Xylitol is effective in plaque reduction, inhibition of plaque acid production, inhibition of the growth and metabolism of the mutans group of streptococci and above all it contributes to the re-mineralization of teeth.

Simons et al (1997) compared the effect of chlorhexidine - xylitol combination and xylitol chewing gum alone on salivary levels of mutans streptococci, lactobacilli and yeasts. They observed that the combination of chlorhexidine-xylitol was effective against mutans streptococci, lactobacilli and yeast where as xylitol alone was effective against mutans streptococci only.

Oxidizing agents; such as hydrogen peroxide and sodium perborate, have also been used, but with little encouraging results.

b. Fluorides

Regarding role of fluorides (details in Chapter 4), it is believed that they inhibit either bacterial growth, polysaccharide formation or acid production. It has been observed that high concentration of fluoride is required to inhibit acid formation. However, polysaccharide production as well as growth of some microorganisms may be reduced by even 10–20 ppm fluoride concentration. Fluorides help in reduction of plaque formation, possibly because the surface of the tooth and the restorative materials contain a number of free charges, which are required for plaque formation and the fluorides are very effective in reducing these free charges. Though the presence of fluorides at the enamel surface is an important cariostatic factor; however, whether fluorides interfere with caries inducing metabolism of the plaque or not, has not been documented.

c. Enzymes

Certain enzymes have been tried which remove dental plaque or reduce the formation of plaque, thereby decreasing the caries incidence. Hydrolytic enzymes, which split the glycoprotein of the saliva and the plaque are effective in caries reduction.

Enzymes like protenase, neuraminidases, lactoperoxidase and other proteolytic enzymes as trypsin and pepsin have been extensively used in various concentrations. It is established that the enzymes in lower concentrations are not very effective and in higher concentrations, they may injure the soft tissues. One protein dissolving enzyme, mutanolysin have shown encouraging results.

Certain polysaccharide-splitting enzymes have the potential of reducing plaque formation; however, they were effective only when given along with diet before the initiation of plaque formation. Certain enzymes act indirectly to reduce plaque accumulation. Dextranase is a hydrolytic enzyme capable of breaking down dextrans in the plaque, subsequently inhibiting its formation. Dextranase incorporated in the diet and/or drinking water has not proved to be effective in removing established plaque; however, it is effective in reducing formation of plaque. Dextranase in mouth washes have been disappointing. The clinical usefulness of dextranase preparations is restricted by the difficulty of maintaining effective concentrations of the enzymes in contact with the plaque which is required for the breakdown of the plaque. A dentifrice containing lacto-peroxidase (an enzyme found in saliva) has an anti bacterial effect towards lactobacilli and streptococci. This enzymes containing dentifrice has a definite cariostatic activity.

d. Enzyme inhibitors

The concept of preventing caries and plaque by blocking microbiological enzyme reaction was studied by various authors using different enzyme inhibitors. From a large number of inhibition tests with different enzyme inhibitors, two substances were finally selected- *Sodium lauryl sarcosinate and Sodium dehydro-acetate*. These substances inhibit dental plaque and were shown to exert an influence on acid production for many hours. Whether, the enzyme inhibitors prevent caries or not, remains controversial.

B. Modification of Caries Promoting Diet

The relationship of diet and caries is an old phenomenon. Diet encompasses everything that is eaten, regardless of its nutritional value whereas nutrition deals with those elements of the diet that are absorbed from the intestinal tract. Dietary factors exert local effects while nutritional factors effect systemically upon dentition.

Sweetness of food and dental caries has long been interrelated. *Pierre Fouchard*, the founder of dental profession, has quoted that 'all sugary foods contribute to the destruction of teeth and those who use sugar frequently, rarely have good teeth'.

It was believed that acids formed from lodgement of food caused caries; and the teeth could be decalcified by placing in a mixture of saliva and sugar. The lactic acid and acetic acid was thought to be responsible for this decalcification.

The famous Miller's theory believes that acids are produced by the interaction of carbohydrates and saliva. This acid leads to the demineralization of enamel causing caries. It is observed that the patient with rampant caries frequently have sucrose containing foods.

Epidemiological Observation of Caries and Diet

General epidemiologic surveys are helpful in determining the possible causes and ways of preventing a disease.

Numerous reports have indicated that Eskimos living on their natural diet had low caries experience; however, their dental health declined after being exposed to high sugar diet.

The children who had different types of sugar containing refined foods had greater caries activity. The sugarcane and unprocessed wheat contained a 'protective agent' that is lost in the refinement of these foods also encourage caries.

It has been observed that the diet received up to 12 years did not confer any protection from caries during subsequent years.

Hereditary fructose intolerance (HFI) is a rare hereditary disease caused by an inborn error of metabolism whereby the patients do not posses liver enzyme (fructose -1-phosphate splitting aldolase) required for digestion of foods containing fructose, causing severe nausea to the patients. On the other hand, starchy foods (not containing fructose) are well tolerated. It has been observed that the teeth of these patients are in extra ordinary good condition unlike an equivalent age group of the general population. Mostly these people are caries free.

The low prevalence of caries in persons with HFI indicates that starchy foods do not produce decay, whereas sugary foods cause caries. Highly significant differences in the proportion of Streptococcus mutans and lactobacillus were found between the plaque of the HFI group and that of the control population.

A few authors have reported high caries incidence in diabetics, (explained by slightly increased salivary glucose levels and reduced salivary flow); however, most surveys have shown a lower caries experience in diabetics. The severe restriction in sugar intake was considered the most likely cause of the lower caries experience in the diabetics.

Workers in sugar industries such as bakeries and candy factories are exposed daily to air polluted with sugar dust. They also consume relatively large amounts of sugar-containing foods during work. The higher caries risk of these workers has been confirmed. Further, the caries experience was higher in production-line workers compared with non production-line workers in the industry.

Phenylketonuria is a rare inherited disorder in which there is a deficiency of the liver enzyme, phenylalanine hydroxylase. These patients have to be given a high carbohydrate diet otherwise severe mental deficiency can occur. Such patient usually exhibit higher caries experience.

Pediatric medicines are usually given in syrup form, which are sucrose based. The children taking such syrups have a higher caries experience than the control ones.

The Vipeholm study was conducted on mentally retarded children to evaluate the effect of sugar and fluorides on dental caries.

The conclusions of the Vipeholm study were:

- Consumption of sugar, if taken up to four times a day at meals and none between meals, is associated with only a small increase in caries increment.
- Consumption of sugar both between meals and at meals is associated with a marked increase in caries increment.
- The increase in caries activity, under uniform experimental conditions varies widely from person to person.
- The increase in caries activity disappears as soon as the sugar intake is withdrawn.
- Carious lesions do occur despite avoidance of sugars.

The effect of substituting sucrose with either fructose or xylitol on dental caries has been evaluated. It is reported that substitution of sucrose by xylitol resulted in a lower caries increment. The plaque organisms are unable to metabolize xylitol to acids. However, substitution of sucrose by fructose does not cause a definite caries reduction.

It is established that substitution of sorbitol in sweets taken in between meals caused a substantial reduction in caries increment. Excessive use of sorbitol sweetened products, however, results in an increased production of acids.

Lycasin, a hydrogenated starch hydrolysate, when substituted with sucrose resulted in reduction in caries activities.

The cariogenic potential of various types of sugars and their pH values were evaluated. It is established that addition of 25% glucose, fructose, lactose or maltose did not produce significantly more caries than starch, while sucrose was much more cariogenic.

The pH of plaque before, during and after intake of food is a guide to the cariogenic potential of that food. Plaque pH studies have been used to differentiate between the potential cariogenicity of different sugars and the different concentrations of sugars. The intake of cheese and sugarless chewing gums after sugary food prevents the fall in plaque pH.

The relative cariogenicity of sweetening agents are given in Table 16.1.

Sucrose has been termed the 'arch criminal of dental caries'. Being the most common constituent in our diet, it is a major cause of dental caries. A property of sucrose, which makes it more cariogenic, is its unique ability to enhance production of extracellular polysaccharides such as dextran in dental plaque. Dextran is not easily metabolized in plaque subsequently making it sticky. It also increases the bulk of plaque.

A few studies have observed sucrose to be more cariogenic while others indicated similar

Table 16.1: Relative cariogenicity of sweetening agents

Compound	Approximate sweetness relative to sucrose
Sugars	
Sucrose	1
Glucose	0.7
Fructose	1.2
Sorbose	1.9
Lactose	0.3
Maltose	0.4
Sugar Compounds	
Glucosylsucrose	–
Maltosylsucrose	–
Tichlorosucrose	2000
Sucralose	600
Sugar alcohols	
Xylitol	1.0
Sorbitol	0.5
Mannitol	0.7
Maltitol	0.75
Lactitol	0.35
Sugar Complex	
Hydrogenated glucose syrup	0.75
Isomalt	0.5
Dipeptide/Polypeptide	
Aspartame	180
Monellin	3000
Thaumatin	4000
Miscellaneous	
Saccharin	5000
Cyclamate	50
Stevioside	200
Acesulfame potassium	130
Glycyrrhizin	50

level of cariogenicity with all sugars. Practically substituting sucrose with glucose, fructose, or maltose for the prevention of dental caries is not much effective. Lactose and galactose are significantly less cariogenic than other dietary sugars.

Relative Cariogenicity of Alternative Sweeteners

Sorbitol and Mannitol

Sorbitol is extensively used in foods manufactured for diabetics and as sweeteners in sugarless syrups. Mannitol is used mainly in chewing–gum. Sorbitol and mannitol are fermented slowly by plaque organisms, much slower than that of sucrose.

Xylitol

Xylitol is used in confectionery and tooth pastes. Xylitol modifies the synthesis of polysaccharides from sucrose in Streptococcus mutans thereby decreasing the ability of the cells to adhere to hard surfaces. Depression of mutans streptococci in plaque and/or saliva has been co-related with the regular use of xylitol. It is established that total substitution of dietary sugar by xylitol resulted in very low caries incidence.

Hydrogenated glucose

Hydrogenated glucose as a syrup is sold under the trade name Lycasin. Lycasin is fermented slowly compared with sucrose and causes minimal depression of plaque pH. It is much less cariogenic than sucrose.

Isomalt

It is sold under the trade name Palatinit. Isomalt causes little acid production when incubated with oral streptococci. It is reported that the use of Isomalt resulted in lower plaque accumulation than sucrose. Further, the intake of snacks containing 100% isomalt in between meals resulted in the decrease of mutans streptococci.

Sucralose

Sucralose is a non-toxic, intensively sweet sucrose derivative that has been shown to be non-cariogenic. Sucralose is not fermentable. Cariostatic effect of sucralose is mainly because of its ability to inhibit Glucosyl transferase (GTF) and Fructosyl transferase (FTF).

Erythritol

Erythritol is the sugar alcohol produced from glucose. It is 70-80% as sweet as sucrose and is also non-hygroscopic. Erythritol is neither used as substrate for the lactic acid production nor for plaque formation. Reduction in caries has been reported using diet containing erythritol as compared to sucrose. Erythritol is a promising sugar substitute from point of view of cariogenicity.

C. Increasing the Resistance of the Teeth to decay

Increasing the resistance of the tooth is considered an important means of preventing caries. Resistance can be increased by many ways such as caries vaccination, lasers and pit and fissures sealants.

CARIES VACCINES

Dental caries is the most common disease of mankind. The prevalence of caries in developed countries is greater than 99.9% and has been increasing in developing countries.

The development of dental caries requires:
a. Presence of cariogenic bacteria that are capable of rapidly producing acid below the critical pH required for dissolving enamel.
b. Sugar in the diet favours colonization of these bacteria to form acid.

This process can be interfered by the presence of an effective immune response.

It is established that mutans streptococci are the primary etiological agent of this disease and that infection is transmissible. A strong association exists between quantity and quality of mutans streptococci and dental caries, although other organisms such as lactobacilli have also been implicated.

It is further established that children become colonized with mutans streptococci between the middle of second year and the end of third year of life during the so called 'window of infectivity'.

The primary source of infection is maternal, although there is evidence that non-familiar transfer can occur when environmental condition favour colonization. Infection is related to maternal dose (higher the level of maternal mutans streptococci infection, the higher the percentage of children getting infected) In case the maternal dose is associated with higher level of sucrose, the children may get infected at an early age.

Oral Immune Environment

The oral immune environment undergoes rapid and early development. Although secretory IgA antibody in saliva and other secretions are essentially absent at birth, mature sIgA is the principal salivary immunoglobin secreted at one month of age.

Bacteria passing through mouth into the stomach and intestine come into contact with specialized lymphatic tissue located in Peyer's patches along with intestinal walls. Certain T and B cells in Peyer's patches become sensitized to these microorganisms. These sensitized T and B cells migrate through lymphatics to blood stream and eventually settle in glandular tissues including the salivary glands. These sensitized cells produce IgA that are secreted in the saliva which are capable of agglutination of oral bacteria, reduced adherence and easy clearance. By six to nine months of age, most children exhibit a more adult like distribution of salivary IgA1 and IgA2 subclasses. Salivary antibody to oral commensal microbiota can be detected in both subclasses at this time. This evidence suggests that significant maturation of the mucosal immune response has occurred by the end of the first year of life. This immunological phenomenon is the basis of caries vaccine.

Characteristics of Dental Caries as Related to Vaccine Development

Dental caries has certain unique characteristics because of which the vaccine against caries is still unsuccessful.

These characteristics are:

i. In dental caries, all the three components, i.e. host, microflora and diet have not only to be present but also keep interacting.

ii. Dental caries starts with the colonization of microorganisms on the outer surface of a tissue which is devoid of blood vessels and tissue fluid. Therefore, natural stimulation of immune system by cariogenic microorganisms takes place mainly via MALT/GALT (mucosa/gut associated lymphoid tissue). Also antibodies mainly work by preventing colonization by microorganisms or interfering with their metabolism. MALT/GALT are exposed to the antigens from these bacteria almost from birth and on a daily basis. This might lead to the development of tolerance and/or systemic hyporesponsiveness.

iii. The hard tissues of the teeth do not shed and the tooth is therefore colonized by a population of microorganisms which are relatively stable especially in retentive pits and fissures. Further in retentive areas, possibilities for immune mechanisms to influence the development of caries are restricted.

iv. Though a strong association between caries and Streptococcus mutans has been proved but a number of other organisms have also been associated with caries.

Effective Molecular Targets for Dental Caries Vaccine

Several stages in the molecular pathogenesis of dental caries are susceptible to immune intervention.

a. Microorganisms can be cleared from the oral cavity by antibody mediated aggregation while still in the salivary phase, prior to colonization.

b. Antibody could also block the receptors necessary for colonization (adhesins) or accumulation (glucan-binding domains of GBPs and GTF) or inactivate GTF enzymes responsible for glucan formation.

c. Modification of metabolically important functions may also be targeted. Antibodies could affect the cariogenicity of Streptococcus mutans by interfering with glucose uptake and acid production. Thus lactate dehydrogenase from Streptococcus mutans has been purified in order to test the possible effect of this enzyme in providing protection against acid producing microorganisms, e.g. streptococci and lactobacilli.

d. IgA antibodies have been found to inhibit the attachment of Streptococcus sanguis to epithelial cells but a corresponding inhibitory effect has not been clearly shown for Streptococcus mutan. This may be because in latter studies the IgA preparation probably did not contain antibodies directed towards relevant cell wall or the analytical methods were not sensitive enough to reveal the effect. The antimicrobial activity of salivary IgA antibody may be enhanced or redirected by synergism with innate components of immunity such as mucin or lactoferrin.

Candidate Antigens

Originally whole cells of Streptococcus mutans were used as antigens, but with the passage of time more specific cell components/cell products have been used. The thrust of the research was to use purified antigen preparations, since the finding that antisera from rabbits immunized with whole cells of Streptococcus mutans contain antibodies which can cross react with human cardiac tissue.

a. Adhensins

Adhesins from the two principal human pathogen, Streptococcus mutans (variously identified as antigen I/II, PAC or PI) and Streptococcus sobrinus (SpaA or Pag), have been purified. Antigen I/II (Ag I/II) were found both in the culture supernatant as well as on the Streptococcus mutans cell surface.

Immunological approaches support the adhesin related function of the Ag I/II family of proteins and their repeating region in Streptococcus. For example, abundant in vitro and in vivo evidence indicates that antibody with specificity for Streptococcus mutans Ag I/II or Streptococcus sobrinus. Spa A can interfere with bacterial adherence and subsequent dental caries.

Numerous immunization approaches have shown that active immunization with intact antigen I/II or passive immunization with monocolonal or transgenic antibody epitopes within this component can protect rodents, primates, or humans from dental caries caused by Streptococcus mutans. Protection in these experiments can be achieved by antibody blockade of initial colonization events or antibody mediated agglutination and cleaning of adhesin-bearing bacteria from the saliva.

b. Glucosyltransferase (GTFs)

Streptococcus mutans and Streptococcus sobrinus, each synthesize several glucosyl transferase. Genes responsible for glucan synthesis in Streptococcus mutans are gtfB, which synthesizes 1,3-linked insoluble glucan, gtfC, which synthesizes glucan with both 1,3 and 1,6 linkages, and gtfD, which synthesis a soluble 1,6-linked glucan. Similarly, the products of gtf1 and gtfS genes of Streptococcus sobrinus synthesize insoluble and soluble glucan products respectively. Mutational inactivation techniques have shown that each of these gene products is important to the cariogenicity of the respective mutans streptococcal strain. For example, insertional inactivation of Streptococcus mutans gtf genes to replace functional wild-type copies of gene markedly reduced caries when gtfB and gtfC genes that coded for GTFs synthesizing water insoluble glucan were inactivated. Similar inactivation of the gtfD gene also resulted in a mutant with lower cariogenicity on smooth surface Streptococcus. In addition, the ability of GTF from initial colonization of Streptococcus mutans to synthesize water insoluble glucan has been correlated with caries incidence in young children.

Antibody directed to native GTF or sequences associated with its catalytic or glucan-binding function interfere with the synthetic activity of the enzyme and with the in vitro plaque formation. Since Streptococcus mutans GTFs bear significant sequence homology active immunization with either Streptococcus mutans or Streptococcus sobrinus, GTFs induced protective immune responses in experimental dental caries rodent models after infection with several mutans streptococcal species. However, a much lower level of mutans streptococcal GTF antibody reactivity was observed with GTFs of other oral streptococci.

Induction of sIgA antibody in humans by oral or topical GTF administration is accompanied by interference with accumulation of indigenous mutans streptococci after dental prophylaxis. Passive administration of antibody to GTF in the diet also can protect rats from experimental dental caries. Thus, the presence of antibody to glucosyl transferases in the oral cavity prior to infection can significantly influence the disease outcome, presumably by interference with one or more of the functional activities of the enzyme.

c. Glucan Binding Proteins

The ability of mutans streptococci to bind to glucans is presumed to be mediated at least in part, by cell-wall-associated glucan-binding proteins (Gbp). Many proteins with glucan-binding properties have been identified in Streptococcus mutans and Streptococcus sobrinus. Each glucan binding protein has the ability to bind 1,6 glucan, although other glucan linkages potentially may impact higher binding constants. Streptococcus mutans secretes at least three distinct proteins with glucan-binding activity, GbpA, GbpB and GbpC.

- GbpA has a greater affinity for water soluble than for water-insoluble glucan.

- Although the function of GbpB in the native environment is as yet unresolved, biofilm formation on plastic surfaces by strains of Streptococcus mutans is directly correlated with expression of GbpB suggesting a role for GbpB in this process.

- The GbpC protein, detected when Streptococcus mutans cultures are stressed during growth, is associated with dextran-dependent aggregation.

Of three Streptococcus mutans glucan-binding proteins, only GbpB has been shown to induce a protective immune response to experimental dental caries. Protection can be achieved by either subcutaneous injection of GbpB in the salivary gland region or by mucosal application by the intranasal route. Saliva samples from young children often contain IgA antibody to GbpB, indicating that initial infection with Streptococcus mutans can lead to natural induction of immunity to this protein. Studies have shown that GbpA appears to be less immunogenic than GbpB and that its ability to induce protective immunity is problematic. Streptococcus sobrinus Gbps have not been evaluated for their protective potential.

d. Lipoteichoic Acid (LTA)

Lipoteichoic acid (LTA) has also been tried but its role is not very certain. LTA has been associated with adherence of group A streptococci to epithelial surfaces, but a similar action for Streptococcus mutans has not been substantiated, though it has been observed that antibodies to LTA from Staphylococcus aureus could inhibit glucose uptake of Streptococcus mutans.

e. Crude Ribosomal Preparation

Crude ribosomal preparation of Streptococcus mutans has also been tried. Anti-ribosomal antibodies have shown to inhibit acid production, growth and glucose photo-transferase activity of virulent Streptococcus mutans. Some preparations do not cross react with human tissues whereas others do.

New Vaccine Strategies

Caries immunization studies in humans have been conducted primarily by oral inoculation and employed Streptococcus mutans cells and cell wall associated glucosyl transferase. In past decade, new strategies have been developed for active as well as passive immunization for caries.

A. Active Immunization

a. Synthetic peptide vaccine: Use of synthetic Streptococcus mutans peptides derived from glucosyl transferase of Streptococcus mutans have shown to inhibit enzyme functioning. Local gingivo-mucosal injection with synthetic peptides from Streptococcus mutans surface proteins has generated protective antibodies both in gingival fluid and saliva.

Synthetic peptide approaches have shown the alanine rich repeat region of Ag I/II to be immunogenic and to induce protective immunity.

Table 16.2: New Vaccine Strategies
Active Immunization Agents
• Synthetic Streptococcus mutans peptides
• Streptococcus mutans antigens coupled to cholera toxin subunits
• Liposome-coated delivery systems
• Fusing Streptococcus mutans genes with attenuated salmonelle
Passive Immunization Agents
• Monoclonal antibodies applied topically
• Immune bovine milk and whey
• Egg yolk antibody

Advantages

 i. Enhanced immune responses

 ii. Avoidance of host tissue reactivity

Disadvantages

 i. Oral inoculation results in rapid break down of proteins/peptides by intestinal enzymes so only a limited proportion of vaccine can be combined with GALT.

b. Coupling Streptococcus mutans antigens to cholera toxin subunits: This has been proved effective in suppressing Streptococcus mutans colonization and reducing caries in rats. Cholera toxin effectively binds to lymphoid cells and functions as an excellent adjunct in inducing an immune response.

Intranasal immunization with Alanine-rich surface protein antigens (PAcA), coupled to cholera toxin B subunit, suppressed colonization of mouse teeth by Streptococcus mutans fusion proteins containing PAcA also inhibited sucrose-independent adhesion of Streptococcus mutans to saliva-coated hydroxyapatite beads. Thus, this Streptococcus mutans adhesin contains multiple functionally based epitopes that are sufficiently immunogenic to be considered for dental caries vaccines. For example, B and T cell epitopes.

c. Fusing Streptococcus mutans genes with attenuated Salmonella: This is an effective vaccine vector genetic recombinant technique which is used to fuse Streptococcus mutans surface protein genes with attenuated salmonella.

Gene fusions of a functionally relevant sequence linked to a mucosal adjuvant sequence can result in chimeric proteins inherently able to enhance immune responses to the functional epitopes.

• Attenuated mutans vectors such as salmonella, which contain plasmids expressing recombinant peptides, can target the vaccine to appropriate inductive lymphoid tissue for mucosal responses. Several of these approaches have successfully induced protective immune response for experimental dental caries by means of chimeric proteins or expressing either adhesin or GTF epitopes.

• Redman and co-workers have shown that oral immunization with recombinant Salmonella typhimusium, expressing surface protein antigen A of Streptococcus sobrinus, was able to induce persistent mucosal immune responses which could confer protection after challenge of Fischer rats with cariogenic Streptococcus sobrinus.

• Other recombinant strategies involving either adhesin or GTF constructs, with or without mucosal adjuvant sequences, have been shown to induce immune responses to these functional domains which could be ultimately protective in caries vaccine applications.

• Constructs involving the attenuated human Streptococcus typhi vector would be expected to have more potential for human vaccine application than would Streptococci Typhimusium, which is a murine pathogen. In this regard, attenuated Streptococci tyhpi (UD908 strains have been prepared to express peptide chimeras in which GTF sequences, associated with the glucan-binding domain, are combined with tetanus toxin fragment C for immunogenicity.

- Defined segments of chromosomal DNA from Streptococcus mutans have been cloned into Escherichia coli. Streptococcus mutans genes for Spa A and glucosyl transferase have been cloned and expressed in Escherichia coli. Bacillus subtilis has also been found to be a suitable host for expression of Streptococcus mutans sucrose genes. This cloned vector bacterium can be introduced orally where it colonizes in a limited time and stimulate lymphoid tissues in GIT to induce an antibody response.

An important advantage of recombinant DNA technique is that it allows production of large quantities of antigen and risk of contamination with human tissues is less.

d. *Liposome delivery system:* Use of dehydrated liposomes to coat the vaccine is a very effective method. Liposomes are microscopic closed vesicles composed of bilayered phospholipid membrane very similar to cell membrane. In rats, use of liposomes doubled the efficacy of orally administered vaccine from 40% to 80%. In an oral immunization study approved by Food and Drug Administration, seven healthy adult volunteers were given Streptococcus mutans glucosyl transferase dehydrated liposomes for three days and substantial increase in salivary IgA antibody was demonstrated.

e. *Conjugate Protein/Peptide with Bacterial Polysaccharide:* Another vaccine approach which may intercept more than one aspect of mutans streptococcal molecular pathogenesis is the chemical conjugation of functionally associated protein/peptide component with bacterial polysaccharides. Added to value of including multiple

targets within the vaccine is that the conjugation of protein with polysaccharide enhances the immunogenicity of the T-cell independent polysaccharide entity.

B. Passive Immunization

Validity of passive immunization was established about 10 years back in experiments on monkeys, in which monoclonal antibodies applied directly to teeth decreased Streptococcus mutans colonization and caries. Since that time there is increasingly active research in passive immunization.

a. *Topical application of monoclonal antibodies:* Recently a marked reduction in Streptococcus mutans has been shown in human subjects after topical application of monoclonal antibodies. Since in this way both systemic and mucosal immune systems are bypassed, so less concern exists about any potential side effects. However, since the recipient is not stimulated to produce any antibodies, continued reapplication is needed.

b. *Immune bovine milk and whey:* Systemic immunization of cows with a vaccine from whole Streptococcus mutans cell generated IgG antibodies in serum and milk. In rats, when this whey was added to a caries promoting diet, there was a substantial decrease in caries production. In humans, use of bovine milk rinses for 14 days resulted in lower percentage of plaque Streptococcus mutans than in both pre-test plaque and control groups' plaque.

c. *Egg-yolk antibodies:* Yolk from eggs of chicken immunized with Streptococcus mutans has been investigated as a source of antibodies. Formalin killed whole cells of Streptococcus mutans were used in one study and cell associated glucosyl transferase as antigen in the other. Caries reduction was seen in both studies.

d. *Transgenic plant antibodies:* IgA antibody has recently been produced in tobacco plant by cross breeding. This IgA is functional against Streptococcus mutans and causes their agglutination. The bovine, egg yolk and monoclonal antibodies produced prior to this are antibodies to IgG. Since IgA antibodies are designed by nature to function on mucosal surfaces and are dominant antibodies in the oral cavity, they have promising capabilities.

Advantages

- Construction of multimeric forms of antibodies because of ease with which genetic material can be exchanged.
- Antibody structure can be manipulated by cross breeding so that specificity of antibody variable region can be maintained while modifying the constant region to humanize the antibody.
- Elimination of concern for cross reactivity that could arise from animal antibodies. Possibility of harvesting monoclonal antibodies on agricultural scale suggesting that they could be made available in almost limitless quantities very cheaply, making even daily use practical.

Use of major food crops such as rice, potatoes and peppers as transformable plants is already being seen as a way to make passive immunotherapy available on a global scale.

Risks Associated with Caries Vaccine

The relatively slow pace of caries vaccine strategies reflects the range of ethical and socio-economic issues attached with the disease; whether such vaccines have any adverse effects have not been documented well. In this age of risk benefit determinations, virtually no adverse effects can be tolerated.

Few manufacturers are interested in vaccine production because profits are small and risks of law suits are great.

Sera of some patients with rheumatic fever shows serological cross reactivity between heart tissue antigens and certain antigens from streptococci. M protein present on surface of the streptococci enables them to resist phagocytosis. Antibodies against M proteins provide antigenic stimulus in susceptible host which could produce autoimmune disease. Some cell wall proteins, glucosyl transferase and ribosomal antigens lack demonstrable cross reactivity, but further research is needed.

Routes of Protective Responses

Mucosal applications of dental caries vaccines are generally preferred for the induction of secretory IgA antibody in the salivary compartment, since this immunoglobulin constitutes the major immune component of major and minor salivary grand secretions.

a. *Oral:* Many of the earlier studies relied on oral induction of immunity in gut associated lymphoid tissue (GALT) to elicit protective salivary IgA antibody responses. In these studies, antigen was applied by oral feeding, gastric intubation or in vaccine containing capsules or liposomes. Although the oral route was not ideal for reasons including the detrimental effect of stomach acidity on antigen, or because inductive sites were relatively distant, experiments with this route established that induction of mucosal immunity alone was sufficient to change the course of mutans streptococcal infection and disease in animal models.

b. *Intra-nasal:* More recently, attempts have been made to induce protective immunity in mucosal inductive sites that are in closer anatomical relationship to the oral cavity. Intranasal installation of antigen, which targets the nasal associated lymphoid tissue (NALT) has been used to induce immunity to many bacterial antigens, including those associated with mutans streptococcal colonization and accumulation.

c. *Tonsillar:* The ability of tonsillar application of antigen to induce immune responses in the oral cavity is of great interest. Tonsillar tissue contains the required elements of immune induction of secretory IgA responses; although IgG, rather than IgA, response characteristics are dominant in this tissue. Nonetheless, the palatine tonsils, as especially the nasopharyngeal tonsils, have been suggested to contribute precursor cells to mucosal effector sites, such as salivary glands. Repeated tonsillar application of particular antigen can induce the appearance of IgA antibody-producing cells in both the major and minor salivary glands of the rabbit.

d. *Minor salivary gland:* The minor salivary glands populate the lips, cheeks and soft palate. These glands have been suggested as potential routes or mucosal induction of salivary immune responses given their short, broad secretory ducts that facilitates retrograde access of bacteria and their products, and given the lymphatic tissue aggregates that all often found associated with these ducts.

e. *Rectal:* More remote mucosal site has been investigated for their inductive potential. The colorectal region as an inductive location for mucosal immune responses in humans is suggested from the fact that this site has the highest zone of lymphoid follicles in the lower intestinal tract.

Mucosal routes of antigen delivery often require additional components which can potentiate aspects of the immune response to induce sufficient antibody to achieve a protective effect. These are:

• Cholera and *E.coli.*
• Heat labile enterotoxins
• Microcapsules and microparticles
• Liposomes

In comparison with parenteral administration, oral route seems to have many advantages.

• Easy to administer.
• Relative absence of side effects.

• Leads to development of IgA antibodies which are found in abundance in oral cavity.

Regulation of IgA system is only partly understood. One interesting observation is that infants who have frequent close maternal contacts in first year have significantly more IgA antibodies against Streptococcus mutans and EB virus. This observation indicates that orally administered antigens can stimulate the development of systemic antibodies as well, especially because antigenic molecules penetrate intestinal epithelial surfaces more easily in infants than in adults. This finding needs more exploration.

Caries Vaccines and Public Health

An important question is whether the research for caries vaccine is justified from public health point of view. This question is very critical as we already have effective means to control the disease. Also, Streptococcus mutans is not the only cariogenic micro-organism and that a series of factors influence the development of caries. So, the question arises, as to what extent successful vaccination against Streptococcus mutans can reduce the incidence of caries?

In a number of studies in Scandinavian countries where children are exposed to caries preventive programs from an early age, it has been seen that considerable caries reduction could be achieved. The successful vaccination directed against Streptococcus mutans could be a valuable adjunct to other caries preventive measures.

In third world countries a rapid increase in caries has been observed both in children and adults. Low dentist: population ratio and lack of organized dental health care system limit the possibility of utilizing conventional caries preventive methods. The existence of basic medical health care system might form a basis for use of caries vaccine as a very useful adjunct.

So the vaccination against dental caries could be a preventive adjunct in some societies and a major public health measure in others. However, the preventive regimen should be thoroughly analyzed including cost-benefit and risk-benefit, if any.

PIT AND FISSURE SEALANTS

Pit and fissure sealants, as the name implies, are the agents, which seal the pits and fissures. Pits and fissures are the potential site for the initiation of caries and are mostly located on occlusal surfaces of posterior teeth, buccal/lingual surfaces of molars and on lingual surfaces of anterior teeth.

The pits and fissures are formed as a result of improper union of developmental lobes during the formation of tooth structure. Occlusal pits and fissures vary in shape but are generally narrow and tortuous with invaginations where bacteria and food debris are retained. The pits and fissures have broadly been classified into four varieties:

- A shallow groove
- Complete penetration of the enamel
- The fissure may end blindly
- The end of fissure may open into an irregular chamber.

Saliva may not readily reach at the base of the fissures. An explorer tip or tooth brush bristle is too large to penetrate into the fissure, therefore the areas cannot be mechanically cleaned.

It has been documented that even fluorides are least effective in the prevention of pit and fissure caries. The possible reasons may be attributed to the inaccessibility of the fluorides to the base of pits and fissures.

Historical Evolution of Sealants

Before the advent of sealers, many techniques and procedures were tried to decrease the vulnerability of pits and fissures to caries.

i. *Extension for prevention:* Earlier authors were of the view that the cavity prepa-

rations should be extended to eliminate non-carious fissures also. The principle known as 'extension for prevention' is still being practiced, though to a lesser extent.

ii. *Prophylactic odontotomy:* Small amalgam restorations were placed in pits and fissures of newly erupted teeth before the appearance of clinical signs of decay.

iii. *Fissure eradication:* The pits and fissures were reshaped into wide non - retentive grooves rather than placing restorations. The dentin exposed by grinding would undergo secondary changes and become resistant to caries. These procedures could not gain popularity because of the reluctance of parents to get operative procedures performed on normal teeth. Further, considering the time and costs involved in such procedures, their applications on community basis were limited.

iv. *Application of impregnating solutions:* Ammoniacal silver nitrate solutions were applied so as to diffuse into enamel (may reach dentin) increasing the resistance of the area. Zinc chloride and Potassium ferrocyanide when applied were also reported to be effective in reducing caries. The impregnating solutions form protein complexes with the organic part of the tooth. The use of impregnating solutions was based on the belief that the primary route for the initiation of caries was by proteolytic action of organisms on the organic part of enamel. However, this concept was not accepted widely in the literature.

v. *Application of non-adhesive dental materials:* Zinc phosphate and Copper cements were used in an attempt to physically block pits and fissures. These materials had limited value due to their high solubility and poor retention on tooth structure.

A low viscosity material is applied to the pits and fissures in order to isolate them from the oral environment. The sealant acts as a physical barrier preventing oral bacteria and dietary carbohydrates from aggregating within the pits and fissures, subsequently the acids resulting in caries.

Requirements of Sealant Material

The sealant is not necessarily required to fill the entire depth of the fissure but it should bond firmly at the fissure orifice. The enamel-sealant interface should not exhibit any microleakage so as to prevent nutrients from diffusing to organisms remaining in the fissures and to prevent new organisms from entering into the fissures. Although, some bacteria seated within the fissures may remain viable for extended periods of time, they can not initiate caries if continuous source of fermentable carbohydrates is not provided.

The requirements of a sealant material are as follows:
* Adhesion to enamel for longer duration.
* Easy manipulation.
* Free flowing, i.e. capable of entering narrow fissures by capillary action.
* Non injurious to oral tissues.
* Rapidly polymerized.
* Low solubility in oral fluids.

Commonly used Sealant Materials

The commonly used sealant materials are:

   i. *Cyanoacrylates:* Methyl-2-cyanoacrylate with or without powdered filler particles has been used as sealant. The clinical studies showed mixed or negative results. The material is relatively unsuitable because of difficult handling characteristics and solubility in oral fluids.

   ii. *Polyurethane:* A polyurethane product, Epoxylite-9070, containing 10% disodium monofluoro-phosphate was used as a sealant. The material showed poor retention and solubility in oral fluids. A polyurethane resin containing amine fluoride is also being used. Even this material was not effective for longer duration.

Commercially available urethane dimethacrylate sealants are: *'Contact seal'* (chemically cured) and *'Helioseal'* (light cured).

   iii. *Bisphenol-glycydyl-methacrylate:* Bisphenol-glycydyl-methacrylate is the resin component of conventional composite resin materials. Bisphenol-glycydyl-methacrylate was diluted with methyl-methacrylate or other co-monomers to improve flow characteristics to be used as a sealant. The mixture undergoes less polymerization shrinkage and has a lower coefficient of thermal expansion than methyl-methacrylate alone and likely to form and maintain firm bonds with enamel.

The commercially available sealants are:
* Concise white sealant
* Delton
* NUVA-Seal I.A
* Oralin pit and fissure sealant
* Prisma-shield
* Visio-seal
* Duraphat
* Glass-ionomer cements

Use of Sealants in Individual Care Programs

Any individual having teeth are at risk of developing dental caries and should be considered for sealant applications. Under certain circumstances patients having caries in pits and fissures are given sealants therapy. Such sealants are referred to as *'Therapeutic sealants'*.

Although the sealants are usually placed in children, it is established that even the adolescent pits and fissures remain at risk. The goal of preventing caries by use of sealants is best accomplished by applying sealants to young teeth and placing *therapeutic sealants* on carious lesions that are limited to enamel.

The following factors affect the decision of sealant placement:

a. *Risk assessment of individuals:* The individuals in the society are assessed for being caries susceptible. Factors contributing for individual to be at risk include history, previous dental care, use of preventive practices in family and systemic problems. The use of sweetened medicines, health status and life style certainly influences an individual's caries risk.

b. *Risk assessment of teeth:* The individual's teeth at risk are to be assessed, e.g. level of caries activity, pits and fissures morphology, caries pattern and life expectancy of primary teeth. The proximal surfaces of the tooth, the eruption status and the ability to isolate adequately are also the key factors required for effective sealing. Further, the distribution of caries provides a clear indication of susceptibility of different teeth. It is suggested that first and second permanent molars are at risk for pit and fissure caries. The decision for pit and fissure sealing depends upon whether the teeth are caries free or exhibiting enamel/dentin caries:

   i. Caries free teeth

   ii. Teeth with enamel caries

   iii. Teeth with dentin caries

      i. **Caries free teeth:** The decision to seal a caries free surface is based upon potential of risk as influenced by pits and fissures morphology, eruption status, caries activity in the mouth and also teeth showing questionable caries.

      Pits and fissures morphology: The morphology of pits and fissures is a significant factor in predicting caries risk. It is stated that teeth with well coalesced pits and fissures and wide grooves do not require sealing. Teeth with deep pits and fissures are ideal candidates for sealants. Permanent molars have the most susceptible pits and fissures. Premolars are much less susceptible to occlusal caries. The need for sealants in first and second deciduous molars is determined by pits and fissures morphology and the life expectancy of the tooth. Sealants may be indicated on deciduous molars with evidence of caries activity or deep and/or stained fissures.

Eruption status: Earlier authors were of the view that the tooth should be sealed immediately after eruption. However, it is suggested that adequate isolation is essential for sealant retention and the success depends upon operator's ability to maintain a dry field. Whenever possible, it is recommended that the sealant placement be delayed until the tooth is sufficiently erupted.

The clinical and epidemiological data shows that the post eruptive age should not be used as a criterion for deciding whether a tooth should be sealed or not. The primary consideration should be the risk of the pit and fissure surfaces to caries coupled with an individual's overall susceptibility to caries.

Caries activity: If the caries activity in the mouth indicates susceptibility to caries, it is advised that the remaining caries free pits and fissures should also be sealed. If an individual demonstrates proximal caries activity, sealant is indicated for non carious occlusal surfaces. The conservation of occlusal surfaces should be considered during restoration of proximal surfaces.

Questionable caries: Many a times it become difficult to distinguish sound pits and fissures, from those with just initiated caries in enamel. Such teeth commonly referred to as *questionable caries*, would be considered at risk and should receive a sealant. A sealant placed over a carious lesion limited to enamel will prevent the progression of undiagnosed caries. Othewise, the sealant is helpful in the diagnosis of questionable caries, proves to be wrong.

ii. **Teeth with enamel caries:** The teeth with enamel caries demonstrate a white opaque appearance surrounding the pits or fissures. Current radiographic methods cannot detect enamel caries in pits and fissures until the lesion has reached the dentine. Sealants can be placed on enamel lesion to restrict the progress.

iii. **Teeth with dentin caries:** The progress of the caries in the dentine usually results in the collapse of at least part of the overlying enamel producing a readily identifiable clinical cavity. However, certain cases exhibit intact surface enamel, thus making it difficult to detect dentinal caries. Pits and fissures with definite caries in dentine should be restored conservatively after caries removal.

Use of Sealants in Communities

The communities often vary with respect to caries levels, treatment resources and the aptitude for prevention. The effective implementation of sealant program in a community involves the following steps.

1. Defining the community: The community means that the basic literacy level, aptitude towards disease and treatment, socio-economic status of the individuals must be known prior to implementing the sealant program.

2. Assessing the need for sealants: After defining the community, the need for sealants can be assessed from the prevalence of untreated pit and fissure caries and the level of control of proximal caries. This assessment can result from an epidemiologic survey or informal observations of the dental surgeons or clinic staff.

3. Assessing support and constraints: After assessing the need, the possible support and constraints should be analyzed. The general constraints are availability of people to work on the project coupled with the necessary funds. The other constraints can be if the state's dental act does not permit dental hygienist or assistant to apply sealants. In such cases, the support of dental surgeons will be required who can devote their time voluntarily.

4. Identifying teeth/tooth surfaces: The tooth surfaces and the individual teeth are to be identified. There are dental conditions that either place them at very low caries risk (e.g. no past caries history combined with well coalesced pits and grooves) or preclude sealant use (e.g. large proximal caries or restorations on all teeth with fissured surfaces). To identify tooth surfaces at higher risk is practically difficult. It is believed that first and second permanent molars are at greatest risk for pit and fissure caries. Although, occlusal surfaces are best suited for sealants applications, buccal pits of lower molars and lingual grooves of upper molars should also be sealed.

5. Implementing sealant program: If there is sufficient need of the sealant in the community, the program can be initiated selecting any of several approaches available for applying sealants in a community and the support and constraints are favourable.

Traditionally, sealant programs are utilized for school children; however, other

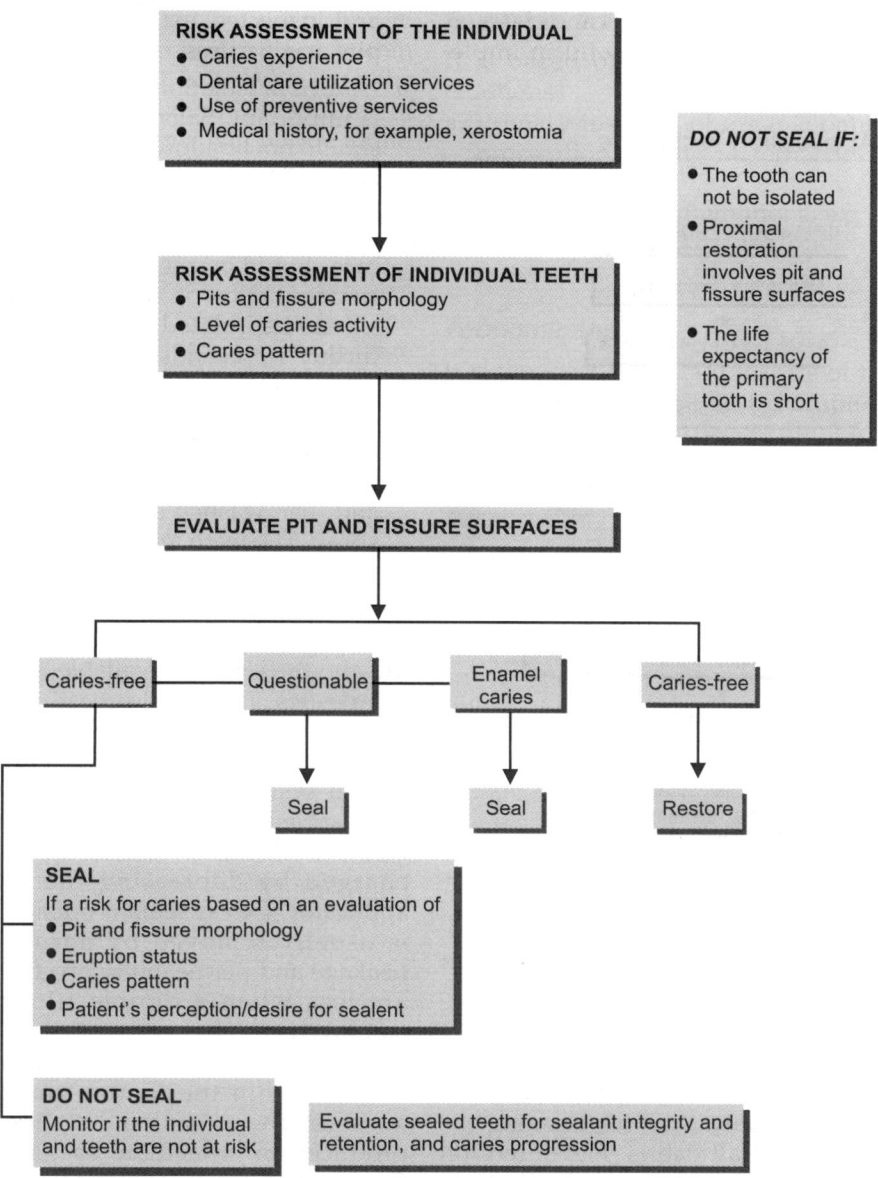

Fig. 16.2: Guidelines for sealant use in individual care programs

population groups may be candidates as well. Mobile van can be useful in implementing such programs.

Sealant Application Technique

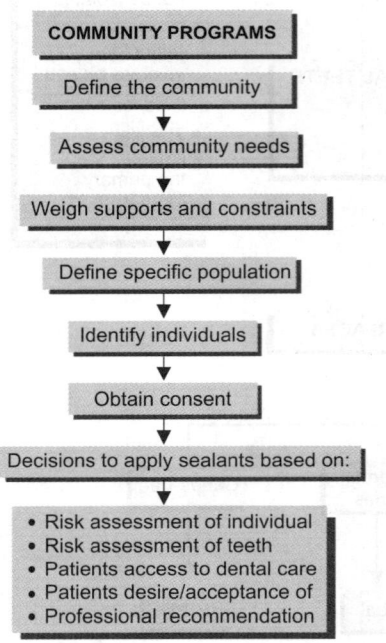

Fig. 16.3: Determinant of sealant use in community programs

The clinical technique for applying sealant involves the following steps:

1. Tooth Preparation

a. Prophylaxis: The fine pumice powder with water is commonly used for cleaning the tooth surface of all debris. Flavoured, oil based or fluoride containing prophylaxis pastes are not recommended since they adversely influence the conditioning of enamel. The pumice slurry can be applied with either the rubber cup or bristle brush rotating at slow speed. After the prophylaxis, the tooth is thoroughly washed and inspected for residual pumice in the pits and fissures.

b. Isolation: Isolation of the concerned tooth is important. Saliva or crevicular exudate should not be allowed to contact the enamel isolated for etching. A rubber dam offers the best means of isolation. Cotton rolls and saliva absorbers can provide a dry field but care should be exercised during change. If contamination occurs accidentally, the site should be isolated, cleaned and etched for further 10 seconds.

c. Acid etching: The isolated teeth are etched for 20-30 seconds with 37% phosphoric acid. The etchant is moved gently over the enamel surface with a cotton pellet or brush and then washed away using an air-water spray. The teeth are dried using an oil-free air spray.

2. Sealant Application

Mostly, the sealants available are light cured composites. The usual procedure is to apply primer first followed by the flowable resin into the pits and fissures. A system, known as Delton system utilizes an applicator with a disposable tube. The applicator tip is applied to the occlusal surface and sealant is discharged by depressing the level of the applicator. Excess sealant outside the fissure is usually removed by normal attrition. Leakage and permeability of a fissure sealant are less when a double film method is employed.

It has been documented that small lesions sealed within the tooth structure do not advance. The etchant and sealing procedure produces an immediate bactericidal effect. Gross reductions occur in the number of viable bacteria in carious dentin of sealed teeth. Chemical and radiographic findings indicate that incipient lesions in sealed teeth will not progress further. Carious teeth, however, should be treated according to conventional operative techniques.

LASER

'LASER' in simple term, is the light (L) amplification (A) of stimulated (S) emission (E) of radiation (R). These are heat producing devices converting electromagnetic energy into thermal energy. They work on the common principle of generation of monochromatic, coherent and collimated radiation by a suitable medium.

The basic difference of the lasers is in their wavelength, which varies with the medium used and the excitation mode. The different wavelengths in lasers can be classified into three groups:

- Ultra Violet (UV) Range : 140-400nm
- Visible Spectrum
  (VS) Range : 400-700nm
- Infra Red (IR) Range : >700nm

Different laser systems are classified according to the medium used and also the mode of their application:

1. Hard Lasers

These are used in surgical applications.

   i. CO_2 Lasers : (Laser Medium: CO_2 gas)

   ii. Nd: YAG Lasers : (Laser Medium: Yttrium Aluminium Garnet crystal dotted with Neodymium)

   iii. Argon Lasers : (Laser Medium: Argon ions)

2. Soft Lasers

These are used in biostimulation and analgesia.

   i. He-Ne Lasers

   ii. Diode Lasers

The newer lasers are:

   i. Pulsed Excimer Lasers

   ii. Q - switched Nd: YAG lasers

All lasers except the CO_2 lasers are transmitted by the glass fibers. The CO_2 lasers are transmitted via mirror systems. Excimer lasers can be transmitted by both systems, i.e. glass fibers and mirrors.

How lasers prevent caries?

The exact reasons for the inhibition of caries by laser pretreatments are still unknown, although the explanations are possible.

The acceptable hypothesis is:

- There is a specific set of laser irradiation that most efficiently and effectively interacts with dental tissues.
- The efficient conversion of light to heat will result in increased resistance of tooth mineral to dissolution by acid.

Initially, lasers were used for drilling and cutting of enamel; subsequently, it was discovered that low energy density lasers partially inhibited caries formation without causing any damage to pulp or oral mucosa. And also lasers decrease the rate of subsurface demineralization in enamel.

The following attributes are desirable for the clinical application of lasers in caries prevention:

a. Minimum energy density to avoid the damages of the soft tissues and the dental pulp.

b. An ability to easily lead the laser beam to the restricted area of the oral cavity by means of a flexible beam guide.

When enamel is exposed to the appropriate dose of routinely used laser irradiation, its surface structure is altered, making it more resistant to acid demineralization. However, because of its high peak power, the laser beam cannot be guided with a conventional optical fiber. Thus, it requires manipulations, which makes it impractical for clinical use.

Use of Nd:YAG laser irradiation lead to increased enamel transparency in the lased area. The lased enamel area showed no subsurface demineralization. The temperature rise at the pulp was 20°C. This system has clinical applications in prevention of dental caries.

The morphology, histology and crystallography of human dental enamel treated with infrared laser radiation were studied. Tetra calcium diphosphate mono-oxide was identified as being a component of the surface reduced carbonate content, when compared to normal surface enamel.

It is reported that Argon laser irradiation of sound root surface significantly increases the resistance of cementum to demineralization.

Summarily, lasers lead to reduced permeability and reduced solubility of enamel.

Unlased enamel has natural and acquired surface defects like cracks, fissures, pores, etc. that act as pathways for demineralizing agents. Lasers, partially fuse or close the enamel surface defects; thereby creating a barrier to demineralizing agents. Irradiation at higher energy densities is more effective than those performed at lower energy densities.

Laser causes dissolution of crystal structure of enamel followed by re-crystallization and growth of hydroxyapatite. It has been observed that lasing in the presence of sodium fluoride was more beneficial since re-crystallization in the presence of fluoride resulted in the formation of fluorapatite, which is less soluble than normal enamel. Laser causes changes in the composition of enamel that reduces its solubility. Laser leads to loss of carbonate and water from enamel, subsequently decrease in enamel solubility. Lased enamel shows protein denaturation and swelling within enamel pores resulting in decreased permeability to acids.

It is established that lased dentin produce superficial sealed layer which make it more acid resistant. The sealed dentin had no tubular structure and the mineral content of the sealed layer was increased. The increase in mineral content was attributed to the burning off of the organic matter from the site.

Laser leads to the formation of craters in dentin. The wall of the crater showed the formation of two radio-opaque layers, one the outer hypermineralized zone and the second the inner hypermineralized zone.

Laser irradiation could be developed into an effective tool for the prevention of dental caries and reducing its rate of progression.

NEWER TECHNIQUES

a. Replacement Therapy

Replacement therapy is a newer modality for prevention of dental caries in which the pathogenic organisms are so mutated as to lose their virulence. The enormous number of bacterial species in oral flora may not lead to frequent manifestations of disease. The host-parasite relationships, which are inherently unstable, become stable over a period of time because of mutations. These mutations results in decreased virulence. In such a state the parasite becomes a part of normal flora after losing its virulence. Similarly, in dental caries the mutations in Streptococcus may make it a organism with no virulence; however, the process may take over thousands of years. In replacement therapy the evolutionary process is speeded-up and the mutations are made in pathogenic organism producing the 'effector strain'. The qualities of this strain are:

- It colonizes same niche in susceptible host tissue that is normally colonized by the pathogen and hence block the attachment sites of the pathogen.
- It will compete with the pathogen for same nutrients so as not to permit the pathogen to grow and survive in the host tissue.
- It should be able to displace the already existing pathogen in the host, so that the therapy can also be used for the treatment of already infected host.
- It should be safe and not predispose the host to any disease.
- Exhibits low pathogenicity.

Earlier also, replacement therapy was tried to treat tuberculosis by using a harmless organism referred to as 'bacto-termo'. Since then, the use of bacteria to fight against bacteria, have been experimented.

In dental caries, according to Miller's acidogenic theory, lactic acid production by Streptococcus mutans is considered the main pathogenic mechanism. So, if a strain is produced which do not possess gene for lactate dehydrogenase (LDH) enzyme, can result in reduced pathogenecity for caries. This approach worked well for Streptococcus rattus, but in Streptococcus mutans the same mutations could not be produced. LDH deficient mutants of various strains of Streptococcus mutans were not found using the same screening methods which were used to isolate the mutants of Streptococcus rattus. However, the exceptionally different strains had some mutations that affected pryuvate metabolism which can be demonstrated by their unusually high production of ethanol, acetate and acetone, when grown in limiting glucose. These strains were mutable to LDH deficiency. In other strains, LDH deficiency was proved to be lethal because of toxic effects of glucose metabolism. This toxic effect can be neutralized by limiting the amount of glucose. It is established that supplemental alcohol dehydrogenase (ADH) activity can complement LDH deficiency. With this knowledge, a mutant of Streptococcus mutans, i.e. BCS3-L1 was created which was deficient in LDH gene with incorporated ADH gene from Zymomonas mobilis. The apparent strains (Streptococcus mutans) used was JH1140. The effector strain so produced, i.e. BCS3-L1 has no measureable LDH activity but 10-fold elevated level of ADH activity.

Another property which BCS3-L1 possess is the production of a bacteriocin called 'mutacin-1140'. Mutacin-1140, a member of a small class of antibiotics called lantibiotics, contains modified amino acids, lanthionine, methyllanthione, didehydroalanine and didehydrobutyrine. For BCS3-L1 to serve as an effector strain for replacement therapy it should be safe and genetically stable. Spontaneous reversion is unlikely because of deletion of LDH gene; however, horizontal transmission f LDH gene is possible, which assures BCS3-L1 its long-term stability.

Advantages

- No need for patient compliance
- Easy to sue
- Spontaneous resistance to mutacin 1140 does not occur readily in sensitive species
- Possibility of bacteremia (in prone patients) can be reduced by directing the cells away from gingival sulcus and any mucosal lesion.
- Vertical transmission of BCS3-L1 is possible so treatment of one generation would lead to protection of future generations.

Disadvantages

- Mutacin production and change in fermentation products resulting from LDH deficiency can upset plaque ecology and can lead to growth of other pathogenic microorganisms.
- Minimal infectious dose has not been determined for any Streptococcus mutans strains in humans.

b. NovaMin Technology

It has been hypothesized that as people age, hydroxyl carbonate apatite (HCA) crystals of enamel become more polarized, resulting in a somewhat more translucent enamel. This allows natural off-white colour of underlying dentin to shine through resulting in yellow/grey colour of teeth. The NovaMin is intended to reverse the effect of age on teeth by employing the rebuilding materials. NovaMin is the only man-made mineral which can lead to formation of essential hydroxyapatite crystals.

NovaMin, available as white powder, is an amorphous, sodium calcium phosphosilicate that was developed to physically occlude dentinal tubules. Reaction of NovaMin particles began when the material is subjected to an aqueous environment. Sodium ions immediately begin to exchange with H^+ or H_3O^+. This rapid release of ions allows calcium and phosphate in particle structure to be released from it. Release of calcium and phosphate continues as long as particles are exposed to aqueous environment. Localised transient increase in pH helps to precipitate calcium and phosphate from NovaMin, as well as saliva to form calcium-phosphate layer. This layer crystallizes to hydroxyl carbonate apatite (HCA) which is chemically and biologically equivalent to normal enamel hydroxyapatite.

Properties

- Odourless
- Biocompatible
- Promotes re-mineralization
- NovaMin helps in tooth whitening by formation of new disorganized HCA crystals.
- It helps to relieve dentinal hypersentitivity.
- When mixed with water, it has a strong antimicrobial action against periodontal pathogens.
- It possesses local anti-inflammatory action, so reduce gingivitis.

c. Bacteriocin Like Inhibitory Substances (BLIS)

The term 'bacteriocin' was initially used to described antibacterial proteins (colocins) produced by some strains of E. coli that inhibits growth of other E. coli.

BLIS was introduced to describe a variety of incompletely characterized proteinaceous inhibitors produced by gram-positive bacteria that are able to kill closely related bacteria by interfering with their metabolic activity, replication or viability.

d. Biotene

It is an oral moistening spray containing five moisturizers, eight amino acids along with milk products to recreate natural protection. It is generally used in xerostomic patients.

PREVENTION OF ROOT CARIES

With the increase in retention of permanent teeth in adults, the problem of root caries is also increasing. The preventive aspects of root caries can be divided into three aspects as in prevention of occlusal caries.

It has been established that the count of 10^6 mutans streptococci/ml of saliva could be considered an elevated risk of root caries. The periodontal treatment also results in exposed root surfaces which can be considered as high risk sites. Depending upon the mutans level, the patients are divided into three categories, i.e. low risk, medium risk and high risk (Tables 16.3 and 16.4).

i. **Low risk group:** Patients with exposed root surfaces without lesions and low salivary mutans streptococci levels fall under low risk group. For these patients, prevention should be accordingly oral hygiene and diet. The use of fluoride tooth paste is sufficient for these patients.

ii. **Medium risk group:** Those patients who have developed a low number of root caries lesions over a relatively long period of time and with low number of mutans streptococci in their saliva. Patients receiving periodontal treatment can be included in these groups. For this group, additional fluoride groups become necessary such as fluoride varnishes.

iii. **High risk group:** This group consists of patients who have several active root caries lesions, which have developed in a short period of time. Even restoration is not successful because new lesions develop at the margins very soon.

For all these patients, the prevention should be intensified and reinforced with the use of chlorehexidine varnishes or gels along with other preventive measures (Table 16.4).

Table 16.3: Distribution of patients into root caries risk groups and appropriate prevention level

Risk Group	Patients Criteria	Prevention Level
Low Risk	Low MS levels of saliva Exposed root surfaces without root caries	Information of the consequences of root exposure Oral hygiene and diet instruction Use of fluoride toothpaste
Medium Risk	Low MS levels of saliva Developing a low number of root caries lesions in a relatively long time Having inactive root caries lesions Receiving periodontal treatment	As for low risk group but with additional fluoride applications.
High Risk	High MS level of saliva Having several active root caries lesions Developing enamel caries Wearing an overdenture supported by natural teeth	As for medium risk group but with applications of chlorhexidine.

Low levels of mutans streptococci in saliva = < 10^6 ml saliva
High levels of mutans streptococci in saliva = >10^6 ml saliva
MS : mutans streptococci

Table 16.4: Caries risk and modalities for prevention

Risk category	Motivation for Child/Adolescent
Low	Good oral hygiene and use of fluoride dentifrices followed by periodic recalls.
Medium	Use of oral hygiene measures Dietary counseling Fluoride mouthrinse Professional topical fluoride Sealants Brush with fluoride dentifrice
High	Use of oral hygiene measures Brush with fluoride dentifrice Sealants Home fluoride (mouthrinse/ 1.1 percent soldium fluoride gel) Topical fluoride application Dietary counseling Antimicrobial agents

Application of fluorides is important, especially immediately after root planning. Fluorides in combination with lanthanides are more affective. Dentinal adhesives also prevent initiation of caries for a prolonged period. Administration of low dose of doxycyclines

(20 mg twice a day) for three months has been reported to reduce gingival crevicular fluid flow, subsequently root caries.

Recently, coverage of root surfaces with connective tissue grafts has shown promising results. Gingival recession as well as caries were prevented.

BIBLIOGRAPHY

1. Acharya, S : Specific caries index : A new system for describing untreated dental caries experience in developing countries. J. Public Health Dent. : 66, 285, 2006.
2. Anderson, M.H., Bales, D.J. and Omnell, K.A. : On the prevention of caries and periodontal disease : results of 15 years longitudinal study in adults. J. Clin. Period. : 18, 182, 1991.
3. Anderson, M.H., Bales, D.J. and Omnell, K.A. : Modern management of Dental Caries : the cutting edge is not the dental bur. J.A.D.A. : 124, 37, 1993.
4. Aranda, M. and Garcia,-Godoy, F. : Clinical evaluation of the retention and wear of a light cured pit and fissure glass-ionomer sealant. J.C. Pediat. Dent. : 19, 273, 1995.
5. Axelsson, P. and Lindhe, J. : Effect of controlled oral hygiene on caries and periodontal disease in adults. J. Clin. Period. : 5, 133, 1978.
6. Autio-Gold, J.T. : Clinical evaluation of a medium filled flowable restorative material as a pit and fissure sealant. Oper. Dent. : 27, 325, 2002.
7. Bader, J.D., Perrin, N.A., Moupome, G., Rindal, B. and Rush, W.A. : Validation of a simple approach to caries risk assessment. J. Public Health Dent. : 65, 76, 2005.
8. Banting, D.W. and Stamm, J.W. : Effect of age and length of residence in a fluoridated area on root surface fluoride concentration. Clin. Prevent. Dent. : 1, 7, 1979.
9. Beighton, D. Lynch. E. and Health, M.R. : A microbiological study of primary root caries lesions with different treatment needs. J. Dent. Res.: 72, 623, 1993.
10. Beiruti, N., Frencken, J.E., Van't Hoff, M.A. and Helderman, P. : Caries preventive effect of resin based and glass-ionomer sealants overtime : a systematic review. Comm. Dent. Oral Epidem. : 34, 403, 2006.
11. Bellini, H.T., Arneberg, P. and Vonder, F.R. : Oral hygiene and caries : A review. Acta. Odont. Scand. : 39, 257, 1981.
12. Benn, D. : Applying evidence based dentistry to caries management : a computerized approach. J.A.D.A. : 133, 1543, 2002.
13. Berkowitz, R.J. : Causes, treatment and prevention of early childhood caries : A microbiological perspective. J. Can. Dent. Assoc. : 69, 304, 2003.
14. Birkhed, D. : Cariological aspects of xylitol and its use in chewing gums – a review. Acta. Odon. Scand. : 52, 1, 1994.
15. Bjarnason, S : High caries levels : problems still to be tackled. Acta. Odont. Scand. : 56, 176, 1998.
16. Bodecker, C.F. : The eradications of enamel fissures. Dent. Items: 51, 859, 1929.
17. Bowen, W.H. : A vaccine against dental caries. A pilot experiment on monkeys. B.D.J.: 126, 159, 1969.
18. Bravo, M., Osorio, E., Garcia-Anllo, I. and Liodra, J.C. : The influence of dft index on sealant success : A 48 months survival analysis. J. Dent. Res.: 75, 768, 1996.
19. Breton, R. and Trahan, L. : Emergence of xylitol-resistant mutans of mutans streptococci from growth at the expense of fructose or sucrose. J. Dent. Res.: 71, 733, 1992.
20. Broadbent, J.M. and Thomson, W.M. : For debate : problems with the DMF index pertinent to dental caries data analysis. Comm. Dent. Oral Epidem. : 33, 409, 2005.
21. Buonocore, M.G. : Principles of adhesive retention and adhesive restoration materials. J. A. D. A. : 61, 382, 1963.
22. Burt, B.A. : Fissure sealants : Clinical and economic factors. J. Dent. Educ. : 48, 96, 1984.
23. Burt, B.A. : Cost effectiveness of sealants in private practice and standard for use in prepared.: J.A.D.A. 110, 103, 1985.
24. Burt, B.A. and Pai, S : Does low birth weight increases the risk of caries : A systematic review. J. Dent. Educ. : 65, 1024, 2001.
25. Carlson, J., Grahnen, H., Johnson, G. and Case, D. : Lactobacilli and streptococci in the mouth of children. Caries. Res. : 9, 339, 1975.
26. Centinaro, R., Puppin-Rontani, R.M., Komati, M. and Baglioni, M.E. : Comparative study of the effectiveness and retention of occlusal

sealing with a fluoroshield and fuji IX. J. Dent. Res. : 79, 1101, 2000.

27. Chalmers, J.M. and Carter, K.D. : Caries incidence and increments in community living older adults with and without dementia. Gerodontology : 19, 80, 2002.

28. Courson, F., Renda, A.M., Attal, J.P., Bounter, D., Ruse, D. and Degrange, M. : In vitro evaluation of different techniques of enamel preparation for pit and fissure sealing. J. Adhes. Dent. : 5, 313, 2003.

29. Deasy, M.J., Singh, S.M. and Kashuba, B. : Antiplaque effects of dentifrices containing triclosan/copolymer/NaF system versus triclosan dentifrices without the copolymer. Am. J. Dent. : 3, 7, 1991.

30. DeForge, H. : Endodontic treatment with Novamin. Proceedings of 11th Annual Veterinary Dental Forum and Veterinary Dentistry 97. October 30-November 2, 1997.

31. Esteves-Oliveira, M., Zezell, D.M., Meister, j., Franzen, R., Stanzel, s., Lampert, F., Eduardo, C.P. and Apel, C.: CO_2 Laser (10.6μm) Parameters for caries prevention in dental enamel. Caries Res. 43, 261, 2009.

32. Fardal, O. and Turnbull, R.S. : A review of literature on use of chlorhexidine in dentistry. J. Am. Dent. Assoc. : 112, 863, 1986.

33. Featherstone, J.D.B. and Nelson, D.G.A. : Laser effects on dental hard tissues. Adv. Dent. Res. : 1, 21, 1987.

34. Feigal, R.J. : The use of pit and fissure sealants. Pediat. Dent. : 24, 415, 2002.

35. Feigal, R.J. and Quelhon, I. : Clinical trial of a self-etching adhesive for sealant application : success at 24 months with prompt L-pop. Am. J. Dent. : 16, 249, 2003.

36. Fejerskov, O. : Recent advances in the treatment of root surface caries. Int. Dent. J. : 44, 139, 1994.

37. Firestone, A.R., Schmid, R. and Muhlemann, H.R. : Effect of the length and number of intervals between meals on caries in rats. Caries Res. : 18, 128, 1984.

38. Fox, J.L., Yu, D., Otsuka, M., Higuchi, W.I., Wong, J. and Powell, G. : Combined effects of laser irradiation and chemical inhibitors on the dissolution of dental enamel. Caries Res.: 26, 333, 1992.

39. Fox, J.L., Yu, D., Otsuka, M., Higuchi, W.I., Wong, J. and Powell, G. : Initial dissolution rate studies on dental enamel after CO_2 laser irradiation. J.D.R. : 71, 1389, 1992.

40. Frentzen, M. and Koort, H.J. : Lasers in dentistry : new possibilities with advancing laser technology. Int. Dent. J. : 40, 323, 1990.

41. Frostell, G., Blomloff, L., Blomquist, T. : Substitution of sucrose by lycasin in candy. Acta. Odont. Scand. : 32, 235, 1974.

42. Gaffar A., Afflitto J., Nabi N., Heries S., Kruger, I. and Olsen, S. : Recent advances in plaque, gingivitis, tartar and caries prevention technology. Int. Dent. J. : 44, 63, 1994.

43. Gustaffson, B.E., Quensel, C.E., Lanke, L., Lundquist, C., Grahnen, H., Bonow, B.E. and Krase, B. : The vipeholm dental caries study. The effect of different levels of carbohydrate intake on caries activity in 436 individuals observed for five years. Acta. Odont. Scand. : 11, 232, 1954.

44. Hallett, K.B. and O'Rourke, P.K. : Social and behavioural determinants of early childhood caries. Aust. Dent. J. : 48, 27, 2003.

45. Hallett, K.B. and O'Rourke, P.K. : Pattern and severity of early childhood caries. Comm. Dent. Oral Epidem. : 34, 25, 2006.

46. Hansel-Petersson, G., Fure, S and Brathall, D. : Evaluation of a computer based caries risk assessment program in an elderly group of individuals. Acta. Odontol. Scand. : 61, 164, 2003.

47. Harris, R., Nicoll, A.D., Adair, I.M. and Pine, C.M. : Risk factors for dental caries in young children : a systematic review of the literature. Comm. Dent. Health : 21, 71, 2004.

48. Hillman, J.D. : Replacement therapy of dental caries. Operative Dentistry Supplement: 6, 39, 2001.

49. Horowitz, A.M. : Dental sealants in the prevention of tooth decay. J. Dent. Educ. : 1, 1984.

50. Ikeda, T., Sandham, H.J., Bradley, E.L. Jr. : Changes in Streptococcus mutans and lactobacilli in relation to the initiation of dental caries in Negro children. Arch. Oral Biol. : 18, 55, 1973.

51. Ismail, A.I. : Determinants of health in children and the problem of early childhood caries. Pediat. Dent. : 25, 328, 2003.

52. Kantola, S. : Laser induced effects on tooth structure in a study of changes in calcium and phosphorous contents in dentin by electron probe analysis. Acta. Odont. Scand. : 30, 463, 1992.

53. Katz, R.V. : Assessing root caries in populations : The evolution of a root caries index. J. Public Dent. Health : 40, 7, 1980.

54. Kawanabe : Non cariogenicity of erythritol as a substrate. Caries Res. : 26, 241, 1992.

55. Keltzens, H., Schacken, T. and Hoeven, H. : Preventive aspects of root caries. Int. Dent. J. : 43, 143, 1993.

56. Kleber, C.J., and Putt, M.S.: Aluminium and dental caries. A review of literature. Clin. Prev. Dent. : 6, 14, 1984.

57. Krasse, B., Emilson, C.G. and Johnberg, L. : An anti-caries vaccine - report on the status of research. Caries Res. : 21, 255, 1987.

58. de Luca-fraga, L.R. and Pimenta, L.A. : Clinical evaluation of glass-ionomer/resin based hybrid materials used as pit and fissure sealants. Quint. Int. : 32, 463, 2001.

59. Lawrence, H.P., Beck, J.D., Hunt, R.J. and Koch, G.G. : Adjustment of the M-component of the DMFS index for prevalence studies in older adults. Comm. Dent. Oral Epidem. : 24, 322, 1996.

60. Locker, D., Jokovic, A. and Kay, E.J. : Prevention Part 8 : The use of pit and fissure sealants in preventing caries in the permanent dentition of children. B.D.J. : 195, 375, 2003.

61. Loesche, W., Rown, J., Straffon, L.H., Loos, P.J. : Association of Streptococcus mutans with human dental decay. Infect. Immunity: 11, 1252, 1975.

62. Lupi-Pegurier, L., Muller-Bolla, M., Betrand, M.F., Fradet, T. and Bolla, M. : Microleakage of a pit and fissure sealant : effect of air abrasion compared with classical enamel preparations. J. Adhes. Dent. : 6, 43, 2004.

63. Lussi, A., Megert, B., Eggenburger, D. and Jaeggi, T. : Impact of different toothpastes on the prevention of erosion. Caries Res. : 42, 62, 2008.

64. Mandel, I.D. : Caries prevention - current strategies, New directions. J.A.D.A. : 127, 1477, Oct. 96.

65. Mandel, Irwin, D. : Caries prevention. Current strategies, New directions. J.A.D.A. : 127, 1477, 1996.

66. Manton, D.J. and Messer, L.B. : Pit and fissure sealants : Another major cornerstone in preventive dentistry. Aust. Dent. J. : 40, 22, 1995.

67. Marja-Leena, M., Paivi, R., Sirkka, J., Ansa, O. and Matti, S : Childhood caries is still in force : a 15-year follow-up. Acta. Odont. Scand. : 66, 189, 2008.

68. Marthalder, T.M. : Changes in dental caries 1953-2003. Caries Res. : 30, 173, 2004.

69. Mattila, M.L., Rantava, P., Aromaa, M., Ojanlatua, A., Paunio, P. and Hyssala, L. : Behavioural and demographic factors during early childhood and poor dental health at 10 years of age. Caries Res. : 39, 85, 2005.

70. Mc Donald, S.P., Cowell, C.R. and Sheiham, A. : Methods of preventing dental caries used by dentists for their own children. B.D.J. : 151, 118, 1981.

71. Mc Ghee, J.R. : Effect of immune bovine milk on Streptococcus mutans in human dental plaque. Arch. Oral Bio. : 36, 41, 1991.

72. Mejare, I., Lingstrom, P., Petersson, L.G., Holm, A.K., Twefman, S. and Kallestal, C. : Caries preventive effect of fissure sealants : a systematic review. Acta. Odontol. Scand. : 61, 321, 2003.

73. Morphis, T.L., Toumba, K.J. and Lygidakis, N.A. : Fluoride pit and fissure sealants : a review. Int. J. Pediat. Dent. : 10, 90, 2000.

74. Muller-Bolla, M., Lupi Pegurier, L., Tardeiar, C., Velly, A.M. and Automarchi, C. : Retention of resin-based pit and fissure sealants : a systematic review. Comm. Dent. Oral Epidem. : 34, 321, 2006.

75. Murray, J.J. and Williams, B. : Fissure sealants and dental caries : A review. J. Dent. : 3, 145, 1975.

76. Nguyen, L., Hakkinen, U., Knuuttila, M. and Jarvelin, M.R. : Should we brush twice a day ? Determinants of dental health among young adults in Finland. Health Econ. : 17, 267, 2008.

77. Oliviera, F.S, Silva, S.M. and Machado, MAAM : Vitremer and Delton as occlusal sealants : retention vs. application technique. J.D.R. : 81, 454, 2002.

78. Plenihakkinen, K., Soderling, E. and Ostela, I. : Comparison of the efficacy of 40% chlorhexidine varnish and 10% chlorhexidine fluoride gel in decreasing the level of salivary Streptococcus mutans. Caries Res.: 29, 62, 1995.

79. Quinonez, R., Santos, R.G., Wilson, S and Cross, H. : The relationship between child temperament and early childhood caries. Pediat. Dent. : 23, 5, 2001.

80. Rajtboriraks, D., Nakornchai, S, Bunditsing, P., Surarit, R. and Iemjaren,P. : Plaque and saliva fluoride levels after placement of fluoride releasing pit and fissure sealants. Pediat. Dent. : 26, 63, 2004.

81. Retlief, D.H., Cleaton-Jones, P.E. and Walker, A.R.P. : Dental caries and sugar intake in South African pupils of 16-17 years in four ethnic groups. B. D. J. : 138, 463, 1975.

82. Ripa, L.W. : The current status of pit and fissure sealants : a review. J. Can. Dent. Assoc. : 5, 367, 1985.

83. Ripa, L.W. and Wolf, M.S. : Preventive restoration : indication, technique and success. Quint. Int. : 23, 307, 1992.

84. Rogers, A.H. : Immunization against dental caries. A review. Aust. Dent. J. : 27, 81, 1982.

85. Scheinin, A., Scheinin, U. and Glan, R.L. : Xylitol induced changes of enamel microhardness in the human mouth. Acta. Odont. Scand. : 51, 241, 1993.

86. Seow, W.K. : Biological mechanism of early childhood caries. Comm. Dent. Oral Epidem.: 26, 8, 1998.

87. Simons, D., Kidd, E.A.M. and Beighton, D. and Jones, B. : The effect of chlorhexidine xylitol chewing gum on cariogenic salivary microflora : A clinical trial in elderly patients. Caries Res. : 31, 91, 1997.

88. Simonsen, R.J. : Glass-ionomer as fissure sealant - a critical review. J. Public Health Dent. : 56, 146, 1996.

89. Simonsen, R.J. : Pit an fissure sealants : review of the literature. Pediat. Dent. : 24, 393, 2002.

90. Slade, G.D. and Caplan, D.J. : Methodological issues in longitudinal epidemiologic studies of dental caries. Comm. Dent. Oral Epidem. : 27, 236, 1999.

91. Sonni, M.W. : The effect of zinc containing chewing gum on volatile sulphur containing compounds in the oral cavity. Acta. Odont. Scand. : 55, 198, 1997.

92. Swift, E.J. : The effect of sealants on dental caries : a review. J.A.D.A. : 116, 700, 1988.

93. Tanzer, M. Jason : Xylitol chewing gum and dental caries. Int. Dent. J. : 45, 65, 1995.

94. Tellesen, G., Larsen, G., Kalighithi, R., Zimmerman, J.G. and Wikesjo, M.E. : Use of chlorhexidine chewing gum significantly reduces dental plaque formation compared to use of similar xylitol and sorbitol products. J. Period. : 67, 181, 1996.

95. Tenovuo, J. and Soderling, E. : Chemical aids in the prevention of dental disease in the elderly. Int. Dent. J. : 42, 355, 1992.

96. Trahan, L. : Xylitol : a review of its action on mutans streptococci and dental plaque and its chemical significance. Int. Dent. J. : 45 (Suppl.), 77, 1995.

97. Tranaeus, Shi, X.Q. and Mansson, B.A. : Caries risk assessment : methods available to clinicians for caries detection. Comm. Dent. Oral Epidem. : 33, 265, 2005.

98. Vachirarojpisan, T., Shinada, K., Kawaguchi, Y., Laungwechaken, P. and Somokote, T. : Early childhood caries in children aged 6-19 months. Comm. Dent. Oral Epidem. : 32, 133, 2004.

99. Vanobbergen, J., Martins, L., Lesaffre, E., Bogaerts, K. and Declerek, D. : Assessing risk indicators for dental caries in the primary dentition. Comm. Dent. Oral Epidem. : 29, 424, 2001.

100. Van Houte, J. : Role of microorganisms in caries etiology. J. Dent. Res. : 73, 672, 1994.

101. Waggoner, W.F. and Seigal, M. : Pit and fissure sealants application updating the technique. J.A.D.A. : 127, 351, 1996.

102. Walker, C. : Efefct of sanguinarine extracts on the microbiota associated with the oral cavity. J. Can. Dent. Assoc. : 7, 513, 1990 (suppl.).

103. Wennerholm, K., Arends, J. and Birkhed, D. : Effect of xylitol and sorbitol in chewing gums on mutans streptococci, plaque and mineral loss of enamel. Caries. Res. : 28, 48, 1994.

104. Westerman, G.H., Hicks, M.J., Flaitz, C.M., Blankenaur, R.J., Powell, G.L. and Berg, J.H. : Argon laser irradiation in root surface caries. J.A.D.A. : 125, 401, 1994.

105. White, B. and Maupome, G. : Clinical decision making for dental caries management. J. Dent. Educ. : 65, 1127, 2001.

106. Zero, D., Fontana, M. and Lennon, A. : Clinical application and outcomes using indicators of risk in caries management. J. Dent. Educ. : 65, 1126, 2001.

17 *Prevention of Malocclusion*

The term malocclusion implies that the physiological occlusion is disturbed leading to abnormal contacts of the teeth. The abnormal contacts, many a times, do not disturb the routine functioning and are only esthetically displeasing. The causes of malocclusion are many and their description is beyond the scope of this book. The management of malocclusion, as the orthodontists have various treatment modalities, the preventive aspects begins with the management of jaw spaces. The pattern of eruption and shedding of deciduous teeth, growth of jaws and the presence/absence of developmental anomalies in any individual is to be assessed before planning for preventive aspects.

The preventive regimen is divided into following three features:

- Preventive orthodonotics
- Interceptive othodontics
- Corrective orthodontics

Preventive Orthodontics

Preventive orthodontics is an action taken to preserve the integrity of the functional occlusion at a specific time. It includes early correction of carious lesions (especially proximal caries) that might change the arch length, early recognition and elimination of oral habits which interfere with normal development of teeth and the jaws, the space maintainers designed to maintain proper positions of contiguous teeth, space regainers, muscle exercises, maintenance of a tooth shedding time and functional analysis. The patients' motivation and education are also a part of preventive orthodontics.

Interceptive Orthodontics

Interceptive orthodontics recognizes and eliminates potential irregularities and malpositions in the developing dentofacial complex.

Interceptive orthodontics includes habit consultation, removal of supernumerary teeth, slicing of mesial surfaces of deciduous cuspids, use of space maintainers, space regainers, labial shields, frenectomies, swallowing exercises and extraction of deciduous teeth as part of serial extraction procedures.

In case of preventive orthodontics, the occlusion is within normal limits where as interceptive orthodontics 'intercepts' a developing malocclusion and the goal is to restore the same to normal occlusion.

Corrective Orthodontics

Corrective orthodontics includes all the technical procedures employed to reduce or eliminate the malocclusion.

The **preventive procedures** vary, depending upon the classification of malocclusion. Angle's classification is followed for convenience. The procedures are as follows:

Class I Type I

- In mild cases slight slicing of the deciduous teeth can be carried out adjacent to erupting permanent teeth.

- Space for first premolar is established by slicing the mesial surface of the second primary molar.
- Separating wires can be helpful on either side of the erupting teeth.

Class I Type 2

Tongue thrusting and sucking are the habits responsible for such types of occlusion.

- The most simple and commonly employed method is the use of oral screen (Fig. 17.1). The oral screen corrects the occlusion and help mouth breathers to refrain from this habit.

  The oral screen is fabricated from plexiglass, fits the vestibule of the mouth and transfers the pressure from the lips to the teeth. Prior to the insertion of screen, the patient should be thoroughly examined for nasal obstruction.
- Another habit breaking appliance is the lingual arch with prongs, which hide the sucking process. The palatal crib with or without spurs are effective and useful measures in stopping thumb sucking. Sometimes bitter lotions are also useful for breaking these habits.

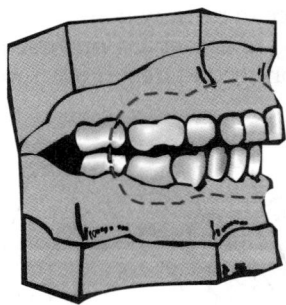

Fig. 17.1: Construction of an oral screen

Class I Type 3

This type of malocclusion can be corrected with the use of inclines (Fig. 17.2a). There must

be adequate space for the maxillary anterior teeth to move labially or for both upper and lower teeth to move reciprocally. The incline planes can be fabricated in acrylic or alternatively steel crowns (Fig. 17.2b) can also be used. The following features affect the success of the treatment:

i. Preferably one or two teeth should be involved.

ii. The initial contact position should be slightly posterior to the fully closed position.

iii. There must be space for the tooth to move.

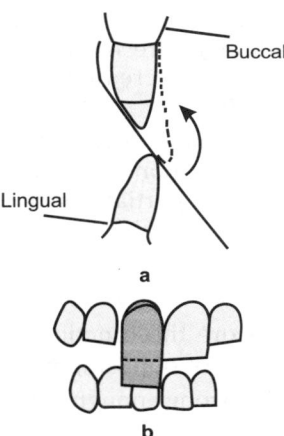

Fig. 17.2a, b: a. Banded incline plane to correct anterior cross-bite; b. Steel crown to correct anterior cross-bite

Class I Type 4

- If both maxillary and mandibular molars contribute to a crossbite, a crossbite elastic fixed with both the molars is utilized to correct it. A band is fixed on the upper molar with a hook to the palatal; and a band on the lower molar with a hook to buccal surface. Thus the teeth are brought back to ideal bucco-lingual relationship. In case, one molar is in crossbite a lingual arch can be used to move the tooth.

Class I Type 5

- Early loss of deciduous teeth can be followed by crowding, impaction or ectopic eruption of permanent teeth. The space maintainers maintain the space and allow widening of the arch, thereby orthodontic therapy can be prevented.

  For prevention and correction of class II and class III malocclusion orthodontic appliances are preferred.

Space Maintainers

Premature loss of deciduous teeth can cause drifting of the adjacent teeth into the space available. This can result in abnormal axial inclination of teeth and even shift in midline. Space maintainers are the devices used to maintain the space created by the loss of deciduous teeth.

The space maintainers can be removable or fixed, functional or non-functional and active or passive. Acrylic partial dentures have also been used as space maintainers.

Requirements of a Space Maintainer

- It must restore the function and prevent over eruption of opposing teeth.
- It should be strong enough to withstand the functional forces.
- It should not exert excessive forces on the adjacent teeth.
- It should maintain the entire mesio-distal space created by a lost tooth.
- It should permit proper oral hygiene.

  Some commonly used space maintainers are:

Band or Loop Space Maintainer

These are the commonest form of space maintaining devices (Fig. 17.3a, b). These are usually used when only one posterior tooth is lost. The tooth distal to the extraction space is banded and a loop of thick stainless steel wire is soldered to it with its mesial end

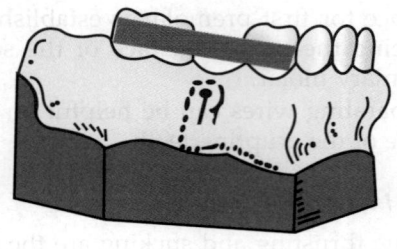

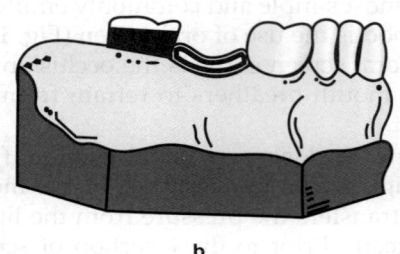

Fig. 17.3a, b: Space Maintainers a. B and bar; b. B and loop

touching the tooth mesial to the extraction space. A stainless steel crown can also be used for the abutment tooth.

Lingual and Palatal Arch Space Maintainers

These are very effective means of space maintenance in the lower arch (Fig. 17.4). The two bands are cemented on first permanent molars or on second deciduous molars which

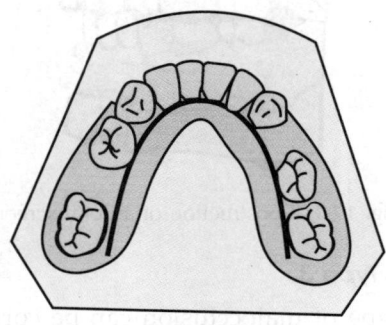

Fig. 17.4: Lingual arch space maintainer

are joined by a stainless steel wire contacting the lingual surfaces of the four mandibular incisors. It is helpful in maintaining the arch perimeter by preventing mesial drifting of molars and lingual tilting of incisors.

Acrylic Partial Dentures

This type of space maintainer is effective where the patient has multiple loss of deciduous teeth. The artificial teeth in the denture restore masticatory functions as well as restrict supra-occlusion of the opposing teeth.

Advantages

- Vertical dimension is maintained
- They can be easily cleaned and allow cleaning of adjacent teeth
- They stimulate underlying mucous membrane thereby facilitating eruption of permanent teeth
- The periodic check up is easy

Disadvantages

- Younger patients may not accept dentures
  Many other modified forms of space maintainers can also be used as the clinical situation warrants.

Planned Extractions of Deciduous Teeth

In certain instances, the deciduous teeth do not shed in stipulated times.

The timely extractions of deciduous teeth lead to proper eruption of permanent teeth. Extraction of deciduous teeth is indicated where they interfere with the eruption of their permanent successors. The crowding of the permanent incisors can be relieved by extracting the deciduous canines. Once the deciduous canines are removed to relieve the crowding of incisors, the first premolars in that arch have to be extracted later in order to provide space for permanent canines. The premolars are extracted as soon as the permanent canines emerge through alveolar mucosa.

Serial Extraction

Serial extraction is a form of modified planned extraction in which certain deciduous teeth are removed in series followed by removal of first premolars. However, this procedure is not followed in skeletal malocclusion and where natural spacing is present. This simplifies the orthodontic treatment, if necessary.

When the upper permanent lateral incisors are emerging, all deciduous canines are extracted so as to align the permanent incisors.

All first deciduous molars are extracted one year later; ideally, when half or more than half of the roots of the first premolars have been formed. The objective is to initiate the eruption of first premolars prior to eruption of canines. The lower permanent canines may erupt before the first premolars and if the first deciduous molars have been extracted, the premolars will become impacted between the canines and the 2nd deciduous molars. It is necessary to remove second deciduous molars in order to allow easy eruption of first premolars. A space maintainer should be given in order to avoid mesial drifting of the first permanent molars.

Advantages

- The method involves physiologic forces guiding the teeth in their normal position
- Better oral hygiene is maintained
- It reduces the total treatment time

Disadvantages

- It requires thorough clinical knowledge. Each patient is to be assessed and planned accordingly
- It is a long preventive regimen (may require 2–3 years)

Muscle Exercises

The occlusion is affected by functioning of adjacent muscles. Usually muscular exercises are indicated in cases of short upper lips and for controlling tongue movements.

- Stretching of the upper lip and keeping it under the incisors is helpful in cases of short hypotonic lips. Alternatively, a paper can be kept in between the lips.

- Also a button can be kept in between the lips and is pulled out by a thread while the lips are kept in position.

- An intra-oral elastic is placed on the tip of the tongue and the patient is asked to raise the tongue and hold the elastic against the rugae and swallow. This exercise corrects the improper positioning of tongue.

- The tip of the tongue and the midpoint of palate is contacted and the mandible is gradually opened leading to stretching of lingual frenum.

BIBLIOGRAPHY

1. Ackerman, I.I. and Proffit, W.R. : Preventive and interceptive orthodontics : a strong theory proves weak in practice. Angle Orthodontist : 50, 75, 1980.
2. Dewel, B.F. : Serial extractions : its limitations and contraindications in orthodontic practice. Am. J. Ortho. : 53, 904, 1970.
3. Ericson, S. and Kurol, J. : Early treatment of palatally erupting maxillary canines by extraction of the primary canines. European J. Ortho. : 10, 283, 1988.
4. Freeman, I.D. : Preventive and interceptive orthodontics : a critical review and the results of a clinical study. J. Preventive Dent. : 4, 7, 1977.
5. Popovitch, F. : The prevalence of sucking habit and its relation to malocclusion. Oral Health : 57, 498, 1967.
6. Richardson, A. : Applicability of interceptive orthodontics in the community. Br. J. of Ortho. : 24, 223, 1997.

18 *Prevention of Oral Cancer*

The menace of oral cancer is posing a challenge to the health professional. The steps taken to prevent oral cancer are limited because the definite causes are unknown. As cancer causes rapid destruction of the tissues, it should be diagnosed and treated as early as possible. The health professional should develop awareness in the masses regarding early signs of the disease. Certain chemical changes in the oral cavity make the environment cancer inducive. The probability of neoplastic event is influenced by the genetic background, age, sex, nutritional status, oral hygiene, intake of alcohol, smoking, tobacco and also the mechanical irritation. The mechanical irritation may be caused by ill-fitting dentures, sharp edges of the teeth, projecting fillings and defective clasps.

Prolonged exposure to an inert substance may lead to malignant change in the oral mucosa. Authors have found cotton as a cause of cancer in 81 year old female who packed sterile cotton daily into both posterior buccal areas for over 30 years to improve the appearance of her sunken cheeks. The lesion was diagnosed as intra-epithelial squamous cell carcinoma of left cheek.

Cancer of the oral cavity is relatively curable being a highly accessible region of the body. 85–90% of oral cancers are of the same type, i.e squamous cell carcinoma. Tongue is most vulnerable followed by palate, floor of the mouth and gingiva. The squamous cell carcinoma can be detected easily and is curable in early stages. Usually the persons of low socio-economic status are at high risk because of habits like tobacco chewing and smoking. More so, these group of people are least concerned with their oral health.

The non-smokers and non-alcoholic individuals are less likely to acquire oral cancer while long term smokers or smoker drinkers are at high risk. The white patches, erythematous zones, petechiae, zones of hypopigmentation and hyperpigmentation and thickening in other susceptible areas should be inspected properly. The dentist should follow the principle *Listen-Look-Examine,* which increases the possibility for detection of an abnormality and improves the diagnosis.

The oral cavity is most vulnerable being in direct contact with the environment. The food, which contain preservatives, additives and fats, have been linked to the development of oral cancer. They may become contaminated by bacteria, fungi and other microorganisms that may produce cancer inducing metabolites. A thorough examination of the oral cavity can reveal cancer lesions in routine. Such lesions can be differentiated from other lesions of the mucous membrane.

Tissues Involved in the Oral Cancer

The oral cancer may involve any tissue of the oral cavity. This involvement can be primary or secondary due to changes in other parts of the body. The common sites are as follows:

Cancer of the Lip

Carcinoma of the lip constitutes about 1.0% of all the neoplasms appearing in human beings; and most of them are squamous cell carcinomas. The lower lip is affected more than the upper lip, both in males and females. Secondary infection is very common with these lesions.

The labial cancers are usually associated with cigarette smoking, smoking of short hot pipes, chronic fissuring of lip, sun exposure, leukoplakia, etc. The prognosis is favourable due to the presence of orbicularis muscle surrounding the lips, difference in lymphatic drainage and vascular input as compared to intra-oral cancer. Most of the lesions are smaller and can be cured by radiotherapy.

Cancer of the Gingiva

Cancer of the gingiva is prevalent both in males and females. Smoking, betel-nut chewing and using snuff in the mucobuccal fold are the common causative agents.

Cancers of gingiva may invade the bone, requiring total or partial removal of the mandible. Radiotherapy and chemotherapy are helpful in curing these cancers.

Cancer of Floor of the Mouth

Cancer of floor of the mouth is prevalent both in males and females. Epidermoid carcinoma is most frequent malignant lesion of the floor of the mouth; however, other malignancies like Adenocarcinoma, transitional cell carcinoma and myxosarcoma, etc. has also been reported. Surgery and radiotherapy are affective in early stages of the disease.

Cancer of the Tongue

Squamous cell carcinoma is the most frequent malignant lesion of the tongue. Males are more frequently involved than females. Treatment includes surgery alone and/or radiotherapy depending upon the condition.

Cancer of the Buccal Mucosa

Cancer of the buccal mucosa is less common than other oral cancers. Males and females are usually equally involved. Usually, the long standing leukoplakia develops into carcinomas. Surgery and radiotherapy, both are effective.

Cancer of the Palate

Squamous cell carcinoma is the most frequent cancer of the palate. Reverse smoking frequently produces this cancer. Chronic sore throat and lump in the neck are associated factors leading to such cancer.

Cancer of the Salivary Glands

Majority of salivary cancers arise from the parotid gland. Males are frequently involved. Radical surgery alone or combination of surgery and radiotherapy are effective treatment regimes.

Diagnosis of Oral Cancer

The commonly employed tests for early detection of oral cancers are
- Self examination
- Sialography
- Toluidine-Blue test
- Oral cytology or Exfoliative cytology
- Biopsy

Self Examination

Self examination by the individual is important to observe any change in colour, contour and texture of the mucous membrane of the oral cavity. Such changes should be brought to the notice of the doctor immediately.

Sialography

Sialography is a technique in which the salivary glands are radiographically evaluated by injecting a radio-opaque dye into the duct.

Specific parenchymal changes are seen in case the gland is cancerous.

Toluidine-Blue Test

The toluidine-blue test is an in-vivo test which indicates the extent of the abnormal changes in the epithelium. The dye stains the altered oral epithelium in the vivid blue colour. However, only the surface epithelium picks up dye and not the underlying tissue. Such a test can be useful aid in determining the best site for a biopsy.

Oral Cytology or Exfoliative Cytology

In this test, the superficial layer of the lesion is scrapped and examined under the microscope. However, biopsy is the preferred procedure as superficial cells might not show the desired changes. Exfoliative cytology is not a substitute of biopsy but valuable where biopsy cannot be carried out due to any reason. This test is preferred for screening large number of people in community basis.

Biopsy

Biopsy is not a primary test for cancer and should be reserved only when malignant disease is suspected. However, whenever the dentist feels the doubt about the normal status of the mucosa biopsy can be taken. It is an important diagnostic aid to confirm or deny the status of cancerous activity in the tissues.

Sequence of Preventive Regime

The preventive regime involves educating and motivating the public regarding menace of oral cancer. A team comprising of the doctor, the hygienist and the nurse can visit the communities and make the people aware of the occurance and subsequent sequelae of the oral cancer.

The posters, charts, slides and movies, etc. can be shown to people to:

– Show the debilitating effects of the disease.
– Explain the sequelae of advanced oral cancer.
– Assure the public regarding the curability of disease if detected earlier.
– Demonstrate the techniques for early detection and diagnosis by the patient as well as dentist.

Further, the community should be informed of the danger signals which can be one or combination of the following:

• Any persistent, scaly white patch.
• Pigmented spot which suddenly increases in size.
• Any non healing ulcer.
• Progressive facial asymmetry.
• Sudden loosening of teeth without history of trauma or blow to the jaw.
• Puffy bleeding gums.
• Paraesthesia, anaesthesia and oral numbness.
• Pain and trismus during jaw movement.
• A lump in the oral tissues, face or neck.
• An extraction wound that does not heal.
• Altered taste in the oral cavity.

The nutritional status of the patient is also important. Though there is no diet that prevents cancer, however vitamin deficiencies may play a role in the occurrence of oral cancers. Chronic vitamin B complex deficiency may induce oral cancer.

It is concluded that improvements in the dental health of communities achieved by the preventive regimes is a welcome step. It is important to maintain this momentum and encourage the wider use of proven preventive strategies in those communities who currently do not receive them.

BIBLIOGRAPHY

1. Aas, J.A., Paster, B.J., Stokes, L.N. and Olsen, T. : Defining the normal microflora of the oral cavity. J. Clin. Microbiol. : 43, 5721, 2005.
2. Barewal, H.S and Schantz, S.S : Emerging role of beta carotene and antioxidant nutrients in prevention of oral cancer. Arch. Otolaryngol Head Neck Surg. : 121, 141, 1995.
3. Benner, S.E., Lippman, S.M., Wargovich, M.J. and Lee, J.J. : Miconuclei, a biomarker for chemoprevention trials : results of a randomized study in oral pre-malignancy. Int. J. Cancer 15 : 59, 457, Nov. 1994.

4. Blot, W., Mchanghlin, J.K. and Winn, D.M. : Smoking and drinking in relation to oral and pharyngeal cancer. Cancer Res. : 48, 3282, 1988.

7. Chamberlain, J. : Evaluation of screening for cancer. Comm. Dent. Health 10(Suppl) : 79, 1993.

8. Clayman, G.L., Chamberlain, R.M., Lee, J.J., Lippman, S.M. and Hong, W.K. : Screening at a health fair to identify subjects for an oral leukoplakia chemoprevention trial. J. Caner. Educ. : 10, 88, 1995.

9. Cowan, C.G., Gregg, T.A. and Kee, F. : Prevention and detection of oral cancer : the views of primary care dentists in Northern Ireland. Br. Dent. J. 11 : 179, 338, Nov. 1995.

10. Downer, M.C., Evans, A.W., Hughes, H.C.M., Jullien, J.A., Speight, P.M. and Zakrzewska, J.M. : Evaluation of screening for oral cancer and precancer in a company headquarters. Comm. Dent. Oral Epid. : 23, 84, April 1995.

11. Early diagnosis and prevention of oral cancer and precancer : Report of symposium III. Adv. Dent. Res. : 9, 134, Jul. 1995.

12. Farah, C.S. and Mc Cullough, M.J. : A pilot case control study on the efficacy of acetic acid wash and chemiluminescent illumination (vizilite) in the visualization of oral mucous white lesions. Oral Oncol. : 43, 820, 2007.

13. Farah, C.S. and Mc Cullough, M.J. : Oral cancer awareness for the general practitioner : new approaches to patient care. Aust. Dent. J. : 53, 2, 2008.

14. Feaver, G.P. : Oral squamous cell carcinoma. Results of screening are encouraging. B.M.J. : 23, 308, April 1994.

15. Garewal, H. : Antitoxidants in oral cancer prevention. Am. J. Clin. Nutr. : 62 (6 suppl), 1410, Dec. 1995.

16. Garewal, H. : Chemoprevention of oral cancer : beta-carotene and vitamin E in leukoplakia. Eur. J. Cancer Prev. : 3, 101, March 1994.

17. Hindle, I., Downer, M.C. and Speight, P.M. : The epidemiology of oral cancer. Br. J. Oral Maxillo-facial Surg. : 34, 471, 1996.

18. Hollows, P., Mc Andrew, P.G. and Perini, M.G. : Delays in the referral and treatment of oral squamous cell carcinoma. B.D.J. : 188, 262, 2000.

19. Holmstrup, P., Vedtofte, P., Reibel, J. and Stoltze, K. : Long-term treatment outcome of oral premalignant lesions. Oral Oncol. : 42, 461, 2006.

20. Horowitz, M., Goodman, S., Yellowitz, A. and Nanejah, A. : The need for Health promotion in oral cancer prevention and early detection. J. Public Health Dentistry: 56, 319, 1996.

21. Lane, P.M., Gilhuly, T. and Whitehead, P. : Simple device for the direct visualization of oral cavity tissue fluorescence. J. Biomed. Opt. : 11, 2006.

22. Lodi, G.L., Sardella, A. and Carrassi, A. : Oral cancer prevention and dentists attitude towards smoking. Eur. J. Cancer B. Oral Oncol. : 31, 153, March 1995.

23. Mathew, B., Sankaranarayan, R., Wesley, R. and Nair, M.K. : Evaluation of mouth self examination in the control of oral cancer. Br. J. Cancer : 71, 397, Feb. 1995.

24. Meurmom, J.H. and Uittamo, J. : Oral microorganisms in the etiology of cancer. Acta. Odont. Scand. : 66, 321, 2008.

25. Oliver, R.J., Bearing J. and Hindle, I. : Oral cancer in young adults : report of three cases and review of the literature. B.D.J : 188, 362, 2000.

26. Peterson, D.E. : Prevention of oral complications in cancer patients. Prev. Med. : 23, 763, Sept. 1994.

27. Reichart, B.R. and Philipsen, H.P. : Oral erythroplakia – A review. Oral Oncol. : 41, 551, 2005.

28. Salaspuro, V. and Salaspuro, M. : Synergistic effect of alcohol drinking and smoking on in vivo acetaldehyde concentration in saliva. Int. J. Cancer : 10, 480, 2004.

29. Scott, S., Grunfeld, E.A. and Mc Gurk, M. : The idiosyncratic relationship between diagnostic delay and stage of oral squamous cell carcinoma. Oral Oncol. : 41, 396, 2005.

30. Scott, S., Grunfeld, E.A. and Mc Gurk, M. : Patient's delay in oral cancer : a systematic review. Comm. Dent. Oral Epidem. : 34, 337, 2006.

31. Scully, E., Hopper, C and Epstein, J.B.: Oral cancer: Current and future diagnostic techniques. : Am. J Dent. 21, 199, 2008.

32. Seitz, H.K. and Becker, P. : Alcohol metabolism and cancer risk. Alcohol Res. Health : 30, 38 & 44, 2007.

33. Silverman, S. Jr. : Oral cancer education and HIV associated malignancies. J. Cancer Educ. : 9, 152, Feb. 1994.

34. Silverman, S. Jr. : Oral lichen planus : a potentially malignant lesion. J. Oral maxillofacial Surg. : 58, 1286, 2000.

35. Slavkin, H.C. : The war on oral cavity and pharyngeal cancer. J. Am. Dent. Assoc. : 127, 517, April 1996.

36. Tagg, R., Asadi-zeydabaddi, M. and Meyers, A.D.: Biophotonic and other physical methods for characterizing oral mucosa. Otolaryngol Cl. North Am. : 38, 215, 2005.

37. Thomas, J.E. and Faecher, R.S. : A physician's guide to early detection of oral cancer. Geriatrics : 47, 58, 1992.

38. Tromp, D.M., Brouha, X.D., De Leeuw, J.R., Hordijk, G.J. and Winnubst, J.A. : Pscyhological factors and patient delay in patients with head and neck cancer. Eur. J. Cancer : 40, 1509, 2004.

39. Voekler, R. : New strategies to fight oral cancer. J.A.M.A. 9 : 276, 1121, Oct. 1996.

40. Winn, D.M. : Diet and nutrition in the etiology of oral cancer. Am. J. Clin. Nutr. : 61 (suppl.), 4375, 1995.

41. Zhang, I. and Rosin, M.P. : Loss of heterozygosity : a potential tool in management of oral premalignant lesion. J. Oral Pathol. Med. : 30, 513, 2001.

19 *Dental Anthropology*

Dental Anthropology is the study of teeth in a perspective beyond the clinical science. It includes the study of dental growth, theories of dental origin, primate dentition and population variation.

TIME PERIODS IN ARCHAEOLOGY

Anthropologists and others have divided the time after advent of stone tools into three 'lithic' (Greek: of stone) time frames. These time periods, defined by material culture are:

1. **Upper Paleolithic (old stone age - Late Pleistocene):** This marks the appearance of fully modern humans in Europe about 35,000 years ago. The hallmark of this time is the commencement of game hunting with an atlatl. It is the last part of the Ice Age, the time of cave art and development of finely made tools.

2. **Mesolithic (middle stone age):** In Europe, it began about 11,000 years ago and is marked by the end of the Ice Age, the extinction of large game hunting with adaptations towards more varied food patterns and earliest pre adaptations for farming.

3. **Neolithic (new stone age):** This time period began about 9,000 years ago in Europe. Plants and animals were domesticated; finely polished stone tools were made; subsequently pottery and village life appeared. The Mesolithic, Neolithic, and the time until today is sometimes called the 'recent' or the 'Holocene' (Greek: recent).

ORGANIZATION OF THE DENTITION

Teeth are calcified structures derived from dermal denticles during the evolution of jaws. Structurally, a tooth consists of a calcified collagenous tissue known as dentin that is covered by a highly calcified layer known as enamel.

The size, shape, number, location and life span of teeth reflect their function and their evolutionary history. The order of eruption, the inter-digitation of the teeth and the replacement of deciduous teeth with permanent successors are few of the patterns to be studied in the organization of dentition.

FEATURES OF VARIOUS DENTITIONS (THE CHARACTERISTICS OF TEETH)

Each family of organisms has different features of dentition. The characteristics of teeth of some of the species are descried below:

1. **Sharks:** They have multiple rows of teeth. As the functional teeth wear off, successional teeth from the lingual aspect replace them. The teeth are essentially similar to the placoid scales that cover the bodies of sharks. The progressive replacement of the teeth is a functional adaptation for these creatures.

2. **Bony Fishes:** In them, additional teeth may appear on the tongue, roof of the mouth, in the throat or on any of the jaw bones of dermal origin. The teeth of bony fishes vary greatly in shape and arrangement.

3. Amphibians and Reptiles: Numerous, simple conical teeth are present on bones of palate and along the jaw margins in them. Also, in Therapsid reptiles (mammalian ancestors), palatal teeth disappear, thus limiting teeth to a single row along the jaws and differentiating them into distinct classes, as present in mammals.

4. Mammals: In mammals, teeth are confined only to the jaw bones. They are having mostly two and sometimes only one functional generation of teeth. Toothless whales and certain edentates even have no functional generation of teeth at all. Despite of the great species diversity in the form of teeth amongst the mammals, their teeth are always socketed. In some of the mammalian species, the teeth are growing continuously. Some of the variations amongst mammalian species are described below:

   i. In carnivores (flesh eating mammals - for example, cats, dogs, lions, tigers, etc.): The fourth upper premolar and the lower first molar have become a shearing apparatus known as *carnassial teeth*. These are maximally developed in lions and tigers. Carnassials are longer and larger than the other teeth and are adapted for cutting instead of tearing.

   ii. In herbivorous mammals (for example, horses, cattle, elephants, etc.): The cusps of their molars often have a crescentic outline or are connected with each other to form ridges. They present a very convoluted surface with ridges on enamel and the clefts filled in between them by a special tissue known as coronal cementum. As a tooth wears away, grinding occurs on a complex surface of dentin, cementum and deeply enfolded enamel. The weared off incisors reveal a complex internal anatomy that can be used to estimate the age of the animal.

iii. In primates (for example, the larger monkeys and baboons): The canine teeth are enlarged to form powerful dagger-like teeth. These are especially prominent in the males. The large canine is used for threatening and intimidation by male baboons.

iv. Hominid Dental Characteristics: Hominids can be divided into three groups according to their origin as follows:

   a. Australopithecines: These are African hominids which include *anamensis, afarensis,* and *africanus* species. They appeared more than four million years ago and seemed to have died out about 2.4 million years ago.

   The dentition of **afarensis** retains primitive apelike features. Their jaws are comparatively large and prognathous. Their maxillary arch is 'omega' shaped and mandibular arch is V-shaped. They had large teeth with canines projecting beyond occlusal plane and diastema distal to the maxillary lateral incisors. Their mandibular premolar is commonly unicuspid.

   In **africanus**, the incisors are spatulate and vertically implanted in the jaws. The canines are short and barely project beyond the occlusal plane. There is no maxillary diastema between the incisors and canines. The dental arch is more curved, like the modern human arch. The mandibular first premolar is 'bicuspid'.

   b. Paranthropus: These are 'robust' African hominids who branched off about 2.7 million years ago. They are known for their large cheek teeth and well developed chewing musculature, often called as *Nutcracker man*. The last of these had become extinct a million years ago.

Dental characteristics of Paranthropus are distinctive. Their incisor teeth are similar to Africanus; however, the cheek teeth are much larger than the anteriors. The premolars are molariform. The cheek teeth also had a thick covering of enamel and were subjected to considerable wear, implying a tough vegetarian diet. The heavy reinforcement of the face and the large attachments for the masticatory muscles confirm the tough diet.

The molars and premolars are enormous when compared to the incisors and canines. They are broad when compared to those of the Australopithecines. Their maxillary third molars display wrinkled enamel, a characteristic seen in the great apes.

c. **Homo:** They evolved in Africa 2.5 million years ago and subsequently spread out around the world. The species are discussed here in chronological order.

Homo habilis is considered to have been a more efficient biped than the Australopithecines. He manufactures and uses stone tools, has greater cranial capacity, less massive jaws with a smaller and less projecting face.

He has parabolic dental arches with small canines and no diastema. The feature peculiar to Homo habilis specimens is the relatively narrower (bucco-lingually) human-like cheek teeth.

Homo erectus is the first hominid having a wide distribution out of Africa into much of the Old World. The dentition of H. erectus is essentially similar to that of modern man. His dental arch is parabolic, having large sized teeth with shovel shaped maxillary central incisors and the more robust canines; cingula are seen around the cheek teeth, and there is some wrinkling of the enamel.

The mandibular second and third molars tend to possess five cusps instead of four cusps.

There is some degree of taurodontism wherein the pulp chamber extends well into the roots.

Neanderthals are also frequently identified as Archaic Homo spaiens.

Their teeth are positioned more anteriorly than ours so that there is retromolar space distal to the third molars and anterior to the anterior border of the ramus. Anterior teeth are comparatively large. Also, the molars are often taurodont.

Homo sapiens present with less robust jaws having smaller teeth. There is a well-documented trend of dental reduction in the past 40,000 years in them.

THE ATTACHMENT OF TEETH

The different types of attachment of a tooth to its surrounding structures are as follows:

Attachment	Description
1. Gomphosis	Teeth are anchored in the alveoli of jaws in a peg in socket joint formed by a fibrous ligament, e.g. in mammals.
2. Pleurodont	Teeth are ankylosed directly to lingual side of jaw, e.g. in reptiles.
3. Acrodont	Teeth are ankylosed directly to the crest of jaw, e.g. in reptiles.
4. Thecodont	Teeth are not ankylosed but have their roots deeply embedded in the sockets; somewhat similar to mammalian sockets, e.g. in alligators and crocodiles.

In mammals (and humans), the tooth socket or alveolus is subjected to continuous remodeling; thus allowing for the eruption and shedding of the deciduous teeth and providing for eruption of permanent teeth. After the permanent teeth come into a functional relationship, the alveolar process constantly remodels itself in life to accommodate the secondary eruption of the teeth as a compensation for occlusal wear. Also, remodeling facilitates physiological mesial drift to compensate for proximal wear. Clinically, this re-modelling response of alveolar bone forms the basis of the orthodontic treatment done by dentists.

TERMS USED IN COMPARATIVE DENTAL ANATOMY AND DENTAL ANTHROPOLOGY

Dentitions are classified into different ways so as to simplify their study, make them more understandable and provide an acceptable terminology for them.

1. Categories of Dentition according to Shape

Teeth are divided into two categories according to their shape:

a. **Homodont dentition:** When all the teeth present in the jaw are uniform and of similar shape in a dentition, it is described as homodont dentition, for example, in alligators, crocodiles, etc.

b. **Heterodont dentition:** Dentition in which the teeth are non-uniform in shape and are specialized regionally into different classes is termed as heterodont dentition. As this dentition is present in mammals and the human beings, so it is described in detail below:

Heterodont Dentition (The Regional Specialization of Teeth)

Many species of animals have teeth that are regionally specialized. In humans and in other mammals, recognized classes of teeth such as incisors, canines, premolars and molars are present. A dentition with such regional specialization is described as heterodont. The different classes of teeth present in human dentition are:

i. *Incisors:* Incisors are the teeth that develop in premaxilla. There are two incisors on each side of jaw; one central incisor and another lateral incisor.

ii. *Canines:* Canines are teeth present adjacent to the incisors in jaws.

iii. *Premolars:* Premolars are defined as cheek teeth having deciduous predecessors.

iv. *Molars:* Molars are cheek teeth distal to premolars that have no deciduous predecessors.

2. Categories of Dentition according to their Generation

Categories of teeth by the generations are as follows:

a. **Anodontia:** This is basically a condition in which all the teeth are absent. American anteater is a species that is without teeth altogether—a vertebrate having no dentition or anodontia.

b. **Monophyodont:** When only single functional generation of teeth is present, then the dentition is known as monophyodont, for example, in toothed whales and seals. In them, a rudimentary deciduous dentition is formed that disappears without eruption.

c. **Diphodont:** Dentition having two generations of teeth is called as diphodont, for example, in humans and most of the mammals. Here, deciduous/milk/lacteal dentition is replaced by the permanent dentition.

d. **Polyphyodont:** The dentition that is replaced more than two times (generally many times) is known as polyphyodont, for example, in reptiles, fishes and amphibians. The succession of teeth occurs throughout the life of an animal and the total number of replacements for each tooth position may be very large, for example, fifty replacements per tooth position in the crocodile.

The replacement teeth erupt from the lingual side. The system is most elegant in sharks where the simultaneous replacement teeth progresses in a 'revolver' fashion with the newly formed teeth arising from the lingual and the exfoliated 'spent' teeth shed from the external or labial side.

3. Categories of Teeth according to their Crown Form

The categories of teeth according to different crown forms are:

a. **Bunodont** (Greek: *mound or hill*) These are low crowned teeth with well developed roots and cone-shaped tubercles; or simple cones in place of developed cusps, for example, posterior teeth in the pig.

b. **Selenodont** (Greek: *the moon*) These are anteroposteriorly elongated teeth having half moon shaped cusps, e.g. cheek teeth of sheep.

c. **Sectorial** (Latin: *secare to cut*) Teeth are blade-like adapted for the cutting of diet into pieces and swallowing them as a whole. A specialized variant of sectorial teeth seen in carnivores are the carnassials which consist of the last premolar in the upper jaw and the first molar of the lower jaw.

d. **Lophodont** (Greek: *crest*) are ridged teeth having transverse ridges as in the tapir . These can be either:

  • **Bilophodont:** Teeth that have two sets of transverse ridges.

  • **Polylophodont:** Teeth that have many ridges as seen in the elephant molar.

e. **Brachydont** (Greek: *short*) teeth have small crowns and well-developed roots, e.g. teeth of human beings.

f. **Hypsodont** (Greek: *height*) teeth have long crowns and short roots as seen in the horse.

It is a functional adaptation for continuous wear sustained by chewing grass, i.e. highly abrasive due to its high silica content.

g. **Haplodont** (Greek: *simple*) teeth have simple crowns and roots, e.g. teeth of dolphin.

Tusks are incisors or canines having continuous growth that protrude beyond the lips when the mouth is closed. The incisors of the Elephant and Hippopotamus; left incisor of the Narwhal and Canines of the Wild Boar are some of the examples of tusks.

ORIGIN OF MAMMALIAN TEETH

The history of origin of teeth with two or more cusps has long interested investigators. Teeth are very useful for studying evolutionary history as they are durable in the fossil record, have clearly discernable anatomic features, and their morphology is under tight genetic control. The similarities of molar teeth in modern humans and our hominid ancestors are readily seen, making them as one of the most useful guides in sorting fossil remains in the field of anthropology. Several theories have been proposed to account for the origin of cusps and molar patterns. The two prominent ones are:

a. **The concrescence theory:** It states that the mammalian teeth originated by the fusion of originally separate reptilian teeth. In the absence of transitional forms as evidence, this theory is pretty much discredited today.

b. **The Differentiation theory/Tritubercular theory:** This hypothesis says that even the most complicated mammalian molar has originated from a simple conical reptilian tooth. It is much more successful in the terms of evolution. This theory is discussed in detail below.

The Tritubercular Theory (Origin of cusps)

The tritubercular theory was first put forth by the American paleontologist *Edward Drinker Cope in 1875* and modified by *Henry Fairfield*

Osborn in 1888, so it is often referred to as the *'Cope-Osborn Theory of Tuberculy'*.

The theory states that the haplodont (Greek: simple), conical teeth of reptiles evolved to form molars which consist of a series of in-line cusps. In reptiles, the upper and lower teeth are arranged alternately in the jaws allowing the jaws to function in a simple hinge fashion. These simple conical teeth can be used for tearing and piercing.

Evolution of Cusps in Maxilla

a. The oldest cusp representing the original reptilian conical tooth is the protocone (Greek: time). To the mesial of the proto-cone, the cusp that appeared is the para-cone (Greek: 'at the side of'). Just distal to the protocone is the metacone (Greek: 'in the midst of or after') (Fig. 19.1)

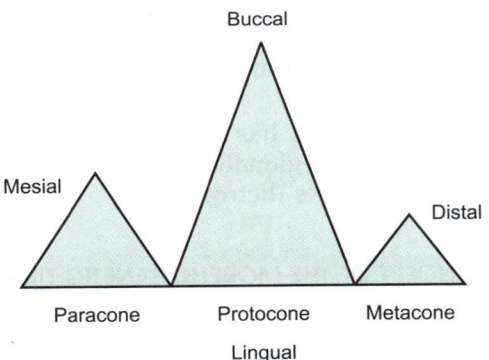

Fig. 19.1: Maxillary molar cusps (initial arrangement)

b. With time, the accessory cusps increased in size and they rotated in relation to the principle cusp to form triangular teeth. They also acquired connecting ridges called lophs (Greek: crest or ridge). The protocone displaced to the lingual with the base of the triangle to the buccal (Fig. 19.2).
c. The upper molar acquired additional cusps, the hypocone on the distal aspect of the molar, completing its appearance as a four-cusped

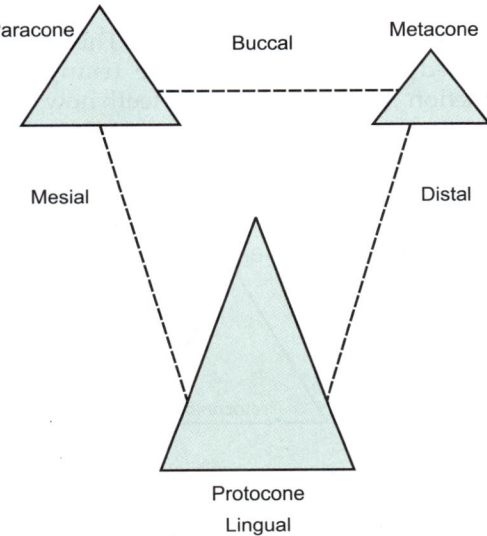

Fig. 19.2: Maxillary molar cusps (final arrangement)

tooth. Small cusp additions to the mesial and distal of the trigon are the protoconule and metaconule. Cusps along the buccal margins can be of different styles as: parastyle, mesostyle, and metastyle. The conules and styles may not be present in all humans.

Evolution of Cusps in Mandible

Similarly, in the lower molars, the cusps are named as protoconid, paraconid, and meta-conid (Fig. 19.3).

While in the lower, the protoconid remained to the buccal with the base of the triangle to

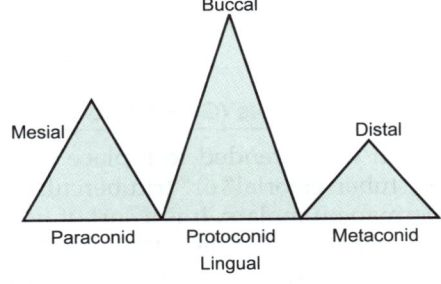

Fig. 19.3: Mandibular/molar cusps (initial arrangements)

the lingual. The triangles were therefore reversed in relation to each other. This allowed inter-digitation between the triangles in function. These trigon/trinid teeth now could function by puncturing food as before and also by the shearing action of the crests acting against each other (Fig.19.4).

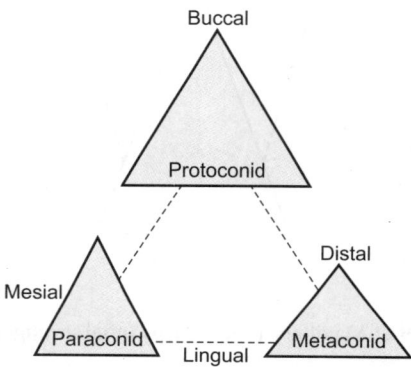

Fig. 19.4: Mandibular molar cusps (final arrangement)

The next step in evolution was the acquisition of the distal talnoid (heel) on the distal of lower molars. This formed a surface for crushing food against the surface of the protocone in the upper. These cuspal pattern form tribosphenic molars, that are ancestral to the cuspal patterns of primate molars, including our own. The fully formed tribosphenic molar probably took an additional 100 million years to develop.

The lower molar talnoid (the heel) gave rise to three cusps, the hypoconid, the entoconid, and the hypoconulid producing a six-cusped molar.

Tribosephnic Molars (Greek Rub or Wedge)

The term was intended to replace the older terms "tubersectorial" or "tritubercular" used for permanent molars. It is a sort of letter 'V' with the open part of the letter facing facially in the upper and lingually in the lower. In occlusion, upper tribosphenic molars are normally located to the midline of their lower molar counterparts.

In humans, in lower second molars, the hypoconulid is lost, producing a four cusp molar. The five-cusp molar occurs in anthropoid apes and man. The Y-5 pattern named after the Y-shaped pattern of fissures separating the five cusps represents vary conservative genetically determined patterns still present in 90% of lower first permanent molars of modern Homo sapiens.

Evolutionary Trends in Mammilian Dentition

Mammilian teeth evolved from reptiles and with evolution there has been a reduction in the number and generations of the teeth. In general, there was a reduction from polyphyodonty to diphyodonty and sometimes to monophyodonty, or in the case of toothless whales, absence of functional generations of teeth at all. The term functional is imperative here because in some animals teeth are not functional. They form, erupt and are shed in utero before birth.

Also, the trend has been changed from homodonty to regionalization of teeth into specialized classes (hetrodonty).

CONCEPT OF THE MORPHOGENETIC FIELD

Heterodonty, the specialization of teeth into classes has raised a number of theoretical questions. In experimental embryology, the early embryo is viewed as a mosaic of 'organization fields' each of which pursues its own unique developmental path. Butler has applied this concept to teeth and determined that a tooth row consists of as three regions - the incisive, canine, and molariform regions. In each region there is a 'best copy', which is the flagship of the group. It is the best illustrated with the canine since there is only one in its class, and it is extremely stable. Dentists find the canine as most consistent tooth in form in the arches.

The 'best copy' of the incisors is the central incisor. It is very stable in form and is seldom missing. Lateral incisors are variable to the point of being peg-shaped. They are sometimes congenitally absent.

In the molariform group, the first permanent molar is the 'best copy' of the group. In modern humans, second and third upper molars are progressively smaller, the distolingual cusp tends to disappear and the tooth retreats from being rhomboidal in shape to heart shape. Going forward in the tooth row, the pattern becomes less clear.

According to Paleontologists humans' 'first' and 'second' premolars are actually the third and fourth teeth of the tooth row. So in a sense, the premolars most distant from the first permanent molar have disappeared from their field altogether.

TEETH AND ANTHROPOLOGICAL STUDIES

Anthropologically, teeth can be studied by metric and non-metric variations that are described as follows:

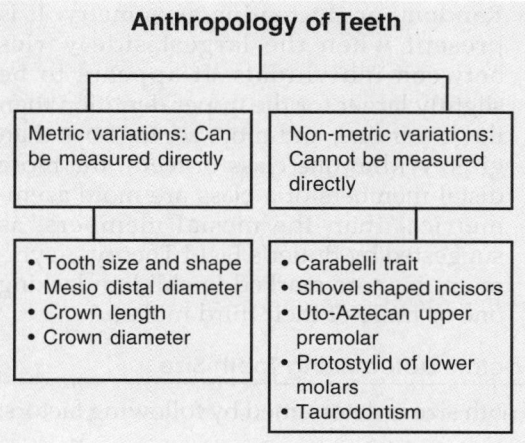

Anthropology of Teeth

Metric variations: Can be measured directly
- Tooth size and shape
- Mesio distal diameter
- Crown length
- Crown diameter

Non-metric variations: Cannot be measured directly
- Carabelli trait
- Shovel shaped incisors
- Uto-Aztecan upper premolar
- Protostylid of lower molars
- Taurodontism

Metric Variations

Metric variations are features that can be measured directly, for example, the mesiodistal crown diameters of teeth. As these features are relatively easy to measure, distribute in a Gaussian fashion, and can be treated statistically, so they have generated a larger literature than any other aspect of dental anthropology. These variations are mainly determined by tooth size which is described as follows:

Tooth Size

Teeth provide an excellent opportunity for anthropological studies as they are preserved in greater numbers than other parts of the skeleton. They are a close reflection of the genotype, are affected by the forces of natural selection and are easily treated by quantitative methods. Dental traits, like nearly all morphological traits, are polygenic in nature and controlled by heredity as well as environmental factors. As teeth develop within the jaws so they are generally unaffected by environment to most extent (with some exceptions, such as trauma or severe nutritional stress). They have a further advantage as they are easy to measure, both in living and in fossil forms.

Human tooth size has undergone a clear-cut reduction during the Upper Paleolithic and the rate of that reduction has accelerated since the end of the last of Ice Age. The reduction began during the Upper Paleolithic period at the rate of roughly 1% per 2,000 years until the end of the Pleistocene about 10,000 years ago. Beginning about 10,000 years ago, the rate of reduction seems to have doubled to about 1% every 1,000 years. When tooth size is considered in relation to body size, the reduction in the dentition is even more dramatic than the reduction in body bulk.

Mechanism of Tooth Size Reduction

There is no single explanation of the mechanisms in dental reduction. Several hypotheses presented to explain the reduction are discussed:

1. **Dental size reduction is a result of facial reduction** and forces do not affect teeth directly.

2. **Smaller teeth conserve precious biological resources** similar to the inability to synthesize Vitamin C. Early primates 'deleted' the ability to manufacture vitamin C as a biological measure, while our ancestors could synthesize it.

3. **As early humans acquired culinary skills, teeth ceased to have survival value and they are just dwindling away due to the Probable Mutation Effect (PME).** This hypothesis attributes the reduction of teeth in size and number to cultural factors. The PME was proposed by Brace in 1963. According to it, food preparation technology may have eliminated the forces that previously maintained tooth size. Initially, the teeth had para-masticatory functions but as more sophisticated techniques like earth oven technique, hot stone boiling, etc. originated for the cooking of meat, the cooked meat become more tender and para-masticatory forces on teeth reduced.

Parameters for Recoding Tooth Size

Usually, the maximum dimensions of the teeth that are commonly used for recording tooth size are:

a. **Mesio-distal diameter (length) of the crown:** This is taken as the greatest mesio-distal dimension taken parallel to the occlusal and facial surface. The measurement is typically taken using calipers with arms machined to a fine point. Teeth with marked occlusal and proximal wear are excluded from the study.

b. **Bucco-lingual crown diameter (breadth):** This measurement is the greatest distance between the facial and lingual surfaces of the crown, taken at right angles to the plane in which the mesio-distal diameter is taken. Bucco-lingual diameters are unaffected by proximal wear, but can become unusable when there is excessive occlusal wear.

c. **Crown height (height):** This is defined as the distance from the tip of the highest cusp to the cervical line on the buccal side. Any occlusal wear at all renders this measurement unreliable; therefore, it is seldom employed.

As an addition to above measurements, any **asymmetry in the crown diameters** can be considered for the anthropological tooth size study. Dental traits ordinarily exhibit a degree of symmetry, but any asymmetry in them might reveal the underlying genetics and developmental biology of teeth.

Two types of asymmetries are relevant in Dentistry are:

a. **Directional asymmetry:** It is the tendency of either left or right side teeth to be consistently larger than the other side within a population. A component of directional asymmetry averaging +/–0.06 mm is common in human dentitions. It varies between teeth not only in the extent of asymmetry, but also in its direction. Thus, the left canine may be larger than the right ones, while first premolars may have right ones larger than the left ones. Different populations may show different patterns within one jaw.

b. **Random, or fluctuating asymmetry:** It is present when the largest side varies between individuals. It appears to be slightly larger for the upper dentition than the lower one; and more so, for boys than girls. Within one class of teeth, the more distal members of a class are more asymmetrical than the mesial members, as suggested by Butler's Field Theory. Asymmetry is more marked in children lacking one or more of their third molars.

Factors Determining Tooth Size

Tooth size is determined by following factors:

i. **Heredity, race and environment:** For one population and a single sex, the mesio-distal and bucco-lingual diameters of each tooth type have normal (Gaussian) distributions. If a tooth from one part of a jaw is large, then teeth from other parts also tend to be large. However, when the anterior teeth are compared with posteriors in groups, it is easily found that their crown diameters are inversely related to each other. Thus, individuals with larger than normal anterior tooth crowns, have correspondingly smaller than normal cheek teeth and vice-versa.

Crown diameter is the result of genetic and environmental factors. Phenotypic characteristics such as crown diameters can have any value within a given range.

Three factors that must be considered in the generation of crown diameter of an individual are:

a. His Genotype
b. Environmental factors within his family
c. Environmental factors that have unique impact on him

Most studies estimate the relative importance of the genotypic and environmental factors by calculating a statistic relationship between them. This relationship is known as HERITABILITY. This is the slope of a regression line and indicates the extent to which children follow their parent.

Crown diameters of different teeth may have different inheritabilities, for example, studies show that the dizygotic twins having different genotype but same environment show a much greater variance in crown diameters than monozygotic twins having same genotype and environment.

Also, in a family, correlation between sister pair was the highest, followed by brother pair, and then by sister-brother. This suggests that at least some of the genes controlling crown diameter are present on the X chromosome. Overall, it is clear that the size of the dentition is part of a complex of features related to a variety of genes located on several chromosomes.

There appears to be a clear relationship between a child's crown diameters and his mother's health during pregnancy, implying that their heritability included shared environmental as well as genetic factors.

ii. **Sexual dimorphism:** The sexual dimorphism of permanent teeth is a well established attribute of primates. The size and distribution of this dimorphism is different in various species and the highest levels are (97% or higher) seen in baboon canines. In many animals, large canines are considered to be visual sexual signs of dominance and rank.

Human dental dimorphism is of the order of 2–6% with mandibular canines showing the greatest dimorphism (up to 7.3%), followed by the maxillary canines. Canines are more prominent and bulkier in males as compared to females. As the canines become larger, the posterior teeth subsequently become smaller in size. Dimorphism in the permanent dentition is variable and it appears to have a substantial inherited component.

Females have a higher frequency of missing teeth and a lesser frequency of supernumerary teeth than do males. Also, females show more shoveling of upper incisors than do males.

iii. **Tooth size related to body size:** Among the primates as a whole, there is a high positive correlation between body size and crown size, at least in males. Within living humans; however, the correlation between body size and crown diameters is low.

iv. **Evolutionary trends of crown diameters and hominid dentition:** There is a decrease in cheek tooth diameters from Homo habilis, to Homo erectus and finally to modern Homo sapiens. The Australopithecines display a high level of dental sexual dimorphism based on crown diameter measurements. In anatomically modern Homo sapiens, if male and female canine mesio-distal diameters are plotted together they show a single, asymmetrical mode, but the distribution for Australopithecines is bimodal.

Non-Metric Variations

These are features are scored visually in terms of presence, absence, degree of development, or form and cannot be measured directly. Non-metric variations are quite complex and require uniform standards for their assessment. This has been accomplished with the use of cast plaster plaques, a process initiated by Dahlberg in the 1940s. Some of the non-metric variations for anthropological studies are described below:

a. The Carabelli Trait

This is the non-metric dental trait, *the tuberclus anomalus* and was first described in 1841 by George Carabelli.

The trait, if present, is located on the mesio-lingual corner of upper first permanent molars and second deciduous molars. The trait is found infrequently in upper second permanent molars. It presents as a cusp of variable sizes, to small pit, furrow or ridge. Sometimes the trait is a sort of lingual cingulum; a similar feature is found amongst the gibbon, chimpanzee, gorilla, and orangutan.

There is a demonstrated relationship between the Carabelli trait and disto-lingual cusp size in upper molars and also between the Carabelli trait and the protostylid of lower molars.

The Carabelli trait has a high incidence of expression in Caucasoid population with a low level of expression of shovel-shaped incisors. Conversely, the Carabelli trait is seldom fully expressed in Mongoloid population, which possesses a high frequency of shovel-shaped incisors.

Thus, it can also be used to estimate times of evolutionary divergence between local races, their ancestry, and migration patterns of populations.

b. Shovel Shaped Incisors

These incisors have very prominent marginal ridges enclosing a deep lingual fossa.

The shoveling is most common in permanent and deciduous upper incisors, but can at times appear in lower incisors also. At time, the shoveling can create a pit on the lingual surface of central incisors. The highest frequencies (greater than 90%) are found amongst Asians and Native Americans and lowest amongst Europeans. Shovel shaped incisors appeared in Homo erectus, suggesting that this is a very ancient trait.

c. Uto-Aztecan Upper Premolar

In the permanent upper first premolar, the buccal cusp may bulge out to the buccal side with a marked fossa in its distal shoulder. The form is seen only in Native Americans, with its highest frequencies in Arizona.

d. Protostylid of Lower Molars

The protostylid is a feature on the buccal side of the lower molar crown ranging from a pit in the buccal grove, through a furrow to a prominent cusp. It is seen especially on the first or third permanent molars or in deciduous lower second molars. It may be present in up to 40% of a population.

e. Taurodontism

The term was coined by Sir Arthur Keith to describe the 'bull-like' condition in cheek teeth in which the tall root trunk encloses a high pulp chamber and short roots. It is best diagnosed in radiographs. In living people, it may appear upto 5% in some populations and it is prominent amongst the Krapina Neandertal specimens.

Other Traits Useful to the Dental Anthropologist

Some of the other traits that are useful to dental anthropologist are:

- Canine ridges
- Metaconule of upper molars, lower premolar cusps
- Cusp number on lower molars
- Molar groove and fissure patterns
- Enamel extensions
- Root number in cheek teeth

EVOLUTION AND AGENESIS

In clinical practice, dentists often assume that teeth which are frequently missing or variable in form are 'on the way out' in evolution. Teeth destined for evolutionary loss anticipate that condition by increased variability in size, shape, and/or agenesis. Supporting evidence would be strong selective pressure toward loss of a tooth in evolution. Another evidence, might be a series of consecutive fossil specimens as evidence of progressive tooth loss.

What is the dental future for humans? It has been suggested that one incisor, one canine, one premolar, and two molars per quadrant; is likely to be the dental profile of future man. This prediction is based on progressive loss of the most distal incisor, premolar, and molar.

If humans are going to undergo great dental reduction then a highly specialized diet will be expected for them. This would seem unlikely for an omnivorous, wide ranging species like humans. Not only is their wide culinary variation within one culture, there are many things eaten in other cultures which one don't even consider as food. So, the future diet patterns, may vary so as to get accustom to the reduced dentition sizes.

20 *Dental Jurisprudence*

The technical training of dental students leaves little opportunity for them to study laws and other legal implications in relation to their profession. An understanding of legal implications is extremely important for a dentist to deal with a variety of circumstances in day to day life. The science that deals with the study of *law* is known as *Jurisprudence*. It is also defined as *the study of the principles and theories on which a legal system is founded*. *Medical jurisprudence* includes application of medical knowledge to question the laws affecting life, certifying the cause of death and proper medical practice, etc. *Dental Jurisprudence* is the science that includes the application of dental knowledge for the purpose of law. It includes elucidation of doubtful legal questions, the state laws and codes covering the legal implications as regard to the practice of dentistry.

The dentist has to serve the law either by helping in identification of the deceased or to be an expert witness to give an opinion regarding any set of situations.

DENTIST AS A WITNESS

Many a times, the dentist himself/herself can be a witness. The witness can be a professional or even a lay witness.

As a lay witness: Any person who is present at the time of the incident and has observed it, or is told about it or has read about it, can be a witness. In case the witness happens to be a dentist, his statement can't be taken as professional or expert opinion. The witness is to respond to the summon of court, whether he/she be a doctor or any other busy professional. Not responding to court summons, quoting being busy in profession, is not an excuse.

As an expert witness: There are certain circumstances which need an expert opinion, e.g. whether the patient's complaint causing the damage is valid technically or not? The extent of disability and likelihood of its continuation is also to be evaluated. A couple of facts may not require an expert witness such as fractured teeth, lacerations, etc.

An expert is called upon to express a professional opinion based on his knowledge in respect to the facts which may and may not be related to the case. The expert is only to give an opinion and not the judgement. It is the duty of the judge and the jury members to compare the specific facts with the standards and then make an appropriate decision.

It is the duty of the dentist to respond to the summons of the court. The court may and may not provide compensation to the dentist. Sometimes, the party which is going to be benefited by the witness pays the dentist, which is considered illegal because it may result in a biased testimony.

An expert opinion is always required in case of a doubt of malpractice. Only an expert view can clarify whether the treatment followed was based on standard principles or not and also the negligence on the part of the dentist, if any.

The expert can change his testimony regarding a case because of any confusion or uncertainty about the facts. The changed opinion affects the decision and may lead to unnecessary delays.

Forensic dentistry, also referred to as *forensic odontology*, is the branch of dentistry which deals with management, examination, evaluation and presentation of dental evidences in criminal or civil legal proceedings in the interest of justice. It is also defined as *the branch of forensic medicine which in the interest of justice deals with the proper handling and examination of dental evidence and with the proper evaluation and presentation of the dental findings.*

Forensic odntology features three major areas:

- Evaluation of injuries to teeth and other tissues.
- Examination of marks which lead to possible identification of a suspect.
- Examination of the dental remains

The most important and common role of forensic dentistry is identification of the deceased individual from the remains recovered at the site.

Dental identification includes:

- Identification is established by comparing post-mortem and ante-mortem records.
- In cases where ante-mortem records are not available, and no clues to the possible identity exist, identification is established by post-mortem records only.

Why to Identify the Deceased

The following situations warrant the identification of the deceased:

- *Criminal:* Investigation in case of criminal death can't begin until the victim has been identified.
- *Marriage:* Individuals from many religious backgrounds can not re-marry unless their partners are confirmed to be deceased.
- *Monetary:* Payments of pension, life insurance and other benefits rely upon positive confirmation of death of an individual.
- *Burial:* Many religions require that a positive identification be made prior to burial in a geographical area.
- *Social:* Correct identity helps preserve human rights and dignity beyond life.
- *Closure:* Identification of individuals missing for prolonged periods can bring sorrowful relief to the family members.

Why Forensic Dentistry Need Special Emphasis

The forensic dentist can help legal authorities by identifying individuals in circumstances like:

- Violent crimes, fires, accidents and natural calamities leading to mass disaster (the cadavers are mostly disfigured to such an extent that identification by a family member or a relative is neither reliable nor desirable).
- Analysis for bite-mark patterns collected from the victim and also the other injured tissues so as to identify whether it is of a human or animal origin.
- Recognition of signs and symptoms which may suggest human abuse.
- Presentations of dental evidence in cases of malpractice and fraud.

Dental evaluation can be carried out in two ways:

Comparative Dental Evaluation

It involves the comparison of ante-mortem with post-mortem records which includes position of individual teeth, their anatomic and pathologic components, patterns of palatal rugae and radiographic interpretation of teeth and paranasal sinuses (especially maxillary and frontal sinus).

Before starting with dental identification, a tentative identification of the deceased is made with the help of clothes and other objects found from body like jewellery, wallet, driving license, etc. It may provide some idea about the residence of the deceased. Missing person's database, if available, can be used to determine the race and the related information. After making a tentative identification, ante-mortem records can be obtained from the dentist who has been dealing with the deceased before death.

The forensic dentist must ensure that the available records are of the person concerned. The name and address of the person and the submitting dentist should be clearly mentioned. An *evidence transfer document* is to be signed, if the jurisdiction so warrants.

The post-mortem records are taken by forensic dentist using photographic and radiographic techniques along with written descriptions of the dental structures. All the records should include the case number, date, demographic and anthropologic information, name of the authority who is requesting for dental examination, location of examination and name of the examining dentist.

Photographs viewing full head and face along with images of upper and lower occlusal arches are taken. Any unusual pathological or restorative findings are recorded followed by appropriate radiographic examination.

Radiographs cannot be taken by regular radiographic procedures in some cases, e.g. in decomposed, dismembered and incinerated bodies; or due to rigor mortis. These cases require soft tissue or jaw resection along with modifications in radiation exposure. The standard settings of impulse and exposure time are reduced to one half for such cases.

Radiographs should be marked to prevent confusion between ante-mortem and post-mortem records. For example, rubber dam punch can be used to make one hole on ante-mortem and two holes on post-mortem films. The post-mortem dentition is depicted in odontogram, showing missing teeth and teeth with restorations. Post-mortem loss of teeth is common in circumstances like mass disasters, drowning cases or if the body is dragged by scavenging animals. When teeth are lost in this manner, the crest of the alveolar bone remains intact without the re-ossification of socket and/or decomposition of the periodontal ligament. To depict the tooth lost in this manner, the abbreviation **MPPA** (Missing Post-Mortem Present Ante-mortem) is used in an odontogram.

After collecting post-mortem and ante-mortem records, a comparative note is prepared with regard to similarities and discrepancies. The discrepancies can be divided in two categories— explainable and non-explainable. Explainable discrepancies normally relate to the time elapsed between post-mortem and ante-mortem records. For example, the number of teeth extracted or restorations placed may vary between part and ante-mortem records. However, unexplainable discrepancies help in exclusion. For example, teeth absent in ante-mortem and present in post-mortem records suggest that the records may not be of the same person.

Depending upon the comparison, four alternate possibilities are:

- *Positive identification:* The ante-mortem and post-mortem data match in sufficient detail, with no unexplainable discrepancies, establishing that they are of the same individual.
- *Possible identification:* The ante-mortem and post-mortem data have consistent features; but, because of certain qualitative, it is not possible to establish positive identity.
- *Insufficient evidence:* The available information is insufficient to draw some conclusion.
- *Exclusion:* The ante-mortem and post-mortem data are definitely inconsistent.

Dental Profiling

When dental records are not available and other methods of identification are also not possible, the forensic expert can produce a 'picture' of general features of the individual's.

This process is known as post-mortem *dental profiling*. A dental profile will typically provide information on the deceased's age, ancestry background, sex and socio-economic status. In some instances it is possible to provide additional information regarding the occupation, dietary habits, habitual behaviors and occasionally on dental or systemic diseases.

The forensic dentist will often work with a forensic anthropologist to help in the identification of an individual or the development of a profile from the remains. The determination of sex and ancestry can be assessed from skull shape and form. Generally, from skull appearance, forensic dentists can determine the race within the three major groups: Caucasoid, Mongloloid and Negroid. Additional characteristics, such as cusps of Carabelli, shovel-shaped incisors and multi-cusped premolars, can also assist in the determination of ancestry. Sex determination is usually based on cranial appearance, as no sex differences are apparent in the morphology of teeth. Microscopic examination of teeth can confirm sex by the presence or absence of Y-chromatin and DNA analysis can also reveal sex.

In developing a profile, dental structures can provide useful indicators to the individual's chronological age. The age of children can be determined by the analysis of tooth development and the subsequent comparison with development charts. Conclusions are usually accurate to approximately ±1.5 years. While eruption dates can be used in determining sub-adult ages, these are highly variable and the actual development stages of the teeth are more accurate.

Other features can be useful in individualizing a profile. The presence of erosion can suggest alcohol or substance abuse, an eating disorder or even hiatus hernia while stains can indicate smoking. Unusual wear patterns may result from pipe stems, cigarette holders, hairpins, carpet tacks or previous orthodontic treatment. The quality, quantity and presence or absence of dental treatment may give an indication of socio-economic status or likely country of residence.

Because of the resistant nature of dental tissues to environmental assaults, such as incineration, immersion, trauma, mutilation and decomposition, teeth represent an excellent source of DNA material. When conventional dental identification methods fail, this biological material can provide the necessary link to provide identity.

OTHER METHODS OF DENTAL IDENTIFICATION

- In some countries, dental prostheses are labeled with the patient's name or a specific number. In case of edentulous patients, the available ante-mortem records may not reflect the current status of the ridge.
- Removable orthodontic appliances can be evaluated for palatal rugae patterns which can be used as identification markings.

ROLE OF DNA IN DENTAL IDENTIFICATION

Since dental tissue is a hard calcified tissue and can resist incineration, immersion, burning, mutilation and decomposition; so it is an excellent material to get DNA. Saliva can also be used to examine DNA. Saliva samples can be taken from clothing if victim or suspect is bitten through garments or directly from the surface of the bite injury.

Two techniques are used to evaluate the fragments of DNA:

- *Restriction fragment length polymorphism (RFLP):* The process requires high molecular weight DNA, which is not present in dental tissue.
- *Polymerase chain reaction (PCR):* This process can be used in dental tissues since DNA

fragments can be produced from small amount of complex template.

The DNA extracted from teeth of an unidentified can be compared with ante-mortem samples (stored blood, hairbrush, clothing, etc.) or with parents or siblings. commonly, genomic DNA (DNA taken out from the nucleus of cell) is used; however, mitochondrial DNA (mtDNA) is more effective. It has an added advantage that because of a high number of mitochondria present in most cells and as it is maternally inherited, it confers the same mtDNA sequence as seen in all maternal relatives. The mitochondrial DNA can be sourced from dentin powder obtained via cryogenic grinding.

Determination of Species and Race

Forensic anthropologist and the dentist can conclude sex and ancestry by examining an individual's skull shape and form. Skull shape can be helpful in differentiating three races– *Caucasoid, mongoloids and negroids*. Additional dental features like cusp of carabelli, shovel shaped incisors, multicuspid pre-molars help in determining race. Sex can not be reliably determined from tooth morphology; but, microscopic examination of teeth can confirm sex by the presence or absence of Y-chromatin from DNA. It has been shown that dentinal fluid contain specific species information. The fluid can be compared using counter-current electrophoresis with artificial antisera. Remnants of cells from fragments of bone or teeth may be examined for the presence of Barr bodies on the sex chromosomes of the cells.

Determination of Age

Dental structures can reveal chronological age upto a certain extent. Age of children can be determined with a variation of ±1.5 years; but, in the middle aged and the elderly, the variation is up to ± 10–12 years.

The radiograph of jaws at death will indicate the extent of mineralization around each tooth, enabling to estimate the age of an individual'.

It is established that the tubules within the root becomes progressively mineralized as age advances. This mineralization alters the refractive index of the dentin, rendering it transparent when examined under a microscope. Such teeth can be compared with the teeth of a known age; and the age can thus be determined at the time of the death.

Recently, more objective methods of age determination are being studied. This depends upon the findings that amino acids are built into the collagen as optically pure enantiomers of the L.aspartic acid type. With the passage of time this L-aspartic acid enantiomer slowly undergoes racemization producing the opposite enantiomer, R-aspartic acid. The rate at which this change occurs is determined and subsequently compared with the teeth of the deceased, which indicates the age of the individual at death.

BITE PATTERN EVIDENCE

Bite pattern taken from the injured tissue or any other objects can be utilized in making the identification of the victim or the culprit, because even the culprit can get bitten by the victim during any aggressive behaviour as a means of self defence.

Bites found on the body of the victim can be of animal or human origin. Animal bites are often avulsive and are of narrower diameters than human bites. Animal bites are generally observed during the postmortem when the body has not been put to last rituals. Self-inflicted bites are observed in Lesch-Nyhan syndrome which is an X-linked, recessively transmitted disease. The individual affected with this disease tends to bite their own forearms or hands in order to prevent themselves from crying when traumatized psychologically. Bite injuries can be seen in children which can be a result of playground altercations. Bite injuries from animals and humans can cause infections like tetanus, tuberculosis, syphilis, actinomycosis, hepatitis B, herpes, cytomegalovirus infections, HIV, etc. Rabies is one of the most serious infection of animal bite.

Bites can be described in an ascending scale of severity, beginning with petechial hemorrhage (erythema), contusion (ecchymosis), abrasion, laceration (incision) and finally avulsion.

The severity of bite injury, in all probability, increases the chance of HIV transmission. As HIV is a predominately blood transmitted virus, so, in order to access the victims blood, a bite must break the skin. Any previous injury or pathological lesion can also present broken skin. In such cases, a superficial bite can allow flow of saliva or oral blood into the injured site.

Characteristics of Bite Marks

Bite mark can be characterized as:
- Individual mark
- Class characteristic

Individual Mark

It is described as the internal characteristic of one bite mark. For example, human incisors make rectangular mark whereas cuspids, depending upon the degree of attrition, can make points or triangular patterns.

Class Characteristic

It is the shape created when the group of teeth from both dental arches are impressed into a tissue or any object. It can be round, ovoid or elliptical. When only one arch is in contact crescent pattern is formed. The diameter of a normal human bite is within a range of 4.0 cm.

Bite mark on an object is reliable; however, when it is recovered from a living tissue (skin or mucous membrane), swelling or shrinkage occurs in them with time which make the mark unreliable. Contusions and area of ecchymosis can be seen along the bitten living tissue while absence of bleeding along the injury indicates that it might be inflicted after death.

Description of a Bite Mark

The demographic information, i.e. name, age, sex and race of victim and examining date should be noted. The bite mark should be described by the forensic dentist as follows:
- Anatomic location of the bite
- Surface, contour and tissue characteristics of bitten area
- Shape, colour, size of bite, type of bite (animal or human bite)
- Relative skin mobility
- Condition of underlying tissues
- Any associated injury like abrasion, laceration, stab or bullet wound which can affect the pattern.

After collection of bite mark pattern, the victim and the suspect are examined thoroughly, which includes intraoral, extraoral, soft tissue and periodontal examination. A dental chart is maintained showing the presence/absence of teeth. Extraoral, intraoral and occlusal photographs at different orientations along with close-up views are taken with a reference scale so that they can be compared with bite pattern photographs. Intentional bite pattern, taken on either a wax sheet or acrylic, are compared with the original bite marks.

All these procedures aid in *Collection of Evidence* about the case.

Range of Bitemark Severity (The Bitemark Severity and Significance Scale)

1. Very mild and diffuse bruising, no individual tooth marks present; may be caused by anything other than teeth (low forensic significance).
2. Complete avulsion of tissue along with some scalloping of the injury margins. The

teeth may be responsible for the injury; however, not an obvious bite injury (low forensic significance).

3. Partial avulsion of tissue, some lacerations present, indicating teeth as the probable cause of the injury (Moderate forensic significance).

4. Obvious bruising and discrete areas associated with teeth; the skin remains intact (moderate forensic significance).

5. Obvious bruising with small lacerations associated with teeth on the most severe aspects of the injury are likely to be assessed as definite bitemark (high forensic significance).

The **lip prints** are also used in isolated cases for human identification. The lip prints are as useful as finger prints.

MASS DISASTER VICTIM IDENTIFICATION

Mass disaster represents one of the most challenging aspects of forensic dentistry. It can occur due to natural, accidental or criminal reasons leading to multiple fatalities which necessitate identification.

Mass disaster includes earthquakes, aircraft accidents, terrorist attacks, volcanic eruptions, fire, storms and floods. Victims are scattered throughout a broad area. Dental offices of that area are also destroyed so one can not get ante-mortem records, which causes even more delay and difficulty in identifications. The dental structures and restorations may be the only part of the body not destroyed and can be utilized for identification.

Identification teams include funeral director, medical examiner, pathologists, forensic anthropologist, forensic dentist, fingerprint specialists and radiographer. Softwares like the FBI-NCIC program, CAPMI-4 version 4.0, winID and Toothpics identification system can be used to assist the team in filing, storing, sorting and matching any of ante-mortem (if available) and post-mortem information.

BIBLIOGRAPHY

1. Aitchinson, J.: Some racial differences in human skulls and jaws. B.D.J.: 116, 25, 1964.
2. Al-Talazani, N., Al-Moussawy, N.D. and Baker, F.A.: Digital analysis of experimental human bitemarks: Application of two new methods. J. Forensic Sci.: 51, 1372, 2006.
3. Atsu, S.S., Gokclemir, K. and Kedici, P.S.: Bitemarks in forensic odontology. J. Forensic Odontostomatol.: 16, 30, 1998.
4. Beckstead, J.W., Rawson, R.D. and Giles, W.S.: Review of bitemark evidence. J.A.D.A.: 99,69,1979.
5. Bell, J.: The current status of lip prints and their use for identification. J. Forensic Odonto Stomatol.: 20, 43, 2002.
6. Bernitz, H., Owen, J.H. and Heerden, W.F. : An integrated technique for the analysis of skin bite marks. J. Forensic Sci. : 53, 194, 2008.
7. Bowers, C.M. and Pretty, I.A.: Expert disagreement in Bitemark casework. J. Forensic Sci.: 54, 2009.
8. Brooks, S.T.: Skeletal age at death : the reliability of cranial and public indications. Am. J. Phys. Anthrop.: 13, 567, 1955.
9. Bushick, R.D.: Forensic Dentistry: An overview for the general dentist. Gen. Dent. : 54, 48, 2006.
10. Dierick, A., Seyler, M. and de Valck, E. : Dental Records: A Belgium study. J. Forensic Odontostomatol.: 24, 22, 2007.
11. Fierstein, M.: Dentistry and the Law. N.Y.J. : 42, 249, 1972.
12. Furness, J.: A general review of bite mark evidence. Am. J. Forensic Med. Pathol.: 2, 49, 1981.
13. Gupta, N. and jadhav, K. : Is re-creation of human identity possible using tooth prints ? An experimental study to aid in identification. J. Forensic Sci.: 192, 67, 2009.
14. Gustafson, G.: Age determination on teeth. J.A.D.A.: 41, 45, 1950.
15. Kittelson, J.M., Kicser, J.A., Buckhingam, D.M. and Herbison, G.P.: Weighing evidence : quantitative measures of the importance of bite mark evidence. J. Forensic odontostomatol. : 20, 31, 2002.
16. Lampe, H. an Roetzscher, K.: Forensic odontology: age determination from adult human teeth. Med. Law : 13, 623, 1994.
17. Leung, C.K.: Forensic Odontology. Hong Kong Dental Bulletin: 13, 16, 2008.

18. Lorensten, M. and Solheim : T. : Age assessment based on translucent dentin. J. Forensic Odontostomatol.: 7, 3, 1989.

19. McKenna, C.J.: Radiography in forensic dental identification – a review. J. Forensic Odontostomatol. : 17, 47, 1999.

20. Neumann, C. and Margot, P.: New perspective in the use of ink evidence in forensic science : Part III. Operational applications and evaluations. J. Forensic Sci.: 192, 29, 2009.

21. Pinchi, V., Forestieri, A.L. and Calvitti, M.: Thickness of the dental (radicular) cementum: a parameter for estimating age. J. Forensic Odontostomatol.: 25, 1, 2007.

22. Pretty, I.A., Anderson, G.S. and Sweet, D.J.: Human bites and the risk of HIV infections. Am. J. Forensic Med. Path. : 20, 232, 1999.

23. Pretty, I.A. and Sweet, D.: A look at forensic dentistry – Part 1. The role of teeth in the determination of human identity. B.D.J. : 190, 359, 2001.

24. Pretty, I.A. and Sweet, D.: The scientific basis for human bite mark analysis – a critical review. Sci. Justice : 41, 85, 2001.

25. Pretty, I.A. : Forensic Dentistry: 1. Identification of human remains. Dent. Update : 34, 621, 2007.

26. Pretty, I.A. : Forensic Dentistry : 2. Bitemark and bite injuries. Dent. Update : 35, 48, 2008.

27. Richmond, R. and Pretty, I.A.: Contemporary methods of labeling dental prosthesis – a review of the literature. J. Forensic Sci.: 51, 1120, 2006.

28. Robinson, F.G., Haywod, V.B. and David, T.J. : Dental practices that aid the general practitioner and forensic dentist. Gen. Dent. : 46, 203, 1998.

29. Rothwell, B.R.: Principles of dental identification. D.C.N.A. : 45, 253, 2001.

30. Sheasby, D.R. and McDonald, D.G.: A forensic classification of distortion in human bite marks. Forensic Sci. Int. : 122, 75, 2001.

31. Stimson, P.G.: Forensic Odontology. J.P.D. : 30, 922, 1973.

32. Sweet, D.: Why a dentist for identification ? D.C.N.A. : 45, 237, 2001.

33. Sweet, D.J.: The wide range of forensic dentistry. Gen. Dent : 50, 8, 2002.

34. Weedu, V.W.: Postmorten identification of remains. Clin. Lab. Med. : 18, 115, 1998.

35. Whittake, D.K., Lcewelyn, D.R. and Jones, R.W. : Sex determination from necrotic pulpal tissues. B.D.J.: 139, 403, 1975.

36. Wright, F.D. and Dailey, J.C. : Human bitemarks in forensic dentistry. D.C.N.A. : 45, 365, 2001.

21   *Ethics in Dentistry*

The strength of any profession revolves around technical knowledge and skill. The medical profession at large and precisely the practice of dentistry, is governed by certain rules and regulations which may not be stated in the law. The society expects the dentists to follow these rules and regulations, which form the foundation of their conduct with the patients and are commonly known as ETHICS. It is mandatory to follow the code of ethics in any profession. Whereas laws are clearly defined, ethical rules may not be clear. Laws are enforced by the government, but ethical rules are enforced only by professional societies.

Ethics and society are interrelated and influence each other. Individuals following ethics make a better society. The gap between general and professional ethics is marginal. There is a difference of degree only and not of quality. For example, 'do not steal', which is a principle in general ethics equally applies to professional ethics.

DEFINITION

The word 'ethics' is derived from the Greek word 'ethos' meaning custom or character. Ethics refer to the philosophy of human conduct or the science of what is morally right. Conduct is a voluntary action carried out without any compulsion and ethics are concerned with evaluating human conduct and judging whether the action is right or wrong.

Ethics form one of the three branches of philosophy (the other two are metaphysics and epistemology) that is concerned with the study of those concepts, which are used to evaluate human activities; especially, the concepts of goodness and obligation. *Ethics may also be defined as a normative study that deals with the conduct of human beings in private or in public.* The study of Ethics is thus, a normative science, not a descriptive one. A descriptive science deals with the factual truths, whereas in a normative science, only moral evaluations are made. Ethics do not teach us what to do, rather they seek to find out what ought to be the basis of our actions and judgements. It is a search for principles that guides our practical conduct and moral perceptions.

The other two branches of philosophy, i.e. metaphysics and epistemology also have a bearing on ethics. *Metaphysics* is concerned with our perception of the ultimate nature of reality. *Epistemology* deals with the conditions under which our claims to knowledge and belief are either valid or invalid. The relation between ethics and epistemology is well described by forensic science, which defines the ethico-legal status of an action on the basis of evidence of facts.

Ethical Dilemmas

The specific problems and moral issues emerged due to changed modern circumstances for dealing with patients are called Ethical Dilemmas. A branch of normative ethics which deals with these specific ethical problems is called *Applied Ethics*; and it includes (a) medical ethics, (b) business ethics, (c) media ethics, (d) legal ethics and (e) environment ethics.

The **principles** that are followed for the making of decisions in the **ethical dilemmas** are listed below:

1. *Analyzing:* Dividing a problem into its leading alternatives.
2. *Weighing:* Assessing the strength and weakness of alternatives by balancing one against the other.
3. *Justifying:* Providing a compelling and sufficient moral reason that appeals to an established moral principle such as to tell the truth.
4. *Choosing:* Selecting alternatives for which some justification can be made.
5. *Evaluating:* Re-examining the choice and the justification based on one's exposure to other similar moral issues.

History of Ethics

The 'Hippocratic Oath' has been regarded as a standard of professional ethics. Various theories have been put forward regarding ethics:

1. Theory of utilitarian ethics: It focuses on utility
2. Theory of deontologic ethics: It focuses on morality of act rather than its consequences. It emphasized that irrespective of the consequence do not compromise with duty.
3. Theory of virtue ethics: It focuses on, how a virtuous person would have reacted in a particular circumstance.
4. Descriptive theories define the meaning of good; may be moral or non-moral characteristics.
5. Prescriptive theories define ethical terms as carrying mandatory force e.g. 'ethical rules for dentists' framed by the Dental Council of India.

Development of Moral behavior: The development of moral behavior occurs in three stages that are:

Stage 1: In this stage, human beings decide what is right or wrong on the basis of inborn tendencies or innate feelings.

Stage 2: Man considers those forms of conduct to be right which were approved by customary modes of behaviour.

Stage 3: Here, it is the individual's conscience with his capacity to judge what is right and what is wrong.

Usually our moral judgements are not decided on the basis of instincts or customs. The transition from customary morality to conscience or reflective morality makes the individual completely responsible for his choice of action.

CODE OF DENTAL ETHICS

A profession consists of a limited group of persons who have acquired some special skill and are able to perform that function in society better than an average normal person. A professional person is expected to have respect for human beings, competence in his chosen field, integrity and primary concern with service rather than with prestige and profit. A systematic set of rules is needed that upholds the dignity and honour of any profession, upgrading its standards and spheres of usefulness. The members of the concerned association should understand their duties and obligations, not only towards their fellow beings but also towards the society. Ethical codes are the result of an attempt to direct moral consciousness of members of the profession to a peculiar problem. Hippocrates wrote the first voluntary code of regulations for the medical profession, protecting the rights of patients and appealing to the finer instincts of physicians. Standards for the protection of human subjects were created in 1947 and are called the **Nuremberg Code**.

In dentistry, the ADA's the (American Dental Association) principles of ethics are followed in routine, labeled as a code of ethics and conduct. This code contains five major sections.

1. Service to public and quality of care
2. Education
3. Governing the profession
4. Research and development
5. Professional announcement

Postulates of Ethics

The different postulates of ethics are:

1. To genuinely differentiate between right and wrong actions.
2. One should know the difference between right and wrong.
3. Knowledge of morality does make a serious impact on human behaviour.
4. Despite certain limitations and constraints one has the capacity/freedom to exercise one's rationality to make moral choices.
5. Order of the temporal lobe of the cerebrum by which actions are carried out in the order of priority.

PRINCIPLES OF ETHICS

There are several ethical principles that health care professionals must be aware of and practise in routine. In one way, these are their duties and obligations towards patients and the society. The important ones are:

1. To do no harm
2. Try to do good
3. Respect for others
4. Justice
5. Truthfulness
6. Confidentiality

To do no Harm

This principle is generally attributed to Hippocrates and is considered to be the foundation of social morality. For example, in dental profession, mistakes like overhanging restorations or failure to sterilize the instruments can cause irreparable damage to the patient's oral health. Such mistakes should be avoided. This principle is more important because of a dual responsibility towards individuals and the community.

Try to do Good

One should try to do good to others. The patients expect better treatment from their care provider. For an epidemiologist, concern is not merely with physical health of subject, but also the potential benefit/harm to the group of community under study. For example, it is unethical to carry out screening in a community where treatment is not possible or is beyond the financial reach of the people.

Respect for Others

The final decision about treatment should be taken jointly by the dentist and the patient after a thorough discussion. The health care professional should respect the patient's capacity in making decisions. However, total autonomy to the patient is to be avoided. It is a breach of ethics and can become a legal problem.

Informed Consent is an essential component of planning a treatment regimen for individuals. The attributes of informed consent are:

- It should be voluntarily given by the patient.
- It should be legally competent.
- It should be informed.
- It should be comprehending.

In certain populations, the concept of individual autonomy may be comprehended. In such situations, informed consent is negotiated with a leader. This can also be followed in cases where persons because of illiteracy or otherwise cannot participate actively. The ethical principles require special justifications before research is conducted on vulnerable individuals. A vulnerable population also includes women who might be subservient to their spouses. Women may or may not be literate, but should participate in the discussion. Illiteracy may not present any problem because informed consent can be taken by talking rather than reading. This empowers women to protect their own interests.

The **Consent Form** is an instrument designed to protect the interests of the investigators and their institutions; and also to defend them against any civil or criminal liability. The informed consent actually consists of two steps. In the first step, the investigator presents whole of the information regarding the procedure to the subject and in the second step, his queries about that procedure are cleared. A list of information conveyed to the prospective subjects includes:

a. A statement that the study involves research coupled with an explanation of the purpose of research and expected duration of the subjects' involvement. A description of the procedure followed should also be identified.
b. A description of any benefit to the subjects.
c. A description of any reasonably foreseeable risks or discomforts to the patient.
d. Whether any medical treatment available during risk.
e. Availability of alternative procedure, if any.
f. A statement highlighting how the confidentiality of records will be maintained.
g. Availability of person(s) for answers to pertinent questions about ongoing research.
h. A statement that participation is voluntary and refusal to participate will involve no penalty or loss of benefits to which the subject is otherwise entitled and the subject may discontinue participation at any time.

These eight elements of test are collectively known as 'Elements of Information' in the informed consent.

Justice

Justice emphasizes that each person should be treated equally without any discrimination of caste, creed, race, etc. It calls for an obligation to protect the weak and to ensure equality in rights and benefits. Practically, it might be difficult to achieve equality between subject rights and benefits so a balance is to be maintained between them. For an epidemiologist, this becomes even more difficult because of the cost and interests of a community, e.g. in some areas priority is for access to water rather than health care services.

Truthfulness

The patient doctor relationship is based on trust. Truthfulness is an ethical principle that one should always follow. Sometimes circumstances can demand the violation of this principle, e.g. physicians often withhold bad news when they believe that would upset the patient. Another example is the use of placebos which is being argued both scientifically and morally. It is established that placebos work in all groups of people; however, ethically, it may be taken as lying to the patient.

Confidentiality

Patients have the right to expect that all communications and records pertaining to their care will be treated as confidential. It can be breached only if it is required in the court of law. Even in epidemiological studies, there should be no violation of confidentiality e.g. The results of an epidemiologic study are generally depicted in tabulated form in which the subject's names are either erased or replaced by a code or another name.

ETHICS AND DENTISTRY

Ethics play a major role in any profession and so too in dentistry. A dentist has some ethical duties not only towards his patients but also towards his fellow dentists. These duties are discussed below:

Duties towards the Patients

The duties towards the patients are:
- A dentist has the ethical obligation to furnish records of the patient to other dentists or to the patients himself either free of cost or after accepting a nominal fee.
- Dentists have an obligation to use their skills, knowledge and experience for general improvement of dental health of the public.
- Dentists should make reasonable arrangements for emergency care of a patient, whether referred or otherwise.
- Dentist shall be obliged to seek consultation, if need be and the referred dentist upon completion of the treatment shall return the patient to referring dentist.

Duties towards another Dentist

The duties towards another dentist are:
a. When informing the patient about his oral health, the dentist should exercise control in that the comments made by him are justifiable, e.g. a difference of opinion to preferred treatment should not be communicated to patient in a manner which may offend him.
b. One should never criticize the fellow dentist in front of other patients.

The following features are considered unethical towards professional colleagues:
- Paying or accepting commissions.
- Undercutting of charges in order to solicit patients.
- If planned treatment is beyond the skills of the dentist and the patient is not referred to a consultant.
- The patient is not sent back after the requisite service of the consultant dentist.

- If consulted dentist accepts charges without request of referring dentist.

LAWS IN DENTISTRY

The laws applicable to the dental practice are same as those applicable to anyone who provides personal services. As a private practitioner, the dentist is governed by **tax laws**, **employment laws** and **law of contract**. The dentist as a professional is also subject to a special statute commonly referred to as **dental law** or **dental practice act**.

The laws that are applicable under the act are as follows:
- The name under which a dentist conducts his practice should not be false or misleading in any respect.
- Use of the name of dentist no longer actively associated with the practice may be continued for a period not exceeding one year.
- A dentist who announces in any means of communication that he/she is certified or a diplomate in an area of dentistry not recognized by DCI, amounts to be making a false or misleading representation to the public.

Laws that are related to third party payments are:
- A dentist who accepts third party payments under a co-payment plan as payment in full without disclosing details to the third party is unethical.
- It is unethical for a dentist to increase the fee to a patient solely because the patient is insured.
- Payments received under a government funded programme or constituent dental society sponsored programme should not be overbilled.
- A dentist who submits a claim form to a third party reporting arbitrary treatment dates so as to assist a patient in obtaining benefits under a dental plan is unethical.

- A dentist who incorrectly describes a dental procedure in order to receive a greater payment or reimbursement is unethical.
- A dentist who recommends or performs unnecessary dental procedures is also unethical.

BIBLIOGRAPHY

1. Beavichamp, T.L. and Childress, J.F. : Principles of biomedical ethics. 51th Ed., 2001, Oxford University Press.

2. Chambers, D.W. : A primer on dental ethics : Part I. Knowing about ethics. J. Am. College of Dentists : 73, 38, 2006.

3. Chambers, D.W. : A primer on dental ethics : Part II. Moral Behaviour. J. Am. College of Dentists : 74, 38, 2007.

4. Shaw, D. : Ethics, professionalism and fitness to practice : three concepts, not one. B.D.J. : 207, 59, 2009.

5. Trathen, A. and Gullaghor, J.F. : Dental professionalism : definitions and debate. B.D.J. : 206, 249, 2009.

22 *Computers in Dentistry*

Advancement is the backbone of progress. Various newer instruments have been added and are still being added to the dental armamentarium. Computer is one such asset to the dental profession that has become a necessity without which survival is difficult. The study of a computer as a machine is mandatory for better understanding of its functioning.

A computer is an electronic machine, which can be equated with a super calculator. Apart from adding and subtracting numbers, the computer can store huge amounts of information for future use. Technically, computer is an electronic device, which accepts data and processes it according to a set of instructions, producing the desired output.

Computer equipment is called 'hardware'. The programs that are operated or run on the computer are termed 'software'. A wide array of computer softwares is available for a variety of applications. One just needs to select the right software as per the requirement. New softwares can also be developed to suit individual demands.

PARTS OF A COMPUTER

A computer is a collection of separate items working together as a team. Some of the components are essential and others make working more pleasant and efficient. Adding extra items expands the variety of tasks one can accomplish with this machine. The computer system is made up of the following:

Basic components
1. System Unit
2. Monitor
3. Keyboard
4. Storage media: The Disk
   a. Floppy Disk Drive
   b. Hard Disk Drive

Optional components
5. Mouse
6. Printer

System Unit

The system unit controls and executes all the information ensuring that the correct information is displayed on the monitor. The unit is available in different shapes.

The 'System Unit' is considered to be the brain of the computer. Inside the unit are components that run various programs. The important components are: CPU (Central Processing Unit), RAM (Random Access Memory), ROM (Read Only Memory) and Interface connections.

The speed of the CPU is measured in megahertz (MHz). A computer has a central clock that keeps all the components in time with each other; One hertz is similar to a clock tick and one megahertz is equal to one million ticks per second. The faster the clock ticks, the faster the computer runs. The present day computers run at the speed of 166MHz, 200MHz or even more.

Monitor

The monitor displays the work done on the computer. The monitors are of various shapes and sizes. They are attached to the main system or can be placed separately.

Keyboard

The keyboard is the main means of giving information to the computer. A computer keyboard is quite similar to that of a typewriter but for some additional keys, which include:

- Arrows and other movement keys (Home, PgUp, PgDn)
- Function keys (F1-F12)
- Text editing keys (Back Space, Del)
- Modifier keys (Shift, Ctrl, Alt)
- Enter key
- Other special keys (Printscreen, Scroll lock, etc.)

Storage Media: The Disk

The computer uses a magnetic disk to store data permanently. The amount of data that can be stored on a disk is measured in kilobytes (one thousand bytes) or megabytes (one million bytes). The various types of disks are :

Floppy Disks

The floppy disk is used to store and move data easily from one computer to another. Floppies of 1.2MB and 1.44MB are available.

Hard Disk

The hard disk is fixed inside the processing unit. The functioning of a hard disk is similar to that of a floppy disk. It also stores information but the storage capacity is much higher. The storage capacity of a hard disks ranges from 20 GB to 600 GB (1GB = 1024MB). Recently, hard disk with the capacity of 1000 GB is also available, community knowns as one Terra bite.

Mouse

A mouse is an important device to point and select objects from the computer screen. Movement of the mouse on the desk controls the movement of the pointer on the screen. The mouse pointer (or mouse cursor) assumes different shapes to indicate different uses. Different types and shapes of the mouse are available. A recent development is the remote controlled mouse.

Printer

As the name implies, a printer is utilized to get prints of data stored inside the computer. Different types of printers are available depending upon mechanism of printing such as inkjet, laser, etc.

DOS (DISK OPERATING SYSTEM)

Using a computer means executing computer programs. Computer programs are sequences of instructions conveyed to the computer to perform in a desired manner. A computer program is usually stored on a disk and then loaded into the computer's main memory.

Operating system is the master computer program that manages the files on the disk file system and executes programs when instructed. The DOS creates new files, reads them, changes them, copies them and deletes them whenever it is required.

DOS provides a common interface between the user and the computer. Because of presence of DOS, the application programs are loaded into the memory and can be executed. By working in a common DOS supported environment, there exists a compatibility between computers. Disk data files and programs that work on one computer will work on another because computers use the same operating system.

What is a file?

The understanding of the concept of file is important. To understand a command it is necessary to know how files are organized and named. Even the programs on a disk working under DOS are arranged in the form of files. The three basic types of commonly used files are as follows:

a. Data files
b. Program files
c. Sub-directory files

a. **Data files** contain records of data which are created, retrieved and modified by application programs. Examples of data files can be letters/documents in a word processor, data base containing records in a word application package, etc.
b. **Program files** are part of a software package. There are mainly four kinds of programs that are stored in disk files. These are files with the extensions EXE, COM, BAT and SYS.
c. **Sub-directory files** are disk files which contain a sub-directory.

Microsoft Windows

Microsoft Windows is the most popular and commonly used software that allows many tasks, which can be performed on a computer. Unlike the text-only interface of DOS, the coloured interface of Windows makes extensive use of pictures to represent information. In Windows, the click of a mouse has replaced lengthy DOS commands. Windows runs several different application programs at the same time. It manages disks and files while using application software without having to quit the application. Windows uses a single menu structure and operating style that is common to all applications.

Once Windows has been installed, the DOS commands are rarely used, but to start Windows, loading of DOS can be preferred.

The common applications of MS Office, a popular software package, can be:

Microsoft Word

Microsoft Word software allows us to write, edit and print text documents. The look of the text can be controlled by changing the font style and size of its characters and by setting such elements as indents, line spacing, gaps and margins. The accuracy of the words can be checked by using the built-in spelling and grammar checkers.

Microsoft Excel

Microsoft Excel allows us to use efficient built-in functions as short cuts for performing mathematical, financial and statistical calculations. These calculations can be as simple as totalling rows or columns of values or as complex as figuring the rate of return on an investment under varying circumstances.

Microsoft Powerpoint

This presentation program puts together slide shows or electronic presentations with professional graphic effects. One can format the slide text in a variety of eye catching ways like charts and pictures.

Microsoft Access

This database stores and organizes information in sets of tables. After creating a database, one can look at the information as a list (in columns and rows), or in a form, as though it was recorded on an index card. One can perform calculations, compute statistics such as total and average, sort information, find specific items and create reports.

In addition to these primary applications, other applications are also provided for instance Microsoft groups, clipart gallery and organization chart, etc.

APPLICATIONS IN DENTISTRY

The computer is becoming increasingly popular in the daily practice of dentistry. Dentists who wish to remain competitive in this new era of technical proficiencies will have to maintain a high level of professional competence. This factor will make the computer an indispensable tool for dentistry. Certain areas have been identified where computers can be of help to the dentists or would be mandatory in the near future:

a. Maintenance of records.
b. Computers in diagnosis.
c. Computers in restorative dentistry.
d. Telecommunication (Internet).
e. Computers in disaster victim identification.

a. Maintenance of Records

The importance of maintenance of records is increasing day by day with patients becoming exceedingly conscious and aware of their rights. Patients' records are also a part of full time office system. This is a collection of patients' data which can be edited, stored, searched and printed as and when the need arises.

Paper records are fragile, susceptible to loss, fire, earthquake and tampering, etc. The drawback of paper records are more important when a subsequent dentist seeks information regarding the patients' previous treatment, etc. or when the original treating dentist is challenged by the patient in court.

Computer based records are more secure than paper records. The electronic patient record should consist of three essential sections: 1. Diagnostic records 2. Treatment records 3. Progress and outcome records. The computer based records can be programmed to display and describe a patient's condition, diagnosis and treatment options to facilitate education, co-diagnosis and informed consent.

Computer records are more transportable than paper records. With the inclusion of e-mail, dentists can now create information links with other dentists, insurers, dental associations, academies, bio-medical libraries, dental suppliers and speciality centres.

Computers also keep the record of financial transactions made in clinics. Interest on overdue accounts can be a big profit item for practitioners. Interest charges allow the doctor to extend credit, charge those patients who pay late and reward those who pay in time. Pay rolls of employees, their bonus, overtime, etc. can also be calculated easily.

Recalls are often very important for any practitioner. Reminders for recall appointments are produced on cards or labels that are mailed to the patients. Referral lists are useful for those offices that want to keep records of individuals who have been referring patients. The total tally of referrals can be "mail merged" with word processing data.

Records also help in evaluating the progress of the clinic in terms of the number of patients, finances, etc. Such evaluations are better feedbacks for better dentistry.

b. Computers in Diagnosis

Computers are helful in diagnosis in the following ways:

i. Computer Assisted Interpretation in Radiographic Diagnosis

The conventional radiography, though an adjunct in diagnosis, may have certain drawbacks such as, limitations of the human eye with regard to minimum perceptible size and contrast, optical illusions, interpretation of visual effects and prior knowledge bias of the observer. Computerized radiography helps in minimizing these drawbacks.

ii. Digital Image Processing

The conventional radiographic film is to be converted into an image that can be stored in a computer. There are two different options in dental radiography. One method is to digitize an existing radiograph using a charged couple device (CCD) camera. The second method uses intra oral direct imaging devices (Radio Visio Graphy (RVG) system). With direct digital radiographic imaging, the step of processing is eliminated and radiation doses are lowered.

After the image has been stored in a digital form in the computer, the next step is to extract features from the image that are, essential for the diagnosis of clinical conditions.

The features are extracted in steps. The first step is to reduce noise. Noise in an image leads to loss of information.

The next step is image enhancement, which enables the observer to recognize the characteristic features more easily. It includes adjusting contrast, enhancing edges of structures and removing background clouding, etc.

This is followed by the image segmentation, which aims at the separation of different regions in the image. For example, a tooth may be segmented into its enamel and dentin regions. Because of the overlap of different parts in a radiograph, the spatial density distribution in the image is not entirely related to the components of the radiographed object. Therefore, practically it is difficult to have image segmentation.

The next step is pattern recognition. This means the different structures or features visible on the radiograph can be isolated. For example, if the operator likes to study only cementum, the same can be isolated. Recognition of a pathologic pattern becomes easier when anatomic or structured noise is removed. Subtraction radiography has proved very effective in this regard.

Texture analysis is recognition of a repeating pattern. At times, recognition of entities is difficult in a single image. In that case, a set of two or more subimages, each representing a specific aspect such as density, contrast or texture is needed.

The computer also has the facility of 'image reconstruction', i.e. it uses data to combine the information of different images into one new image. For example, a three-dimensional representation of an object may be produced by images of two dimensions.

iii. Computer Aided Image Analysis

The computer uses data from various sources. After putting the same to a computer program

called interpretation, the 'analysis' can be arrived at.

The clinician enters the data of a patient and the program compares the data with facts in the knowledge base. When the program encounters an interpretation that has a reasonably high probability, the program displays the same to the clinician together with other likely probabilities.

The system can also suggest additional tests to improve upon the reliability of the diagnostic outcome and can provide scientific references with regard to the diseases and pathologic conditions.

iv. Computer Assisted Dental Diagnosis

After image analysis, the complete information is fed to computer for possible diagnosis of the disease. A computer can efficiently store and retrieve large amounts of data which can be executed, when required. The process of diagnosis by the computer involves a certain set of procedures or programs.

These set of programs are known as 'modules'. Modules 1 and 2 are used to diagnose symptomatic dental conditions and module 3 provides a differential diagnosis of a soft tissue lesion. Module 4 provides definitions for terms used in the program. Module 5 allows the user to bypass the diagnostic sequences of the modules 1 and 2 and directly access a treatment plan.

c. Computers in Restorative Dentistry

Innovations in technology have created some exciting possibilities in restorative dentistry. Computer Aided Design and Computer Aided Manufacturing (CAD/CAM) has been able to provide us restorations of high precision with less time required for manufacturing. The CEREC was the first commercially available CAD/CAM system.

Restoration fabrication either by traditional lost wax casting technique or high technology

CAD/CAM system utilizes three functional steps:
  i. Data acquisition
  ii. Restoration design
  iii. Restoration fabrication
  i. Data acquisition is the process of gathering information from the patient, i.e. the shape and size of the prepared tooth, the location of the proximal contacts, and the static and dynamic positions of the occluding teeth. This information is gathered by a specialized camera, a laser system or a miniature contact digitizer. The system projects an image of the preparation and surrounding structures on a monitor, allowing the dentist or auxiliary personnel to design the restoration. This is known as computer surface digitization. There are other techniques for computer surface digitization, which include:
  • Photogrammetry
  • Moire
  • Laser scanning
  • Computer tomography scanning
  • Magnetic resonance imaging
  • Ultrasound
  • Contact profilometry
  ii. Restoration design is carried out by the computer automatically or with interactive help from the user. The operator must input and/or confirm the boundaries of the restoration such as the position of the gingival margin and the proximal contacts.
  iii. Restoration fabrication includes machining with computer controlled milling machines, electric discharge machining and sintering. This stage includes micromilling procedures. The computer guides a milling machine to mill a restoration out of a block of high quality ceramic.

The CEREC 2 system, an improved version, provides improved accuracy of fit, an automatically generated occlusion, free unrestricted cavity design and automated and simplified operation.

Advantages

• Eliminates the need for impression making, temporary restoration and multiple appointments.
• Time saving for both the patient and the dentist.
• More precise restoration.
• Better quality material.
• Computer fills up the undercuts automatically.

Limitations

• Failures may be due to fracture at the margins and even bulk fractures.
• With any CAD/CAM system, precision is demanded when the cavity is prepared. Smooth walls and well defined margins are required to capture as accurate an 'impression' as possible.
• With the CEREC system, no occlusal anatomy or occlusal relationships are treated; they are established by the dentist with a handpiece after the restoration is cemented.
• Esthetics is also a limitation since most CAD/CAM systems are fabricated from a block of material that is only of one shade.

Some commercial CAD/CAM systems are as follows:
• CEREC
• SOPHA
• CICERO
• DentiCAD
• Procera

d. Telecommunication (Internet)

The internet is simply a 'global network of networks', a system that links computer networks all over the world so that anyone can communicate with others.

The various tools for use on the internet are as follows:

i. Electronic mail
ii. News groups
iii. FTP sites
iv. World Wide Web (WWW)

i. Electronic Mail/E-mail

This service allows users who are members to transfer almost any kind of data, be it text, pictures, video, sound and even computer software through the network. This service is generally provided free to the subscribers.

Electronic mail is much faster in transferring data limited only by the speed of the modem and the connection rate provided by the phone line. Using e-mail can significantly reduce the cost of postage and telephone charges especially when sending large amounts of data.

In dentistry, digitized clinical pictures or radiographs in addition to histologic sections, etc. can be transferred to the referring colleagues in addition to routine letter writings.

ii. News Groups

This is the place where one can chat, discuss, as well as enquire about certain topics. It is like throwing a question into the internet to get a response.

One can use a discussion group for modes of examination, diagnosis and treatment of rare conditions and also evaluating and assessing treatment options for specific conditions. It also provides the opportunity to evaluate new trial materials in the market through the responses of those who have already tried them.

iii. FTP Sites

FTP refers to File Transfer Protocol, which is for the basic download (retrieval) and upload (transfer) of data throughout the internet. FTP serves to provide free limited access to retrieve information such as texts, pictures, or computer software from a huge data base. For complete functions, FTP software is generally required. Most web browsers will only be able to download data but not upload it. Since most servers or databases require an access code to upload for security reasons, such software is the most important tool if one wants to start and maintain a web page on WWW.

iv. World Wide Web (WWW)

The WWW is the biggest global network as it combines different networks that are available for access.

Search for specific sites or any of the related topics can be carried out by using one of the numerous search engines. Through this connection, doctors as well as patients can have access to any information. The patients can be more knowledgeable not only in the matters of public health and hygiene, but also in other aspects of dental practice.

The biggest limiting factor, however, is the resistance to change. Simply using a computer may be a big hurdle for some. Furthermore, some knowledge about the hardware and the dial-up-networks is a prerequisite to setting up such a system to get connected to the internet, apart from joining a service provider.

e. Computers in Disaster Victim Identification

Recently, a program called DAVID (Disaster and Victim Identification) has been conceived with the idea of taking the help of computers for identifying disaster victims. The incidences of natural disasters, such as Tsunami and earthquakes led to the need for the development of such computer programs.

BIBLIOGRAPHY

1. Bener, F., Schweigher, J. and Edelhoff, D. : Digital dentistry : an overview of recent developments for CAD/CAM generated restorations. B.D.J. : 204, 505, 2008.

2. Clement, J.G., Winship, V., Ceddia, J., Al-Amad, S., Morales, A. and Hill, A.J. : New software for

computer assisted dental data matching in disaster victim identification and long term missing persons investigations : 'DAVID Web'. Forensic Science International : 159, 524, 2006.

3. Ewers, R., Schicho, K., Undt, G, Truppe, M. and Seemann, R. : Basic research and 12 years of clinical experience in computer assisted navigation technology : a review. Int. J. Oral Maxillofacial Surg. : 34, 1, 2005.

4. Forsell, M., Haggstrom, M., Johansson, O. and Sjogren, P. : A personal digital assistant application (Mobil Dent) for dental fieldwork data collection, information management and database handling. B.D.J. : 205, E17, 2008.

5. Fortin, T. and Coudert, J.L. : Computer assisted dental implant surgery using computed tomography. Computer Aided Surgery, 1, 53, 1995.

6. Hikmet, U. : Clinical decisions making using computers : opportunities and limitations. Dental Clinic North Am. : 46, 521, 2002.

7. Ireland, A.J., McNamara, O.C., Clover, M.J., House, K., Wenger, N., Barbour, M.E., Zhang, L. and Sandy, J.R. : 3D surface imaging in dentistry – what we are looking at. B.D.J. : 205, 387, 2008.

8. Kojima, T., Sohmura, T., Nagao, M., Wakabayashi, K., Nakamura, T. and Takahashi, J. : A preliminary report on a computer assisted dental cast analysis system used for prosthodontic treatment. J. Oral Rehab. : 30, 526, 2003.

9. Lewis, C. : Win ID2 versus CAPM14 : two computer-assisted dental identification systems. J. Forensic Sci. : 47, 536, 2002.

10. Mc Crivney, J. and Fixott, R.H. : Computer assisted dental identification. Dental Clinic North Am. : 45, 309, 2001.

11. Reynaulck, P.A., Harper, J., Mason, R., Cox, M.J. and Eaton, K. : An intricate web-designing and authoring a web-based course. B.D.J. : 204, 519, 2008.

12. Rosenberg, H., Grad, H.A., Matear, D.W. : The effectiveness of computer-aided self instructional programs in dental education : a systematic review of the literature. J. Dent. Educ. : 67, 524, 2003.

13. Ross, S., Fasbinder, D. and Reiss, B. : Computer application in dental diagnosis. Int. J. Comput. Dent. : 1, 9, 1998.

14. Tan, J., Leung, D. and Tay, P. : The use of the internet in dentistry. B.D.J. : 182, 191, 1997.

15. Tinschert, J., NaH, G., Hanenpfluq, S. and Spiekermann, H. : Status of current CAD/CAM technology in dental medicine. Int. J. Comput. Dent. : 7, 25, 2004.

16. Watzinger, F., Birkfellner, W., Millesi, W., Sinko, K. and Bergmann, H. : Positioning of dental implants using computer aided navigation and an optical tracking system : case report and presentation of a new method. J. Craniomaxillofacial Surg.: 27, 77, 1999.

17. Wenzel, A. : Computer aided image manipulation of intraoral radiographs to enhance diagnosis in dental practice : a review. Int. Dent. J. : 43, 99, 1993.

18. Jonathan, Tan., Dominic Leung and Peter Tay : The use of internet in dentistry. Br. Dent. Journal : 182, 5, 1997.

19. Rhodes, P.R. : The computer based oral health record. Journal of Dental Education, 220, 60, 1996.

20. Rekow, E.N. : High-technology-innovations and limitations - For restorative dentistry. Dental Clinics North Am., Vol. 37, July 1993.

21. Tsutsumi, S., Umino, K. and Kaneko, T. : A development of dental CAD/CAM system. Quintessence : 10, 135, 1991.

22. Vander Stelt, P.F. : Computer assisted interpretation in radiographic diagnosis. Dental clinics of North America. Vol. 37, No. 4, Oct. 1993.

23. Vander Zel, J.M. : Ceramic fused to metal restorations with a new CAD/CAM system. Quintessence Int. 24, 769, 1993.

24. Walmsley, A.D. : Caught in the web. Br. Dent. J. : 180, 435, 1996.

23

Psychology and Public Health

'Psychology' is derived from two different Greek words – 'psyche' means soul and 'logos' means science. Thus, literally psychology means science of soul. Since soul is scientifically non-existent, it cannot be regarded as a base for any scientific study and research.

As the concept of soul failed, the scientists tried to define the term in different ways, viz. 'science of mind', 'study of mental activity' and 'science of conscious experience', etc. However, the most accepted and realistic definition of psychology is by Watson, who defined it as *the science of behaviour*. It was later improved as *the scientific study of behaviour of an organism in relation to its environment*.

Psychology, in simple words, is the subject that explains human mind and behaviour and seeks to understand thoughts, emotions and behaviour.

HEALTH PSYCHOLOGY

Health psychology is concerned with understanding how biology, behaviour and social context influence health and illness.

Health and illness are viewed as products of a combination of factors including biological (genetic), behavioural (life style, stress etc.) and social (cultural, family and social support) conditions.

Many health psychologists provide clinical services as a part of their duty, while others perform non-clinical roles, primarily involving teaching and research.

Health psychology is further divided into four disciplines:

i. **Clinical health psychology:** A division of health psychology, reflecting the clinical aspect of health psychology.

ii. **Occupational health psychology:** The division is related to occupation. It is concerned with identifying psychosocial characteristics of work places that give rise to health related problems.

iii. **Public health psychology:** The division is concerned with the general population. Psychologists present research proceedings to educators, policy makers and health care providers in order to promote better public health.

iv. **Critical health psychology:** It deals with social justice and right to health for all; making achievements in balancing health inequalities.

Public health psychology, also known as community psychology, deals with the relationship of individuals to communities and the society at large. The quality of life of individuals in a society is to be understood so as to provide them with better health services. Community psychology makes use of various perspectives to address issues of communities and the relationship within them. It takes a public health approach and focuses on prevention and early intervention as a means to solve problems in addition to treatment. Sociology, social psychology and community development are all interrelated disciplines.

The values of community psychology have been continuously analyzed. The changing environment may have an impact on individuals; but an understanding as to how humans behave is also important. Four principles have been suggested.

- Adaptation, whereby individuals relay according to the surrounding environment.
- Succession implies understanding the history of current structures, norms, attitudes and other related features, which affect the environment.
- Cycling of resources means identification of the possibilities of new resources and taking advantage of existing sources in a better ways.
- Interdependence, as regards the relationship between one setting and the others, thereby anticipating the impact of intervention.

One of the goals of community psychology involves empowerment of individuals that have been marginalized by the society. Empowerment is viewed as a process by which people in a community gain mastery over their lies. Community psychologists often advocate equality for all and policies that allow for the well being of the community as a whole, particularly the marginalized individuals.

Community psychology is like social psychology in taking a systematic approach to human behaviour, but it is more concerned with using psychological knowledge to resolve social problems. It focuses on the problems of workers as to opposed solely the goals of the management. It is mainly concerned with enhancing the abilities of relatively powerless social groups such as minorities, children and the elderly.

The community perspective looks at the whole ecological system including political, cultural and environmental influences. It realizes that the 'interaction' between a person and the environment may have an effect on his/her behaviour. The community approach emphasizes the effects of stress and social support and the possibility of prevention and self-help.

Concepts of Psychology

The various concepts as regard to psychological studies are:

- *Structural:* The structural concept visualizes psychology as the science of conscious experience that is dependent upon the person having the experience.
- *Functional:* The functional concept established the fact that consciousness contributed to the survival of human kind by learning and gaining experience. Instead of the structure of consciousness, it is the functioning of the human mind that forms the basis of psychology.
- *Behaviouristic:* The behaviouristic concept argues that a healthy human being can be influenced to have any type of personality by manipulating the environment.
- *Pyscho-analaytical:* The concept is based on the fact that a healthy individual and a psychologically imbalanced one behave separately in the same environment. The human behaviour is the result of different instinctual impulses viz. sex, frustration and depression etc.
- *Individual psychology:* The concept advocates that every individual is driven by the desire of power and dominance, which may be due to a sense of inferiority or otherwise. The concept is not valid at the community level.

Psychology in Dental Treatment

The concept of psychology and its implications start functioning the moment a patient enters the dental clinic. The psychological aspects start even as the patient asks for an appointment over the telephone. Before the start of the treatment, the dentist assesses the patient by his/her clothes, conversation, previous dentist visited, overall hygiene, taste of colours, shoes, etc. The patient also makes his/her own assessment of the dentist regarding his/her outlook, clinic, cleanliness of the clinic, equipment, his way of the first intro-duction, etc. Most patients want to know if the dentist is quick in alleviating pain, others may enquire about the fee and many others may be worried about availability of time. Very few may be interested in the nationality, marital status and even the political affiliation of the dentist. Few patients consider their dentist as a neutral object and few dentists may regard their patients as a set of teeth and gums with a tongue, cheeks and lips which are parts of a profitable business.

Psycho-therapeutic Alliance

The patient's feelings towards the therapist and vice-versa are important for better alliance between the two. The alliance is considered either positive, that is of love and respect or negative, if it is marked by hatred and a lack of trust. The feeling of patient is called 'transference', and the therapist's feelings are known as 'counter-transference'. This is a two way relation present between the doctor and the patient. The outcome of the relationship can be considered a therapeutic alliance. Usually all combinations give either positive or negative therapeutic alliances.

For example, a female patient may start liking the young dentist. She wants to be treated again and again and for that purpose she may go to the extent of dislodging her fillings to get noticed frequently. She may even pose with an emergency toothache. The dentist also enjoys treating her because she is pretty, talks sweetly, but her appearances and erotic looks may not allow the dentist to work properly. This results in a positive trans-ference and positive counter-transference, but resulting in a negative therapeutic alliance.

In some instances, the patient and the dentist dislike each other, as a result the treatment carried out is usually of inferior quality. This is a negative transference, negative counter-transference and negative therapeutic alliance. Careful manipulations by the dentist can help in improving the patient's attitudes and feelings, and consequently the therapeutic alliance.

The relationships of understanding can benefit both the doctor and the patient. Usually the dentist's role is active and the patient's role is passive in these relations. There is always a scope for beneficial change with the dentist encouraging the patient to take active part in the treatment planning. The difference between a psychiatrist and a dentist is that the psychiatrist spends more time in talking to the patients while the dentist emphasizes more on mechanical efforts. Dominance is an important factor in dentist-patient relationships. A balance is to be maintained between the dominance of the dentist and the acceptance of the patients. Active involvement of patients in his or her treatment is very essential. A patient who arrives with a clean mouth encourages the dentist to do better work. Dentistry cannot be performed with the patient's resistance but with his consent and co-operation.

Many a time, the dentist or the patient can have obsessional qualities. Patients with obsessional qualities will arrive right on time and narrate their problems in detail. They will report with even minor problems and will expect the dentist to give them his/her full time.

In psychology, it is understood that all of us have our own set of ideas for others. For example, we want our tailor to be like this, our priest to behave in that manner, our physician to act in a certain way and so also for the dentist. The patient is constantly making judgements about the dentist throughout the treatment. A well dressed dentist who greets the patient in a civilized manner wins the confidence of the patient. A dentist's confidence during work makes the patient more comfortable.

Communicative Psychology

Communication skill is very important for the dentist to inculcate confidence in the patient.

Sympathetic attitude towards the patient's personal problems and gentle behaviour can go a long way in bringing confidence in patients. The instructions to the patient may be casual for the dentist but for the patient, these are very important, since that might be new for them. The best communication is achieved with a slow and humble approach, illustrated with examples without using technical words. Written instructions can also be given to the patients to whom any attendant can explain the same. Ideally, the combination of verbal and written instructions is fruitful and always has a synergistic action on the patient's memory.

Generally, patients do not disrupt procedures and the dentist carries out the treatment. The expectations of both the dentists and the patients are reasonably taken care of. The discrepancies, if any, between the ideal and actual behaviour depend upon the level of communication. The gap in communication between the dentist and the patient, may lead to frustration on both the sides. The dentists should be trained, as far as communication skills are concerned.

Any communication between the doctor and the assistant or between the doctor and any other person during the treatment procedure should be avoided. The nervous patient can be reassured by verbal encouragement. The tone of the voice coupled with a personal touch can be as effective as a tranquilizer. It is always better to prepare the patient mentally for pain of a short duration. Most patients accept this and become cooperative. So much so, the verbal communication is very effective when giving general anaesthesia. While giving local anaesthesia, the dentist and the assistant should be careful not to talk, since the patient usually presumes that there is no regulation on the quantity of local anaesthesia and more or less than the required quantity of anaesthesia may be given.

In psychology, the analytical observation of human behaviour has led to a number of mechanisms being recorded by people who defend themselves in a number of ways. In the early years, a child tries to act in the same manner as his/her father or one of the teacher. However, many children live in their own world of fantasy.

We try to justify whatever we do in life. This is the rationalization which, by simple meaning, justifies what we have done in order to maintain our self esteem. For example, dentists working in government run teaching institutions where private practice is not allowed but doing private practice at their respective houses would justify themselves by asking what is the harm in doing some extra work after the government working hours? Persons, who are running practices right in the hospital premises would say, "So what, who doesn't do anything to earn extra." At least we are giving something to the patient and then charging, where as there are so many departments where they charge by hook or by crook and still do nothing." Those who are not doing any type of practice will justify themselves saying, "we are full-time employees of the government and get a non-practicing allowance-why do private practice". There is always an emotional element to the way in which the explanation is offered. The other aspect of rationalization is projection in which the blame is projected on to other people. For poorly finished amalgam restorations, if pointed out by someone, a dentist would tend to say that today's materials are not up to the mark. This phenomenon is called displacement. Displacement means than the emotional expression is detached from the intended object and then attached to another person to whom it is safer to shift the blame.

Stress is one phenomenon common among all professionals. Most of the members claim that they work in adverse conditions and are continually subjected to stress. All these hazards are mostly psychological in origin. Dentists usually work in confined areas with constant tension and many of them find little time for exercises. Physical labour is involved with the work of dentists. Disorders such as rheumatoid arthritis, parkinsonism, etc. may affect a dentist.

Alcohol in any amount should be avoided by the dentists since it may lead to fumbling and tremors which are always embarrassing. In recent years, attention is being paid to designs of the dental operatory, making the dentist more comfortable. Auxiliary help can eliminate routine problems and allow the dentist to practice in a better way. When the morale is good, staff related problems are minimal and when the environment and work conditions are fine there would be minimum stress and tensions. A short break during practice is necessary to refresh the mind. Working environment and freshness of mind always speaks on the quality of work.

HYPNOSIS

In the early 18th century, magnetic healing force was utilized to induce anaesthesia and control phobia in dental patient. Later, it was modified as 'Hypnosis', which was accepted by the medical fraternity. They were of the view that hypnosis can be induced without sleeping. The concept of hypnosis became popular and many investigators used this technique even in major surgeries.

Although general anaesthesia was popular, yet hypnosis was routinely utilized in psychotherapy. Psychotherapy is not at all a new way of healing. Around 1960, hypnosis was recognized as a specialized psychiatric procedure.

Techniques of Hypnosis

Hypnosis is the art of altering the concentration of human beings resulting in behavioural changes and, subsequently some sort of sedation or even unconsciousness. The patient is asked to concentrate on one spot.

Alternatively, the patient is asked to think deep at some point, which produces hypnotic effects. The techniques of inducing hypnosis should be performed with patients lying or sitting comfortably in a quiet room away from distractions. The patient feels the eyelids falling and finally close. The generally accepted use of the term hypnosis is to define an area of research and treatment that uses complex and systematically arranged suggestions to produce desired results. These sets of suggestions, usually along with traditional usage, are termed hypnotic induction procedures. Hypnotized individuals can be distinguished externally by a sleepy appearance, fixed glassy stare, psychomotor retardation, sensory distortion and even amnesia. Many authors have produced results as effective as hypnotizing with such techniques as relaxation, contemplation and task motivating instructions. It is indicated that phobics are readily modifiable with hypnosis in which therapeutic strategies are applied.

The suggestions in hypnosis have shown to distort perceptions, induce sensory changes and modify expectations in both phobics and others. The study of hypnosis is beneficial even if it is not practiced. With this awareness, the presence of counter-suggestions can be identified and controlled in the day to day practice of the dentist.

The most frequent reason for non-use of hypnosis in dentistry is that the procedure takes too much time. The criticism probably arises from the section which tries to hypnotize all the patients. The clinicians can use hypnotic susceptibility tests as a screening device that can be turned into a hypnotic induction. Highly hypnotizable patients usually require a very short time to respond. A more efficient and time saving device is group hypnosis. Many clinicians prefer group hypnosis to prepare phobic and fearful patients.

The multiple hypnotic technique is commonly used these days. Few researchers have focused on systematic desensitization and others on reciprocal inhibition. The clinicians can combine any number of these techniques with hypnosis to suit the needs of each phobic patient. A combination of methods is always helpful for those who are otherwise non-responsive to hypnosis.

It has been established that long term effects of trauma in childhood can lead to phobia of a different nature. Many patients suffer from emotional difficulties, including phobia, which in turn may or may not be of traumatic origin. Hypnosis is contraindicated in patients with impairment of the thought process. As a general rule, hypnosis should be used for relaxation and the dentist should modify the behaviour of the phobic in the office.

It is further observed that effectiveness of hypnotic treatment is related to characteristics of the subject sample. In studies where the sample sought treatment for phobia, there was a clear superiority of hypnosis. It is clear that the level of fear as well as the degree of hypnotizability are important indicators of hypnotic strategies.

There are plenty of case reports whereby hypnosis has been helpful in alleviating fear in the patient's mind. In one such case, the author, with hypnosis, was able to treat a patient who required extraction of all the remaining natural teeth, claimed to be allergic to all anaesthetic agents, was intensely fearful and used to have convulsions even on entering the dental office. The author started with hypnotic relaxation and desensitization along with non-verbal induction, thereby completely controlling the patient.

Most people can be hypnotized provided they wish to be. They should also have the ability to concentrate and cooperate. Electro-encephalographic studies have shown that hypnosis is a state of increased susceptibility to suggestion. The degree of susceptibility can be gauged by giving some suggestions and observing if the patient complies. A positive response to the suggestions suggests a susceptible patient. Hypnosis, though a very good technique, should be carried out selectively by the dentists and they should undergo training for the same.

Hypnosis is a useful adjunct in dentistry; however, it is not widely used among dental practitioners.

CHILD PSYCHOLOGY

Over the years, study and research on child psychology has gained significance, making it one of the valuable disciplines of psychology. In order to study the behaviour, the growth and development of the child is important as it affects the overall personality.

Child psychology is a sub-branch of psychology that studies the social, physical and mental growth of human beings from conception to adolescence. Right from birth, the sensory, motor, perceptual, learning, emotional, reasoning, intellect and speech development is studied until the child reaches adolescence. The prenatal and postnatal development, process of maturation is also evident in mental development.

Child psychology implies physical and mental development of the child from the very beginning of life, coupled with the effect of the environment on the child's growth and developmental pattern. It also provides the norms for social, emotional, cognitive and intellectual development of the child at different ages.

The study of child psychology helps the dentist to understand the behaviour of the child along with parent-child relationships and the effect of the home environment, if any, on the child. It also helps in understanding and catering to the needs of children of all age groups.

Behaviour

The manner in which an individual responds to a particular stimulus is called behaviour.

The stimulus may be pleasant or unpleasant. It is an observable act and usually varies amongst different individuals. Behaviour Science deals with the observation of human actions and reactions in various physical and social environments.

The child's behaviour is broadly classified into two:

- Cooperative (Positive behaviour)
- Uncooperative (Negative behaviour)

The child showing cooperative behaviour will not be apprehensive and understand the procedure in a congenial environment. The child may need motivational words from the receptionist or the dentist, which makes the child cooperative. Such children are called 'potentially cooperative'.

The uncooperative child shows tantrums such as crying loudly and resisting opening the mouth. Certain children are shy and because of this factor, they do not cooperate properly. Such children can be motivated by verbal interactions or showing them videos of the dental procedures.

Child's Behaviour in Dental Clinic

A child's behaviour in the dental clinic is best explained by Frankel's Behaviour Rating Scale.

Rating	Behaviour
1. Definitely negative (- -)	Refuses treatment and cries forcefully. Such behaviour is usually associated with fear.
2. Negative (-)	Reluctant to accept treatment and displays evidence of negativism.
3. Positive (+)	Accepts treatment, but may become uncooperative if anything unpleasant

Contd...

Rating	Behaviour
	happens during treatment.
4. Definitely positive (+ +)	Understands the importance of dental care and accepts the treatment.

Factors Affecting Child's Behaviour in the Dental Clinic

The factors affecting a child's behaviour in the dental clinic are categorized as:

I. Factors under control of the dentist

II. Factors out of control of the dentist

III. Factors under control of the parents

I. Factors under Control of the Dentist

a. Environment of Dental Clinic

- The environment in the dental clinic should be calm, comfortable and simulate a homely environment. A pleasant environment helps allay the anxiety of children and makes them feel relaxed.
- A dental clinic should have a separate entry and exit so that child patients do not come across other treated patients.
- The waiting room should be lively, having posters, T.V., story books and toys, etc. Aquarium and computers are also helpful in allaying the fear of a child.
- The auxiliary staff should be kind and cooperative with children and should treat them with love and care.
- The operating room should also be decorated. Cartoons and light music make the child comfortable.
- Children should be given an early appointment. An appointment during the nap time of a child may be avoided. Children should

not be kept waiting for too long in the waiting area.

b. Effect of Dentists Activity and Attitude

The dentist should behave in a friendly manner with the child. The conversation should be fluent and in simple words. He/she should avoid jerky and quick movements.

The categories of features by which a dentist can enhance cooperation with the child patients are:

- The information about the child, his upbringing and also the status of the parents should be gathered prior to the treatment. The behaviour of the child is observed with patience as he enters the dental office, at the time of waiting and also during history taking.
- The child should be familiarized with and made to accept certain protocols in the dental clinic. The implications of the treatment coupled with the benefits should be clearly explained to the child.
- The child's attention is deviated from the sensations associated with the dental treatment. It is carried out by the following means:
  - o By diverting his/her attention towards pleasant features like cartoon films, music, etc.
  - o By involving the child in any game or pleasurable task. However, the child should not be allowed to talk too long, since that may interfere with the treatment procedure.
- The dentist should understand the feelings of the child patient and modify the treatment procedures accordingly.
- The dentist should be flexible in attitude. For example, during the first visit, the dentist can perform simple treatment procedures and later, once the confidence of the child is gained, other procedures can be carried out.

- The dentist should educate both child and parent about the importance of good oral health and its impact on general health.

c. Presence of Parents in Operatory

Infants generally need their mother's presence, while older children can be treated alone. The fearful child can be treated in presence of the mother.

II. Factors Out of Control of the Dentist

Genetics, coupled with family environment and schooling constantly affect the behaviour of a person. The other factors beyond the control of the dentist are:

a. Growth and Development

i. *Prenatal:* Any injury, trauma, infection or deficiency during pregnancy can adversely retard the physical and/or mental development of the child. For example, Rubella infection during the first trimester of pregnancy leads to severe mental retardation of the newborn.

ii. *Post natal:* Any aberrant physical growth can affect the behaviour of the child. For example, a physically handicaped child suffers from psychological trauma due to rejection by other children. And also, certain neurological disorders like epilepsy, cerebral palsy, autism, etc. make the child mentally handicapped.

Children less than 3 years of age, generally lack the intellectual development and behave negatively; however, with advancing age their behaviour improves.

b. Nutritional Factors

Nutrition plays an important role in the development of behaviour. Nutritional deficiencies or excess can lead to various physical and developmental malformations, which affect the overall behaviour of the child.

c. Past Experience

An unpleasant past experience is generally associated with the child's negative behaviour.

d. Socio-economic Status

Children from low socio-economic status families usually do not get proper attention. Such children may develop a kind of resentment and remain tense and irritable.

However, the children from high socio-economic status families may show a normal attitude or Spoilt/Stubborn behaviour.

III. Factors under Control of the Parents

Parents have a definitive role in shaping a child's personality and behaviour. The factors affecting the child's behaviour are:

a. **Home environment:** An affectionate environment in the home coupled with the mothers's attitude affects the child's behaviour. It is the home where the child first learns to walk, talk, play etc. Parent's affection is required during that period. In case where parents are separated, the child may feel insecure, inferior, apathic and depressed.

b. **Peer influences:** Paternal attitude towards the child and his status in the family affect the child's behaviour. A younger sibling may imitate the older one or may behave in the opposite manner depending upon their relationship.

c. **Mother's attitude:** The attitude of the mother affects the development of the child in many ways:

During the prenatal period the factors influencing the fetus are:

- The nutritional status of the mother affects growth.
- The neurohormonal system of the mother facilitates the development of emotions in the foetus.
- Intake of alcohol, smoking etc. during pregnancy affects the child's development.

The physical and emotional behaviour of the mother affects the overall personality of the child. In case the mother exaggerates these features, the behaviour is described as over-protective. Mothers usually do not allow their children to take decisions and are actively associated with their day-to-day activities. Such mothers provide everything to one child who in turn become dependent on the mother. The causes of mothers being overprotective are:

- The child is born after a long gap.
- An only or sick child
- Physically or mentally handicapped child

The over protected child may be:

- Cooperative and polite
- Shy, submissive and anxious
- Lacking self confidence
- Not knowing how to cope with the circumstances.

The management of such children is usually not difficult. The commonly employed 'Tell-Show-Do Technique' familiarizes the child with the dentist, dental auxiliaries and the treatment procedure. The dentist and the auxiliary build confidence in the child and the child starts accepting the treatment.

In certain cases, the mother does not bother for the child. Lack of a mother's love and care lead to uncooperative behaviour. Such children are usually timid and lack confidence.

The causes of mothers being under-affectionate are:

- Being emotionally disturbed
- Unwanted child
- Too busy in profession or social activities
- Living alone because of divorce or husband's death

Such children are weak emotionally. They need personal attention and care. Love and affection showered on these children help overcome the psychological complex.

In some cases, the under-affectionate attitude of the mother takes the shape of total neglect, physical violence and verbal ridicule. Being continuously neglected makes the child disobedient and aggressive. The severe form of such behaviour is known as the *Battered Baby Syndrome*. Such children are sensitive and emotionally very weak.

In certain cases, the mother's behavior is 'authoritarian'. The mother strictly follows definite norms for the child. She keeps criticizing him/her and the child becomes evasive and consequently shows slow reflexes.

Such children need affection and can be managed with love and care in the dental clinic.

Behaviour shaping on the other hand is the procedure which helps in developing the desired behaviour by continuously inculcating the characteristics of the behaviour.

Behaviour Management

The treatment of children needs a lot of patience, love and affection coupled with a firm approach as needed. A balance is to be maintained as regard dental treatment and managing the behaviour of the child. Behaviour Management includes the modalities by which the dentist and the team effectively and efficiently perform dental treatment after instilling a positive attitude towards dental procedures. The dentist should be able to shape and manage the behaviour of the child and, at the same time, allay fear and anxiety as regard dental treatment.

The different approaches for behaviour management are:

i. *Audioanalgesia:* Auditory stimulus such as pleasant music has been used to reduce stress and pain. A sound stimulus is provided to the child or any other patient so that the patient's mind is deviated from the fear of being treated.

ii. *Humour:* Jokes certainly help to elevate mood of the child, thus helping him relax. Humour motivates the child and relieves anxiety of both the parent and the child. It also helps in improving the relationship of the dentist with the child and the parents.

iii. *Relaxation:* The child is asked to take a few deep breaths. Certain other exercises are also helpful in relaxing the child or the parents.

iv. *Coping:* It is a mechanism by which the child copes up with the environment. Such methods reduce stressful situations and the child feels relaxed.

A simple example of coping is when the dentist asks the child to raise his/her hand as a signal whenever he/she is uncomfortable. This method is commonly used even for adult patients.

v. *Voice Control:* The dentist modifies the pitch and intensity of his voice in an attempt to dominate the interaction with the child. Generally, the dentist deals gently and softly with the child. However, if he/she doesnot fully cooperate, the dentist can change his/her tone to one of firmness so that the child understands the limit of misbehaviour.

vi. *Hypnosis:* It is one of the most effective non pharmacological therapies used with children. It is an altered state of consciousness which produces desirable behavioural and physiological changes.

vii. *Physical restraints:* It is used only for children showing extremely negative behavior. The child is controlled physically by the dentist or the team.

The dentist must obtain parental consent in written for hypnosis and using physical restraints.

The routinely used physical restrainted techniques are:

i. *Hand-Over-Mouth Exercise (HOME):* It is a commonly used technique in which the dentist firmly places his hand over the mouth of the child; narrates the treatment procedure in the ear and asks for co-operation. When the child indicates his willingness to cooperate, the dentist removes his hand and performs the procedure.

Indications

- Child showing extremely negative behaviour.
- Child in the age group of 3–6 years.

Contraindications

- Child less than 3 years of age.
- Handicapped and mentally sick child.

Precautions

- The child's airway should not be restricted while performing HOME.
- The whole procedure should not last for more than 20–30 seconds.

ii. *Hand over mouth with airway restricted (HOMAR):* In rare circumstances, the same procedure can be modified by restricting the air spaces also for a few seconds. This is known as 'Hand over mouth with airway restricted (HOMAR)' technique.

The advantage of airway restriction is that the child remains quiet for sometime till breathing is normal. The dentist in the meantime can easily proceed with the treatment. However, airway restriction should be needed only as the last resort.

iii. *Certain other physical restraint used are:*

- The child is seated in his/her mother's lap and one of the mother's hands is placed on the child's forehead while the other is used to hold the child's wrists.
- Mouth blocks and tongue blades are also used to keep the mouth open.

FEAR AND ANXIETY

Fear of the dental treatment and the dental clinic is quite common. The thought of an injection prick evokes fear. The sight of surgical equipments and instruments, etc. and also the sound of air rotors are common causes of fear in children. Anxiety is a psychological and physiological state, which is a combination of somatic, emotional and behavioural components. These components create an unpleasant feeling associated with uneasiness, fear and worry.

The various types of fear observed in the dental clinic are:

- *Subjective fear:* Fear transmitted to children from family experiences and peer groups.
- *Objective fear:* Fear due to previous unpleasant events, injury or seeing patients in acute pain.
- *Innate fears:* Fear without any stimuli or previous experience. Developmentally the child may be fearful.

Anxiety can be due to:

- The child experiences uncertainty due to delay in the start of the procedure or seeing patients sitting in the reception area and discussing dental procedures.
- The child may be anxious due to previous experiences narrated by friends and others.

The response of fear depends upon various factors and occurs at different psychological levels. Every child responds differently. Sometimes, the child is ready to accept the situation and face the perceived difficulties. Alternatively, he/she many take the situation as a challenge in response to a fight he/she may here had with a friend or sibling.

Prevention of Fear

The following features help in preventing or eliminating fear.

- By gradually familiarizing the child with the dental operatory.
- Reassurance combined with practical demonstration.
- By deviating the child's attention from a fear stimulus by alternating it with pleasant ones.
- The presence of someone with whom the child gets confidence.

ANGER

Anger is a negative emotional state which starts from the stage where the individual's desires are not fulfilled or the other person is not reacting according to expectations. It ranges from minor irritation to intense rage.

Anger can be evoked due to many reasons viz. interferences or restrictions of any type owing to personal, physical or social causes. The conflict over activities of interest to the child may lead to the development of anger.

Infants and young children generally respond in a primitive manner but as they grow, the response becomes symbolic.

Anger should be channelized in socially acceptable ways rather than being suppressed or repressed.

PHOBIAS

Phobia is derived from the Greek word 'phobos', which means fear. Phobia or morbid fear is an irrational, intense, persistent fear of certain situations or activities. The phobia is baseless fear and is involuntary. It can affect individuals of any age group. Usually the following features are seen in such individuals:

- Tendency to avoid or escape the threat.
- An emotional reaction anticipating or encountering the threat.
- Existence of perceived obsession that is held in mind.

Classification of Phobias

Phobias can be classified into the following three types, which are based on the causative factors.

1. *Simple phobia:* An isolated fear of a single situation or object leading to its avoidance is called simple phobia. For example:

Acrophobia	Phobia of height
Agoraphobia	Phobia of open space
Arachnophobia	Phobia of spiders
Aquaphobia	Phobia of water
Astraphobia	Phobia of lightning
Claustrophobia	Phobia of closed spaces
Cyanophobia	Phobia of dogs
Zoophobia	Phobia of animals
Nyclophobia	Phobia of darkness
Pyrophobia	Phobia of fire
Xenophobia	Phobia of strangers

2. *Social phobia:* It is the fear of being noticed or 'looked at'. The person feels shameful in the presence of others. For example, public speaking, public meetings etc.

3. *Situational phobia:* The fear of public transport, tunnels, being alone at home or being away from home.

Phobias in Childhood

A child shows different phobias at different ages. For example:

Phobia of	*Age*
Animals	Usually at 2–4 years, may extend upto ten years
Darkness	Between 4–6 years
School phobia	School going age
Social phobia	In adolescent age

Phobics are unable to apply logic to a problem. Only 'suggestion' and 'persuasion' can help. The procedure can change the emotions within the phobic individual to some extent.

BIBLIOGRAPHY

1. Ailen, K.D. and Kuhn, B.R. : Expanding child behaviour management technology in pediatric dentistry – a behavioural science perspective. Pediat. Dent. : 16, 13, 1994.
2. Angner, E., Ray, M.N., Kenneth, G. and Auism, J. : Health and happiness among older adults : A community based study. J. Health Psychol. : 14, 503, 2009.

3. Berggren, J. and Carlsson, S.G. : Psychometric measures of dental fear. Comm. Dent. Oral Epidem. : 12, 319, 1984.

4. Boswell, S. : Immersion : building a foundation for long term patient relationship. J. Calif. Dent. Assoc. : 8, 37, 1996.

5. Brand, H.s., Gortzak, R.A. and Abraham, I.L. : Anxiety and heart rate correlation prior to dental check up. Int. Dent. J. : 45, 347,1995.

6. Burke, F.J. and Freeman, R. : Psychological aspects of patient management in dental practice. Dent. Update : 21, 148, 1994.

7. Certo, M.A. and Bernat, J.E. : Parents in the operatory. N.Y. State Dent. J. : 61, 34, 1995.

8. Chellapah, N.K., Vignesha, H. and Milgrom, P.L. : Prevalence of dental anxiety and fear in children in Singapore. Comm. Dent. Oral Epidemiol. : 18, 269, 1990.

9. Forgione, A.G. : Hypnosis in the treatment of dental fear and phobia. Dent. Clin. North. Am. : 32, 745, 1988.

10. Gatchel, R.J. and Ingersoll, B.D. : The prevalence of dental fear and avoidance : a recent survey study. J. Am. Dent. Assoc. : 107, 809, 1983.

11. Hakeburg, M. and Berggren, U.F. : Dimensions of the dental fear survey among patients with dental phobia. Acta. Odont. Scand. : 55, 314, 1997.

12. Howe, J.A.M. : Beyond psychobiography : Towards more effective synthesis of psychology and biography. Br. J. Psychology : 88, 235, 1997.

13. Huber, M.T., Freeman, R., Humphris, G., MacGillivary, S and Terzi, N: Empirical evidence of the relationship betwen parental and child dental fear: a structured review and meta-analysis. International J Pediat. Dentistry 20, 83, 2010.

14. Johnsson, P. and Berggren, U. : Assessment of dental fear. A comparison of two psychometric instruments. Acta. Odont. Scand. : 50, 43, 1992.

15. Linberg, G. and Hwang, C.P. : Children's dental fear picture test (CDFP), a projective test for the assessment of child dental fear. ASDC. J. Dent. Child. : 61, 89, 1994.

16. Kent, G., Rubin, G., Getz, T. and Hamphris, G. : Development of a scale to measure the social and psychological effects of severe dental anxiety : social attributes of the dental anxiety scale. Comm. Dent. Oral Epidemiol. : 24, 394, 1996.

17. Lee, M. : the hidden history : finding out what's really troubling your patient. Compendium. : 15, 466, 1994.

18. Locker, D., Shapiro, D. and Liddel, A. : Negative dental experiences and their relationships to dental anxiety. Comm. Dent. Health : 13, 86, 1996.

19. McMillan, D.W. and Chavis, D.M. : Sense of community : A definition and theory. American J. Comm. Psychol. : 14, 6-23, 1986.

20. Ogden, J., Bavalia, K., Bull, M., Frankum, S., Goldie,C. and Gosslau, M. et al : 'I want more time with my doctor' : A quantitative study of time and the consultation. Family Practice: 21, 479, 2004.

21. Rao, A., Sequire, P. and Peter, S. : Characteristics of dental fear amongst dental and medical students. Int. J. Dent. Res. : 8, 111, 1997.

22. Resnicow, K., Jackson, A., Blissett, D., Wang, T., McCarty, F., Rahotep, S. and Periasamy, S. : Results of the Healthy Body Healthy Spirit Trial. Health Psychol. : 24, 339, 2005.

23. Riger, S. : What's wrong with empowerment ? Am. J. Comm. Psychol. : 21, 279, 1993.

24. Ronis, D.L. : Updating a measure of dental anxiety : reliability, validity and norms. J. Dent. Hyg. : 68, 228, 1994.

25. Sharman, S.J., Garry, M., Jacobsen, J.A., Loftus, E.F. and Ditto, P.H. : False memories for end-of-life decisions. Health Psychol. : 27, 291, 2008.

26. Soo, H. and Lam, S. : Stress management training in diabetes mellitus. J. Health Psychol. : 14, 933, 2009.

27. Tolendano, M., Osorio, R., Aguilera, F.S. and Pegalajar, J. : Children's dental anxiety : Influence of personality and intelligence factors. Int. J. Paed. Dent. 5, 23, 1995.

28. Veerkamp, J.S., Gruythuysen, R.J. and Van Amerongen, J. : Treating fearful children : does a patient's view of the child's fear change ? A.S.D.C. J. Dent. Child. : 61, 105, 1994.

29. Weiss, J. and Diserens, K. : Health behaviour of dental professionals. Clin. Prevent. Dent. : 2, 5, 1980.

30. Williams, J.A. : Translating research in the social and behavioural sciences for more effective use in community dentistry. J. Public Health Dent. ; 36, 155, 1976.

31. Zimmerman, M.A. : Empowerment Theory : Psychological, Organizational and Community Levels of Analysis. Handbook of Community Psychology : 43-63, 2000.

24   *Health Agencies*

Health and public health are interrelated. Health at the individual level can only be achieved if the society at large is healthy. The goal 'Health for All' is achievable, though seems difficult. Certain agencies, may be at government or semi-government or non-government level, are working for this goal. The important agencies are:

WORLD HEALTH ORGANIZATION (WHO)

The WHO is a specialized, non-political agency of United Nations which directs and coordinates the international matters of health and public health. It provides information and advice in the health related issues and matters through the channel of its publications.

The WHO constitution was drafted by the 'Technical Committee' under the chairman-ship of Dr. Rene Sand of Brussels.

It came into force on 7th April, 1948 with headquarters at Geneva. Dr. Brock Chrisholme was the first Director General of the WHO. This day is celebrated every year as the World Health Day. A World Health Day theme focuses attention on specific aspects of public health.

The sole objective of the WHO is the attain-ment of the highest level of health by all people.

Its membership is open to all the countries. Each member state contributes yearly to the budget and is entitled to the services of the organization.

Structural Organization of WHO

It consists of the following:

a. The Parliament (World Health Assembly): The parliament is the principle constituent of the WHO. It decides the policy, approves the budget and various methods for achieving the targets. The WHO has its own governing bodies, its own membership and its own budget. It's session takes place once in year, usually in the month of May in Geneva. It is attended by delegations of Member States and representatives from other international bodies as well as non-government organizations.

The First World Health Assembly decided Geneva as the headquarter of the WHO and English and French as working languages with addition of Chinese, Russian and Spanish as official languages.

b. The Cabinet (Executive Board): It is com-prised of 34 individuals, technically trained in the field of health. The World Health Assembly elects these members out of Member States. The Board meets at least twice a year. Main meeting is normally in January in which agenda, for forthcoming health assembly is agreed upon while second shorter meeting is in May for administrative decisions. The main function of Board is to give effect to the decisions and policies of Health Assembly and facilitate its working.

c. The Secretariat (Civil Service): The staff of WHO (both regional offices and Head office) is known as 'The Secretariat'. The Director General (appointed for a five year term by assembly) heads the Head office while Regional Directors are appointed at regional offices.

Regionalization of WHO

The concept of regionalization/decentraliza-tion of WHO was decided and the whole world was divided into six regions. The WHO has six regional organizations, each consisting of a Regional Office, Regional Director and the Regional Committee. The overall control including finances, etc. lies with the Head office. The regional offices are:

Country	Headquarters
South-East Asia Region	New Delhi, India
Eastern Mediterranean Region	Alexandria, Egypt
Region of Americas	Washigton D.C., USA
Western Pacific Region	Manila, Phillipines
African Region	Brazzaville, Congo
European Region	Copenhagen, Denmark

Regional Office of South East Asia (New Delhi, India) was the first regional office set up by the WHO with its headquarters at New Delhi. Its regional committee consists of eleven member states of South East Asian region that are named below (in the sequence of their joining from first to last):

• Thailand
• India
• Burma (Myanmar)
• Sri Lanka
• Indonesia
• Nepal
• Mongolia
• Islands of Maldives
• Bangladesh
• Democratic People's Republic of Korea
• Bhutan

Functions of WHO

The WHO has specific responsibilities for establishing and promoting international standards in the field of health, which comprises:

i. **Prevention and control of specific disease:** The global eradication of small pox is an outstanding example of international health cooperation and now with same spirit, the WHO is fighting the global battle against AIDS. An important activity of the WHO is the epidemiological surveillance of the communicable disease.

The WHO is actively participating in the fields of immunology, quality control of drugs including biological products, drug evaluation and health laboratory technology. The monitoring is also a part of the WHO activity.

ii. **Development of comprehensive health services:** The main function is to promote and support national health policy and the development of comprehensive national health programmes. The appropriate technology for health (ATH) is the new programme launched by the WHO to encourage self-sufficiency in solving health problems.

iii. **Family health:** One of the activity of the WHO is family health. It is broadly divided into maternal health, human reproduction, nutrition and health education.

iv. **Environmental health:** The WHO advises governments on national programmes for the provision of basic sanitary services. The services include quality of air, water and food, radiation protection and early identification of new hazards originating from technological developments.

v. **Health statistics:** The WHO has been concerned with dissemination of a wide variety of morbidity and mortality statistics relating to health problems. The data is published in (a) weekly epidemiological record, (b) quarterly world health statistics and (c) annual world health statistics.

vi. **Biomedical research:** The WHO stimulates and coordinates research work. It has established a worldwide network of Centres, which promote research, besides awarding grants to research workers.

vii. **Health literature and information:** The WHO library is one of the satellite centres of the Medical Literature Analysis and Retrieval System (MEDLARS) of the US National Library of Medicine. The WHO has a public information service at headquarters and each of the six regional offices.

viii. **Cooperation with other organizations:** The WHO collaborates with other specialized agencies and maintain healthy working relationships.

UNICEF (UNITED NATIONS INTERNATIONAL CHILDREN'S EMERGENCY FUND)

The UNICEF was created by the United Nations General Assembly on December 11, 1946 to provide emergency food and health care to children in countries that had been devastated in wars. In 1953, the name was modified to United Nation Children's Fund. The head office is in New York city. Various governments and private agencies contribute towards finances. The main goal of UNICEF is to develop community level programmes for promoting health and well-being of children.

The Organization

More than 200 countries carry out UNICEF's mission through mutual cooperation and head office assistance. The supply division is based in Copenhagen, which is the primary point of distribution for essential items such as life saving vaccines and other medicines for children and their mothers.

The 36 member executive board guide and monitor all activities of the UNICEF including administrative functions. The board members are usually government representatives elected by United Nations economic and social council, for three years term.

Recently, the UNICEF, has started with world class athletes to promote the organization's work and to raise funds.

The UNICEF research centre was established in 1988 to strengthen the research capabilities and to support its advocacy for children worldwide. The main goals are:

- Generation and communication of strategic and influential knowledge on issues affecting children and the realization of their rights.
- Support of the UNICEF policies and programmes.
- Securing and strengthening financial basis.
- Knowledge exchange.

Functions

i. **Child Health:** The UNICEF supports and helps any programme for the welfare of the children anywhere in the world. It has supported India's BCG Vaccination Programme. Two plants for manufacturing triple vaccine and iodised salt were established in India with UNICEF help.

ii. **Child Nutrition:** The UNICEF is aiding 'Applied Nutrition' programmes in association with food and agriculture organization.

iii. **Motivation:** The UNICEF is to improve the care of children through motivation, parent education, day care centres, child welfare and youth agencies.

iv. **Education:** In collaboration with UNESCO, UNICEF is assisting India in the expansion and improvement of teaching science in India. Currently UNICEF is promoting a campaign, GOBI to encourage four strategies for a 'Child Health Revolution'.

G – Growth charts to monitor child development

O – Oral rehydration for mild and moderate dehydration

B – Breast feeding motivation

I – Immunisation against Measles, Diptheria, Polio, Pertussis, Tetanus and Tuberculosis.

The UNICEF is also participating in Urban Basic Services (UBS) to improve the quality of survival and development of the children of low income families of urban areas.

UNDP—THE UNITED NATIONS DEVELOPMENT PROGRAMME

The UNDP was founded in 1965 combining expanded programme of technical assistance and the United Nations Special Fund.

The organization has office in 166 countries with head office at New York. The UNDP tries to meet developmental challenges and achieve Millenium Development goals.

The basic objective of the UNDP is to help poor nations to develop their human and natural resources. It helps countries develop strategies to combat poverty by expanding access to economic opportunities and resources. The UNDP projects cover agriculture, industry, science and education, health and social welfare, etc.

FAO—THE FOOD AND AGRICULTURE ORGANIZATION

The Food and Agriculture Organization was founded in 1945 with its headquarters in Rome. The main aims of FAO are:

• To help nations to raise their living standards.
• To improve the nutrition of people.
• To increase the efficiency of farming, forestry and fisheries.
• To better the condition of rural people.

To increase the production of food, FAO is running its own Technical Cooperation Programme (TCP). Food quality control and greenhouse technology for forticulture are some of the TCP projects which are in progress in India.

ILO—INTERNATIONAL LABOUR ORGANIZATION

The International Labour Organization is an agency of United Nations that deals with labour issues. The ILO was established in 1919 to improve the working and living conditions of working individuals all over the world. The international labour organization has a tripartite governing structure, which represents government, employer and the worker. The governing body is composed of 28 government representatives, 14 workers' group representatives and 14 employers' group representatives.

International Labour Conference is held in June every year in Geneva. The purpose of ILO are:
• Setting international labour standards.
• To contribute to the establishment of lasting peace by promoting social justice.
• To improve, through an international action, labour conditions and living standards.
• To avoid child labour (child labour is defined as work that deprives children of their childhood, their potential dignity and that is harmful to physical and mental development).
• To avoid forced labour.
• To promote economic and social stability.
• Also helps in prevention of HIV/AIDS.

CARE— THE COOPERATIVE FOR ASSISTANCE AND RELIEF EVERYWHERE

It was founded in North America in the wake of Second World War in 1945. It is one of the largest international relief and humanitarian organization with head office at Geneva. It provides emergency aid and long term development assistance.

The primary objective of CARE in India was to provide food for children in the age group of 6–11 years.

CARE-India focused its development programmes in the area of health and income supplementation. In India, it is helping in the following projects:

- Integrated nutrition and health
- Better health and nutrition
- Anaemia control
- Improving women's health
- Improved health care for adolescent girls
- Child survival.

CARE campaigns in the fight against global poverty include:

- World hunger campaign
- Education to improve quality and accessibility of basic education.
- Victory over poverty.
- Provides educational programmes to eradicate HIV/AIDS.

USAID (UNITED STATES AGENCY FOR INTERNATIONAL DEVELOPMENT)

The US Government presently extends aid to India through USAID.

A USAID mission functions in New Delhi. The US has been assisting in a number of projects designed to improve the health of India's population such as:

- Malaria Eradication
- Medical Education
- Nursing Education
- Health Education
- Water Supply and Sanitation
- Control of Communicable Diseases
- Nutrition
- Family Planning.

INTERNATIONAL RED CROSS

The term International Red Cross is actually a misnomer as no official organization exists

bearing this name. The movement consists of several district organizations that are legally independent from each other and are also united through basic principles and objectives. The different movements are:

- The International Federation of Red Cross and Red Crescent Societies.
- National Red Cross and Red Crescent societies in each country.

The emblem and the red cross flag were officially approved in 1863.

Collectively, it is a non-political, non-official international humanitarian organization devoted to the service of mankind in peace and war. It was founded by a young swiss businessman Henry Dunant.

In 1919, the League of the Red Cross Society was created with headquarters in Geneva to coordinate the work of the national societies. The first President/Chairman is Henry Davison.

Role of Red Cross

- In the beginning, its role was largely confined to humanitarian service on behalf of the victims of war.
- Later, its role was extended to help the victims of natural disasters.
- The Red Cross also has a major role in service to first aid and nursing, health education, maternity and child welfare services.

Indian Red Cross

The Red Cross Society in India was established by an act of the Indian Legislature in 1920. The objectives are:

- Improvement of health
- Prevention of disease
- Mitigation of suffering

In peace time, the society provides military hospitals with newspapers, periodicals, musical instruments and other comfort goods.

The Red Cross Home at Bangalore for disabled ex-servicemen is one of the pioneer institutions of its kind in Asia. Disaster services comprises distribution of milk, medicine, vitamin tablets, codliver oil and other items to needy people.

The Junior Red Cross gives an opportunity to lakhs of boys and girls all over India with activities such as Village Upliftment, First aid, antiepidemic work and promoting international friendliness, understanding and cooperation.

THE WORLD BANK

It is combination of International Bank for Reconstruction and Development (IBRD) and the associated institutions and International Development Association (IDA). It is the specialized agency of UN that helps the underdeveloped countries to raise the living standards of their people. It provides financial assistance in the form of loans for different projects that will enhance the economic development of underdeveloped and developing countries, e.g. projects concerned with electricity, water, health, agriculture, etc. The International Bank for Reconstruction and Development (IBRD) has 186 member countries while the International Development Association (IDA) has 168 members.

THE COLOMBO PLAN

It was established during Common Wealth Foreign Ministers Conference held in 1956 at Colombo with the objective of co-operative economic development of South-East Asian Countries.

It comprises of 20 regional members, i.e. countries of South-East Asia including India and six non-regional members – Australia, Canada, Japan, New Zealand, USA and UK.

All India Institute of Medical Sciences, New Delhi was established by the Colombo Plan with financial assistance from New Zealand.

Functions

It provides assistance to its member countries in following fields:
• Agricultural development
• Industrial development
• Health promotion

THE ROCKEFELLER FOUNDATION

This was founded in 1913 by John D. Rockefeller for the promotion of well-being of human populations all around the world.

Functions

Initially, the foundation was limited to the field of medical and public health education; later on fields of life sciences, agricultural sciences, social sciences and humanities were also included.

India and the Rockefeller Foundation in India

The foundation has been working for the benefit of Indian population. Some of its work are:
• A project for control of hookworm infections.
• Helps in establishment of All India Institute of Hygiene and Public Health, Kolkata.
• Helps in training competent research workers by providing them international scholarships, financial aid, research materials, etc.
• Financial assistance to teaching institutions.
• Setting of libraries in medical institutions.

THE FORD FOUNDATION

The Ford Foundation was established in 1936 by Edsel Ford (son of Henry Ford – founder of Ford Motors). Its headquarters is at New York.

Functions

The main aims of the Ford Foundation are:
- To strengthen democratic value
- To reduce poverty and injustice
- To promote international cooperation
- Advance human achievements.

Ford Foundation in India

The Ford Foundation in India was established in 1952. This office also serves Nepal and Sri Lanka.

Initially, the foundation focused only on agricultural and rural development. Presently the foundation is working for:
- Agriculture and rural development
- Forest and natural resource management
- Human rights

- Higher education and scholarship
- Art and culture
- Regional cooperation and international security.

The Foundation carried out various projects in India. A few are:
- Establishment of Orientation Training Centres providing training courses in field of public health.
- Establishment of Research and Action Projects for the maintenance of environmental sanitation.
- Establishment of National Institute of Health Administration and Education.
- Coordinating Water Supply and Drainage System of Kolkata.
- Supporting Research in field of Family Planning.

School Dental Health

Health is defined as a state of complete physical, mental and social well being and not merely an absence of disease or infirmity. In recent years, the definition of health is modified as being—the study of human beings to lead a socially and economically productive life.

Health education is the combination of planned learning experiences designed to facilitate voluntary actions conducive to health. It is the means of providing health information to people in a simple understandable way, which they apply to their everyday living. The comprehensive definition of health education including dental health education can be standardized as follows:

'A process with intellectual, psychological and social dimensions relating to activity which increases the abilities of people to make informed decisions affecting their personal, family and community well being. This process, based on scientific principles, facilitates learning and behavioural changes in any individual.'

School health program is defined as an organized set of policies, procedures, and activities designed to protect and promote the health and well-being of students and staff members of the school by providing adequate health services, a healthy school environment, and health education.

SCHOOL BASED HEALTH CENTERS

Dental health education, promotion, and preventive programs have traditionally comprised a significant portion of dental public health activities. Health promotion provides the education, access and availability of a known preventive method to the population.

A school-based health center provides comprehensive preventive and primary health care services to students on a school campus. While the procedures at school-based health centers may vary to meet the community's needs, there are certain general characteristics of all school-based health centers, which are enumerated below:

a. The school-based health centers are designed to serve all students, focusing mainly on socio-economically weaker sections.

b. An advisory board representing parents, youth and family organizations should pan and oversight the working of health center.

c. The school-based health center should include a multidisciplinary team comprising physicians, social workers, psychologists, nutritionists, dentists, dental hygienists and nurses.

d. The school-based health center works cooperatively with school nurses, coaches, faculty members and other supporting staff to assure that the center is an integral part of the school.

e. Written consents signed by parents are required before services can be provided in the school-based health center.

f. The school-based health center provides a comprehensive range of services that specifically meet general medical as well as dental and oral care.

Advantages of a school-based health center The various advantages of school-based health center are:

a. It attends to health care needs of the school children, especially when they need it.
b. It supports students by providing a safe site for discussing sensitive issues like depression, family problems, relationships, etc. related to their lives.
c. It supports the school environment by helping children to address health problems that may intervene in their learning process.
d. It also supports families by allowing parents to stay at their work while attending to their child's routine health care needs.
e. It saves money by keeping children out of hospitals and physician's clinics.
f. It strengthens the relationship between a community and the school.

Staff of School-based Health Center

Each school-based health center is staffed by a multi-disciplinary team of health care professionals. The staff includes a physician/ medical director, nurse practitioner or physician's assistant, registered nurse, school nurse, social worker, psychologist, licensed professional counsellor and receptionist. Some school-based health centers also employ dental providers including dentists, dental hygienists and dental assistants. The school-based health center can also have linkages with a hospital and/or other providers to accept referrals for complex health problems and to provide services to students during hours when the school-based health center is closed.

SCHOOL HEALTH PROGRAMS

School health program is defined as an organized set of policies, procedures, and activities designed to protect and promote the health and well-being of students and staff members of the school by providing adequate health services, a healthy school environment, and health education.

The school health programs originated around the beginning of the 20th century to help fight infections; for screening needs of physically disabled; for screening nutritional deficiencies and for first aid administrations.

The brief **history** of the progressing health programs is as follows:

a. In the 1930s and 1940s children were provided nutritional supplements, eye examinations, health education, smallpox vaccinations and in some cases oral health services.
b. In the early 1950s, school based fluoride regimens were introduced in the form of multiple manual applications of neutral sodium fluoride solution and as school water fluoridation programs.
c. In the 1960s access for rapid immunization of total school populations against poliomyelitis, and almost universal establishment of nursing services within the school system to deal with day-to-day accidents and illnesses, was a legacy for the attainment of early school health objectives.
d. At the approach of the 21st century, school health services also included or attempted to address major societal health issues like alcohol, drugs and tobacco use, sex, HIV, AIDS and other sexually transmitted diseases; gang violence and child abuse; and self esteem, depression, homicide and suicide as well as health problems of dysfunctional families.
e. Many states also include oral health as objective of oral health. Each state department of health has at least one person responsible for directing health education.

Importance of School Dental Health Program

The importance of School Dental Health Program is commonly as follows:

a. It is an economical and powerful means of raising community health.
b. It is the most logical and practical place to implement large scale school dental health program.
c. 5–16 years of age group comprises 30% of total population so a part of population is being targeted.
d. Health patterns can be easily modified and altered at this age.
e. As school environment is more conducive to learning, therefore dental health education and motivation is more effective.

Aims of School Dental Health Program

A school dental health program aims to:

a. Inform about the relationship between dental health and general health to the students.
b. Encourage strict observation of oral and dental care procedure and to avail professional care regularly.
c. Emphasize on the importance of balanced diet and harmful effect of bad oral habits.
d. Introduce students about the harmful effects of bad oral habits.
e. Provide complete provision of information regarding preventive and curative measures to be followed for adequate oral health.
f. Correlate dental health activities with the overall school health program.
g. Motivate dental surgeons to provide maximum dental health care to infants and children.
h. Follow "Tell Show and Do" approach to teach "Home dental care" to children.
i. Prepare "orodental health" and "learn about your teeth program".

Objectives of School Health Program

The objectives to be achieved by school health program are:

a. To evaluate the dental health status of students and school staff.
b. To counsel students, parents and teachers regarding dental health status finding.
c. To educate and motivate children for the correction of curable defects.
d. To identify, educate and motivate the handicapped children.
e. To prevent and control diseases.
f. To provide emergency services.

Necessity of School Health Programs

School-age children, especially younger ones are mostly dependent on parents and/or on school based programs for oral health education. However, many teachers believe that oral health instructions should be the sole responsibility of parents and health educators – not the teachers of academic subjects. This belief might be legitimate if, universally, parents were able to care for their children's oral health. But in a developing country like India, we generally see that a child reared by uneducated and financially weak parents is often dentally neglected. In these homes, parental involvement in the oral health care of a child frequently begins with seeking help to relieve pain. Some may not be able to feed their family properly; however, oral health remains a priority in their lives. Also, many working mothers and single parents cannot participate in school activities and tend to relinquish responsibilities to the school authorities. In addition, behavioural change may be more difficult to achieve at home under parental guidance than under the teacher. In other words, many parents themselves do not know how to help their child help themselves and need help from school health program. Still, whenever possible, the parent must be included in a school-based oral health program. Parents can provide strong positive reinforcement, either through role modeling or verbal messages that support the behavioural and attitudinal changes promulgated in the school setting. Ideally, parent education should parallel child education, in this way, parents can learn to improve their own oral health as well as have the guidelines to assist their children.

Professional Volunteerism

Professional involvement in school programs has a significant role along with parental involvement. The involvement of oral health care providers (Dentists, dental hygienists and dental students) in a dental program is known as professional volunteerism. It helps in:

a. Identifying teaching-learning resources, speaking to students, faculty, and parent-groups.
b. Providing in service training to faculty and administrators.
c. Assisting the schools on special occasions, such as career day and health fairs.
d. The support of the professional community enhances a program's credibility, improves the image of dentistry and dental hygiene and is a particular builder for participating providers.

Dentists, dental hygienists and dental students can and should play major role in school health programs. Their involvement may range from taking the lead in planning a comprehensive oral health program and implementing it; to participate by providing education to the students, treatment or preventive services. Whatever the role one plays, it requires the provider to be knowledgeable about the needs of the students in the school. It requires current scientific knowledge about the prevention of oral diseases and conditions identified among the targeted school children.

Important Elements of School Dental Health Program

A school dental health program should:

a. Improve relationship between school and community
b. Conduct dental examination
c. Provide proper health education
d. Perform specific dental health programs like:
   • Classroom based fluoride program
   • School water fluoridation program
   • Tooth brushing programs
   • Nutrition as a part of school preventive dentistry program
   • Sealants placement
   • Science fairs
e. Have provision for referral for dental care (An important part of School Dental Health program especially for places where it is not possible to provide all the required treatment and care).

Advantages of School based Program

A combined educational, promotional and preventive dental program in the school would greatly reduce the amount of classroom time lost in travelling to a treatment facility. Comprehensive school programs also would obviate the loss of study time due to pain and apprehension before and after treatment.

Advantages of a comprehensive school-based program are:

1. Students are available for preventive or treatment procedures.
2. School-based clinics are less threatening than private clinics.
3. School dental programs increase the effectiveness of teaching oral health subjects.
4. Dental services supplement the school nursing services by providing total health care for school children.

DIFFERENT ASPECTS TO BE COVERED IN SCHOOL HEALTH PROGRAMS

The needs of students in a particular school or district coupled with available resources – human, equipment, and financial – will dictate necessary preventive and treatment services, education and policies.

Dental Caries

Students should be taught that dental caries is an infectious disease with a multi-factorial etiology. Also, they need to know that the disease can be prevented, arrested and even reversed by re-mineralization.

Fluorides

Students should be provided knowledge about various types of fluorides and their method of action. They should be taught about the dietary and topical fluorides, the frequency and duration of different application procedures; and about the need and benefits of using them as dietary supplements, topically and in water fluoridation programs.

Pits and Fissure Sealants

School dental health programs should describe the nature, need, mode of action and the need for the re-application of the sealants.

Gingivitis

Gingivitis is the most common oral disease occurring in children. So students should be explained about:

a. The nature of dental plaque and its role in oral diseases.
b. The frequency and techniques of tooth brushing and flossing for the plaque removal.
c. The different types of tooth brushes available in the market.
d. The sequale of untreated gingival diseases.

Oral-Facial Injuries

Since children are in their play group age and are prone to facial injuries so they should be taught about:

a. Use seat belts at all times, and their bags when possible.
b. The use of mouth guards and head gears.
c. To use their play equipment safely in playground.
d. To wear helmets when riding bicycles and motorcycles.

Diet and Nutrition

Students should be told about the balanced diet and its role in their proper physical and mental development. They should be made to understand that the sugar consumption, especially sticky sweets and refined carbohydrates are key components of the caries progression. The best message about sweets is that if one consumes sugars, it should be consumed along with the meals.

Schools should also provide an environment that promotes avoidance of excessive sugar consumption.

Oral Cancer

Though rare in children a brief knowledge about risk factors, signs and symptoms, protective factors, need for clinical examination and recommended frequency of the examination procedure can be provided to students.

LEVELS OF COMPREHENSIVE ORAL HEALTH CARE PROGRAMS

Level 1

Level 1 includes the comprehensive oral health curriculum with the minimal participation of teachers or health educators in the program. The programs included in Level I are:

School Water Fluoridation Program

It is used only if the school has an independent water supply (usually in consolidated rural schools).

The recommended concentration of fluoride for school water supplies is 4.5 ppm. It has been found that up to a 40% reduction in the incidence of dental caries occurred after 12 years but its installation cost is relatively high and workers should be trained to operate, monitor, and maintain the water fluoridation unit.

Fluoride Mouth Rinsing Programs

These are the most popular school-based fluoride regimen and are supervised by classroom teachers or other adult volunteers. Caries reduction in this program ranges from 20–25%.

Fluoride mouth rinse regimens, as originally introduced, consisted of mixing pre-weighed packet of fluoride powder with a specified amount of water in a container with a calibrated plastic pump to dispense 5 to 10 ml of solution (it would yield a 0.2% neutral sodium fluoride rinse). After mixing, the solution is dispensed into paper cups for the use by the students. Nowadays, most of schools order premixed solutions that are available in individual containers.

Students are requested to put the solution in their mouth and to rinse vigorously for 60 seconds. Then students are asked to empty the contents of their mouth back into the cups and blot their lips with a napkin. The waste products are then put into a plastic bag for disposal. Generally, this procedure is not recommended for children before first grade unless extensive training is provided to the children so as to ensure that they do not swallow the contents of the cup.

Dietary Fluoride Tablets Program

The use of fluoride tablets in school is a method of administering systemic fluoride to children. This self-applied fluoride regimen is used in communities with deficient fluoride in water supply. This program is carried only with the parental consent. A teacher first dispenses the fluoride tablets to participating students and instructs them to put the tablet in their mouths and chew it for 30 seconds. The resultant solution is then vigorously swished between the teeth for 30 seconds before swallowing the solution. Advantages of fluoride tablets are:

- Both topical and systemic benefits are acquired by this approach.
- 20–30% reduction in the incidence of carious lesions has been reported by this approach.
- A daily fluoride tablet is more effective than a weekly rinse, as effect occurs daily and it is also easy to remember daily schedule as compared to weekly one.

The comparison of School-based Self-applied Fluoride Regimens is described below:

Fluoride mouth rinse	Fluoride tablets
Safe and effective	Safe and effective
Inexpensive	Inexpensive
Easy to learn and do	Easy to learn and do
Non-dental personnel can supervise	Non-dental personnel can supervise
Well accepted by participants	Well accepted by participants
Time required– 5 minutes	Time required – 3 minutes
Provides topical benefits	Provides systemic and topical benefits
Waste materials need to be disposed	No waste materials
	Suitable for pre-school children

Level 2

In level 2, participation of school dental health staff is accompanied by a dental hygienist. A dental hygienist is educated to plan and participate in the school programs that include oral prophylaxis, use of a variety of methods of fluoride application to foster re-mineralization, teaching oral hygiene procedures, diet counseling, placement of pit and fissure sealants and screening and referral for suspected oral pathologies for definitive diagnosis and treatment.

Many school districts or public health agencies have dental trailers that are used to provide prophylaxis and screening programs for students. Others use portable equipment that is set up in a room designated for the purpose by the school authorities.

Dental trailers may be used by hygienists for the placement of dental sealants. Sealant placement when coupled with a follow-up gel application of fluoride helps to provide protection to the whole tooth.

Level 3

Level three consists of requirements of level 1 and 2 programs along with addition of a treatment delivery option.

This level of a comprehensive school oral health program involves the ability to identify and refer all the discerned pathologies for treatment as early as possible. To achieve this level, an annual screening is indicated for all children and a semi-annual screening for children classified as high risk.

The objective of whatever level of preventive care program is selected is that it should be affordable, and accessible to everyone (with a priority for high-risk students). Once the primary preventive dentistry procedures have reduced the incidence of oral disease of that of the annual treatment workload, the number of extractions for a school population should approach to zero.

Some of the school dental health programs are enumerated below:

1. Texas statewide preventive dentistry Tattletooth program.

2. Tattletooth 11 (A new generation program). It was developed in early 1970's by Texas education agency and the Texas Department of Health.

3. Tattle Tooth 11 (A new generation 'Super-brush' preschool curriculum).

4. Crest's first grade oral health education program developed by Procter and Gamble in 1963.

5. ASKOV Dental demonstration (1949-57) (checkups and demonstration to prevent dental caries).

6. School Health Additional Referrals Program (SHARP) in Philadelphia.

TEXAS STATEWIDE PREVENTIVE DENTISTRY PROGRAM

Tattletooth Program

a. This program was developed in 1974 as a cooperative effort between health professional organizations, the Texas Department of Health and the Texas Education Agency through a grant from the Department of Health and Human Services to the Bureau of Dental Health.

b. It was pilot tested in 1975 and field tested in 1976 for schools within the state.

c. In 1985, the Texas legislature mandated that the essential elements for comprehensive health education curricula should be identified in the School Health Education Evaluation Project and incorporated into the school curriculum statewide so as to be taught to the state's school children.

d. In May 1987, an advisory committee recommended that a new program should be developed to replace the existing Tattletooth program. The model was developed according to a systematic process of educational development that began with recognition and analysis of needs. An educational model was developed, the program was conceptualized and materials were designed accordingly.

Tattletooth II Program

a. This comprehensive oral health curriculum targets students from preschool to grade 12.

b. Three videotapes were produced as part of the teacher-training package. The first videotape familiarizes teachers with the lesson format and content of the lessons. A second videotape, "Brushing and Flossing" was developed for the dual purpose of teacher training and as an educational unit to be used by the teacher with the students. A third videotape provides teachers with additional background information as a means of preparing them to teach lessons.

c. To facilitate bilingual education, the program has also been translated into Spanish for preschool children (grade 3).

d. Its curriculum includes scope and sequence charts that present the teacher what he or she is to teach and what the teacher in the previous grade level should have taught. It also tells the teacher what the students will have to learn the next year.

e. The students in grade 3, 5, 7, 9 and 11 are given the Texas Assessment of Academic Skills (TAAS) by the Texas Education agency to assess their performance.

f. Each grade level has five core lessons and two enrichment lessons.

g. Hygienists instruct teachers, using videotapes designed for teacher training and provide them with a copy of the curriculum.

h. In 1993, with funds appropriated by the State legislature, the Texas Bureau of Dental Health Services employed approximately 20 dental hygienists and dental assistants to promote the program statewide.

i. Teachers are encouraged to invite a dental professional to demonstrate brushing and flossing in the classroom. A field trip to a dental office is strongly recommended for nursery children.

j. Bulletin board suggestions, a book list, films and videotapes are available for each grade.

k. Annually, approximately 76,000 children are incorporated by this program with aid from the Texas Dental Hygienists Association.

This is the one program that matches subject matter with grade level, provides teachers with guidance information, and is available in two languages to target major minority groups of the state. To obtain the program for their classroom, teachers must attend in service training provided by a state regional dental hygienist.

SCHOOL DENTAL HEALTH PROGRAM IN INDIA

A School Dental Health Program ongoing in India is described below:

Bright Smile Bright Future Program

It is developed by the Colgate oral pharmaceuticals. Both the IDA and Colgate have been partnering for over 25 years for awareness generation program. Latest in the series was *The Bright Smiles, Bright Future*, which started in July 2003, targeting 45 lakh school children across India.

It accomplishes:

- Free dental screening and treatment referrals
- Oral health education
- Scholarships and grants
- Research and training.

To involve communities, families, or individuals in assuming responsibility for their own oral health, many ingredients are necessary. These include but are not limited to knowledge, skill, motivation, access to preventive agents and treatment services and safe and healthy environment.

Further, decision makers and teachers must be willing to include health education and health promotion in schools. Finally, government policies are also important. Smoke-free schools are a result of a policy that bans the use of tobacco products in school campuses.

BIBLIOGRAPHY

1. Books, C., Miller, L.C., Dane,J., Bullock, L., Libbus, M.K., Johnson,P and Vanstone, J.: Program evaluation of mobile dental services for children with special health care needs. Spec Care Dentist. 22, 156, 2002.

2. Carr. B.R., Isong, U and Weintraub. J.A: Identification and description of mobile dental program- A brief communication. J. Public Health Dentistry 68, 234, 2008.

3. Douglas, J M.: Mobile dental vans: planning considerations and productivity. J. Public Health Dentistry. 65, 110, 2005.

26 *Health Education*

Health education implies educating people about health. It encompasses environmental health, physical health, social health, emotional health, intellectual health, and spiritual health. It can be defined as *the principle by which individuals and groups of people learn to behave in a manner conducive to the promotion, maintenance, or restoration of health*. However, as there are multiple definitions of health, there are also multiple definitions of health education. The Joint Committee on Health Education defined Health Education as *any combination of planned learning experiences based on sound theories that provide individuals, groups, and communities the opportunity to acquire information and the skills needed to make quality health decisions*. The World Health Organization defined Health Education as *comprising of consciously constructed opportunities for learning, which involves some form of communication designed to improve health literacy, including improving knowledge, and developing life skills which are conducive to individual and community health*.

Education for health motivates people to improve upon their living conditions. Its aim is to develop a sense of responsibility for health conditions as individuals, as members of families, and as communities. In communicable disease control, health education includes an appraisal of what is known about a disease, an assessment of attitudes of the people and the presentation of specific means to overcome the deficiencies.

Health education not only teaches prevention and basic health knowledge, but also provides ideas that re-shape everyday habits of people with unhealthy lifestyles. This type of conditioning affects the recipients of such education and the future generations will also be benefitted from the improved ideas about health. Moreover, health education can help people deal with situations of extreme stress, anxiety, depression or other emotional disturbances in a better way. Health education can be carried out at individual level, in small groups or even in masses.

Aims and Objective

- Informing people about health and disease.
- Increasing awareness regarding importance of healthy life.
- Disseminating scientific knowledge regarding availability of preventive modalities.
- Motivating people to change their lifestyle and eating habits.
- Motivating people to inculcate habit of exercising daily.
- Encouraging people to adopt preventive measures judiciously and wisely.
- Encouraging people to seek medical help immediately in case, signs of disease appear.

The Health Educator

A health educator is 'a professionally competent individual, trained to use appropriate educational methods to facilitate the development of policies, procedures and systems conducive to the health of individuals and communities'. The qualification and training of health educator is not defined.

The process by which the qualification of licensed professionals or educators is determined is known as *credentialing*. Accreditation and certifications are all forms of credentialing.

The society for Public Health Education (SPHE) started the process of certification of health educators. Prior to this, there was no certification for individual health educators.

Health education teaching consists of a curriculum, which helps students achieve desirable attitudes and practices related to critical health issues. The desirable attitudes are: emotional health and a positive self image; care of the human body and its vital organs; physical fitness; issues related to misuse of alcohol, tobacco, etc.; health misconceptions and myths; effects of exercise on the general well-being; nutrition and weight control; sexual relationships; aspects of community and ecological health; effect of communicable and degenerative diseases and factors affecting population's environmental health.

Code of Ethics for Health Education

The 'Code of Ethics' for health education is a document that will continue to meet the challenges of the future health problems.

The Health Education profession is dedicated to excellence in the practice of promoting individual, family, organizational, and community health. The Code of Ethics provides a framework of shared values within which Health Education is practised.

- The ultimate responsibility is to educate people for the purpose of promoting, maintaining, and improving individuals, family, and community health. When a conflict of issues arises, health educators must give priority to those who promote quality of living.
- Health Educators are responsible for their professional behaviour and for promoting an ethical conduct among their colleagues.
- Health Educators are accountable for their professional activities and actions.

- Health Educators respect their rights, dignity and confidentiality by adapting strategies and methods to the needs of the communities.
- Health Educators contribute to the health of the population and to the profession through research and evaluation activities.
- Those involved in the training of Health Educators have an obligation to accord learners the same respect by providing quality education that benefits the profession and the public.

National Health Education Standards

The National Health Education Standards (NHES) are written expectations for what student should know and be able to promote personal, family, and community health. The standards provide a framework of instructions and student assessment in health education. The standards are:
- Students will comprehend concepts related to health promotion and disease prevention to enhance health.
- Students will analyze the influence of family, peers and media technology on health behaviours.
- Students will be able to access valid information to modify health habits.
- Students will be able to use communication skills to promote healthy life.
- Students will be able to use decision-making skills to enhance health.
- Students will be able to use goal-setting skills to improve health.
- Students will be able to manage behaviour leading to better health.
- Students will advocate for community as well as individual's health.

Principles of Health Education

The principles of health education are basically the principles of education. There are no set rules for teaching or disseminating knowledge amongst population. However, information, education and communication are the three fundamental principles of education. For convenience, the principles followed in health education are:

- The education should be at psychological level, i.e. active participation of the public along with topic of their interest is mandatory. Interesting subject makes the public receptive.
- The dissemination of knowledge or education starts at the level the people understand. The level of understanding of the population dictates the instructor to modify the teaching material accordingly.
- Repeated information along with convincing communication is important in health education. The so-called 'booster dose' is required to refresh the minds of the people. It has been established that repeated advertisements, posters, etc. have definite impact on the population.
- The population groups should be involved thoroughly in educative programs. In case the participants learn by doing themselves, it must have the better effect.
- The education should be conveyed to the population at their psyche level. Every individual might not be able to accept what is being told to him/her.
- The instructor should command respect from the public. He/she should be a recognized figure and must be friendly with the public. The instructor's attitude matters a lot in disseminating knowledge amongst the masses.

ORAL HEALTH EDUCATION

Oral health education is described as *any process which enables individuals or communities to increase control over the features, which determine their oral health*. It should be noted that the phrase 'dental health education' was commonly used during the early nineties; later the term 'oral health education' was widely adopted, reflecting a greater emphasis on the health of the whole oral cavity.

The dental team has long been encouraged to educate their patients in order to promote good oral health, and prevent dental disease. Major improvements in the oral health of individuals have been achieved over the past couple of decades.

Changes in Oral Health Education

- The drastic change in education methods stresses upon involvement and participation in learning experiences.
- In the past, oral health education has increasingly sought inputs from the fields of sociology and psychology.
- Oral health education is striving to modify attitudes and behaviour of the communities towards oral health.
- Oral health education has become more specific, and has increased the number of target groups.
- A major change has been that of accountability, the need to evaluate what is achieved at every stage.

Limitations of Oral Health Education

- It is presumed that health education, which targets the whole population may increase inequalities in health.
- Changing personal health behaviour appears to be more difficult for some groups than others; this may result in blaming the victim for not making the appropriate behaviour changes.
- There is no evidence of effectiveness of educative programs aimed at caries reduction, unless fluoride agents are judiciously used.
- Oral health promotion is effective in increasing knowledge levels; but, there is no evidence that such changes are related to changes in behaviour.

• The habit of consuming sweet foods and drinks is generally not satisfactorily changed.

Kay and Locker's (1997) statement 'Despite hundred of studies involving thousands of individuals, we know remarkably little about how best to promote oral health', seems justified. Summarily, it is observed that education has been of limited value till date.

To overcome the limitations of oral health education, some consistent guidelines, as well as effective teaching methods, should be developed. However, the question remains as to whether the dentist or other members of the dental team, are suited to fulfill the patient education role.

The National Institute for Clinical Excellence (NICE) put preventive advice on priority while educating people regarding oral health. The effect of oral hygiene, diet, fluoride use, tobacco and alcohol, etc. on oral health is to be understood by everyone in the community.

The effectiveness of such advice may depend upon:

• The frequency with which it is delivered
• The attentiveness of the patient
• The age, sex and occupation, etc. of the patient
• Who delivers the advice

There is need for more consistent advice to be offered by dentists to their patients. It emphasizes the 'simplicity of the message' because in the past, there has been a lack of consistency in providing the preventive information to the patients. It advocates a two tier approach:

 i. All patients should be advised properly regarding their general and dental health, not just those thought to be 'at risk'.
 ii. For those patients about whom there is greater concern (e.g. those with medical conditions, those with evidence of active disease and those for whom the provision of reparative care is problematic), more intensive actions are required.

To be successful for delivering better oral health education, following features are considered.

• Information for patients needs to be understandable, relevant, non-authoritarian, and given with conviction.
• Try to make a specific 'preventive diagnosis' and offer advice, which is aimed at solving the current dental problem.
• Avoid repeated phrases such as 'brush your teeth better'. Specific advice, with an evaluation component to assess patient progress will be sensible and fruitful.
• Be realistic about the advice and the timings. The knowledge should be built gradually.
• Practical demonstrations involving the patient will make education more interesting.

COMMUNICATION IN HEALTH EDUCATION

Education is primarily a matter of communication. The health educator must know how to communicate with the audience. The purpose of communication is to transmit information from one person or group of persons to other persons with a view to bring about behavioural changes.

Elements of Communications

The basic elements of communication are:
a. Communicator
b. Message
c. Audience
d. Medium

a. **Communicator:** The communicator is the originator of the message. The effective communicator should have clearly defined objectives. The language used should be simple and lucid so as to make the public receptive.

b. **Message:** It is the information a communicator wishes his audience to receive, understand, accept and act upon. A good message must be chosen keeping in mind the needs of the audience. The message should be clear and appealing.

c. **Audience:** The consumer of the message is the audience. The audience may be the total population or a specific group within the population.

d. **Medium:** The choice of the medium is an important factor in the effectiveness of communication. It has to be carefully selected, bearing in mind, its ability to deliver the message, its cost and availability. Communication should be adjusted to the local cultural patterns (folk media) of the people.

Media

The term 'media' includes all vehicles for communication.

Media are usually understood to be the specific tools used for formal teaching, other than human voice. These tools are best grouped in two categories:

A. Audio-visual aids (used in teaching individuals or small groups)

B. Mass media (used in teaching the large gathering)

The other media can be:

C. Lectures and Group Discussions

D. Symposium and Workshops

E. Demonstrations and Role playing

A. Audio-Visual Aids

Audio-visual aids are increasingly being used in modern education. They bring information of specialized nature to a selected audience, without assimilation and representation on the part of the teacher. Audio-visual aids involve techniques which are attractive for audience participation.

These are classified into three groups - auditory, visual and a combination of both auditory and visual.

a. *Auditory aids:* These comprise tape recorders, microphones, amplifiers, earphones, etc. The tape recorders are extensively used as teaching aids.

b. *Visual aids:* Visual aids are further categorized as:

i. Not requiring projection: For example, black board, flannel graph, exhibits, models, specimens, posters, etc.

ii. Requiring projections: For example, are, slides, film strips, epidiascopes, overhead projectors, silent films, etc.

c. *Audio-visual aids:* These comprise slide-tape combination, sound films, closed circuit television, etc.

B. Mass Media

The modalities of mass media are used to educate general public or the population as a whole. The examples are:

a. *Radio:* Radio is a potent instrument of education. FM Radio has further revolutionized the media approach. It is available in every house, even in remote villages. The talk or the message through radio should be simple and direct. It should be within 5-8 minutes.

b. *Television:* Television has become the most potent of all media. The public attitudes can be molded through television. The television being the cheapest media of mass education, it can be utilized for rural population also.

c. *Press:* Newspaper is the most important channel of communication to the people. The newspapers are read by most of the families. The articles and features published in newspapers have great impact on the public.

d. *Health magazines:* The health magazines can be an important channel of communications. The material needs expert presentation. The advertisements, etc. in the health magazines are well read by the people.

e. *Films:* Films are usually expensive source of communication. Further, it is difficult to produce films suitable to the local audience.

f. *Posters:* Posters are widely used for dissemination of information to the general public.

The posters should be attractive in order to invite attention of the public. The message should be clearly displayed so as the same may be understood easily.

Mass media are generally less effective in changing human behaviour than individual or group methods because communication is 'one way'. For effective health education, mass media should preferably not be used alone, but in combination with other methods.

C. Lectures and Discussions

Lectures are mostly used for the population group, whose literacy level is better. Since communication is one-way and the participation from the other side is negligible, it is not considered a good method for general public. General Discussion, however, are 'two-way' communication, where people learn by exchanging their views and experience. This method is useful when the groups have common interests and similar problems.

For an effective group discussion, the group should comprise less number of participants not exceeding 20 people. There should be a group leader who initiates the subjects, helps the discussion in the proper manner, prevents side conversations, encourages everyone to participate and sums up the discussion in the end.

Panel discussion is also an effective way of communication, wherein 4–6 persons who are qualified on the subject speak in front of a large group or audience.

The panel comprises a chairman and a moderator along with speakers. The chairman opens the meeting, welcomes the group and introduces the panel speakers. He introduces the topic briefly before inviting the panel speaker. Each cards can be displayed (summary of the topic printed on the card) for the public.

D. Symposium and Workshops

Symposium constitutes a series of speeches on a selected subject. There is no discussion among the symposium members unlike in panel discussion. In the end, the audience may raise questions and contribute to the symposium. The chairman makes a comprehensive summary at the end of the entire session.

The workshop consists of a series of meetings, with emphasis on the subject in depth. Workshops are designed to react at individual level within the groups.

E. Demonstrations and Role playing

A demonstration leaves a visual impression on the mind of the people and is more effective than the lectures, etc. People are shown the tooth brushing methods and the use of other preventive aids. Role playing is based on the assumption that communication can be more effective if the situation is dramatized by the group. Role playing is followed by a discussion of the problem.

Barriers of Communications

Certain barriers of communications pose problems for effective implementation of education modalities to the public. The barrier can be physiological (hearing disturbance), psychological (emotional problems) or even cultural/religious beliefs.

These barriers should be identified and removed, for achieving effective communication.

BIBLIOGRAPHY

1. Blinkhorn, A.S. : Dental health education : what lessons have we ignored ? British Dental Journal : 184, 58-59, 1998.
2. Chien, Wai-T : Improving health education through information technology : a commentary on Bond (2007). Int. J. Nursing Studies : 44, 1279, 2007.
3. Cottrell, R.R., Girvan, J.T. and McKenzie, J.F. : Principles and Foundations of Health Promotion and Education. New York. Benjamin Cummings, 1997.
4. Evans, W.D. What social marketing can do for you ? British Medical Journal : 332, 1207, 2006.

5. Hubley, J. : Principles of Health Education. British Medical Journal : 289, 1054, 1984.

6. Kann, L., Brener, N.D. and Allensworth, D.D. : Health education : Results from the School Health Policies and Programs Study 2000. J. School Health : 71, 266, 2001.

7. Kay, E.J. and Locker, I. : Effectiveness of oral health promotion : a review. London Health Education Authority, pg.1-5, 1997.

8. McKenzie, J., Neigher, B. and Thackeray, R. : Health Education and Health Promotion. Planning, Implementing and Evaluating Health Promotion Programs. 5th Edition, San Francisco, CA: Pearson Education, Inc., 2009.

9. Mertz, E. and Mouradian, W.E. : Addressing children's oral health in the new millennium : trends in the dental workforce. Acad. Pediatrics : 9, 433, 2009.

10. Mouradian, W.E. : The face of a child : Children oral health and dental education. J. Dent. Educ. : 65, 821, 2001.

11. Mouradian, W.E. : Ethics and leadership in children's oral health. Pediat. Dent. : 29, 64, 2007.

12. Nash, D.A.: Adding dental therapist to the health case team to improve access to oral health care for children. Acad. Pediatrics : 9, 447, 2009.

13. Orme, J., Viggiani, N.D., Naidoo, J. and Knight, T. : Missed opportunities ? Locating health promotion within multidisciplinary public health. Public Health : 121, 414, 2007.

14. Seale, N.S., McWhorter, A.G. and Mouradian, W.E. : Dental education's role in improving children's oral health and access to care. Academic Pediatrics : 9, 440, 2009.

15. Thorpe, A., Griffiths, S., Jewell, T. and Adshead, F. : The three domain of public health : An internationally relevant basis for public health education. Public Health : 122, 210, 2008.

16. Watt, R.G. and Marinho, V.C. : Does oral health promotion improve oral hygiene and gingival health ? Periodontology 2000 : 37, 35, 2005.

27   *Dental Manpower*

Over the years, the dental patient is becoming professionally oriented. The dentists and the other allied professionals are striving hard to satisfy the increasing demands of the patients. The new research and technology, coupled with patient's awareness are giving momentum to the dental profession. However, in order for the dental profession to continue to evolve, adapt, and meet the needs of the communities, increased manpower will be mandatory.

The concept of teamwork in dentistry has been gradually raising its profile. The key to meet the needs of the public lies in having a responsive, competent and elastic workforce. Oral health status and the prevalence of oral diseases vary substantially between countries, and also between different population groups and regions in the same country. Dental care delivery systems also differ amongst these regions. Variation in oral health needs and demand for oral health care require different size and configurations of manpower. The number and composition of dental manpower definitely influence the future of dentistry.

Dental manpower refers to the number, distribution, and characteristics of dentists, dental auxiliaries, and other supporting staff involved in providing oral health care at the community level. Dental auxiliaries or dental ancillaries are a generic term for all persons who assist the dentist in treating patients.

The dentist is the key figure in the dental team. The dentist is responsible for the treatment and care of patients and liable for self committed actions and also of the employees.

The dental auxiliaries/ancillaries are designated according to their training, the tasks they are expected to undertake and the legal restrictions regarding their working. These can be classified as:

- Operating auxiliaries
  - Dental nurse.
  - Dental therapist.
  - Dental hygienist.
- Non-operating auxiliaries
  - Dental assistant.
  - Dental secretary or receptionist.
  - Dental laboratory technician.
  - Dental heath educator.

Dental Nurse

The dental nurse is effective in executing oral health care modalities. The nurse supports and assists the dentist before, during and after the treatment procedure. The nurse prepares the dental surgery and ensures that the working area and the equipments are sterile. The nurse will make the patient comfortable and record the preliminary observations. Some patients are nervous about dental treatment; in such cases, the nurse motivates and helps the patient feel relaxed. The nurse helps the dentist during surgery by holding suction devices, adjusting lights and also providing requisite armamentarium as and when required. The dental nurse also provides post-operative care to the patient and advice accordingly. A nurse with good organizational skill is an asset in dental operatory.

Dental Therapist

A dental therapist is a licensed dental auxiliary who specializes in treating children's teeth and taking care of their oral hygiene. The duties of a therapist vary in different regions. Local dental regulations, usually determine the duties of a therapist. The therapists, under the prescription of a dentist, are licensed to examine children's teeth, administer restricted techniques of local anesthesia, take radiographs, provide sealants, perform scaling and cleaning, restore simple lesions and undertake vital pulp treatments in children.

Dental Hygienist

The dental hygienist is a member of the dental team whose primary goal is to aid in prevention of dental diseases. The hygienist must have a license to practice dental hygiene under the laws of the concerned state or province. The dental hygienists work under the supervision of dentists.

Dental hygienist conducts interviews and collects preliminary dental information. During examination they wear mask and gloves to avoid infections. They inspect the teeth, gums and related tissues and take radiograph, if necessary. The initial assessment and diagnosis is recorded and reported to the dentist. A major part of their work involves scaling and root planning. Hygienists also instruct patients on how to achieve and maintain good dental health. They demonstrate proper brushing and flossing techniques and also advice on nutrition.

Duties and Responsibilities

- Take medical and dental history.
- Record and document the initial findings.
- Examine the teeth and gums for the presence of any abnormality.
- Examine the mouth and tongue for signs of soft tissue lesions.
- Take radiographs, if necessary.
- Apply fluoride and sealants to the teeth.
- Perform scaling, root planning and polishing.
- Take impressions and make study models.
- Guide patients to carry out proper oral hygiene.
- Develop dental health programs for community.

Dental hygienists should have good interpersonal skills to work with patients, especially those who may be nervous about dental procedures. The communication skills help explaining good health practices to patients. Dental hygienists should have excellent manual dexterity and good observation skills. A trained hygienist help the dentist organize the dental operatory in a better way and also advise the patient as regard post operative care.

Dental Assistant

Dental assistants help the dentist and the other dental auxiliary providing efficient dental treatment. The assistant prepares the patient, sterilizes instruments, passes instruments during the clinical procedures, holds a suction device, and also carry out other non-specialized tasks. With the help of an assistant, the dental operator can focus exclusively on the treatment aspect. The dentist along with the assistant effectively manages the patient with four hands.

Dental Secretary or Receptionist

The secretary takes care of the secretarial work and also acts as a receptionist. Dental secretaries arrange appointments for the patients on phone or e-mail, etc. They make sure that the patient who needs immediate care should consult the dentist with minimal delay.

The duties of the dental secretary/receptionist vary from office to office. It also depends upon the dentist who decides the limit of powers to the secretary.

The duties in routine can be as follows:
- Attend phone calls
- Meet and greet patients with a 'ready to help' attitude
- Schedule patients' appointments
- Maintain patient records
- Manage office administrative work
- Maintain income-tax records, patients' billing/receipt, etc.
- Maintain records of purchases and utilization of materials, etc.

Dental receptionists need to be caring, understanding, and sensitive to the needs of people of all ages, cultures and lifestyles. They need to have a mature and confident outlook. They should be observant and vigilant. They must understand and respect the confidentiality of the patient.

Dental Laboratory Technician

A dental laboratory technician or a dental technologist is a member of the oral health care team who assists the dental surgeon for all the laboratory work, whether dentures, orthodontic appliances, crowns, etc. The technician uses a wide range of materials for dental appliances. He/she should have detailed knowledge of the make up and use of these materials in order to design and make these appliances. A qualified technician with technical skill and an artistic aptitude helps greatly in a successful dental practice.

Denturism is defined as 'the practice by denturists of making artificial dentures and fitting them to patients.' Denturism is a recognized profession throughout the world, in which a denturist provides duplicate dentures and dental appliances directly to the public. Denturism is legislated and practiced in couple of western countries.

Dental Health Educator

The dental health educator is a person who instructs the community regarding preventive dental modalities and in selected cases permitted to apply preventive agents. They provide information to individuals and communities in an effort to promote, maintain and improve healthy lifestyles. They are also responsible for collecting and analyzing data for the purpose of research, design and presenting preventive oral health care programs. The main objective of a dental health educator is to inculcate behaviour changes so as the communities can adopt preventive regimes on priority basis.

DENTAL MANPOWER: A GLOBAL ASPECT

It is estimated that the World's population is approximately 660 crores. Out of this, a quarter is children under 15 years of age and 10% may be over the age of 65 years. The dental health professionals in proportion to given population should increase to cope up with increasing demands of the public.

Global oral health trends have changed over the last few decades. While dental diseases declined in developed countries; and polarized to the extent that 80% of the diseases remain concentrated in 20% of the population, the same was not the case in developing countries. The decline in oral diseases in developing countries has occurred only in urban areas. The factors that have led to an improvement in oral health include awareness towards oral health, fluoridated toothpastes, better oral hygiene and balanced diet.

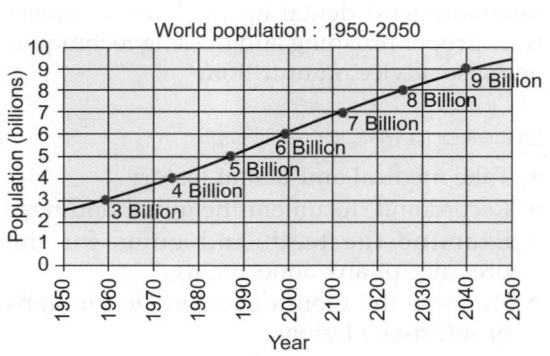

The lack of sufficient dental manpower is the matter of concern for many developing countries. In these countries, changing expectations by the public and a greater demand for sophisticated services by patients has led to a shortfall in the dental workforce. The growth of private dental colleges has widened the access but only in urban areas. There might be an overall increase in availability of dental professionals, but unfortunately the rural population could not gain from these. In Ethiopia, there are only 52 qualified dentists for a population of 63 million people; a dentist to population ratio of 1 : 1.2 million. Contrast to this, UK has one dentist to every 2,100 people.

The World Health Organization has stated that 'All people should have at least such a level of health that they are capable of working productively and also capable of participating actively in the social life of their community'. Following this, the Primary Health Care approach was planned, which allows equitable distribution of services and provide appropriate oral health at the community level.

DENTAL MANPOWER: INDIAN ASPECT

India is a country of diverse geographic character, varying culture and religion, with 16 official languages. The population (about 1,160,000,000) represents over 15% of the world's inhabitants. It occupies 2.4% of the world's land area and ranks among the highest population densities on Earth. The Indian population is distributed among 28 states, 7 union territories, 5564 tehsils/talukas, 640,000 villages, and 5161 towns and cities. India is predominantly a rural nation, as over 72% of its people continue to live in rural areas.

Indian economy is growing at 7-8% for the last couple of years. Foreign trade has also increased from 23.7% of GDP in 2003/04 to 35.5% in 2007/08.

Health of any population depends on two major factors:

i. Health care delivery system
ii. Socio-demographic profile of its population.

i. Health Care Delivery System

The health care delivery is based on the principle of providing *health for all* through primary health care approach, which is the foundation of rural health care system. According to the National Family Health Survey conducted by the Ministry, one-third of India's households are in urban areas, and two-thirds in rural areas. The World Bank has also reported that the poor are concentrated in rural areas especially in the north, where they are predominantly engaged in agricultural activities. The poor, normally are less literate and have less access to oral health facilities; subsequently suffering from oral diseases.

The Indian healthcare system is still affected by infrastructural deficiencies and great variations in the quality of care delivered.

Since independence, India never had oral health status data and it was a great problem for policy makers in making assessment of the need of oral health services.

An integrated network of sub-centers, primary health centers, community health centers, district hospitals and multi specialty tertiary care hospitals provide different levels of care to the population as shown in the flow chart below:

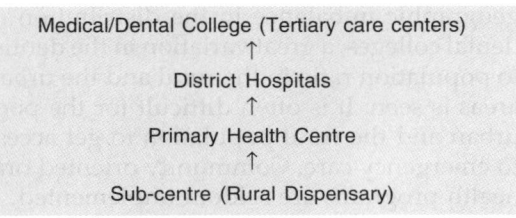

Medical/Dental College (Tertiary care centers)
↑
District Hospitals
↑
Primary Health Centre
↑
Sub-centre (Rural Dispensary)

Rural health infrastructure has been well designed to cover rural population through 136,815 sub-centers (SCs), 26,952 primary health centers (PHCs), and 3708 community health centers (CHCs).

ii. Socio-demographic Profile of its Population

It includes socio-economic status, literacy rate, human development index and health indicators such as maternal and infant mortality rate, life expectancy at birth, etc.

Oral healthcare delivered through primary health care infrastructure is of limited resources and dental manpower. The country is presently producing approximately 18,000 dentists per annum in a rough estimate, the dentist/population ratio is 1:10,000 in urban areas and 1:2,50,000 in rural areas. The WHO recommends dentist to population ratio as 1:7500. The distribution of dentists is grossly uneven with more than 90% of doctors available in urban settings and only 10% available for 72% of rural population. In most of the states, the dentists are not posted at the level of CHC and PHC. Government hospitals and establishments cater to a small part of the population, while the majority seek treatment through private clinics. Besides this, there is an acute shortage of equipment and material and other essential facilities to run the minimal curative services for such a vast population.

Dentistry is facing serious problems regarding accessibility of its services to everyone. The major missing link causing this unfortunate situation in a country like India is the absence of a primary health care approach in dentistry. Due to significant geographic imbalance in the distribution of dental colleges, a great variation in the dentist to population ratio in the rural and the urban areas is seen. It is often difficult for the poor urban and the rural population to get access to emergency care. Community oriented oral health programs are seldom implemented.

There are several reasons for this contradiction, the main being:

1. Geographical variations
2. Uneven dentist : population ratio
3. Poor specialist : generalist ratio
4. Poor dentist: auxiliary ratio
5. Low priority given to oral health

MANPOWER PLANNING

The manpower planning implies evolving oral health strategy implementing at the community level, and gathering feedback for the benefit of the population. The strategy should clearly define the immediate need of the population and also the possible needs of the future. The type of dental services required for the community at large should also be defined.

The main emphasis of dental manpower development is the prevention and management of disease process, improving community based services and better integration of allied health care services.

The planning can be executed in five steps:

1. Defining the Plan

The rationale of planning process and the reasons for initiating the plan; for example, who will be involved in the planning process and what the plan aims to achieve, are to be clearly defined. However, before starting the planning process, it is important to analyze the possible forces, which may act for the success/failure of the plan.

The decisions of the planning organization are to be evaluated thoroughly that may influence the plan. The decision making involves visioning possible scenarios based on an analysis of current trends.

The scope of the plan includes the structure of the plan, the timescale, geographic areas, services and staff to be included to ensure development of the organization. It is important that the scope of plan should not be too narrow to miss essential features; and also, it should not be too wide, which may make it unmanageable.

2. Vision for the Future

The vision involves looking at future events, both within and outside, and considering how these events may affect the service to be delivered. If these events are understood at the outset, there will be an opportunity to plan change, modification or addition of any other event so that the objectives can be achieved.

Developing a vision of what the dental service/manpower will look like in future is generally an excellent way of ensuring trust on the team. This way every one will work together as a team to help achieve the desired goals.

The goals of the plan are to be clearly defined. The success of the plan depends upon clear and concise goals, which encourages the associates work together. Defining the goals will also enable the desired changes to be described in a way that can be clearly identified, monitored and recorded. The goals can differentiate between intended and other possible outcomes of the plan conceived.

Once the goals have been identified and a vision of the future created, these can be used during situations like what next? or what if? types of possibilities. It is advisable to keep these scenarios relatively simple at this stage; adding complexities may deviate the plan.

3. Assessing Demand

The demand implies the numbers, types, skill and competence of people needed to deliver the planned service. The numbers should not be identified on the basis of current needs; which will restrict the demand to today's model of working. Demand will have to be worked up keeping in view the future scenarios. A couple of areas may need additional manpower while changing responsibilities in certain areas may solve the problem.

The following information will help identifying the future needs.
• People in need of oral health
• Quality of the needs
• Provision of services already existing

Community mapping data is required to enable identification of the characteristics of the population. It also establishes whether any up-to-date data currently exists concerning the oral health needs of this population. The mapping data includes the following features:
• Demographic statistics such as population, ethnicity and unemployment, etc.
• Information as regard dental caries, periodontal disease and oral cancers, etc. as well as general information viz. smoking and alcohol consumption, etc.
• Information regarding the use of services from the service providers.
• Availability of all service providers and also knowledge relating to the accessibility of these services.

Once the characteristics of the population and the accessible services are defined, it will be easy to identify the treatment needs. It is necessary to understand the requirements of the population before developing service pathways. The service pathways so established, are analyzed to see the possibility of improvement so as to meet the changing needs of the population.

The organization need to achieve better activity for a given manpower. It implies increasing productivity by motivation and inculcating sense of sincerity.

To increase the productivity of a specific staff group, it is advised to use the skills of that group more effectively by transferring the relevant tasks amongst them. The staff at any level may spend most of their time undertaking tasks that do not require their level of training or skill. These tasks can often be transferred to other workers. When the transfer is amongst the existing staff, this is referred to as changing the 'skill mix'. The transfer may also require new manpower.

An important characteristic of manpower supply is the flow of workers into and out of the organization. An understanding of this flow is needed in order to control the supply and forecast the future needs. The number of workers at any time should be a balance between the one who are leaving and the one who are joining.

The performance of existing staff is evaluated periodically. In case of non-performance, radical changes can be planned. The continuity of staff should have to be performance based.

The number of staff (whether existing or new) required for each specific function can now be planned. However, it is important that the skill, knowledge and competence required by the service are identified separately. The focus should remain on the needs of the patient. The number and type of dental professionals once identified, the training process of the whole team is to be continued to improve upon skill and competence.

4. Developing an Action Plan

Once the supply and demand assessments have been planned, the possible erupting gaps will have to be identified. On this basis, actions will be prioritized so that the gaps that present the highest risk receive the greatest focus. The gap is to be reduced by increasing supply, reducing demand or a combination of both.

The following features are considered:
– Utilizing the skill of people in the particular field.
– Reducing demand by reviewing the traditional staff.
– Increasing productivity of the existing staff.

The list of options for increasing supply or reducing demand once established, the likely impact of these options on the plan is assessed. The cost for the proposed solutions should also be considered.

A number of scenarios can be used to test the plan. It is essential to analyze the plan under varying circumstances. An action plan is established that will allow adjustments in response to influencing factors from time to time. The plans are usually flexible that can be changed and adapted depending upon the circumstances. The flexibility allows adaptation

and changes to meet the challenges encountered during the implementation process.

5. Implementation and Review

At the beginning of the planning process, the plan's goals were defined. The goals at that stage seemed to have measurable outcomes. The plan once implemented, it becomes necessary to ensure that the progress towards the goals is actually measured. This will ensure that if the plan deviates from the desired goals, the requisite changes can be thought of.

Realistically, no plan is likely to be perfect given the number of uncertainties that may hamper the implementation. The effective monitoring processes can provide early warnings. It is important to review these warnings carefully within the plan.

If the problem has been spotted early, it may be possible to adjust the actions within the plan. In case new working strategies are implemented, an assessment may be made concerning the level of resistance to change in the organization. If the problem is so severe that adjustments cannot be made to bring the plan back on course, the only option left is radical revision of the plan. A clear systematic approach is to be followed to revise the plan. Each step of the existing plan is reviewed to find out which part of the planning process was flawed.

The review process is not simply about producing an updated plan but is also a learning exercise. By undertaking a methodical approach, a better understanding will be achieved concerning what worked well and what did not. This learning can be utilized developing the modified plan.

Future Needs in Dentistry

The coming era promises plenty of new opportunities and challenges, and the dental profession should gear up to address the unmet needs of the community in the new millennium. In a society that steadily increases its consumption of health services, increasing workforce is needed. The immediate need is an oral health care system that uses existing health care infrastructure with an emphasis on community-oriented prevention at an affordable price. The emphasis should be on multidisciplinary approach that maximizes the use of clinical skills, facilitates the development of new professional roles, and increases system capacity. Dental education must emphasize the professional ethics and moral responsibility of graduating professionals to efficiently address community needs.

BIBLIOGRAPHY

1. Beazoglou, T., Bailit, H. and Brown, L. J. : Selling your practice at retirement. Are there problems ahead? J. Am. Dent. Assoc. 131, 1693, 2000.

2. Beehr, T.A. and Newman, J.E. : Job stress, employee health, and organizational effectiveness : a facet analysis, model, and literature review. Pers Psychol. : 31, 665, 1978.

3. Bourassa, M. and Baylard, J.f. : Stress situations in dental practice. J. Can Dent. Assoc. : 60, 65, 1994.

4. Bolin, K.A. and Shulman, J.D. : Nationwide survey of work environment perceptions and dentists' salaries in community health centers. J.A.D.A. : 126, 214, 2005.

5. Brown, L.J. : Dental Work Force Strategies during a period of change and Uncertainty. J. of Dent. Educ. : 65, 14, 2001.

6. Collins, R.J., Broderick, E.B. and Herman, D.J. : Dental manpower planning in the Indian health services. J. Public Health Dentistry : 53, 109, 2007.

7. Dixit, S. : Dental manpower status in Nepal. Journal of Nepal Dental Association : 10, 1, 2009.

8. Jolanta, A. and Vilma, B. : An assessment of dental treatment need : An overview of available methods and suggestions for a new comparative summative index. J. Public Health Dentistry : 69, 24, 2009.

9. Khader, Y.S., Airan, D.M. and Al-Fariri, I. : Work stress invent tory for dental assistants development and psychiatric evaluation. J. Public Health Dentistry : 69, 56, 2009.

10. Mahal, A.S. and Shah, N. : Implications of the growth of dental education in India. Int. Dent. Education : 70, 884, 2006.

11. Russel, B. : A new day coming ? A productive discussion on Dental Workforce Change. J. Public Health Dentistry : 68, 125, 2008.

12. Sengupta, A. and Nundy, S. : The private health sector in India. B.M.J. : 331, 1157, 2005.

13. Shah, N. : Oral health care system for elderly in India. Geriatric and Gerodontology : 4, 162, 2004.

14. Smith, E.B. : Dental Therapist in Alaska : Addressing Unmet Needs and Reviving Competition in Dental Care. Alaska Law Review : 24, 105, 2007.

15. Solomon, S. : Dental workforce. Dent. Clin. North Am. 53, 435, 2009

16. Wendel, O.T. and Glick, M. : Lessons learned : Implications for workforce change. J.A.D.A. : 139, 232, 2008.

28 *Dental Practice Management*

Dentistry too, like many other professions, needs business acumen. Management deals mainly with the business aspect of dentistry. Management is indeed a very wide subject and cannot be concluded in a couple of pages. However, understanding the basics in management enables budding dentists to become better professionals and also businessman.

Dental practice management is defined as *the process of utilizing inputs (human and economic resources) by planning, organizing and controlling for the purpose of producing outputs (services provided), so that the objectives are achieved*. Management starts with planning the location of the dental set up including the layout and the format of clinical chairs, sitting rooms and laboratories, etc. The next step is the input, which includes purchase of equipments and materials as well as the recruitment of staff to carry out routine procedures of the profession. Management also deals with how to control finances, tax liabilities and maintaining the records for future needs. The feedback of the practice envisages the satisfaction of the patient as regards treatment and payments, appointments and waiting. It also includes the remedial actions to be taken after thoroughly analyzing the psychological aspects of the patient and the behavior of the staff. Conflicts, if any, can be resolved before the remedial action is initiated.

The following chart classifies the steps in managing a dental practice.

Planning
- Location
- Format
- Chamber layout
- Discipline/Decorum

Inputs
- Equipment
- Material
- Manpower
- Interior designing

Staff
- Recruitment
- Training
- Motivation
- Team spirit

Control
- Income
- Records
- Practice analysis
- Counseling

Feedback
- Practice analysis
- Staff evaluation
- Remedial action
- Resolving conflicts

The following features play a vital role in managing the dental practice.

PHILOSOPHY OF PRACTICE

The philosophy of practice is the approach of the dentist as regards his/her principles and beliefs concerning the profession. This philosophy usually reflects the views of the dentist. These views should be clearly defined and understood by the auxiliary staff. The persons attached with the organization must have clear understanding of the policies, desire and expectations of the dentist. The same is true, or rather more important, in group practices.

Once the philosophy is specified, practice objectives should be clearly spelt out. Practice objectives are the basis for making any managerial decisions. These should be understood by all the members working in that institution. The practice objective provides:

- Basis to allocate resources
- Means to evaluate effectiveness in practice
- Guidance to the persons working in the institution
- Strength to achieve goals
- Motivation to achieve effective and resourceful practice

Practice policies should be clear to every staff and auxiliary in the dental organization. Preferably the policy should be in writing, since the written policy minimizes misunderstanding amongst staff members. The policy regarding dental practice should be flexible and be updated periodically. A flexible policy helps accommodate changes in the market vis-à-vis the attitude of the patient towards the treatment and its cost. Policy should not be viewed as rules. Rules dictate set direction for action while policies are guidelines.

Location of Practice Set-up

The choice of a practice location is important, since the dentist is to spend his/her prime time there. The location cannot be changed frequently; therefore, selection of a place for the practice is to be thoroughly investigated. Certain factors influence decision making. The first and foremost is the personal factor. The dentist may have some sort of choice for his clinic. The basis of preference can be climatic, geographical, or even presence of schools, etc. Certain people prefer small towns, while others prefer metros. Both have advantages

and disadvantages. Many dentists avoid hectic activities of the cities and prefer a calm life.

The second factor is the professional factor. Professional factor includes revenue earnings and growth. Availability of adequate facilities, types of patients in and around that area, and opportunities for referral practice, etc. influence the choice of the location of the practice.

The third factor is the economic factor, which influences the selection of a site for practice. The economic viability of a location is determined by its compatibility with the dentist's financial status and the prosperity of the resident community. In an area inhabited predominantly by affluent individuals, the practice can be established quickly and if services are properly provided, economic growth can be seen within no time. The patients' paying capacity plays an important role in deciding the location.

Certain additional factors also influence the choice of location of the practice. The availability of physicians around it is important; in case of an emergency and also because the physician can refer patients. A patient is usually convinced about dental treatment if referred by a physician.

Design of the Clinic

The design of the clinic involves the total surface area for the reception, operatories, sterilization room and laboratory. On an average approximately 800–1000 sq.ft. area is sufficient to start the dental clinic. Initially, two to three operatories are sufficient. Later on, as the practice is established, more operatories can be added.

The reception area should provide sufficient space for 8–10 persons to sit comfortably along with the front office manager. The décor of the room should be fine enough as to attract patients. The facilities of water, tea and toilets, etc. should be provided to the visitors.

The operatories should be identical in size and shape. Usually 80–100 sq.ft. area is sufficient for each operatory. The support equipments should also be standardized in each operatory. The operatory for the dental hygienist should be as good as the one for the dentist.

The flow of staff and patients from the reception to the operatory and from the laboratory to the operatory, etc. should be without any hindrance. As the number of operatories increases, the complexity of their relationship increases. The path should be the shortest for the patient to travel from one operatory to another. Two different paths can be created for convenience; one, for the movement of the supporting staff and the other for the patients. Usually the staff corridor is provided at the back of the operatories.

The operatories should be connected to each other and also to the reception, sterilization room, laboratory, etc. for better communication amongst staff members. Sound systems including bells and intercom devices can be provided in each operatory.

Selection of Equipment/Instruments

The equipment/instruments in the dental clinic should be selected keeping in view the latest technology and the comfort of the patient. The dental chair is available in different forms. The dentist is to select the chair depending upon the type of work in that operatory. For example, if oral surgical procedures are to be carried out, light cure unit and ultrasonics may not be required. The adjacent stool should be comfortable to the operator as well as can be adjusted according to the need of the patients. The assistant should also be provided with a stool.

Other diagnostic instruments viz. high and low speed handpieces, evacuation system, light cure units, ultrasonics and prepared trays should be selected carefully and be changed as and when required.

The equipment required in the sterilization room and also the dental laboratory should be purchased keeping in mind the establishment of the practice and also the type of practice.

Selection of Staff and Auxiliary

The activities that compose the selection process of staff and auxiliary are job analysis and application, interviews, references, medical examinations and financial negotiations. Job analysis implies the process of determining which work can conveniently be carried out by which member of the organization. The dentist should balance duties and responsibilities amongst various staff members. Specific duties are assigned to the selected members attached to the organization. These are known as job duties.

The job duties should be specified and clearly written. These duties are to be performed daily, weekly or even monthly. The emotional components of the job should also be looked into. These can be working at late hours and during holidays or working in an environment where the noise level is high and so on. The job specification implies the decision making ability of the employee. All these factors are to be taken into account while fixing accountability for not being efficient of any staff members.

The recruitment of employees should be given top priority. Only qualified, dynamic employees 'willing to work' attitude are to be recruited. Advertisements are one of the best methods. These advertisements should provide detailed information to potential aspirants. Unspecific advertisements may invite inquiries from the people who are not fit for the job. The advertisement should be comprehensive; it should include working hours, vacations, salary and promotions/incentives, etc. Direct recruitment can also be helpful in case one or two persons are to be employed. Acquaintances can recommend a person; or the dentist might know someone for a sufficient amount of time to deem him/ her a suitable candidate for the post.

Selection implies a process by which the employee is chosen from a group of qualified applicants. Once the applications are collected, the candidates with the requisite qualification are separated. Usually in a resume, all positive points are described. The screened candidates, are then asked to fill a form which projects their views about strengthening the organization and how best their manpower can be utilized for revenue earnings. This would further help the dentist to screen potential candidates. These candidates can now be invited for personal interviews. Interview itself is an art. This is a device to screen applicants for a specific job. The questions can be asked regarding personal skills and attitude towards the profession. An informal interview prior to the formal interview has advantages. An informal chat in the reception, once amongst the candidates themselves and also with the front office manager may lead to some conclusions prior to the formal interview. In some instances, stress interview is helpful. During stress interview the applicant is asked to solve problems on the spot. Alternatively, the dentist keeps silent for a couple of minutes. The silence usually agitates the applicant. It is found that those who are comfortable with silence, usually manage patients in a better way. They are also capable of managing conflicts amongst staff members, if any. Senior members who have been working in the organization for many years should also be involved in the interview process. This instills confidence in the senior employees and also their experience is utilized in selecting the most capable candidate. In case more than one candidate qualify or hold the same position, a practical test can be given. The body language with the working environment plays an important role in selecting the most suitable candidate for the post.

Once selected, the candidate(s) should be thoroughly examined medically for any disease unsuitable to the public and also which disqualify the candidate keeping in view the working conditions. Dental examination is also important as any employee with poor oral hygiene is not suitable for a dental organization. A one month or a two month period can be designated as probation period, which should include training of the employee.

MARKETING OF DENTAL SERVICES

Marketing is the art of selling. In dentistry and medical fields, services are being sold. The motto is to deliver dental services in a better way in today's competitive market.

The National Health Surveys have pointed out that almost 10% of the population has no natural teeth and other 30% have one or more missing teeth. Periodontal disease and caries affect almost every person. The problems should be adequately analyzed, efficiently planned and dental services should be effectively provided to the public.

Marketing is defined as *a system of interacting business activities designed to plan, promote and distribute products and services to potential customers.*

Marketing Research

Satisfaction of the customers is the main aim of any business organization. Marketing research is undertaken to evaluate the inclination of the customers, the financial status of the population and also the ongoing trend.

Marketing research is defined as 'the study of product design, coupled with activities such as physical distribution, advertising and sales leading to upgradation of the business.'

Marketing research provides valuable information which helps in arriving at a decision. It fills the communication gap between the producers and a consumers. It studies the details of the habits of consumers, their preferences, needs and opinions, etc. Customers' attitude is a very important aspect of marketing research.

Marketing research involves the systematic methodology in collecting, processing and interpretation of marketing data. The process is carried out step-wise as:

a. The aim should be clearly defined.
b. The researcher should understand the nature and scope of the aim.
c. The cost estimates and preparations of budget should be planned.
d. The data may be collected from direct questionnaires of the public or from government publications, etc.
e. The collected information is analyzed thoroughly and a report is prepared.

The objectives of marketing research are:
• It provides a basis for planning policies and program of any organization.
• It provides ways and means to minimize incidental expenses.
• It determines the price policy keeping in view the competitors in mind.
• It studies the likes and dislikes of consumers.
• It provides information with regard to new developments and technical changes.
• It studies the impact of external forces working against the organization.

Advantages

• It keeps informing the institution about the changes and preferences of the consumer/patients.
• It looks into the possibility of adding new customers.
• It acts as a sales booster as it establishes direct relation with the consumer thereby knowing their requirements.
• Modus operandi of the competitors can be studied.
• Quality of services can be improved by continuing meeting the public.

Limitations

• Large finances are involved, so small organizations cannot afford it.

• The inferences drawn may not be correct for all times since human psychological behaviour keeps changing.
• The collected data may not be reliable.
• The expectations of the consumers may be too much as to be accepted by the organizations.

Publicity and Advertisements

Publicity and advertising is one of the major aspects of marketing. It means 'turning the attention of the public towards the product or the organization.' It is a form of communication through diverse media such as hand bills, newspapers, magazines, bill boards, radios, televisions and motion pictures. The basic aim of advertisement is to popularize the organization.

In medical profession and dentistry, although advertisements are not allowed ethically, yet in today's competitive world, no one can deny their importance. Advertisements in local newspapers, pamphlets, etc. are always useful for nursing homes/clinics. Any cost effective advertisement medium can be selected.

Direct Mail

A message is sent to the customers by mailing them letters, booklets, calendars, etc. containing detailed information. The written part should be attractive and impressive. This method is effective since some sort of secrecy is also maintained in this method. This type of advertisement is quite suitable for doctors, but the drawback of this method is that only those patients who have already visited the doctor are covered.

Newspapers and Magazines

Newspapers and magazines are the most effective and powerful media of advertising. The message can be conveyed easily through regional language newspapers. Newspapers offer the widest circulation and have a universal appeal. The cost of advertising is also less as compared to other mediums.

Newspapers suffer from certain drawbacks. These are not suitable for illiterate people. Secrecy is also not maintained in this type of advertising. Most people read newspapers casually. Magazines, on the other hand are read with more interest. Advertisements given in the magazines are more descriptive and attractive, but the cost of advertising is higher as compared to the newspapers. The circulation is also limited.

Radio and Television

These types of advertisements are rarely used in the medical profession because of ethics and also because of the high cost of the advertising medium. This is suitable only for large organizations.

The text of the advertisement is very important. This is the heart of advertising and should be drafted with utmost care. This is known as advertisement 'copy'. The copy in an advertisement is defined as the written material including headlines, advertiser's name and address as well as the main body of the message. This is the total structure relating to the message which the advertiser wants to convey by using any medium of advertisement. The salient features of an advertisement 'copy' are given below:

- It should be written in simple and lucid language.
- Criticism of others institutions should be avoided.
- It must attract the reader's attention. It should be presented in such a manner that it attracts the consumer immediately. Headlines should be short, attractive and properly framed. Attractive borders can be inserted around the advertisement copy.
- It should have an everlasting impression on the reader. The arguments should be convincing.

- It must educate the people. The copy should contain certain information with regard to the services available in the institution. Nothing should be concealed therein.

In any organization, salesmanship is one quality which can boost the business at any level. The words 'salesmanship' means the art of convincing customers to buy the products or to avail the services. It is an art of enhancing sales by establishing personal contact between the buyer and the seller.

The advertisements must provide complete information to the patient regarding the product or the services. The consumer deserves to know every aspect of the institution before a rational choice of the services can be made. Advertisements that indicate the type of services provided by the dentist are usually considered unethical.

Delivery of Dental Services

The dental care delivery system should provide the following:

- An efficient and cost effective dental service.
- The best health care delivery system.
- The best possible manpower and facilities.

Various internal and external factors affect the delivery of dental services. The dentist is to choose from the available choices given below.

FIXED vs MOBILE CLINICS

A dentist is to decide whether to have a fixed or a mobile clinic. A fixed clinic is preferred where the population base is permanent and the demand and need is sufficient. In private practice, the mobile dental clinic can be effectively utilized to provide services to scattered groups of people especially in rural areas. The cost of operation, maintenance and transportation is higher with mobile clinics, however, higher cost is justified in providing service to the people at remote areas.

Selection of Practice

The most important decision a dentist makes in his career is where, how and when to set up a practice. He/she must first decide if the practice will be general, special, solo, partnership, group, institutional, salaried or private. The characteristics of different types of practice are:

Solo Practice

This is the most prevalent type of practice. The individual dentist does everything. He is his own boss, sets his own office hours, fee structure, vacation schedule, etc. A considerable financial investment is necessary. The disadvantages of this type of practice is liabilities of book keeping, income tax, dental insurances and other formalities, which are to be kept updated. This requires more manpower and subsequently more expenses.

Partnership Practice

The partnership practice envisages practice by two or more persons. Each partner is responsible for the other's financial commitments and legal liabilities. Partnership practice can be best started with equal investments by each dentist or percentage thereof.

Group Practice

In this practice, the dentists agree to the joint use of equipment and personnel with a centralized administration. Emergencies can be treated by all or any dentist available. In such practices, distribution of salaries should be decided at the beginning to have harmony and satisfaction among members. Members of the group are equally liable for lawsuits and financial liabilities. In such practices one administrator controls the overall functioning.

Salaried Practice

Working in any clinic/hospital/institution and getting salary is called salaried practice.

Many dentists opt for a salaried practice because of problems of finances, experience, etc. Initially, a dentist may earn a salary from charitable hospitals, small organizations or working under some experienced doctor.

DENTAL PAYMENTS

Payments can be made in cash or by cheque as convenient to the patient. Dental insurance and third party payments are gaining importance in Asian countries.

Third-party payment: This means that the payment for dental treatments would be borne by the insurer, the third party.

Budding dental professionals can incorporate themselves in the panel of these associations. The public can subscribe yearly or monthly basis to become a member so as to avail the benefit of free dental treatment. Usually four parties are involved in a prepaid dental care system:

a. The patient
b. The insurer
c. The government
d. The dental office staff

The Patient

The patient is the most important entity in any dental organization. Treatment can only be successful if the patient is concerned for the treatment and maintenance of oral health. Sometimes, especially in case of third party payments, the patient may opt for dental treatments just to maintain insurance records.

The Insurer

The insurer helps to pay for whatever level of care the patient needs. Many a time, the insurer does not cover costly treatments like bridges, orthodontic work, etc. The patient may analyze the validity of such a system and opt for other alternatives.

The Government

Dentistry is considered to be beyond the approach of peple from lower socioeconomic groups. Therefore, the government's help is mandatory to provide dental health care to this class of population. This is possible only in government hospitals.

The Dental Office Staff

The dental staff provides the best possible treatment working as a team. A balance must be maintained between providing patients with the best possible care and the money they spend on that. The patients in third party involvement must understand the proposed treatment and the cost from the very beginning. The patient in any case must be thoroughly examined and informed accordingly.

RECORD KEEPING

Record keeping is one of the major components in practice management. Records includes comment form, diagnosis and treatment planning for appointment schedule, photographs and radiographs, diagnostic casts and also the medical laboratory tests, if any.

A comment form is the basic need of the dental clinic. The comment form should be written in clear words and in two or three languages (at least one local language) so as to enable the patient to understand the text properly. The diagnosis and treatment records are sometimes mentioned on the comment form itself or can be made separately. All the paper-work records are to be separated from the casts, etc. These days, computers can best be utilized for the purpose.

Certain records are designated as problem-oriented records. Such records are more important because of their possible medico-legal implications. The exact time and date of patient arrival, initial photograph, treatment carried out, medicines prescribed and also the appointment schedule should be clearly written and witnessed. These records should be kept in a way that they can be easily retrieved whenever required. In Most cases accident victims need to have problem-oriented records.

Computer storage is simple and quick. Otherwise paper storage should be categorized as 'active' and 'inactive' records. For example, a record after five years, become inactive. In computers, softwares are available which simplify the work of the operator.

FINANCIAL IMPLICATIONS

The Actual and accurate financial records are necessary for any organization. Financial records are required to review, analyze and properly maintain the cash flow. This affects the practice and also helps the dentist add more resources, if required. In the beginning, a bank account is opened in any bank in the name of the organization. The transactions can be made by the dentist himself or two persons can be made responsible for signing the cheques, etc. Preferably, all payments should be made through cheques. Everyday receipts and expenditure are noted in the computer by the front office staff and an accountant should recheck the same. Once or twice a week, the money is deposited in the bank. The bank statement, month-wise or quarterly is rechecked with the records available in the office.

All the financial records for the year should be collected, clearly labeled and saved. Bank statements and other statements of loans, insurances, etc. should be kept handy, so that the same can be retrieved easily.

PRACTICE FEEDBACK AND ANALYSIS

Practice feedback and analysis are important for every practitioner, whether new or established. Growth in practice is indispensable and depends upon various variables.

Usually two aspects are considered important. One is financial and the other non-financial. The financial aspect basically concerns revenue earnings and non-financial implies quality assurance, staff behavior, patient recalls and appointment schedule, etc.

The key here is financial analysis. The revenue earnings of the practice should increase uniformly and should be maintained. Budget estimates for any establishment are necessary for any given year. A budget should be prepared for salaries, incidental expenses, materials and maintenance. Most dental clinics, especially initially, run on bank loans. Monthly instalments should also be considered. Monthly income and expenditure charts should be ready for reference and self motivation. The expenses are divided into controllable and non-controllable. The controllable expenses should be carefully dealt with. Revenue earnings are not sufficient, manpower can be decreased, sequentially, decreasing the overall expenses on salaries.

The second aspect of practice analysis is also important. A feedback proforma may be circulated amongst patients and thoroughly evaluated after receiving responses. The analysis of various aspects is necessary, such as quality of the treatment, behavior of the receptionist, waiting time and the comfort in the waiting area, appointment schedule and also the patient recall system. The other areas which should also be explored is that of the patient's expectations. The patient's preference of recent technology in treatment affects the success of the clinic.

In conclusion, the dentist should be willing to make changes, if warranted. Analysis is a continuous process, which starts from the first patient in the clinic and ends only if the practice is closed.

BIBLIOGRAPHY

1. Arnbjerg, D., Soderfeldt, B. and Palmquist : Factors determining satisfaction with dental care. Comm. Dent. Health : 9, 295, 1992.
2. Ashurov, G.G. : The marketing of dental goods and services. Stomatologia : 76, 70, 1997.
3. Ball, R. : Practical marketing for dentistry - Buyer's behaviour. B.D.J. : 181, 66, 1996.
4. Ball, R. : Practical marketing for dentistry - The core concept of marketing. B.D.J. : 180, 427, 1996.
5. Ball, R. : Practical marketing for dentistry - Marketing communicating tools. B.D.J. : 181, 214 and 217, 1996.
6. Harris, N.O. and Crabb, L.J. : Ergonomics : Reducing mental and physical fatigue in the dental operatory. Dent. Cl. North Am. : 22, 331, 1978.
7. Kemy, D.J., Nugent, G.J. and Pakozdi, G.J. : Guidelines for dental associate ships. J. Can. Dent. Assoc. : 41, 94, 1975.
8. Komensley, A.M. : Ownership and maintenance of dental records. J.A.D.A. : 97, 44, 1978.
9. Masalin, K. : Motivating your patients - marketing dental services. Int. Dent. J. : 40, 18, 1990.
10. Pau, A.K. and Goucher, R. : A dental practice placement scheme : benefits for practitioners an undergraduates. Eur. J. Dent. Educ. : 5, 155, 2001.
11. Rippon, R. : Marketing Dentistry. B.D.J. : 181, 198, 1996.
12. Somer, D. : Marketing the value of dentistry. J. Can. Dent. Assoc. : 62, 549, 1996.

29

National Oral Health Policy

The Government of India has made a commitment to Health. Inspite of natural calamities and economic constraints, the face of the Health Map of India is fast changing for the better.

In the past, oral health did not find its appropriate place in the national and state health planning perhaps due to the following misconceptions:

a. Lack of awareness in the masses about the prevalence and severity of dental diseases.

b. Oral diseases are not life threatening or severely debilitating.

c. The fact that oral diseases are almost preventable by simple and low cost means is not in the knowledge of authorities responsible for formulating the National Oral Health Policy

NEED FOR A NATIONAL ORAL HEALTH POLICY

Increasing Prevalence and Severity of Dental Diseases

Over the last four decades a number of point prevalence studies on dental caries, periodontal diseases, oral cancers and malocclusion have been conducted in India. A fact emerged from these studies that dental caries has been increasing both in prevalence and severity over the last three decades. In the years 1940-50, its prevalence reported was 40 to 50 percent with an average DMFT of 1.5. In 1980–90 the point prevalence has increased to about 80 percent in children with the average DMFT (average number of decayed, missing and filled teeth in an individual) being 5 in urban areas and 4 in rural areas at the age of sixteen years. Periodontal disease prevalence has already been in the range of 90–100 percent in the various age groups and it has already been established that the initiation of this disease (gingivitis) also starts very early in life. The above facts have been substantiated and the need for urgent intervention has been stressed by a number of national level workshops.

Dentist-population Ratio

There are a total of about 1,35,000 dentists serving the entire population of over 110 crore. Out of these, 90% are clustered in cities while only 10% are in rural areas with a population of over 75%. The dentist/population ratio is 1:2,50,000 for rural and 1:3000 for urban population. In order to bring down the disease prevalence and severity, it is important to implement organized oral health preventive programmes at community level as has been demonstrated in a number of western countries where the increasing trend of dental caries has been totally reversed. In the early nineties, the average DMFT in Norway was 12.5, in New Zealand 10.7, and in Sweden 14.1, but within a decade with the stringent implementation of organized preventive measures in the community, reversal in the trend of dental caries has started and it has already declined by almost 70–80 percent. In India it is still increasing rapidly.

Crippling Nature of Oral Diseases

Almost 85 percent of our children and 95 to 100 percent of our adult population is suffering from periodontal disease which is initially painless and self destructive leading to gradual tooth loss. Mostly people accept it as the disease of old age.

Dental caries is consistently increasing in its prevalence and severity, especially in children and today according to a number of investigators, 80 to 85 percent of children suffer from these diseases and the average number of decayed, missing and filled teeth per child at the age of 16 years is about 4 in rural areas and 5 in urban areas with almost no dental restorative help available. If this disease keeps on increasing at this pace, there is a possibility that the oral cavities in the young adults may be crippled with no functional molars left for mastication of food within the next 10 to 15 years leading to aggravation of health and nutritional problems. In addition to the crippling of oral cavities, the oral diseases can also have adverse effects on the vital organs of the body. The pus oozing pockets of periodontal disease of adults act as a focus of infection for other vital organs of body such as kidney, heart, lungs, brain, etc. Dental caries with its crippling effect on the functional component of oral cavity can lead to more malnutrition as the young adults would not be able to chew any coarse food available to them.

35% of all body cancers are oral cancers. Most of these are preventable. About 35% of the children suffer from malaligned teeth and jaws affecting proper function.

Oral manifestations and spread of infections related to HIV, hepatitis and tuberculosis are on the increase.

Impelling Economic Reasons for Early Recognition and Prevention of Oral Diseases

Besides the above mentioned health related reasons necessitating the early recognition of these diseases in order to be able to prevent not only the diseases but also the pain, so as to make oral health services more relevant in the field of health, there is also an impelling economic reason as the comprehensive oral health care system that has been developed in highly industrialised countries is extremely expensive.

Dental caries is an expensive disease, which causes economic losses both to the individual and to the country. In the USA alone, $4,383,000,000 were spent in 1970 for dental caries with the major expenditure going towards restoration of the carious teeth. This expenditure is increasing every year. This sum was approximately one percent of the total national income and 10 percent of the nation's health bill. In the UK, in the financial year 1977, approximately 250 million pounds were spent in England on dental treatment within the general dental services section for the national health service. In addition, it is estimated that loss of time from schools by children visiting dentists is roughly 51 million hours per year. Children suffering from pain of dental origin can cause their parents to lose hours of sleep with debilitating effects.

India is a developing country and spends approximately 1 to 1.5 percent of the total national budget on health and as such there is no separate allocation for oral health, so we in India can not afford to spend on the highly expensive dental restorative treatment.

Cost Effectiveness	
On the average, DMFT (average no. of decayed teeth/child)	= 4.5
Population of India	= 1100 million
Child population	= 440 million (40% of adult)
The cost of filling one tooth	= Rs. 100
If every child clamours for one filling	= Rs. 100 × 440 million
	= Rs. 4,4000 million

Prevention of Oral Disease—The Only Alternative

When the oral health situation worsened in the western countries inspite of their spending almost 1 percent of the total national income (United States - 1970) on restorative oral health, the condition kept on deteriorating and the expenditure kept on increasing. About 10 years back DMFT in USA was 11.6, Norway 12.5, Sweden 14.1, England and Wales 10.5, New Zealand 10.7 and Japan 8.7. This upward trend of dental caries could be effectively checked by the implementation of organized oral health preventive programmes at the community level. By means of stringent implementation of the preventive measures during the last decade, the upward trend has been achieved to the tune of 60–80 percent.

In India with limited resources and manpower, once such a situation develops, there would be no going back. This is a historic juncture at which our country is standing. Even in the face of such a grim situation, there is no national oral health policy and the country is without any plan to provide even the minimum coverage to the rural masses.

There is an urgent need to prevent the dental diseases in India. The method used for primary prevention of dental caries also achieves primary prevention of periodontal disease and oral cancer. Hence, in the National Oral Health Policy for India, there is a great need for emphasis on prevention.

The above facts amply justify the need for a National Oral Health Policy.

EXISTING ORAL HEALTH SERVICES

At present Oral Health Services exist at District, Sub Division and Tehsil level hospitals and in about 20% of Community Health Centres in our country. There is practically no paradental infrastructure at the said levels. There are no Oral Health services available in rural communities of India as the Dentist/Population ratio is 1:2,50,000 in the rural areas.

At present, there are a total of 1,25,000 registered dentists comprising both 'A' and 'B' class serving the entire population of 110 crores. 'A' class registered dentists are those who are professionally qualified from a recognized dental institution. 'B' class registered dentists are those who otherwise do not possess any professional bachelor's qualification in dentistry but are practising dentistry because of their experience or having some technical qualification in dentistry (Technicians) or are otherwise registered dental practitioners (RDS). If 'A' class and 'B' class registered dentists are combined for calculation of dentist population ratio, then a population of approximately 25,000 comes under a single dentist for catering to the dental treatment requirements of the public. If, however, only 'A' class registered dentists are considered, a population of approximately 30,000 comes under the purview of each dentist. 10% of total dentists in the country are posted in rural areas, where 75 percent of the population lives.

Urban Areas

Out of a total of 1,35,000 dentists in India 90% dentists are working in urban areas in medical/dental colleges, hospitals and in private practice. Hence in urban areas, at least, the services of a dental specialist are available to the masses.

INTEGRATION OF ORAL HEALTH SERVICES INTO THE EXISTING HEALTH INFRASTRUCTURE

Integration of Oral Health services into the existing Health Infrastructure is given in Tables 29.1 and 29.2.

The principal unit of administration in a State in India is a district with an average population of about 3.5–4 million. There are a total of 439 districts. The districts consist of blocks known as community development blocks. Each block comprises of approximately 80,000-1,20,000 population in about 100 villages. The health services in rural areas are being administered through Community Health Centres (CHCs)/ Primary Health Centres (PHCs) which are proposed to be set up, one in each block. Earlier, the health services in the rural areas were being administered through PHCs covering a population of 80,000-1,20,000, i.e. one development block. However the Central Council of Health at its meeting held in January 1983 proposed reorganization of PHC system and has proposed one CHC for every 80,000-1,20,000 population and one PHC for every 30,000 population. The new proposed set up is diagrammatically detailed in Tables 29.1 and 29.2.

As of date about 2328 CHCs have already been established by upgrading the primary health centres:

Rationale

At present, no oral health cover is being given to rural population; it is therefore intended to introduce preventive and promotive oral health services from the village level onwards. At the village level it is intended to give special training in oral health to Anganwadi workers and village health guides in preventive infant dental care and promotion of oral health in mother and child. At the sub-centre level the male and the female health worker/multi-purpose workers should be given training in oral health for prevention of diseases in the community, oral health education to the community, relief of pain and appropriate referrals to the Dentist.

At the Primary Health Centre, there is a need for the appointment of one Dental

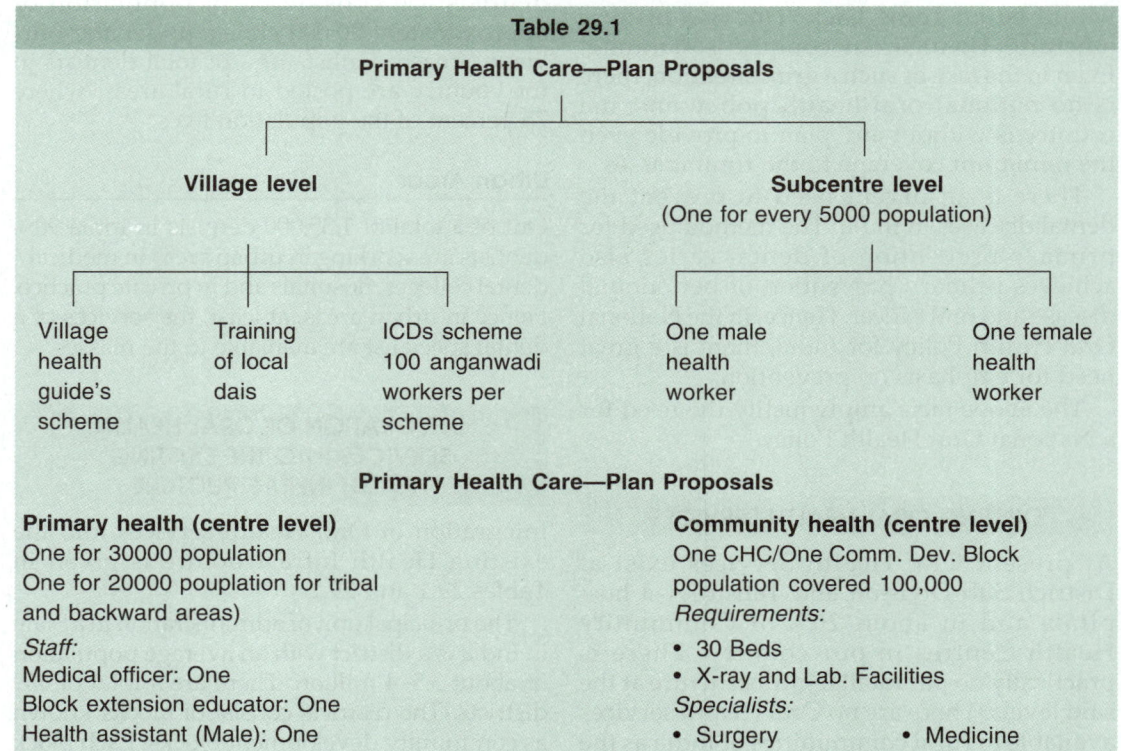

Table 29.1

Primary Health Care—Plan Proposals

Village level			Subcentre level (One for every 5000 population)	
Village health guide's scheme	Training of local dais	ICDs scheme 100 anganwadi workers per scheme	One male health worker	One female health worker

Primary Health Care—Plan Proposals

Primary health (centre level)	Community health (centre level)
One for 30000 population	One CHC/One Comm. Dev. Block
One for 20000 pouplation for tribal and backward areas)	population covered 100,000
	Requirements:
Staff:	• 30 Beds
Medical officer: One	• X-ray and Lab. Facilities
Block extension educator: One	*Specialists:*
Health assistant (Male): One	• Surgery • Medicine

Contd...

Health assistant (Female): One	• Obstetrics & Gynaecology
Supporting staff: One	• Paediatrics • Non-Medical Post
(Compounder, Driver, Lab., Ancillary Staff)	*Referrals:*
	• State level hospital
	• Medical college hospital

Table 29.2

Primary Health Care

Plan Proposal for the Integration of Primary Oral Health Centre into the existing health infrastructure

Levels	Available Infrastructure		Recommendations
Village for population of approximately 1000	1. Village Health Guide:	One	**Village Health Guide and/or**
	2. Locally trained Dai:	One	**Anganwadi Worker**
	3. Anganwadi worker: under ICDS scheme	One	would be trained and function for:
			(i) Preventive Infant Oral Health Care
			(ii) Promotion of Oral Health Care in mother and child care
Sub-Centre for every group of villages with total population of approximately 3000-5000	1. Multipurpose Health Worker Male:	One	**Multipurpose Health Workers** both male and female after suitable training will also function for
	2. Multipurpose Health Worker Female:	One	(i) Prevention of oral diseases
			(ii) Oral health education
			(iii) Relief of pain
			(iv) Referral to dentists
Primary Health Center (One for 30000 population) (One for 20000 population in hilly, tribal and backward areas)	1. Medical Officer:	One	**Additional Requirements:**
	2. Block Extension Educator:	One	Dental Surgeon: One
	3. Health Assistant Male:	One	Health Assistant: One
	4. Health Assistant Female:	One	(Dental Chairside)
	5. Supporting Staff - (Compounder, Driver, Lab asstt., Ancillary Staff)		
Community Health Center	Specialists:		**Additional Requirements:**
	– Surgery		Dental Surgeons: two (with one specialist)
	– Medicine		Health Assistants (Dental): Two
	– Obstetrics & Gynaecology		Dental Hygeinists: Two
	– Paediatrics		Dental Mechanic: One

Surgeon to render curative aspects and also look after the referrals, in addition to guiding preventive and promotive strategies in oral health at PHC, sub-centre and village level. There is also a need for appointment of one Health Assistant (Dental) who would supervise the Oral Health component of the male and female health workers at the sub-centre, and also at the village level. In addition to the supervisory role he would assist the Dental Surgeon at the PHC in the various procedures.

At the Community Health Centre, there is a need to appoint two Dental Specialists to deal with the vast range of dental problems in the whole of the community development block. These two Dental Specialists would also need two Chair-side Assistants and the other necessary infrastructure, such as Operation Theatre facilities and ward servants. One dental mechanic with requisite training is also required with adequate Dental Laboratory facilities.

Oral Health Services at the District and State Level

At this level, four Dental Specialists with postgraduate qualifications in different specialities of Dentistry are needed to provide the speciality services to the entire district. In addition there should be one Chief Dental Officer and One Programme Officer to look after and co-ordinate the oral health programme of the entire district upto the village level.

State Level

At the State level there would be sufficient number of Dental Colleges as per the requirements of the individual State, which in addition to looking after the dental education, both at the undergraduate and postgraduate level, would also cater to the difficult referral cases from the region/state. At the Directorate level, there should be a Director of Oral Health Services with an independent charge and budget with requisite infrastructure provided under the rules.

Central Level

At the central level or national level, it is recommended that there should be:

1. Additional Director General Oral Health with an independent charge and budget with requisite infrastructure provided under the rules.
2. National Oral Health Commission: A National Oral Health Commission should be constituted in the Health Ministry at the Central Level to co-ordinate, monitor and evaluate the goals achieved in the National Oral Health Programme in the country.

The Commission should comprise of the following members :

a. Additional DGHS (Oral Health)
b. Dental Advisor, Govt. of India
c. A representative of the National Dental Association
d. A representative from the Dental Faculty of the Universities.
e. A representative from the Dental Council of India
f. A representative from the Armed Forces Dental Corps
g. Directors (Dental) from all the States

PLAN OF EXTENDING MINIMUM ORAL HEALTH CARE TO THE ENTIRE INDIA

Health has been declared as a fundamental human right. This implies that the state has a responsibility for the health of its people. Oral health is an integral part of general health, rather oral cavity can rightly be called a gateway to the body. The sequelae of crippled oral cavity have already been stressed under the title "Crippling nature of oral diseases : and its effect on the general health". Evaluation of the existing oral health services warrants the following valid criticism.

a. Predominantly urban oriented
b. Mostly curative in nature
c. Accessible mainly to a small part of the population, i.e. privileged ones.

The implementation plan would be discussed under the following two heads:

Plan for Rural India

As has been discussed earlier, the rural areas are virtually without any dental coverage. The services of a specialist are not available even for the need of emergency services. It has therefore been planned to deliver the minimum oral health cover to the entire rural population utilising the existing health and educational infrastructure: Multipurpose workers, Health Assistants, Health Guides and School teachers are the focal key persons for the delivery of primary preventive strategies at the periphery and village level and medical doctors and other associated staff at the CHC/PHC. The whole health team should be trained in various oral health care strategies by the dentists who have been specially trained for conducting these training programmes in specially created centres for this purpose (details discussed subsequently).

The implementation plan for whole of the rural population is as follows:

Strategies to provide primary prevention to the population and handling of emergencies.

This would be discussed under the following heads.

A. Preventive package
B. Methodology of instituting primary prevention
C. Training of trainers. (National training center)

A. Preventive Package

Most of the common oral diseases and oral health problems including dental caries, periodontal diseases, oral cancers and some forms of malocclusion are largely preventable. About 50–60 percent of the oral diseases can be prevented by early detection and primary prevention, which is not merely prevention of initiation of diseases, but also the reversal of the diseases in their initial stages. The primary prevention package for oral health to be delivered to the rural community should comprise of:

i. Oral health education
ii. Plaque control (proper cleaning of the teeth to remove dental plaque)
iii. Use of chemico prophylactic and therapeutic agents
iv. Dietary counselling.

i. Oral Health Education

MPWs (Multipurpose Workers), Anganwadi workers, Health Guides, school teachers and occasionally the doctors employed at the CHC and PHC should impart oral health education to the various groups of the community, viz. children of various age groups, e.g. upto 5–6 years along with mothers/parents, 7–10 years, 11–15 years and 16 years and above/adult community. The above age groups have been formulated keeping in view the fact that the mental calibre, understanding level and the assimilation and capabilities differ in children of various age groups. These education programmes should be made a part and parcel of all other health education programmes, e.g. family planning, eye care, health care, etc. However, an effort should be made that some of these sessions be exclusively devoted to oral health, especially delivered by school teachers and various health workers and medical officers. The lectures can be imparted with the help of audio-visual aids to small groups of individuals in the community, held at regular intervals in different areas of villages with maximum participation of people. These programmes would be reinforced by school teachers and by person to person talks between various members of the community and the health workers when they visit the families for carrying out various health programmes. The oral health education should be a part of training programme of various categories of health workers and anganwadi workers. Doctors with appropriate oral health information should act as leaders of the whole health team. Oral health education should include education on the various oral hygiene measures for the removal of dental plaque, which is the causative agent for both dental caries and periodontal diseases; education on restriction of eating anything sweet to not more than three times a day preferably with meals, to be followed by suggesting alternative in between snacks and regarding the use of fluorides for the prevention of dental caries.

Oral cancer and potentially pre-cancerous lesions

The oral health education must also include emphasis on early recognition of pre-cancerous and cancerous lesions, their prevention and referrals. The community, through MPWs/health workers, school teachers and anganwadi workers should also be cautioned about the ulcers in mouth which do not disappear in one or two weeks. In such a case the individual should be referred to a dentist. The health workers should also educate that betel leaves, pan, pan masala, reverse smoking, etc. are not good as these can lead to cancer and are the most common cause of oral cancer. These habits can lead to development of some ulcers, precancerous or cancerous lesions in the oral cavity as well as of some other parts of the body. The individuals with these habits should regularly check-up their mouths for the presence of any ulcer, red swollen area, fibrous bands in the mouth or tongue with difficulty in opening the mouth or red patch, etc.

Infant dental care

Special emphasis on infant dental care should be given while imparting training to various health workers and anganwadi workers, who in turn should disseminate the information while delivering oral health education lectures to the community. The main components of infant dental care should be:

1. Information about importance of nutrition and well balanced diet for pregnant women, for the healthy body with healthy teeth and gums.

2. Pregnant mothers must be informed that they should not take any medicine without consulting a qualified doctor and must always tell the health care provider about the pregnancy so that an antibiotic-tetracycline which causes yellowish brown discoloration of the teeth of infant/baby is not prescribed to her during pregnancy.

3. The newly born babies mouth is free of bacteria. The germs in the baby's mouth are transferred from parents during normal cuddling, kissing, etc. So it is very important for parents to keep their mouths clean if they want their baby's mouth to be free from disease and if possible restrict direct mouth to mouth contact.

4. Health workers must teach the mothers and demonstrate to them how to clean the gum pads of the infants with a pre-boiled wet cotton cloth or gauze piece after every feed.

5. When first tooth erupts in the mouth of a child, a soft baby tooth brush must be introduced or otherwise teeth/mouth along with gum pads must be cleaned routinely with pre-boiled, wet cotton cloth or gauze piece.

6. Children must be encouraged to get into the habit of chewing even before teeth erupt, e.g. chewing of rusks, a long piece of carrot, apple, etc. must be encouraged.

7. It is very important to take care of deciduous/milk teeth since healthy, decay free milk teeth create a healthy environment for permanent teeth.

Geriatric dental care

It is also important to impart training to health workers to take care of the oral health of the elderly people.

1. People must be told that poor oral health/ periodontal disease or loss of tooth is not age related. If proper care is taken, one can have healthy teeth and gums throughout the life span of an individual.

2. Even elderly people need preventive and restorative oral health care, as in case of young adults, so they must be given advice on prevention of oral diseases and referred to specialists for restorative care if need be.
3. Edentulous elderly should have dentures (complete or partial) in order to avoid potential nutritional deficiency problems.
4. Till the time edentulous elderly people own their dentures, they must clean their ridges with pre-boiled, clean, wet cotton cloth/gauze piece.
5. Care of denture: The dentures must be brushed, cleaned with soap and water after every meal. The ridges also should be taken care of as advised earlier.

Dento-facial injuries due to accident

Contact sports, the increasing number and velocity of vehicles on the roads, injuries to children at play and adults in the house and the high costs involved in restoring function and aesthetics requires the use of preventive measures; as much as maintaining pulp vitality, promoting completion of root growth, managing complications and restoring functions and facial appearances. It also involves intersectional cooperation in the promotion of safety rules for helmets, mouth-guards, seat-belts, etc. and setting up of trauma units at designated places.

ii. Plaque Control (Proper Cleaning of Teeth to Remove Plaque)

In small groups, children and parents should be demonstrated the plaque in their mouths; the knowledge which has already been given in the oral health education programmes. The method of proper brushing can be demonstrated and each member of the group can be encouraged to brush their own mouth and each other's mouths. Frequency of brushing should be stressed as three times a day after every meal.

The families who cannot afford tooth brush and tooth paste can be taught the proper use of chewing stick (dattan) three times a day.

iii. Use of Chemico Prophylactic and Therapeutic Agents

Fluoride has been proved beyond doubt as an anti-caries agent and should be used to prevent dental caries in its topical forms.

iv. Dietary Counselling

Adults and children should be educated that sugar in diet is fermented by bacteria in the mouth leading to the production of acids which make cavities in the teeth.

• Rural masses should be educated to reduce the sugar food stuffs (sweet lollies, biscuits, cold drinks and other sweets) to not more than three times a day.
• Avoid taking snacks in between meals, and if at all required, then substitute sugary snacks with salted protein containing snacks, e.g. grams, groundnuts and soya-beans, etc.
• Avoid retentive sugars such as gachak, rewari, etc.
• Avoid hidden sugar as well—such as cough syrup, tonics, etc.
• Total diet exposures not to exceed five times a day.
• Government should issue instructions to put statutory warning on all sugar snacks such as chocolates, toffees and sweets that "eating sweets leads to decay of teeth".

B. Methodology of Instituting Primary Prevention

The multipurpose workers, health assistants, medical officers, health guides, health volunteers and school teachers can be trained for primary prevention in rural areas as stated earlier.

i. They can be given knowledge about the use of fluorides, the benefits derived, and some knowledge on mode of action of fluorides in the prevention of dental caries.

All the categories of health workers can be given practical knowledge about the preparation and use of daily family mouth rinse—an alternative to fluoride toothpaste.

Practical knowledge and technical know-how can be given to auxiliaries especially school teachers, regarding the preparation of fluoride solutions for mouth rinses in schools and topical application and how fluoride application has to be done in children every six months.

ii. The whole medical team and school teachers can be educated about plaque. Plaque can be demonstrated to them in their own mouths by disclosing it and then the correct method of brushing can be demonstrated so as to remove the plaque. The health workers can further teach and demonstrate it in small groups in the community and teachers to the school children in schools.

iii. *Handling of dental emergencies:* the whole of the medical team including health auxiliaries can be trained to handle various types of minor dental emergencies and referrals.

iv. *Diagnosis of oral cancer:* The health auxiliaries, i.e. the whole medical team can be trained in the early detection and diagnosis of a possible oral cancer, precancerous condition and such cases to be referred to PHC/CHC/medical doctors or specialists.

C. National Training Center Training of the Trainer

It is important to calibrate the trainers, viz. dentists from the various states and union territories, who would be assigned the duty of training the various health teams, posted at the PHC/CHC in their respective states. A union Government can identify a center which would have the capacity of training the existing health infrastructure, i.e. doctors, multipurpose workers, health guides, school teachers, etc. for this purpose and also would standardize the various education materials, courses, evaluation criteria for the training of different categories of health workers. The education materials for the education of community by the health guides and multipurpose workers, school children in various age groups by the school teachers have also to be prepared and standardized.

Provision of at least One Dentist at PHC with Efficient Equipment

The present dental manpower situation in the country is such that presently, there are about 1,35,000 dentists available for a population of 11000 million and only about 10–12 percent of these dentists are serving in the rural population which constitutes about 75% of total population. Thus, in the rural areas the dentists population ratio is 1:2,50,000.

Projections for 2020 indicate that at the present 2% rate of increase in population per year, the population of India would be about 1500 million. Considering the number of dental graduates passing out every year, it is estimated that by 2020, there would be about 1,75,000 dentists bringing the dentist population ratio to 1:20,000.

There is need to stress for more provision of dental hygienists and other auxiliary oral health workers. The role of the dental surgeons should be broadened. They need to devote time to work as leaders of oral health care team in the communities.

The distribution of one of the various dental personnel should be as detailed below as per DCI workshop of September 1991.

1. Sub Centre

Oral Health Worker - 1 under public
health dentist or

a trained dental surgeon for 3000–5000 population.

2. **Primary Health Centre**

Dental Surgeon	- 1
Dental Hygienist	- 1
Chairside Assistant	- 1 (for a population of 30,000)

3. **Community Health Centre**

Dental Surgeon	- 2
Dental Hygienist	- 2
Chairside Assistant	- 2
Dental Technicians	- 1

4. **Upto 100 Bedded Hospitals or Referral Centres at Sub Division Level**

Dental Surgeons	- 3 with one specialist
Dental Hygienists	- 2
Dental Technician	- 1
Health Assistants	- 4 (Chairside)

5. **District Hospital**

Dental Specialist Surgeons (including one Chief Dental Surgeon)	- 4
Dental Hygienist	- 3
Dental Technician	- 2
Health Assistant (Dental Chairside)	- 1

6. **Referrals/State Hospitals/Medical College Hospitals/ Deptt. of Dental Surgery (750 or more beds)**

Dental Surgeons (Specialist)	- 9
Dental Hygienist	- 4
Dental Technician	- 3
Health Assistant (Dental Chairside)	- 12

7. **State Directorate:** Director-Dental Health Services with other hierarchical staff with independent charge and separate budget head.

8. **Central Health Ministry:** Additional Director General Oral Health with independent charge and separate budget head.

Mobile Dental Clinics

In order to provide dental health curative and restorative services along with primary prevention of dental diseases, it is proposed that there should be well equipped mobile dental clinics so that the services can be rendered to the rural masses at their doorsteps, more so in various remote and inaccessible areas. There should be at least 3–4 mobile dental clinics at each district level catering to a population of 4,50,000 to 5,00,000. Each mobile dental clinic should have two dental chairs and units, each with airturbine, micromotor, ultrasonic scalers and other equipment. There should be three dental surgeons posted with each mobile dental clinic, with one dental technician and three chairside assistants. Two dental surgeons should look after the restorative and curative work of the patients, whereas one should devote time on the primary prevention of dental diseases through organizing lectures, participating in discussions using audio-visual aids to educate and motivate the rural masses to follow the primary preventive measures.

Continuing Dental Education Programme in each State

Each state under the directorate of health services (dental) must identify one or two training centers in the state. The directorate must conduct at least one CDE programme every 6 months. This CDE programme must be compulsory for each dental surgeon serving in the state health services. Through these CDE programmes the dental surgeon's knowledge must be updated regarding the most recent concepts of dental procedures as well as on the various methods and approaches of preventive and curative aspects of the dental diseases. The directorate must ensure not only compulsory attendance of dental surgeons but also their active participation through group discussion/panel discussion/practical training, etc. so that they participate with interest. The directorate should evolve a system to objectively evaluate (some point system) the active participation of the dental surgeons in these CDE programmes. The directorate should also make arrangements to conduct such like CDE programmes for private practitioners.

Role of Dental Colleges

Each dental college should be given the responsibility to adopt one whole district so as to take care of the preventive oral (dental) health services to the rural and the urban communities of the district effectively using the internship programme. The interns working in the dental colleges should be posted compulsorily for 6 months in the community so as to get oriented to train the school teachers, parahealth workers and anganwadi workers in delivering the oral health preventive packages to the masses. Dental colleges can explore and utilize the special provision of funds available with the planning commission for such like projects for adoption of one district by a dental college community.

Strategies of Oral Health Care in Urban Areas

The dentist population ratio in urban areas is approximately 1:3,000 as compared to 1:2,50,000 in rural areas. However, if the prevalence of dental diseases in urban and rural areas is compared, the average number of decayed, missing and filled teeth per child by the age of 16 years in urban areas is approximately 5.0 as compared to 4.0 in rural

areas, reported by a number of investigators. Almost 85–90 percent of children and 100 percent adults in both urban and rural areas suffer from gingival and periodontal diseases, respectively. This clearly indicates that even though the services of dental specialists are available to the masses in the urban areas but in reality the oral diseases prevalence has not decreased and is rather high. This is probably due to lack of awareness and motivation of the public as well as the dentists in the primary prevention of the oral diseases. It has been seen in a number of developed countries, e.g. Sweden, USA, UK, etc. that by institution of organized preventive measures in the community, the dental caries could be reduced by almost 50–70% over a period of 10–15 years. So, there is a need to change the attitude of the public as well as the dentists and also to make them aware that the oral diseases are preventable and reversible in the initial stages. To achieve this the following needs to be done:

i. Involvement and reorientation of the dentists working in urban areas.

ii. Implementation of primary prevention package through the school health schemes in the different urban areas.

iii. Involvement, education and motivation of the teachers in the various schools/colleges and other educational institutions in the urban areas.

iv. Exploration and involvement of other voluntary (Rotary Club, Lion's Club, YMCA, YWCA, Neo's and neats, etc.) organizations working in different urban areas in achieving the oral health targets.

i. Involvement and Reorientation of Dentists in Urban Areas

First of all there is a need to involve the dentists, teaching staff posted in the dental colleges, hospitals as well as private practitioners. Two month refresher courses in the concept and implementation of primary protection from oral diseases should be started at some recognized institutions in the country to reorient them.

This can be started after the training of the dentists from various states for the implementation of the National Oral Health Policy in the rural areas is completed, i.e. over a period of 1–1/2 years. After that a group of 15 dentists from the various dental colleges and the private practitioners from urban areas of the country can be trained at the centre identified for this purpose. This can be a continuous programme. The dentists so trained can further train the dentists in their own states. All the teaching aids and material can be made available to them.

ii. Implementation of Primary Preventive Package through the School Health Schemes in the different Urban Areas

Since very little organized health system is operative in urban areas, it is important to explore all the possible avenues to implement minimum oral health coverage to the urban population. The dentists of the school health schemes are operative in a large number of urban areas. The dentists of the school health program after proper training, can form a good nucleus for the delivery of preventive package.

iii. Involvement, Education and Motivation of the Teachers in the various Colleges and other Educational Institutions in the Urban Areas for the Delivery of Primary Preventive Package to the School/College going Children and Young Adults

Education is one of the most organized systems prevalent in the urban areas. Hence, the utilisation of this system and involvement of teachers at various levels starting from small school children to young adults in the colleges and universities would be ideal to create awareness and to motivate the population in the formative years towards developing habits leading to prevention of oral diseases. The dentists employed in school health schemes and other hospitals, after proper training can be instrumental in the training of preventive component, i.e. teachers in the delivery of the preventive package.

iv. Exploration and Involvement of other Voluntary (Rotary Club, Lions Club, YMCA, etc.) and Health Organizations Working in different Urban Areas in Achieving the Oral Health Targets

A number of other health workers, such as family planning workers, social health workers, anganwadi workers and number of voluntary organizations such as Rotary Club, Lion's Club and other health organizations such as child welfare are operating and active in the various urban areas. These are potential sources which can be utilised for the delivery of the preventive package.

UTILISATION OF THE MASS MEDIA

Since there is a widespread network of radio television, press and cable network in our country, the proper utilisation of this media will help ensure not only spreading the right message but would also lend authenticity to what the various type of workers would be propagating in the field. For this purpose, with the help of the Ministry of Mass Communication, two to three minute films can be projected on television at peak hours along with clearly defined messages and flashes on radio.

REORIENTATION OF DENTAL EDUCATION IN INDIA

Community Dentistry component in each dental college should be made more dynamic, active and viable. Special funds can be allocated to each dental college from the planning commission for adopting one district to implement oral health care programmes, but these programmes would have to be standardized, monitored, evaluated and reported. Basic dental curriculum should be preventive and community need based.

There would be a need to reorient some of the dental education programmes in the various dental colleges according to the national oral health policy. As already envisaged in the plan, two teachers (dentists) from each dental college would be given the training in the center identified for this purpose, who in turn will be responsible for conducting the reorientation programmes in their own colleges. One of the important components should be that out of the one year internship, six months are to be spent in the rural areas.

Involvement of other Allied Departments

The department of education and social welfare should be involved to impart correct oral health promoting information to school children at an early age, which would help to develop proper attitude in them. It would be preferable to include chapters giving adequate knowledge about oral diseases and their prevention in the text books of class 4th, 7th and 9th.

SETTING UP OF APEX BODIES OF DENTAL EDUCATION AND RESEARCH

To give a proper lead to the total health care systems in the country, it is important to set up apex bodies of national importance in post graduate dental education and research on the pattern of NIDR (National Institute of Dental Research) in the USA and the AIIMS (All India Institute of Medical Sciences) in New Delhi and the P.G.I., Chandigarh in India. In the beginning, at least one such institute of national importance ought to be set up on oral health where meaningful research applicable to Indian conditions can be carried out systematically on a longitudinal basis.

OUTLINE OF PLAN OF ACTION

A plan of action aiming at achieving the above mentioned objectives should consist of the following:

A. Detailed activities
B. Targets

A. Detailed Activities

Activities within the Sole Responsibility of the Ministry of Health, Government of India

a. The Ministry of Health, Government of India, would set up a time schedule for implementation of the National Oral Health Policy. The preferable time schedule would be starting of the plan of action as soon as possible.

b. Oral Health would be made an integral part of the curriculum of multipurpose workers and other health auxiliaries as well as the Medical Doctors.

c. In order to implement the National Oral Health Policy, the Ministry should set up a National Training Care Center, which would be strengthened and augmented and would be charged with the responsibility of:

 • Preparation of teaching aids for all training programmes.
 • Preparation of pre and post evaluation training criteria and systems
 • Preparation of standardized oral health education programmes for education of the community; expecting mothers, small children under 6 years, 6–10 years, 10–16 years and above 16 years and the adult community and also development of teaching aids for the above mentioned programmes.
 • The center to be responsible for training at least 6 dentists from each state and two from each dental college in order to implement national oral health policy in a standardized and efficient manner.

- The center could also run reorientation and continuing education programmes for the dentists in government service and private sector (optional).

d. The Union Government should send the requisite information regarding the National Oral Health Policy to all the State Governments.

e. The Union Government should guide the State Governments about making those trained dentists responsible for training the various health auxiliaries and the medical doctors at the PHC's for the implementation of preventive package to the community. The dentists who are trained from the Dental colleges are to be made responsible for training the doctors and the other personnel in Medical/Dental colleges.

f. There should be a statutory warning on the wrappers of all sweets, chocolates and other retentive sugar eatables "Eating sweets leads to decay of the teeth".

g. Toothbrush and fluoride toothpaste and 10 mg sodium fluoride tablets are most essential components in prevention of dental caries and periodontal diseases (prevalence >90%). The government should take adequate steps to get at least one standardized tooth brush, one fluoride tooth paste and 10 mg sodium fluoride tablets manufactured by one of the Government of India's own company such as I.D.P.L. and remove all taxes on these three items so that these can be made available at very cheap rates to the whole of the Indian population (appropriate Ministry to be contacted).

h. Media like Television, Radio, etc. should be used to create awareness among the people about oral health. For this purpose, with the help of the Ministry of Mass Communication, two or three minute films can be projected on TV at peak hours and also clearly defined radio messages should be standardized at the centre identified by the government so that the right type of message, directed at specific goals, be conveyed.

i. There should be an oral health care chapter in school books of 3rd, 7th and 9th classes elaborating on the common dental diseases, their causes and stressing on the ways and means to prevent these by self help. Writing of these chapters would be the responsibility of the Centre identified, for inclusion of this material in text books - the Department of Education should be contacted.

j. Dental treatment should be made available to low income groups by rendering subsidized dental services and providing insurance to workers.

k. No sales tax or excise duty on equipment and materials for dentists setting up private practice in rural areas.

l. The cost of dental treatment should be brought down by reducing excise duty, customs duty and taxes and categorizing all dental instruments and materials under the category of 'Dentistry' (Ministry of Commerce and Finance).

m. Every primary health center should have the services of the dentists available for the community with efficient equipment. Gradually, each of these dentists should be provided with four dental hygienists in order to launch effective preventive measures in the community and for the supervision of the other health auxiliaries for this purpose.

n. There should be a regular posting of dental students in the rural areas and out of one year internship, six months should be spent in rural areas.

o. Since the responsibilities of the Union Government are quite a few towards the implementation of the National Oral Health Policy and also there is not even a single doctor in oral health presently employed in the Directorate of Health Services; therefore, it is high time that a post of Additional Director General Health Services (Oral

Health) be created in the Directorate of Health Services who should be responsible for looking after the oral health of the country.

p. Dental Advisory Committee under the Dental Advisor, Govt. of India.

Activities within the Responsibility of Ministry of Health within the State Governments

a. The State governments and union territories under the Direction of the Central Government would start serious implementation of the National Oral Health Policy within a stipulated time schedule and would adopt the National Oral Health Policy as a part of their health planning.

b. The State Governments would depute or especially employ 4 dentists for training in the dynamics of implementation and strategies of national oral health at the centre identified by the Union Government. They would also send 2 representatives from each dental college for such training.

c. The State Governments would make the 4–6 dentists from their States who have been trained, responsible to train the various health teams at PHCs in the implementation of National Oral Health Policy at the periphery, i.e. at the village level and also in various urban areas.

d. There would be reorientation programmes in each of the dental college towards the National Oral Health Policy to be conducted by the dentists trained from each dental college.

e. Each State Government would appoint within the next 5 years one dentist at each CHC and then at each primary health centre and if in any state dentists are already available at the PHCs, efforts would be made to equip them with efficient and sufficient equipment.

f. Each State Government would train more hygienists/dental technicians and dental auxiliaries and in a phased manner post 4 dental hygienists with each dentist.

g. Oral Health would become an integral part of the health package being implemented by the health team, i.e. medical doctors, health auxiliaries, multipurpose workers, etc.

h. Each State Government would get dental health education material published and printed and make it available for mass education at the level of Primary Health Center and the various dentists and other hospitals. The education material for samples would be provided to the States by the training centre.

i. The State Government would implement all the activities being listed under the Union Government such as inclusion of oral health care chapters in the text books of different grades of school children, etc., as would be applicable to the States from time to time.

B. Targets

The action plan of the National Oral Health Policy will have the following targets to be achieved within the stipulated period for a meaningful action plan.

a. Within one year, the Government of India would have appointed the required focal points within the Ministry of Health as recommended in detailed activities especially for oral health.

b. Within one year, the Union Government would have adopted the National Oral Health Policy as an integral part of the National Health Policy.

c. Within one year, the Government of India would have identified, augmented and supported a National Center for the various tasks assigned under the section of detailed activities for preparing of training manuals and teaching aids for the implementation of National Oral Health Policy. The training centres would start conducting the required training of dentists from various States within the 2nd year.

d. Within one year, each state of India will have adopted the National Oral Health Plan operation in their respective states.

e. Within 5 years, each state of India would have appointed one dentist in each Primary Health Center of their own state and would have equipped each clinic with efficient and sufficient equipment.

f. Within 3 years, all the Medical Health Teams working in all the Primary Health Centers of various states of India would have been trained by dentists in the delivery of the preventive care to the community.

g. These dentists varying in number between 4–6 depending upon size of the state would have already undergone training at the National Training Centre in implementation of strategies of National Oral Health.

h. Each state would appoint a programme officer responsible for organisation and supervision of oral health programmes within the second year of the action plan. The programme officer should preferably be at the level of Joint Director in the Directorate of Health in each state.

i. The Union Government would provide the initial speed and money for implementation of action plan of the National Oral Health Policy within their states.

j. Each State would provide the necessary funds for creating additional support or augmenting the existing oral services within their states.

k. The National Oral Health Policy would be fully operational in all the states and union territories of India within 5 years.

l. The Advisory Committee—under the Dental Advisor to the Ministry of Health and Family Welfare, Government of India would be entrusted with the task of directing the implementation of National Oral Health Policy, its monitoring, review, required changes and will supervise and guide the working of all the National Centres set up for Oral Health under the Ministry of Health, Government of India.

COST OF TECHNICAL IMPLEMENTATION

Identification and establishment of a National Centre to act as a focal point for the implementation of training manuals and standardized teaching aids for the implementation of National Oral Health Policy.

It will be preferable if the centre is identified in a dental college or institute which is involved in such activities, like research which can be identified with the help of ICMR. In such as case the centre would only need augmentation or strengthening and a lot of cost effectiveness can be achieved.

Development of the Health Infrastructure with the integration of Oral Health in the General Health, will strengthen the Institutional and Physical infrastructure of the country and will help build up the critical man of managerial, technical and scientific competence required to strengthen the socio-economic development as India goes with renewed health and strength into the 21st Century.

30

Dental Council of India and Dentist Act

The institution governing the growth and development of dental education and dental health in India, known as the Dental Council of India came into being on the 12th of April, 1949 after the Dentist Act was enforced on 29th March, 1948. This act was a real milestone in the history of dental profession in India.

Dentistry was an integral part of medical science. However, it was only in the early 19th century that medical education based on modern system of medicine was started by the East India Company, because their primary aim was to have some medical helpers for their doctors who were stationed in India. This way medical teaching was started in India. In 1920, course of dentistry was introduced for the first time at Calcutta. The first full fledged autonomous dental college was founded at Calcutta by the late Dr. Rafuddin Ahmed—rightly known as the father of Dental Education in India. The college was started with a one year diploma course (L.D.Sc) and in 1922, the duration of the course was raised to two years. In 1923, another dental college, the Punjab Dental College was started in Lahore by Dr. Satya Pal. In 1926, American Dental College was started in Karachi by Dr. M. K. Patel. In 1928, another dental institution under the name of Andhra Dental College and Hospital was founded at Bezwada by Dr. H. M. Rao and in 1933, the college was renamed as American Dental College and Hospital, Madras. In 1932, City Dental College and Hospital, was started at Calcutta and upto 1940, 114 graduates were granted the degree of L.D. Sc. Admission requirements in that year was 'matriculate'. In 1933, Bai Yamunabai L. Nair Hospital Dental College was started with one year course for medical licentiates and two year course for matriculates. The diploma awarded was L. D.Sc. In 1946, the college was taken over by the Bombay Municipal Corporation. Dr. V.M. Desai was the first dean.

In 1933, Dr. Montmorency Dental College and Hospital was inaugurated at Lahore with Dr. V.S. Malik and Dr. M.L. Watts at the helm of affairs. This was also one of the pioneer institutions which awarded the MDS degree. Dr. K.L. Shourie was the first to be awarded MDS degree after doing research on caries. Another private dental college started functioning at Bombay in around 1938. Dr. A.M. Malaowalla was the first to qualify the 4 year BDS degree awarded by the Bombay University. Same college was later taken over by the government with the name Govt. Dental College, Bombay.

With the establishment of many dental institutions, the Govt. of India appointed a committee "Health Surgery and Development Committee" under the chairmanship of Sir Joseph Bhore, to make a broad survey of the existing system as regard to health and make recommendations for further development of health education and profession. Earlier than that two dental journals, namely Indian Dental Journal was founded in 1925 by Dr. R. Ahmed and the Indian Dental Review was started in 1927 by Dr. M. K. Patel. The West Bengal Government, in 1934, appointed a committee called the Dental Education and Registration enquiry committee which recommended a standard curriculum and enactment of Dentists Act.

Dr. S.K. Majumdar was the pioneer in starting the All India Dental Association. He founded the All India Dental Association in 1946 with its headquarters in New Delhi. Dr. R. Ahmed was elected its first president and Dr. N. N. Bery was the General Secretary. Dr. Bery on behalf of the Indian Dental Association presented the draft to the Government which was ultimately shaped into the Dentist Act.

In the meantime Bhore's Committee Report was also tabulated. The dental section of the committee consisted of C.D. Marshall Bay, Dr. R. Ahmed and Dr. V.M. Desai. The Bhore Committee, concluded and recommended as follows:

a. Dentistry is a neglected subject in almost all Indian Universities.

b. Post graduate training in Dentistry doesn't exist.

c. Extreme shortage of qualified dental surgeons.

d. Profession of dentistry is unorganized and no legal provisions exist for its regulations.

e. Dental surgeons be employed in state's own dental hospitals.

f. Three types of dental personnels should exist:
   i. Dental Surgeon
   ii. Dental Hygienist
   iii. Dental Mechanic

g. 25 new dental colleges should be established with 100 admissions in each institution.

h. The education of dentistry should be uniform and standardized.

i. Master of Dental Surgery (MDS) should be started.

j. Dental wing should be attached with every medical college and the dispensaries at the state/district levels.

k. State and national dental councils be created and the legislation should be enacted for the dental profession.

THE DENTIST ACT 1948

The Dentist Act made provisions for the regulation of the profession of dentistry and for that purpose to constitute Dental Councils. The bill for its regulation was referred to the Select Committee, consisting of eminent personalities like Raj Kumari Amrit Kaur, M.L. Chattopadhya, Deshbandhu Gupta and seven more. The committee submitted its report on 28th January 1948 and was placed before the constituent assembly on 25th February, 1948. The bill was debated thoroughly, with the then union health minister, Raj Kumari Amrit Kaur advocating for its favour. Later it was passed on 26th February, 1948 and received the president's consent on 27th March, 1948.

For the purpose of regulating the standards of dental education in the country, the Dentist Act, 1948, empowered the Dental Council of India to:

1. Inspect any dental institution imparting dental courses, such as BDS, MDS, Dental Mechanic and Dental Hygienist courses. The powers to appoint inspectors for this purpose are vested in the executive committee of the council.

2. It can recommend the recognition and derecognition of the various dental institutions to the government.

3. To lay down regulations in curriculum for the various courses in dentistry such as BDS and MDS, to ensure uniformity and maintain standards of dental education in the country.

4. To lay down code of ethics for dental surgeons in their professional behaviour.

5. The council is entrusted with the task of maintaining an All India Dentists Register.

For the first five years, the act provided that the president of the council would be nominated by the central government. Accordingly, Dr. K.C.K.E. Raja, the then Director General of Health Services was the first to be nominated. Dr. Lt. Col., C.K.Lakshmanan who succeeded Dr. Raja was then nominated as the president of the council. Dr. R. Ahmed was the first elected president of the council who was elected on 5th November, 1954. The President and secretary of the Dental Council of India for the last decade are tabulated as follows:

President	Dr. R.K. Bali	17.01.98 to 03.10.2004
	Dr. Anil Kohli	25.10.04 to till date
Secretary	Sh. A. L. Miglani	25.02.94 to 30.04.02
	Sh. S.S. Arora	01.02.02 to 13.04.07
	Maj. Gen. (Retd)	
	P.N. Awasthi	14.11.0 to till date

The Dentist Act, 1948 was enacted as follows:

Introductory

1. 1. This Act may be called the Dentists Act, 1948.
   2. It extends to the whole of India except for the state of Jammu and Kashmir omitted by act 42 of 1972.
2. In this Act, unless there is anything repugnant in the subject or context:
   a. "the Council" means the Dental Council of India constituted under section 3;
   b. "dental hygienist" means a person not being a dentist or a medical practitioner, who scales, cleans or polishes teeth, or gives instruction in dental hygiene;
   c. "dental mechanic" means a person who makes or repairs denture and dental appliances;
   d. "dentistry" includes:
      i. the performances of any operation on, and the treatment on any disease, deficiency or lesion of, human teeth or jaws, and the performance of radiographic work in connection with human teeth or jaws or the oral cavity; under anaesthesia.
      ii. the mechanical construction or the renewal of artificial dentures or restorative dental appliances;
      iii. the performance of any operation on, or the giving of any treatment, device or attendance to, for the purpose of, or in connection with, the fitting, inserting, fixing, constructing, repairing or renewing of artificial dentures or restorative dental appliances, as is usually performed or given by dentists;
   e. "dentist" means a person who practises dentistry;
   f. "medical practitioner" means a person who holds a qualification granted by an authority specified or notified under section 3 of the Indian Medical Degrees Act, 1916, or specified in the Schedules to the Indian Medical Council Act, 1956 or specified in any other law for the time being in force in any State, or who practises any system of medicine and is registered or is entitled to be registered in any State medical register by whatever name called;
   g. "prescribed" means prescribed by rules or regulations made under this Act;
   h. "State Council" means a State Dental Council constituted under section 21, and includes a Joint State Council constituted in accordance with an agreement under section 22;
   i. "register" means a register maintained under this Act;
   j. "recognized dental qualification" means any of the qualifications included in the Schedule;
   k. "recognized dental hygiene qualification" means a qualification recognized by the Council under section 11;
   l. "registered dentists", "registered dental hygienist" and "registered dental mechanic" shall mean, respectively, a person whose name is for the time being registered in a register of dentists, a register of dental hygienists and a register of dental mechanics.
   [2A. Any reference in this Act to a law which is not in force in the State of Jammu and Kashmir shall, in relation

to the State, be construed as a reference to the corresponding law, if any, in force in that State.]

3. The Central Government shall, as soon as may be, constitute a Council consisting of the following members, namely:

   a. One registered dentist possessing a recognized dental qualification elected by the dentists registered in Part A of each state register;

   b. One member elected from amongst themselves by the members of the Medical Council of India;

   c. Not more than four members elected from among themselves, by:

      i. Principals, Deans, Directors and Vice-Principals of dental colleges in the States training students for recognized dental qualifications:
      Provided that not more than one member shall be elected from the same dental college;

      ii. Heads of dental wings of medical colleges in the States training students for recognized dental qualifications;

   d. One member from each University established by law in the States which grants a recognized dental qualification, to be elected by the members of the Senate of the University, or in case the University has no Senate, by the members of the court, from amongst the members of the Dental Faculty of the University or in case the University has no Dental Faculty, from amongst the members of the Medical Faculty thereof;

   e. One member to represent each State, nominated by the Government of each such State from among persons registered either in a medical register or a dental register of the State—In this clause, "State" does not include a Union territory;

   f. Six members nominated by the Central Government, of whom at least one shall be a registered dentist possessing a recognized dental qualification and practising or holding an appointment in an institution for the training of dentists in a Union territory, and at least two shall be dentists registered in Part B of a State register;

   g. The Director General of Health Services, ex Officio; Provided that pending the preparation of registers the State Governments may nominate to the first Council members referred to in parts (a) and (e) and the Central Government members referred to in part (f) out of persons who are eligible for registration in the respective registers and such persons shall hold office for such period as the State or Central Government may, by notification in the Official Gazette, specify.

4. The Council shall be a body corporate by the name of the Dental Council of India, having perpetual succession and a common seal, with power to acquire and hold property, both movable and immovable, and shall by the said name sue and be sued.

5. Elections under this Chapter shall be conducted in the prescribed manner, and where any dispute arises regarding any such election, it shall be referred to the Central Government whose decision shall be final.

6. 1. Subject to the provisions of this section an elected or nominated member shall hold office for a term of five years from the date of his election or nomination or until his successor has been duly elected or nominated, whichever is longer: Provided that a member nominated under clause (e) or clause (f) of section 3, shall hold office during the pleasure of the authority nominating him.

2. An elected or nominated member may at any time resign his membership by writing under his hand addressed to the President, and the seat of such member shall thereupon become vacant.

3. An elected or nominated member shall be deemed to have vacated his seat if he is absent without excuse, sufficient in the opinion of the Council, from three consecutive ordinary meetings of the Council or, in the case of a member whose name is required to be included in a State register, if his name is removed from such register, or if he has been elected under clause (c) of section 3, if he ceases to hold his appointment as the Principal, Dean, Director or Vice-Principal of a dental college, or as the Head of the dental wing of a medical college, or if he has been elected under clause (b) or (d) of section 3, if he ceases to be a member of the Medical Council of India or the Dental or Medical Faculty of the University, as the case may be.

4. A casual vacancy in the Council shall be filled by fresh election or nomination, as the case may be, and the person elected or nominated to fill the vacancy shall hold office only for the remainder of the term for which the member whose place he takes was elected or nominated.

5. Members of the council shall be eligible for re-election or re-nomination.

6. No act done by the Council shall be called in question on the ground merely of the existence of any vacancy in, or defect in the constitution of, the Council.

7. 1. The President and Vice-President of the Council and until the President is elected, a members thereof among themselves: Provided that on the first constitution of the Council and until the President is elected by the member of the Council nominated by the Central Government in this behalf shall discharge the functions of the President: Provided further that for five years from the first constitution of the Council, the President shall, if the Central Government so decides, be a person nominated by the Central Government who shall hold office during the pleasure of the Central Government, and where he is not already a member, shall be a member of the Council in addition to the members referred to in section 3.

2. An elected President or Vice-President shall hold office as such for a term not exceeding five years and not extending beyond the expiry of his term as member of the Council, but subject to his being a member of the Council, he shall be eligible for re-election.

8. 1. The Council shall:
   a. Appoint a Secretary who may also, if so decided by the Council, act as Treasurer;
   b. Appoint such other officers and servants as the Council deems necessary to enable it to carry out its functions under this Act;
   c. Require and take from the Secretary or from any other officer or servant such security for the due performance of his duties as the Council considers necessary; and
   d. With the previous sanction of the Central Government, fix the fees and allowances of the President, Vice-President and other members of the Council, and the pay and allowances and other conditions of service of officers and servants of the Council.

2. Notwithstanding anything contained in clause (a) of sub-section (1), for the

first four years from the first consti-tution of the Council, the Secretary of the Council shall be a person appoin-ted by the Central Government, who shall hold office during the pleasure of the Central Government.

9. 1. The Council shall constitute from among its members an Executive Committee, and may so constitute other Committees for such general or special purposes as the Council consi-ders necessary for carrying out its functions under this Act.

2. The Executive Committee shall consist of the President and Vice-President ex officio and the Director-General of Health Services ex officio, and five other members elected by the Council.

3. The President and Vice-President of the Council shall be Chairman and Vice-Chairman, respectively, of the Executive Committee.

4. A member of the Executive Committee shall hold office as such until the expiry of his term of office as member of the Council but, subject to his being a member of the Council, he shall be eligible for re-election.

5. In addition to the powers and duties conferred and imposed on it by this Act, the Executive Committee shall exercise and discharge such powers and duties as may be prescribed.

10. 1. The dental qualifications; granted by any authority or institution in India, which are included in Part I of the Schedule shall be recognized dental qualifications for the purposes of this Act.

2. Any authority or institution in India which grants a dental qualification not included in part I of the schedule may apply to the Central Government to have such qualification recognized and included in that Part, and the Central Government, after consulting the Council, and after such inquiry, if any, as it may think fit for the purpose, may, by notification in the Official Gazette, amend part I of the schedule so as to include such qualification there in, and any such notification may also direct that an entry shall be made in Part I of the Schedule against such dental qualification declaring that it shall be a recognized dental qualification only when granted after a specified date.

3. a. The dental qualifications, granted by any authority or institution outside India, which are included in Part II of the Schedule shall be recognized dental qualifications only for the purposes of the regis-tration of citizens of India when the register is first prepared under this Act.

b. Where any dental qualification granted by any authority or institu-tion outside India, and held by a citizen of India, is recognized for the purposes of the register when it is first prepared, after the commence-ment of the Dentists (Amendment) Act, 1972, the Central Government may, after consultation with the Council, by notification in the Official Gazette, amend Part II of the Schedule so as to include therein the dental qualification so recognized.

4. a. The dental qualifications granted by any authority or institution outside India, which are included in Part III of the Schedule, shall be recognized dental qualifications for the pur-poses of this Act, but no person possessing any such qualification shall be entitled for registration unless he is a citizen of India.

b. Where any dental qualification granted by any authority or insti-tution outside India, and held by a citizen of India, is recognized, except on reciprocal basis, after the commencement of the Dentists (Amendment) Act, 1972, the Central Government may, after consultation with the Council, by notification in the Official Gazette, amend Part III of the Schedule so as to include therein the dental qualification so recognized.

5. The Council may enter into negotiations with any authority or institution in any State or country outside India which, by law of any such State or country, is entrusted with the maintenance of a register of dentists, for the setting of a scheme of reciprocity for the recognition of dental qualifications and in persuance of any such scheme, the Central Government may, by notification in the Official Gazette, declare that any such qualification granted by any authority or institution in any such State or country, or such qualification, only when granted after a specified date, shall be a recognized dental qualification for the purpose of this Act, and any such notification may provide for an amendment of the Schedule and may also direct that any such dental qualification as is specified in the notification shall be entered in the Schedule as so amended.

6. The Central Government may, after consultation with the Council, by notification in the Official Gazette, amend the Schedule by directing that an entry be made therein in respect of any dental qualification declaring that it shall be a recognized dental qualification only when granted before a specified date].

11. Any authority in a State which grants a qualification for dental hygienists may apply to the Council to have such qualification recognized, and the Council may, after such inquiry, if any, as it thinks fit, and after consulting the Government and the State Council of State in which the authority making the application is situated, declare that such qualification, or such qualification only when granted after a specified date, shall be a recognized dental hygiene qualification for the purposes of this Act.

12. The Council may prescribe the period and nature of an apprenticeship or training which shall be undergone and the other conditions which shall be satisfied by a person before he is entitled to be registered under this Act as a dental mechanic.

13. Notwithstanding anything contained in any other law, but subject to the provisions of this Act,

a. Any recognized dental or dental hygiene qualification shall be a sufficient qualification for enrolment in the appropriate register of any State;

b. No person shall, after the first registers are compiled under this Act, be entitled to be enrolled in any register as a dentist or dental hygienist unless he holds a recognized dental or dental hygiene qualification or as a dental mechanic unless he has undergone training which satisfies the prescribed requirements referred to in section 12.

14. Every authority in a State which grants any recognized dental or dental hygiene qualifications shall furnish such information as the Council may from time to time require as to courses of study and training and examinations to be undergone in order to obtain such qualification, as to the ages at which such courses of study and examinations are required to be undergone, and generally as to the requisites for obtaining such qualification.

15. 1. The Executive Committee may, subject to regulations, if any, made by the Council appoint] such number of Inspectors as it deems necessary to attend at any examinations held by authorities in the States which grant recognized dental or dental hygiene qualifications and to inspect any institution recognized as a training institution.

    2. Inspectors appointed under this section shall not interfere with the course of any examination but they shall report to the Executive Committee on the sufficiency of every examination at which they attend and of the courses of study and training at every institution which they inspect, and on any other matters with regard to which the Executive Committee may require them to report.

    3. The Executive Committee shall forward a copy of such report to the authority or institution concerned and shall also forward copies with remarks, if any, of the authority or institution concerned thereon to the Central Government and to the Government of the State in which the authority or institution is situated.

15A.1. The Council may appoint such number of Visitors as it may deem necessary to attend at any examination held by any authority or institution in a State which grants recognized dental qualification and to inspect any institution training students for recognized dental qualifications.

    2. Any person, whether he is a member of the Council or not, may be appointed as a Visitor under this section, but a person who is appointed as an Inspector under section 15 for any inspection or examination shall not be appointed as a Visitor for the same inspection or examination.

3. The Visitor shall not interfere with the course of any examination but shall report to the President of the Council on the sufficiency of every examination at which he attends and of the courses of study and training at every institution which he inspects, and on the adequacy of the standards of dental education including staff, equipment, accommodation and other facilities prescribed for giving dental education, and on any other matters with regard to which the Council may require him to report.

4. The report of a visitor shall be treated as confidential unless in any particular case the President of the Council otherwise directs: provided that if the Central Government requires a copy of the report of a visitor, the Council shall furnish the same.

16. 1. When upon report by the Executive Committee it appears to the Council:

    a. That the courses of study and training or the examinations to be undergone in order to obtain a recognized dental hygiene qualification from any authority in a State, or the conditions for admission to such courses or the standards of proficiency required from the candidates at such examinations are not in conformity with regulations made under this Act or fall short of the standards required thereby, or

    b. That an institution does not satisfy the requirements of the Council, the Council may send to the Government of the State in which authority or institution is situated a statement to such effect, and the State Government shall forward it, along with such remarks as it may think fit, to the authority or institution concerned with an intimation of the period within which the authority or institution may submit its explanation to the State Government.

2. On receipt of explanation, or where no explanation is submitted within the period fixed, then on the expiry of the period, the State Government shall after consulting the State Council, forward its recommendations and those of the State Council, if any, to the Council.

3. The Council, after considering the recommendations of the State Government and the State Council and after such further inquiry, if any, as it may think fit to make, may declare that the qualification granted by the authority or institution shall be a recognized dental hygiene qualification only when granted before a specified date.

4. The Council may declare that any recognized dental hygiene qualification granted outside the States shall be recognized as such only if granted before a specified date.

16A.1. When, upon report by the Executive Committee or the visitor, it appears to the Council:

   a. That the courses of study and training or the examination to be undergone in order to obtain a recognized dental qualification from any authority or institution in a state, or the conditions for admission to such courses or the standards of proficiency required from the candidates at such examinations are not in conformity with the regulations made under this Act or fall short of the standards required thereby, or

   b. That an institution does not, in the matter of staff, equipment, accommodation, training and other facilities, satisfy the requirements of the

Council, the Council shall send a statement to that effect to the Central Government.

2. After considering such a statement, the Central Government may send it to the Government of the State in which the authority exercises power or the institution is situated, and the State Government shall forward it, along with such remarks as it may think fit to make, to the authority or institution concerned, with an intimation of the period within which the authority or institution may submit its explanation to the State Government.

3. After considering the explanation, or where no explanation is submitted within the period fixed, then, on the expiry of that period, the State Government shall make its recommendations to the Central Government.

4. The Central Government may, after considering the recommendations of the State Government and after making such further inquiry, if any, as it may think fit, by notification in the Official Gazette, direct that an entry shall be made in Part I of the Schedule against the qualification granted by the authority or institution declaring that it shall be a recognized dental qualification only when granted before a specified date or that the said recognized dental qualification if granted to students of a specified college or institution affiliated to any university shall be a recognized dental qualification only when granted before a specified date or, as the case may be, that the said recognized dental qualification shall be a recognized dental qualification in relation to a specified college or institution affiliated to any university only when granted after a specified date.

17. All declarations under section 11 or section 16 shall be made by a resolution passed at a meeting of the Council and shall forthwith be punished in the Official Gazette.

17A.1. The Council may prescribe standards of professional conduct and etiquette or the code of ethics for dentists.

2. Regulations made by the Council under sub-section (1) may specify which violations thereof shall constitute infamous conduct in any professional respect, that is to say, professional misconduct, and such provision shall have effect notwithstanding anything to the contrary contained in any other law for the time being in force.

18. 1. The Council shall maintain a register of dentists to be known as the Indian Dentists Register and consisting of the entries in all the State registers of dentists.

2. Each State Council shall supply to the Council twenty printed copies of the State register as soon as may be after the 1st day of April of each year, and each Registrar shall inform the Council without delay of all additions to and other amendments in the State register.

19. 1. The Council shall furnish copies of its minutes and of the minutes of the Executive Committee and an annual report of its activities together with an abstract of its accounts to the Central Government.

2. The Central Government may publish in such manner as it thinks fit any report, copy or abstract furnished to it under this section.

20. 1. The council may, with the approval of the Central Government, by notification in the Official Gazette, make regulations not inconsistent with the provisions of this Act to carry out the purposes of this chapter.

2. In particular and without prejudice to the generality of the foregoing power such regulations may:

a. Provide for the management of the property of the Council;

b. Prescribe the manner in which elections under the chapter shall be conducted;

c. Provide for summoning and holding of meetings of the Council and the Executive Committee, the times and places at which such meetings shall be held, the conduct of business threat and the number of members necessary to constitute a quorum;

d. Prescribe the functions of the Executive Committee;

e. Prescribe the powers and duties of the President and Vice-President;

f. Prescribe the tenure of office and the powers and duties of the Secretary and other officers and servants of the Council, and Inspectors, and Visitors appointed by the Council;

g. Prescribe the standard curricula for the training of dentists and dental hygienists, and the conditions for admission to courses of such training;

h. Prescribe the standards of examinations and other requirements to be satisfied to secure for qualifications recognition under this Act;

i. Any other matter which is to be or may be prescribed under this Act: Provided that regulations under clauses (g) and (h) shall be made after consultation with State Governments.

3. To enable the Council to be first constituted, the Central Government may make regulations for the conduct of the elections to the Council, any regulation so made may be altered or rescinded by the Council in exercise of its powers under this section.

4. Every regulation made under this section shall be laid, as soon as may be after it is made, before each House of Parliament, while it is in session, for a total period of thirty days which may be comprised in one session or in two or more successive sessions, and if, before the expiry of the session immediately following the session or the successive sessions aforesaid, both Houses agree in making any modifications in the regulation or both Houses agree that the regulations should not be made, the regulation shall thereafter have effect only in such modified form or be of no effect, as the case may be; so, however, that any such modification or annulment shall be without prejudice to the validity of anything previously done under that regulation.

State Dental Councils

21. Except where a Joint State Council is constituted in accordance with an agreement made under section 22, the State Government shall constitute a State Council consisting of the following members, namely :

   a. Four members elected from among themselves by dentists registered in Part A of the State register;

   b. Four members elected from among themselves by dentists registered in Part B of the State register;

   c. The heads of dental colleges, if any, in the State which train students for any of the recognized dental qualifications included in Part I of the Schedule, ex officio;

   d. One member elected from amongst themselves by the members of the Medical Council or the Council of Medical Registration of the State, as the case may be:

   e. Three members nominated by the State Government; and

   f. The Chief Medical Officer of the State, by whatever name called, ex officio: Provided that in the State of Saurashtra, as it existed before the 1st November, 1956, the State Dental Council constituted under Saurashtra Ordinance 25 of 1948, as amended by Saurashtra Ordinance 40 of 1949, shall be deemed to be the State Council constituted under this Act.

22. 1. Two or more State Governments may enter into an agreement to be in force for such period and to be subject to renewal for such further periods, if any, as may be specified in the agreement, to provide:

   a. for the constitution of a Joint State Council for all the participating States, or

   b. for the State Council of one State to serve the needs of the other participating States.

   2. In addition to such matters as are in this Act specified, an agreement under this section may:

   a. provide for the apportionment between the participating States of the expenditure in connection with the State Council or Joint State Council;

   b. determining which of the participating State Governments shall exercise the several functions of the State Government under this Act, and the references in this Act to the State Government shall be construed accordingly;

   c. provide for consultation between the participating State Governments either generally or with reference to particular matters arising under this Act;

   d. make such incidental and ancillary provisions, not inconsistent with this Act, as may be deemed necessary for expedient for giving effect to the agreement;

3. An agreement under this section shall be published in the Official Gazettes of the participating States.

23. A Joint State Council shall consist of the following members, namely:

    a. two members elected from among themselves by dentists registered in part A of the register of each of the participating States;

    b. two members elected from among themselves by dentists registered in part B of the register of each of the participating States;

    c. the heads of dental colleges, if any, in all the participating States which train students for any of the recognized dental qualifications included in Part I of the Schedule, ex officio;

    d. one member elected by the Medical Council or the Council of Medical Registration, of each participating State as the case may be;

    e. two members nominated by each participating State Government;

    f. the Chief Medical Officer of each participating State, by whatever name called, ex officio;

24. Every State Council shall be a body corporate by such name as may be notified by the State Government in the Official Gazette or, in the case of a Joint State Council, as may be determined in the agreement, having perpetual succession and a common seal with power to acquire and hold property, both movable and immovable, and shall by the said name sue and be sued.

25. 1. The President and Vice-President of the State Council shall be elected by the members from among themselves: Provided that for five years from the first constitution of the State Council, the President shall, if the State Government so decides, be a person nominated by the State Government who shall hold office during the pleasure of the State Government, and where he is not already a member, shall be a member of the State Council in addition to the members referred to in section 21 or 23, as the case may be.

    2. The President or Vice-President shall hold office as such for a term not exceeding five years and not extending beyond the expiry of his term as a member of the State Council, but subject to his being a member of the State Council, he shall be eligible for re-election.

26. Elections under this Chapter shall be conducted in the prescribed manner, and where any dispute arises regarding any such election, it shall be referred to the State Government whose decision shall be final.

27. 1. Subject to the provisions of this section, an elected or nominated member shall hold office for a term of five years from the date of his election or nomination or until his successor has been duly elected or nominated, whichever is longer: Provided that a member nominated under clause (e) of section 21 or clause (e) of section 23, shall hold office during the pleasure of the authority nominating him.

    2. An elected or nominated member may at any time resign his membership by writing under his hand addressed to the President, and the seat of such member shall thereupon become vacant.

    3. An elected or nominated member shall be deemed to have vacated his seat

       a. if he is absent without excuse, sufficient in the opinion of the State Council, from three consecutive ordinary meetings of the State Council, or

b. in the case of a member whose name is required to be included in any State register, if his name is removed from the register, or

c. where he has been elected under clause (d) of section 21 or under clause (d) of section 23, if he ceases to be a member of the Medical Council or the Council of Medical Registration of the State as the case maybe.

4. A casual vacancy in the State Council shall be filled by fresh election or nomination, as the case may be, and the person elected or nominated to fill the vacancy shall hold office only for the remainder of the term for which the member whose place he takes was elected or nominated.

5. Members of the State Council shall be eligible for re-election or re-nomination.

6. No act done by the State Council shall be called in question on the ground merely of the existence of any vacancy in, or defect in the constitution of, the State Council.

28. 1. The State Council may, with the previous sanction of the State Government,
   a. appoint a Registrar, who shall also act as Secretary and if so decided by the State Council also as its Treasurer;
   b. appoint such other officers and servants as may be required to enable the State Council to carry out its functions under this Act;
   c. require and take from the Registrar or from any other officer or servant such security for the due performance of his duties as the State Council considers necessary;
   d. fix the salaries and allowances and other conditions of service of the

Registrar and other officers and servants of the State Council;
   e. fix the rate of allowances payable to members of the State Council;

2. Notwithstanding anything contained in clause (a) of sub-section (1), for the first four years from the first constitution of the State Council, the Registrar of the State Council shall be a person appointed by the State Government, who shall hold offices during the pleasure of the State Government.

29. 1. The State Council shall constitute from among its members an Executive Committee consisting of the President and Vice-President ex officio and the Chief Medial Officer of the State or the States concerned, by whatever name called, ex officio and such number of other members elected by the State Council as may be prescribed.

2. The President and Vice-President of the State Council shall be Chairman and Vice-Chairman, respectively, of the Executive Committee.

3. A member of the Executive Committee shall hold office as such until the expiry of his term of office as member of the State Council, but subject to his being a member of the State Council, he shall be eligible for re-election.

4. The Executive Committee shall exercise and discharge such powers and duties as may be prescribed.

30. 1. The State Council shall furnish such reports, copies of its minutes and of the minutes of the Executive Committee, and abstracts of its accounts to the State Government as the State Government may from time to time require and shall forward copies of all material so furnished to the State Government to the Council.

2. The State Government may publish in such manner as it thinks fit any report,

copy or abstract furnished to it under this section.

Registration

31.
1. The State Government shall as soon as maybe cause to be prepared in the manner hereinafter provided a register of dentists for the State.
2. The State Council shall upon its constitution assume the duty of maintaining the register in accordance with the provisions of this Act.
3. The register of dentists shall be maintained in two Parts, A and B, persons possessing recognized dental qualifications being registered in Part A and person not possessing such qualifications being registered in Part B.
4. The register shall include the following particulars, namely:
    a. The full name, nationality and residential address of the registered person;
    b. the date of his first admission to the register;
    c. his qualification for registration, and the date on which he obtained his degree or diploma in dentistry, if any, and the authority which conferred it;
    d. his professional address; and
    e. such further particulars as may be prescribed.

32.
1. For the purpose of first preparing the register of dentists, the State Government shall, by notification in the Official Gazette, constitute a Registration Tribunal consisting of three persons and shall also appoint a Registrar who shall act as Secretary of the Tribunal.
2. The State Government shall, by the same or a like notification, appoint a date on or before which application for registration, which shall be accompanied by the prescribed fee, shall be made to the Registration Tribunal.
3. The Registration Tribunal shall examine every application received on or before the appointed date, and if it satisfied that the applicant is qualified for registration under section 33, shall direct the entry of the name of the applicant on the register.
4. The register so prepared shall thereafter be published in such manner as the State Government may direct, and any person aggrieved by a decision of the Registration Tribunal expressed or implied in the register as so published may, within thirty days from the date of such publication, appeal to an authority appointed by State Government in this behalf by notification in the Official Gazette.
5. The Registrar shall amend the register in accordance with the decisions of the authority appointed under sub-section (4) and shall thereupon issue to every person whose name is entered on the register a certificate of registration in the prescribed form.
6. Upon the constitution of the State Council, the register shall be given into its custody, and the State Government may direct that all or any specified part of the application fees for registration in the first register shall be paid to the credit of the State Council.

33.
1. A person shall be entitled on payment of the prescribed fee to have his name entered on the register when it is first prepared, if he resides or carries on the profession of dentistry in the State and if he:
    a. holds a recognized dental qualification, or
    b. does not hold such a qualification but, being a citizen of India has been

engaged in practice as a dentist as his principal means of livelihood for a period of not less than five years prior to the date appointed under sub-section (2) of section 32:

Provided that no person other than a citizen of India shall be entitled to registration by virtue of a qualification

a. specified in Part I of the Schedule unless by the law and practice of\the State or country to which such person belongs persons of Indian origin holding dental qualifications registrable in that State or country are permitted to enter and practise the profession of dentistry in such State or country, or

b. recognized, in pursuance of a scheme of reciprocity, under sub-section (5) of section 10

Provided further that a person shall be entitled to registration by virtue of a qualification specified in Part II of the Schedule only if he is a citizen of India: Provided further that for the purpose of the first preparation of the register of dentists under this Act, a person shall be entitled to have this name entered in the appropriate part of the register without payment of any registration fee,

a. in the State of Saurashtra, as it existed before the 1st November, 1956, if he is registered on the register of dental practitioners maintained under Saurashtra Ordinance No. 25 of 1948, as amended by Saurashtra Ordinance No. 40 of 1949; or

b. in the State of Travancore-Cochin as it existed before the 1st November, 1956, if he is registered on the register of dental practitioners maintained under the Travancore Medical Practitioners Act, 1119 or

c. in the State of Jammu and Kashmir, if he is registered on the register of dental practitioners maintained under the Jammu and Kashmir Dentists Act, 1958.

2. A person domiciled in a state shall be entitled on payment of the prescribed fee to temporary registration as a dentist for a period of five years, if he has been engaged in practice as a dentist as his principal means of livelihood for a period of not less than two years during the five years prior to the date appointed under sub-section (2) of section 32, and a person so registered shall be entitled to permanent registration if for a period of five years from the date of his temporary registration he has been engaged in practice as a dentist.

34. 1. After the date appointed under sub-section (2) of section 32 a person shall, on payment of the prescribed fee, be entitled to have his name entered on the register of dentists, if he resides or carries on the profession of dentistry in the state and if he

   i. holds a recognized dental qualification, or

   ii. does not hold such a qualification but, being a citizen of India, has been engaged in practice as a dentist as his principal means of livelihood for a period of not less than two years before the date appointed under sub-section (2) of section 32 and has passed, within a period of ten years after the said date, an examination recognized for this purpose by the Central Government:

Provided that no person other than a citizen of India shall be entitled to registration by virtue of a qualification

a. specified in Part I of the Schedule unless by the law and practice of the state or country to which such person belongs persons of Indian origin holding dental qualifications registrable in that state or country are permitted to enter and practice the profession of dentistry in such state or country, or

b. recognized, in pursuance of a scheme of reciprocity, under sub-section (5) of section 10;

Provided further that a person registered in Part B of the register shall be entitled to be registered in Part A thereof, if within a period of ten years after the date of his registration in Part B he passes an examination recognized for the purpose by the Central Government.

2. Notwithstanding anything contained in sub-section (1)

a. A State Council may during the period of two years immediately after the commencement of the Dentists (Amendment) Act, 1955, permit for sufficient reasons the registration in the State register of any displaced person who does not hold a recognized dental qualification but has been actually practising the profession of dentistry as his principal means of livelihood from a date prior to the 29th day of March, 1948. Explanation—In this clause "displaced person" means any person who, on account of the setting up of the Dominions of India and Pakistan or on account of civil disturbances or fear of such disturbances in any area now forming part of Pakistan has, after the 1st day of March, 1947, left or been displaced from, his place of residence in such area and who has since then been residing in India;

aa. the State Council may, during the period of two years immediately

after the commencement of the Dentists (Amendment) Act, 1972, permit, for sufficient reasons, the registration in the State register of any displaced person or a repatriate who does not hold any recognized dental qualification but has been actually practising the profession of dentistry as his principal means of livelihood from a date prior to the 29th day of March, 1948.

Explanation-In this clause,

i. "displaced person" means any person who, on account of civil disturbances or fear of such disturbances in any area now forming part of Bangladesh, has, after the 14th day of April, 1957 but before the 25th day of March, 1971, left, or has been displaced form, his place of residence in such area and who has since then been residing in India;

ii. "repatriate" means any person who, on account of civil disturbances or fear of such disturbances in any area now forming part of Burma or Ceylon, has, after the 14th day of April, 1957, left or has been displaced from, his place of residence in such area and who has since then been residing in India;

b. A person other than a citizen of India, holding a reputable dental qualification and employed for teaching or research in a dental institution situated in any of the states may be permitted temporary registration in the state register of dentists for the period of his employment or for a period of five years, whichever is shorter:

Provided that he does not practice the profession of dentistry for personal gain and his application for registration is approved by the President of the Council.

35. 1. After the date appointed for the receipt of applications for registration in the first register of dentists, all applications for registration shall be addressed to the Registrar of the State Council and shall be accompanied by the prescribed fee.

2. If upon such application, the Registrar is of opinion that the applicant is entitled to have his name entered on the register, he shall enter thereon the name of the applicant: Provided that no person, whose name has under the provisions of this Act been removed from the register of any state, shall be entitled to have his name entered on the register except with the approval of the State Council from whose register his name was removed.

3. Any person whose application for registration is rejected by the Registrar may, within three months from the date of such rejection, appeal to the State Council, and the decision of the State Council thereon shall be final.

4. Upon entry in the register of a name under this section, the Registrar shall issue a certificate of registration in the prescribed form.

35A.1. Notwithstanding anything contained in this chapter, the Registrar may, by order in writing, amend the register by deleting therefrom the name of any person who by reason of the formation of the State of Andhra, has ceased to reside or carry on the business or profession of dentistry in the State of Madras:Provided that the Registrar shall, before passing an order, make such inquiry as he deems necessary.

2. Any person aggrieved by an order under sub-section (1) may appeal to such authority and within such time, as may be specified in this behalf by the State Government of Madras; and such authority shall pass such order on the appeal as it thinks fit.

3. An order of the Registrar under sub-section (1), or where an appeal has been preferred against it under sub-section (2), the order of the appellate authority shall be final.

4. The provision of this section shall cease to be in force from such date as the State Government of Madras may by notification in the Official Gazette appoint.

36. 1. The State Government may, by notification in the Official Gazette, direct that the State Council shall maintain a register of dental hygienists or a register of dental mechanics.

2. The provisions of section 35 shall, so far as they may be made applicable, apply in respect of applications for registration in a register referred to in this section.

37. A person shall be entitled on payment of the prescribed fee to have his name registered on the register of dental hygienists, if he resides in the State and holds a recognized dental hygiene qualification: Provided that for the purposes of the first register of dental hygienists, a person shall be entitled to be registered, if he has been engaged as a dental hygienist as his principal means of livelihood for a period of not less than two years prior to the date of notification under sub-section (1) of section 36.

38. A person shall be entitled on payment of the prescribed fee to have his name entered in the register of dental mechanics, if he satisfies the prescribed requirements referred to in section 12: Provided that for the purposes of the preparation of the first register of dental mechanics a person shall be entitled to be registered, if he has been engaged as a dental mechanic as his principal means of

livelihood for a period of not less than two years prior to the date of notification under sub-section (1) of section 36.

39. 1. The State Government may, by notification in the Official Gazette, direct that for the retention of a name in a register after the 31st day of December of the year following the year in which the name is first entered in the register, there shall be paid annually to the State Council such renewal fee as may be prescribed in respect of each register, and where such direction has been made, such renewal fee shall be due to be paid before the 1st day of April of the year to which it relates.

    2. Where a renewal fee is not paid before the due date, the Registrar shall remove the name of the defaulter from the register: Provided that a name so removed may be restored to the register on payment in such manner as may be prescribed.

    3. On payment of the renewal fee, the Registrar shall issue a certificate of renewal and such certificate shall be proof of renewal of registration.

40. A registered dentist shall on payment of the prescribed fee be entitled to have entered in the register any further recognized dental qualification which he may obtain.

41. 1. Subject to the provisions of this section, the State Council may order that the name of any person shall be removed from any register where it is satisfied, after giving that person a reasonable opportunity of being heard and after such further inquiry, if any, as it may think fit to make—

    i. that his name has been entered in the register by error or on account of misrepresentation or suppression of a material fact, or

    ii. that he has been convicted of any offence or has been guilty of any infamous conduct in any professional respect or has violated the standards of professional conduct and etiquette or the code of ethics prescribed under section 17A, which in the opinion of the State Council renders him unfit to be kept in the register, or

    iii. that he having been permitted temporary registration under clause (b) of sub-section (2) of section 34 has, on such registration, been found to practise the profession of dentistry for personal gain.

    2. An order under sub-section (1) may direct that any person whose name is ordered to be removed from a register shall be ineligible for registration in the State under this Act either permanently or for such period of years as may be specified.

    3. An order under sub-section (1) shall not take effect until the expiry of three months from the date thereof.

    4. A person aggrieved by an order under sub-section (1) may, within thirty days from the date thereof, appeal to the State Government, and the order of the State Government upon such appeal shall be final.

    5. A person whose name has been removed from the register under this section or under sub-section (2) of section 39 shall forthwith surrender his certificate of registration and certificate of renewal, if any, to the Registrar, and the name so removed shall be published in the Official Gazette.

    6. A person whose name has been removed from the State register of dentists under this section or under sub-section (2) of section 39 shall not be entitled to have his name registered in the register of dentists in any other State register of dentists except with

the approval of the State Council from whose register his name has been removed.

42. The State Council may at any time, for reasons appearing to it sufficient and subject to the approval of the State Government, order that upon payment of the prescribed fee the name of a person removed from a register shall be restored thereto.

43. No order refusing to enter a name in a register or removing a name from a register shall be called in question in any Court.

44. Where it is shown to the satisfaction of the Registrar that a certificate of registration or a certificate of renewal has been lost or destroyed, the Registrar may, on payment of the prescribed fee, issue a duplicate certificate in the prescribed form.

45. As soon as may be after the 1st day of April in each year, the Registrar shall cause to be printed copies of the registers as they stood on the said date and such copies shall be made available to persons applying therefore on payment of the prescribed charge, and shall be evidence that on the said date the persons whose names are entered therein were registered dentists, registered dental hygienists or registered dental mechanics, as the case may be.

46. 1. Any reference in any other law to a person recognized by law as a dentist shall be deemed to be a reference to a dentist registered under this Act.

    2. No certificate required by or under any other law from a dentist shall be valid unless the person signing it is registered as a dentist under this Act.

    3. After the expiry of three years from the date appointed under sub-section (2) of section 32, a person who is not registered in Part A of the State register of dentists shall not, except with the sanction of the Central Government or the State Government hold any appointment as dentist in any dispensary, hospital or other institution which is supported wholly or partially from public or local funds:

    Provided that the provisions of this subsection shall not apply to any such person who is holding such an appointment immediately before the said date.

    4. After the expiry of two years from the publication of a register of dental hygienists in a state, no person whose name is not entered in that register shall hold appointment as dental hygienist in any dispensary, hospital or other institution in the state which is supported wholly or partially from public or local funds.

    5. Any person who is a registered dentist, registered dental hygienist or registered dental mechanic in a state may practice as such in any other state.

46. a. Where a dentist registered in one state is practicing dentistry in another state, he may, on payment of the prescribed fee which shall not exceed the renewal fee for registration in such other state, make an application in the prescribed form to the Council for the transfer of his name, from the register of the state where he is registered, to the register of the State in which he is practicing dentistry, and on receipt of any such application, the Council shall, not with standing anything contained elsewhere in this Act, direct that the name of such persons be removed from the first-mentioned register and entered in the register of the Second-mentioned State and the State Councils concerned shall comply with such directions:
    Provided that such a person shall be

required to produce a certificate to the effect that all dues in respect of his registration in the former State have been paid: Provided further that where any such application for transfer is made by a dentist again whom any disciplinary proceeding is pending or where for any other reason it appears to the Council that the application for transfer has not been made bona fide and the transfer should not be made, the Council may, after giving the dentist a reasonable opportunity of making a representation in this behalf, reject the application.

Miscellaneous

47. If any person whose name is not for the time being entered in a register falsely represents that it is so entered, or uses in connection with his name or title any words or letters reasonably calculated to suggest that his name is so entered, he shall be punishable on first conviction with fine which may extend to five hundred rupees, and on any subsequent conviction with imprisonment which may extend to six months or with fine not exceeding one thousand rupees or with both.

48. If any person,
   a. not being a person registered in a register of dentists, takes or uses the description of dental practitioner, dental surgeon, surgeon dentist, or dentist, or
   b. not being a person whose name is entered on a register of dental hygienists, takes or uses in a State where such register has been published, the title of dental hygienist, or
   c. not being a person whose name is entered on a register of dental mechanics, takes or uses in a State where such register has been published, the title of dental mechanic, or
   d. not possessing a recognized dental qualification, uses a degree or a diploma or an abbreviation indicating or implying a dental qualification, he shall be punishable on first conviction with fine which may extend to five hundred rupees, and on any subsequent conviction with imprisonment which may extend to six months or with fine not exceeding one thousand rupees or with both.

49. 1. After the expiry of three years from the date appointed under sub-section (2) of section 32 in the case of dentists, and in the States where a register of dental hygienists or dental mechanics has been prepared under section 36 from such date as may be specified in this behalf by the State Government by notification in the Official Gazette, in the case of dental hygienists or dental mechanics, no person, other than a registered dentist, registered dental hygienist or registered dental mechanic, shall practice dentistry, or the art of scaling, cleaning or polishing teeth, or of making or repairing dentures and dental appliances, as the case may be, or indicate in any way that he is prepared to do practice: Provided that the provisions of this section shall not apply to:
   a. practice of dentistry by a registered medical practitioner;
   b. the extraction of a tooth by any person when the case is urgent and no registered dentist is available, so however that the operation is performed without the use of any general or local anaesthetic;
   c. the performance of dental work or radiographic work in any hospital

or dispensary maintained or supported from public or local funds.

2. If any person contravenes the provisions of sub-section (1), he shall be punishable on first conviction with fine which may extend to five hundred rupees, and on any subsequent conviction with imprisonment which may extend to six months or with fine not exceeding one thousand rupees or with both.

50. If any person whose name has been transferred from a register fails without sufficient cause forthwith to surrender his certificate of registration or certificate or renewal, or both], he shall be punishable with fine which may extend to fifty rupees per month of such failure and in the case of a continuing offence with an additional fine which may extend to two rupees per day after the first day during which the offence continues.

51. 1. Except as hereinafter provided, the profession of dentistry shall not be carried on by a company or other corporate body.

2. The provisions of sub-section (1) shall not apply to:
   a. A company or other corporate body which carries on no business other than the profession of dentistry or some business ancillary to the profession of dentistry and of which the majority of the directors and all the operating staff are registered dentists;
   b. the carrying on of the profession of dentistry by employers who provide dental treatment for their employees by registered dentists otherwise than for profit;
   c. the carrying on of the profession of dentistry by any hospital or dispensary or institution for the training of dentists or dental hygienists or by any local authority or other

body authorized or required by law to provide dental treatment: Provided that any company or other corporate body carrying on the profession of dentistry immediately before the date appointed under sub-section (2) of section 32 may continue so to do until the expiry of three years from such date.

3. If any person contravenes the provisions of sub-section (1), he shall be punishable with fine which may extend on, first conviction to five hundred rupees, or on any subsequent conviction with imprisonment which may extend to six months or with fine not exceeding one thousand rupees or with both.

52. No court shall take cognizance of any offence punishable under this Act except upon complaint made by order of the State Government or the State Council.

53. The State Council shall before the end of June in each year pay to the Council a sum equivalent to one-fourth of the total fees realised by the State Council under this Act during the period of twelve months ending on the 31st day of March of that year.

53A.1. The Council shall maintain appropriate accounts and other relevant records and prepare an annual statement of accounts including the balance sheet, in accordance with such general directions as may be issued and in such form as may be specified by the Central Government in constitution with the Comptroller and Auditor-General of India.

2. The accounts of the Council shall be audited annually by the Comptroller and Auditor-General of India or any person appointed by him in this behalf and any expenditure incurred by him or any person so appointed in connection with such audit shall be payable

by the Council to the Comptroller and Auditor-General of India.

3. The Comptroller and Auditor-General of India and any person appointed by him in connection with the audit of the accounts of the Council shall have the same rights and privileges and authority in connection with such audit as the Comptroller and Auditor-General of India has in connection with the audit of Government accounts, and in particular, shall have the right to demand the production of books of accounts, connected vouchers and other documents and papers and to inspect the office of the Council.

4. The accounts of the Council as certified by the Comptroller and Auditor-General of India or any person appointed by him in this behalf, together with the audit report thereon, shall be forwarded annually to the Central Government.

5. A copy of the accounts of the Council as so certified together with the audit report thereon shall be forwarded simultaneously to the Council.

54. 1. Whenever it appears to the Central Government that the Council is not complying with any of the provisions of this Act, the Central Government may appoint a Commission of Enquiry consisting of three persons, two of whom shall be appointed by the Central Government, one being the Judge of a High Court, and one by the Council; and refer to it the matters on which the enquiry is to be made.

2. The Commission shall proceed to enquire in a summary manner and report to the Central Government on the matters referred to it together with such remedies, if any, as the Commission may like to recommend.

3. The Central Government may accept the report or remit the same to the Commission for modification or reconsideration.

4. After the report is finally accepted, the Central Government may order the Council to adopt the remedies so recommended within such time as may be specified in the order and if the Council fails to comply within the time so specified, the Central Government may pass such orders or take such actions as may be necessary to give effect to the recommendations of the Commission.

5. Whenever it appears to the State Government that the State Council is not complying with any of the provisions of this Act, the State Government may likewise appoint a similar Commission of Enquiry in respect of the State Council to make enquiry in like manner and pass such order or take such action as specified in subsection (3) and (4).

55. 1. The State Government may, by notification in the Official Gazette, make rules to carry out the purposes of Chapters III, IV and V.

2. In particular and without prejudice to the generality of the foregoing power, such rules may provide for:

   a. The management of the property of the State Council, and the maintenance and audit of its accounts;

   b. the manner in which elections under Chapter III shall be conducted;

   c. the summoning and holding of meetings of the State Council, the times and places at which such meetings shall be held, the conduct of business threat and the number of members necessary to form a quorum;

   d. the powers and duties of the President and Vice-President of the State Council;

e. the constitution and functions of the Executive Committee, the summoning and holding of meetings thereof, the times and places at which such meetings shall be held, the number of members necessary to constitute a quorum;

f. the term of office and the powers and duties of the Registrar and other officers and servants of the State Council, including the amount and nature of the security to be given by the Treasurer;

g. the particulars to be stated, and the proof of qualifications to be given in applications for registration under this Act; (gg) the form of application for transfer of registration from one state to another;

h. the charge for supplying printed copies of the registers, and the fees payable for:

i. registration or renewal of registration;

ii. supplying a duplicate certificate of registration or renewal; and

iii. transfer of registration from one State to another;

i. the forms of certificates of registration and renewal;

j. any other matter which is to be or may be prescribed under Chapters III, IV and V, except sub-sections (1), (2), (3) and (4) of section 54.

3. Every rule made by the State Government under this section shall be laid, as soon as may be after it is made; before the State Legislature.

THE DENTISTS (AMENDMENT) ORDINANCE, 1992

Whereas parliament is not in session and the President is satisfied that circumstances exist which render it necessary for him to take immediate action;

Now, therefore, in exercise of the powers conferred by clause (1) of article 123 of the Constitution, the President is pleased to promulgate the following Ordinance :

1. 1. This ordinance may be called the Dentists (Amendment) Ordinance, 1992.

2. It shall come into force at once.

2. After section 10 of the Dentist Act, 1948 (hereinafter referred to as the principal Act), the following-sections shall be inserted, namely:

10A.1. Notwithstanding anything contained in this Act or any other law for the time being in force:

a. no person shall establish an authority or institution for a course of study or training (including a post-graduate course of study or training) which would enable a student of such course or training to qualify himself for the grant of recognized dental qualification; or

b. no authority or institution conducting a course of study or training (including a post-graduate course of study or training) for grant of recognized dental qualification shall;

i. open a new or higher course of study or training (including a post-graduate of study or training) which would enable a student of such course or training to qualify himself for the award of any recognized dental qualification; or

ii. increase its admission capacity in any course of study or training (including a post-graduate course of study or training),

Except with the previous permission the Central Government obtained in accordance with the provisions of this section.

Explanation 1: For the purpose of this section, "person" includes any University or a trust but does not include the Central Government.

Explanation 2: For the purpose of this section, "admission capacity", in relation to any course of study or training (including a post-graduate course of study or training) in an authority or institution granting recognized dental qualification, means the maximum number of students that may be fixed by the Council from time to time for being admitted to such course or training.

2. a. Every person, authority or institution granting recognized dental qualification shall, for the purpose of training permission under sub-section (1), submit to the Central Government a scheme in accordance with the provisions of clause (b) and the Central Government shall refer the said scheme to the Council for its recommendation.

   b. The scheme referred to in clause (a) shall be in such form and contain such particulars and be preferred in such manner and be accompanied with such fee as may be prescribed.

3. On receipt of a scheme by the Council under sub-section (2), the Council may obtain such other particulars as may be considered necessary by it from the person, authority or institution concerned, granting recognized dental qualification and thereafter, it may.

   a. If the scheme is defective and does not contain any necessary particulars, give a reasonable opportunity to the person, authority or institution concerned for making a written representation and it shall be open to such person, authority or institution to rectify the defects, if any, specified by the Council;

   b. consider the scheme, having regard to the factors referred to in sub-section (7) and submit the scheme together with its recommendations thereon to the Central Government.

4. The Central Government may, after considering the scheme and the recommendations of the Council under sub-section (3) and after obtaining, where necessary, such other particulars as may be considered necessary by it from the person, authority or institution concerned, and having regard to the factors referred to in sub-section (7), either approve (with such conditions, if any, as it may consider necessary) or disapprove the scheme and any such approval shall be a permission under sub-section (1): Provided that no scheme shall be disapproved by the Central Government except after giving the person, authority or institution granting recognized dental qualification a reasonable opportunity of being heard.

   Provided further that nothing in this sub-section shall prevent any person, authority or institution whose scheme has not been approved to submit a fresh scheme and the provisions of this section shall apply to such scheme, as if such scheme has been submitted for the first time under sub-section (1).

5. Where, within a period of one year from the date of submission of the scheme to the Central Government under sub-section (1), no order passed by the Central Government has been communicated to the person, authority or institution submitting the scheme, such scheme shall be deemed to have been approved by the Central Government in the form in which it had been submitted, and accordingly, the permission of the Central Government required under sub-section (1) shall also be deemed to have been granted.

6. In computing the time limit specified in sub-section (5), the time taken by the

person, authority or institution concerned submitting the scheme in furnishing any particulars called for by the Council or by the Central Government shall be excluded.

7. The Council while making its recommendations under clause (b) of subsection (3) and the Central Government, while passing an order either approving or disapproving the scheme under subsection (4) shall have due regard to the following factors, namely:

   a. whether the proposed authority or institution for grant of recognized dental qualification or the existing authority or institution seeking to open a new or higher course of study or training, would be in a position to offer the minimum standards of dental education in conformity with the requirements referred to in section 16A and the regulations made under sub-section (1) of section 20;

   b. whether the person seeking to establish an authority or institution or the existing authority or institution seeking to open a new or higher course of study or training or to increase its admission capacity has adequate resources;

   c. whether necessary facilities in respect of staff, equipment, accommodation, training and other facilities to ensure proper functioning of the authority or institution or conducting the new course of study or training or accommodating the increased admission capacity have been provided or would be provided within the time-limit specified in the scheme;

   d. whether adequate hospital facilities, having regard to the number of student likely to attend such authority or institution or course of study or

training or as a result of the increased admission capacity have been provided or would be provided within the time-limit specified in the scheme;

   e. whether any arrangement has been made or programme drawn to impart proper training to students likely to attend such authority or institution or course of study or training by persons having the recognized dental qualifications;

   f. the requirement of manpower in the field of practice of dentistry; and

   g. any other factors as may be prescribed.

8. Where the Central Government passes an order either approving or disapproving a scheme under this section a copy of the order shall be communicated to the person, authority or institution concerned.

10B. 1. Where any authority or institution is established for grant of recognized dental qualification except with the previous permission of the Central Government in accordance with the provisions of section 10A, no dental qualification granted to any student of such authority or institution shall be a recognized dental qualification for the purpose of this Act.

   2. Where any authority or institution granting recognized dental qualification opens a new or higher course of study or training (including a post-graduate course of study or training) except with the previous permission of the Central Government in accordance with the provisions of section 10A, no dental qualification granted to any student of such authority or institution on the basis of such study or training (including a post-graduate course of study) or purposes of this Act.

   3. Where any authority or institution granting recognized dental qualification increases its admission capacity

in any course of study or training (including a post-graduate course of study or training) except with the previous permission of the Central Government in accordance with the provisions of section 10A, no dental qualification granted to any student of such authority or institution on the basis of the increase in its admission capacity shall be a recognized dental qualification for the purpose of this Act.

Explanation - For the purpose of this section, the criteria for identifying a student who has been granted a dental qualification on the basis of such increase in the admission capacity shall be such as may be prescribed.

10C.1. If after the 1st day of June, 1992 and on and before the commencement of the Dentists (Amendment) Ordinance, 1992 any person has established an authority or institutions for grant of recognized dental qualification or any authority or institution granting recognized dental qualification has opened a new or higher course or study or training (including a post-graduate course of study or training) or increased admission capacity, such person, authority or institution, as the case may be, shall seek, within a period of one year from the commencement of the Dentists (Amendment) Ordinance, 1992, the permission of the Central Government in accordance with the provision of section 10A of the principal Act.

2. If any person or, as the case may be, any authority or institution granting recognized dental qualification fails to seek the permission under sub-section (1) of this Ordinance, the provisions of section 10B of the Principal Act shall apply, so far as may be, as if permission of the Central Government under section 10A has been refused.

3. In section 55 of the principal Act, in sub-section (2), after clause (f), the following clauses shall be inserted, namely : "(fa) the form of the scheme, the particulars to be given in such scheme, the manner in which the scheme is to be preferred and the fee payable with the scheme under clause (b) of sub-section (2) of section 10A; (fb) the criteria for identifying a student who has been granted a medical qualification referred to in Explanation to sub-section (3) of section 10B."

31 Indian Dental Association

Dr. S.K. Mujumdar, created an association for dental professionals in 1946 in the name of 'The All India Dental Association'. Dr. Rafiuddin Ahmed became its first President. Dr. V. M. Desai became the second President in 1948. Col. N.N. Berry was appointed secretary in the year 1948, who later took over as President in 1950. The association was formed to unite dental professionals across India and to foster education and improve awareness as regards dentistry. Later, the All India Dental Association became the 'Indian Dental Association', as it is known today.

Indian Dental Association has more than 30,000 dental professionals as its members. It effectively harnesses its vast resources aimed at attaining professional excellence of the dentists in their day to day activities and ensures optimal oral health for all.

The **objectives** of IDA are:

1. To be actively involved in and to help in the promotion, encouragement and advancement of the dental and allied sciences.
2. To encourage IDA members to undertake measures for the improvement of public oral health and dental education in India.
3. To main the dignity and honour of the dental profession.
4. To protect the rights and interests of the members of the Association.
5. To foster friendship, co-operation and co-existence amongst members of the association and to implement well formulated schemes for the social security of members of the Association.

For the attainment and furtherance of the above objectives, the association may:

a. Hold periodical meetings, conferences and trade exhibitions for the members of the association and for the dental profession in general.
b. Publish and circular journals/newsletters which shall be the official voice of the association, being especially adapted to the needs of the dental profession in India and which shall undertake publicity and propaganda work of the Association through its columns.
c. Maintain an association office or offices as herein afterwards provided.
d. Encourage the opening of libraries in Head office, state and local branches and procure other relevant material, books etc. out of the funds of the association and from donations it receives.
e. Publish from time to time papers embodying dental research, conducted by members independently or under the auspices of the association.
f. Encourage research and continuing dental education in the dental and allied sciences, with grants from the funds of the association, by establishment of research centers and related foundations etc. and scholarships, prizes or awards, in such manner as many from time to time be determined by the Association. Maintain contact with national and international associations having similar objectives.
g. To set up trust/research centre/foundation, oral cancer and oral health educational initiatives, etc., to carry out public charitable and educational activities.

h. To set up educational institutions.

i. Conduct an education campaign amongst the masses of India on the matter of oral hygiene, by co-operating with different public bodies working with similar objectives.

j. Consider and express views on all questions pertaining to the Indian Legislation affecting public health, dental profession and dental education and take such steps from time to time regarding the same, as shall be deemed expedient and necessary.

k. Grant the "IDA Seal of Acceptance" to oral health products, dental instruments, equipment and material, etc., with regard to their safety, efficacy and quality, in the interest of the dental profession and the public. This authority is vested with the Central Council only.

l. Represent the interest of the dental fraternity, to plead for and to protect its rights, to secure all benefits for its members, to defend their rights and also to liaison with Central Government/State Government and various appropriate bodies.

m. Do all such things as are cognate to the objectives of the association or are incidental or conducive to the attainment of the above objectives.

n. Safeguard the professional interest and social security of the individual member as a consumer.

o. Cooperate with other specialty societies and associations having similar objectives.

p. Start and run charitable dental clinics by itself or by co-operating with other charity organizations or government/semi-government bodies.

q. All activities of the association shall be carried out in India. However, the association can collaborate globally with regard to oral health program and scientific activities.

r. To conduct voluntary CDE accreditation points program.

s. To formulate base minimum standards to set up dental clinic and have voluntary dental practice accreditation program.

t. Liaise with Government, National and International bodies, Associations, Organization, etc.

The commonly used **abbreviations** are:

a. "IDA" means the Indian Dental Association.

b. "CC" means Central Council of IDA

c. "EC" means Executive Committee of state/local/defence branches

d. "HSG" means Honorary Secretary General (Head Office)

e. "AGM" means Annual General Body Meeting

f. "EOGM" means Extra Ordinary General Body Meeting

g. "CDH" means Council on Dental Health

h. "CDE" means Council on Dental Education

The benefits of association are open to all members irrespective of caste, creed, religion and sex etc.

IDA EMBLEM

The significance and the rationale behind the Emblem design which projects the image of our association is as follows:

1. **Head of the elephant:** It represents sega-ciousness or thoughfulness.

2. **Tusks of the elephant:** They denote the dental profession and were used as far back as the Egyptian culture. Denotes beauty of teeth.

3. **The staff of aesculplus:** Stand for the captor of authority and represents the professional authority of the association.

4. **Serpents entwined around the staff:** In 300 B.C. the God of Medicine and Healing of the Romans was Aescupius who used serpents and a rod for healing. The Greek philosopher, Hippocrates, adopted this as a symbol of healing. It has since been associated with the medical science. Our emblem has two serpents entwined around the staff in opposite directions.

5. **Wings on the staff:** Represent the spread of knowledge according to the Greek mythology wherein God Hermes had wings on his legs.

The Emblem has six small and three large divisions on the wings on either side of the staff.

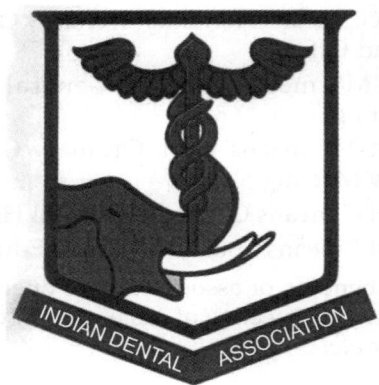

Fig. 31.1: IDA Emblem

Types of Membership

Members can be enrolled under the following categories:

A. Annual member - A dental surgeon who pays the annual subscription.

B. Silver member - A dental surgeon who pays membership fee for a period of five years

C. Gold member - A dental surgeon who pays membership fee for a period of ten years

D. Life member - A dental surgeon who pays a one-time subscription fee

E. Student member - An undergraduate from a dental institution

F. Affiliate member - A dental surgeon residing outside India

G. Honorary member - A dental surgeon of high scientific or literary standing having rendered valuable services to the IDA. Usually the honorary member is nominated by the Central Council.

Eligibility

A. Dental Surgeon should apply for membership in the prescribed application form and shall confirm to the following conditions and prerequisites:

a. He/she should be a dental surgeon registered under Part A of the Indian Dentists' Act, 1948 (Graduates).

b. A dental surgeon with Part-B Registration of the Indian Dentists Act 1948 and who is already a member in good standing, as on 31st January 1998, without any arrears shall continue to be a member. There shall not be any further admission of Part-B Registered Dental Practitioners in local/state branches and Head Office.

c. An applicant should not have been convicted by any competent court of law for any cognizable offence; and should not be of unsound mind or insolvent. He/she should not have been engaged in any activity detrimental to the interest of association. While joining he/she should sign a declaration to that effect in the application form.

d. The application should not be involved in any illegal activity.

e. In the case of student membership, he/she should be an undergraduate student, studying up to internship from a dental institution/college, recognized/approved by the Dental Council of India. The application form should bear the Principal's signature and the stamp of the institution.

f. In the case of Affiliate Members, the non-resident dental surgeon must provide his/her professional credentials, which must be endorsed by a dental body of that country.

Subscription

General Rules

The Association shall reserve the right to revise the subscription from time to time.

a. All subscriptions are payable in advance on the first day of January, every year.

b. The annual year for subscription shall be from 1st January to 31st December every year.

c. The last date of receipt of subscription towards renewal of membership shall be 31st January at the Head office. For convenience, subscription should be received by 15th December at the local branch and by 31st December at the state branch.

d. In case the annual fees of any member do not reach the Head office on or before 15th February every year, his/her membership will be automatically terminated. Such member can enroll again as a member by paying admission fee and the necessary subscription.

e. Any Annual/Silver/Gold member shall pay his/her entire amount of subscription directly either only to Head office or State Office or Local branch.

The Annual/Silver/Gold/Life/Student/Affiliate membership fee and admission fee prescribed may be reviewed from time to time, as recommended by the Central Council and approved by AGM/EOGM.

Subscription Fee

a. **Annual Member**

Admission fee: Those joining for the first time or seeking readmission shall pay an entire entrance fee of Rs.300/- to the admitting local/state/defence branch or Head office.

Annual fee: They shall pay a uniform entire subscription of Rs.650/- either at local/state/Defence/Head Office.

Renewal fee: They shall pay a uniform entire subscription of Rs.650/- either at local/state/Defence branch or Head Office.

b. **Silver Member (Membership for 5 years)**

Admission fee: Those joining for the first time and seeking readmission shall pay the entire entrance fee of Rs.300/- to the admitting Local/State/Defence/Head Office.

Membership fee: Shall pay at a time the entire fee of Rs.3250/- for five years either only at Local/State/Defence/Head Office.

c. **Gold Member (Membership for 10 years)**

Admission fee: Those joining for the first time or seeking readmission shall pay the entire entrance fee of Rs.300/- to the admitting local/state/defence branch or Head office, either only at Local/State/Defence/Head Office.

d. **Life Member**

Admission fee: Those joining for the first time shall pay the entrance fee of Rs.300/- to the admitting local/state/defence branch or Head Office.

Life Membership Fee: A one-time fee of Rs.10,650/- either at Local/State/Defence/Head Office.

e. **Student member:** Consolidate fee (for the period of the undergraduate course including internship) –The uniform subscription of Rs.1000/- for tenure of their undergraduate course, either to the Local/State/Head Office. However, Student Member may pay yearly rupees 200/- depending upon the year in which he/she becomes student member.

f. **Affiliate member:** The entire annual subscription of US $100 directly to the Head Office.

g. **Affiliate life member:** A one-time fee of US$350 directly to the Head Office.

h. **Honorary members:** Not to pay any subscription fee.

Admission of Member

Annual/Silver/Gold/Life

a. A dental surgeon who wishes to apply for membership of the IDA has to first completely fill and submit the application form. He/she shall have to submit the application form along with the prescribed fee and supporting documents/credentials to the local branch/state branch/ Head Office for approval.

b. The Hon. Secretary of the Head Office/state branch/local branch/Defence branch shall have the authority to scrutinize the application form and other supporting documents. If the Secretary has any doubts or reservations, he shall refer the case to the Central Council or the Executive Committee for their decision. He cannot reject the membership without the consent of the Central Council or Executive Committee.

c. Applications received at each branch office must then be submitted to the Central Council/Executive Committee for their approval subsequently. After verification, if all documents are found to be in order and to the satisfaction of the Secretary/ Central Council/ Executive Committee, the application shall be passed and the member should be informed and enrolled subsequently.

d. After approval, the subscription amount shall be deposited accordingly.

e. The original application forms, along with the photograph shall be dispatched to Head office for its record immediately. The local branch shall forward two copies of the application to the state branch after admission and the state branch shall forward one copy to Head Office.

f. In the event of false information, the application shall automatically get cancelled.

g. In the Branch Executive decides with a 2/3rd majority not to admit the applicant in the larger interest of the branch, the application shall be rejected and the applicant be intimated. In case the applicant appeals to state branch/ Head Office, the decision of Central Council shall be final.

h. The decision of granting or rejecting membership by Central Council is final and cannot be canvassed in any court of law. The decision of Central Council regarding granting or rejecting membership to any applicant/member shall be binding on State, Local, Defence branches.

i. By becoming member of the local or state or Defence branch, a member shall automatically become member of the central organization, i.e. Indian Dental Association subject to receipt of his/her subscription share by Head Office.

j. Head Office shall process the form and only Head Office can issue the identity/membership card to members. State and Local branch shall not issue any identity/ membership card to members.

Direct Member

a. A dental surgeon who wishes to become a member of the IDA but does not reside or practice within the area of a state/local branch can directly apply to Head Office as Direct Member.

b. Persons residing or practicing within the jurisdiction of a state branch but in a place where no local branch exists shall be admitted to the respective State branches, as direct members.

c. The Head Office/State Office shall reserve the right to accept or decline an application for direct membership as may be applicable.

Honorary Member

a. For an Honorary Member to be admitted, he/she should be proposed by at least twenty-five members of the Association or ten members of the Central Council.

b. The election shall take place at a meeting of the Central Council, where the voting will be done by secret ballot after due discussion.

c. The person shall be considered elected as Honorary Member if 2/3 of the members who are present and who cast their vote in his or her favour. Such members shall continue as Honorary Member for life.

Student Member

a. An undergraduate student studying up to internship from any dental institution, recognized/approved by the Dental Council of India, shall be admitted as student member, on submission of an application form, duly signed by the Principal and no payment of the prescribed fees.

Affiliate Member

a. A non-resident dental professional, interested in becoming member of the Indian Dental Association, shall apply for affiliate membership directly to Head office , by paying the annual/life membership fees.

b. He/she should be a member of the National Dental Society/Association of his/her country and should produce a certificate to that effect.

c. All affiliate members shall apply for membership to Head Office only an shall be attached to Head Office only.

Transfer of Membership

Transfer of membership from one branch to another shall be done at the time of membership renewal, i.e. November/December/January and on production of proof of IDA membership in the previous year. Once the subscription is paid to respective Local branch/State branch/Defence branch/ Head Office for current year, membership will only be transferred in the following year with fresh request. However for communication purpose mailing address will be changed with written request.

Membership Privileges

a. All members excepting student members shall be supplied with a copy of all the publications of the Association, free, or at such rates as the Central Council may fix from time to time.

b. All members shall be entitled to the use of the library and the Association rooms, if any, set apart for the use of the members.

c. All members can attend CDE programs, conferences, lectures and demonstrations, organized by the Association, according to the terms as laid down by the Association.

d. Only annual/silver/gold and life members who have paid subscription before 31st July shall have the right to attend the AGM/EOGM of Central Council and of State branch and of Local branch and vote on all resolutions put forward at the meetings and vote for elections of Office Bearers and other posts. Those who have paid the subscription after 31st July can only attend the AGM/EOGM but cannot vote on any resolution or vote in any election.

e. Student, affiliate and honorary members shall have no right in the working of the Association.

f. All members shall enjoy any other privileges that may hereafter be conferred by the Central Council.

g. Only Annual/Silver/Gold and Life Members shall be eligible to contest and hold offices; i.e. office bearers of Local branch/State branch/Defence branch/Head Office and Members of State EC without portfolio/Representative to the Central Council/Representative of Local Branch to State EC/Local branch of EC member, provided they are members in good standing.

h. Members in good standing is one who's subscription share has been received by Head office on or before 31st January.

Termination of Membership

A. Resignation: A member wishing to resign from membership may do so by tendering the resignation in writing to the Head Office with a copy to the state/local branch.

B. Non-payment of Fee: The membership of a member, whose subscription remains unpaid after 15th February at Head Office, every year, will be automatically terminated.

C. Undesirable Conduct

a. If the conduct of any member is deemed by the Central Council/ state/local Executive Committee, prejudicial to the interest of the Association or calculated to bring the dental profession or the Association into disrepute, in violation of the rules and regulations of the Association or who is creating obstacles and hurdles in the working of the Association, that member shall be asked to submit a written explanation as to why disciplinary action should not be taken against him/her for his/her conduct.

b. In the event of the explanation being found unsatisfactory, the member may be asked either to apologise or to resign from the association. If the member is agreeable, his/her apology or resignation shall be accepted. In case of a branch member, the matter shall be referred to the Central Council through the State branch, giving details of the case for further reference.

c. In the event of the said member refusing either to apologise or to resign, an EOGM of his parent branch shall be convened to consider the case and notice of at least 7 days, in case of a local branch, 14 days in case of a state branch and 21 days in case of Head Office, shall be given to the member concerned. The member shall give an opportunity to explain his/her conduct.

d. If at the meeting 60% of the total strength of members who are eligible to vote and present at the meeting and who record their votes, vote in favour of removal of the member's name from membership, the resolution shall be sent to the Central Council through the state branch for confirmation. The member's name shall be removed from the register of membership of the local branch/state branch/ Head Office, only after receipt of the confirmation from Central Council.

e. Before the Central Council gives its final decision, the member shall have the right to appeal. However in the meantime, the member shall be suspended from all privileges of membership.

f. In case of direct members, the state and Head Office shall follow the same procedure as the case may be.

D. No authentic qualification/certificates

a. A member who is not qualified but who has secured admission on misrepresentation shall automatically cease to be a member on the same day.

b. If any member does not possess the requisite qualifications to join as a member in a state/local branch or Head Office but has been admitted by the state/ local branches, such information shall be brought to the notice of the Central Council and a detailed enquiry will be conducted by the Secretary regarding the member's credentials and the facts placed before the Central Council.

c. If the Central Council decides that the concerned member is not qualified to become a member of the association, an explanation shall be sought from the concerned member, giving 15 days time for the member to justify his/her case.

d. If the member prefers to appear before the Central Council and explain his/her case, he may be given an opportunity. After receiving the member's explanation or after hearing the member, if the Central

Council is convinced that the member does not possess the requisite qualification to be admitted as member, be/she shall be removed from the rolls of the state/local branch and Head Office forthwith and it shall be intimated to the member and the local and state branch.

e. In the event of the member's not responding to the letter sent by Head Office, by registered post, in due time before the last date mentioned in the letter, the decision of the Central Council shall be final and binding on the member.

E. Forming a parallel dental association

a. If any member floats/forms another dental association parallel and detrimental to the IDA at a regional or All India level, he/she shall be removed from the membership of the IDA.

b. Any member of the IDA joining the parallel Association shall also be removed from membership of the Association. This does not apply to specialty societies. While removing, the procedure as laid in Sub Section 7.C in the article membership (Undesirable Conduct) shall be followed.

F. Refund of Subscription: No member shall be entitled to ask for any refund of the membership fees, either in whole or part thereof once the subscription is paid to Local branch/State branch/Defence branch/Head Office.

Re-admission as Member

a. Members who have ceased to be members under clauses 7.A and 7.B of Article Membership, can be re-admitted as new members, upon fresh application, subject to approval by the Executive Committee / Central Council and upon payment of admission fees, annual fees and any dues outstanding against them except annual fee as on the date when they had ceased to be members.

b. The Central Council shall however have the power to write off a part or whole of any outstanding dues against such members on the recommendation of the branches concerned, or in the case of direct members, on its own initiatives.

c. Members, whose names have been removed under clauses 7.C and 7.E of Article Membership, may be re-admitted subject to the decision and approval of the Central Council, on the expiry of two years or thereafter, provided their application for re-enrolment, supported by ten members of the Association testifying to their good conduct during the intervening period, is accepted.

d. But the member who has resigned under clauses 7.C and 7.E of Article Membership, can be re-admitted on submitting a written apology acceptable to the Central Council and or on the recommendation of the state/local branch concerned, by majority vote and he/she shall be charged an admission fee as a new member.

e. On all matters of re-admission, the decision of the Central Council shall be final and binding on the members.

Central Council

The Central Council shall be the national level governing body of the Association having its jurisdiction within the territory of India. The Central Council shall control and regulate the management and general affair of the Association. The Central Council shall oversee all State branches, Local branches, Defence branch and Membership of the IDA.

Management of Indian Dental Association

The general management of the Head Office (HO), as a whole, shall be vested with the Central Council. Nobody in receipt of salary or an honorarium from the funds of the association can be elected as an office bearer of the association.

Composition:

a. Central Council Office Bearers

Post	Tenure
1. President	One Term
2. President Elect	One Term
3. Four Vice-Presidents	One Term
4. Honorary Secretary General	Five Terms
5. Honorary Joint Secretary	Five Terms
6. Honorary Assistant Secretary	Five Terms
7. Honorary Treasurer	Five Terms
8. Editor of the Journal	Five Terms
9. Chairman – Council on Dental Health	Two Terms
10. Chairman – Council on Dental Education	Two Terms
11. Immediate Past President	One Term
12. Chairman – International Committee	Two Terms
13. Vice-Chairman, International Committee	Two Terms
14. Chairman – ICCDE Indian Division	Two Terms
15. Secretary – ICCDE Indian Division	Two Terms
b. *Representatives* from State Branches to Central Council	One Term

Functions and Powers

The Central Council shall direct and regulate the general affairs of the Association, and its decision in all matters shall be final and binding, on matters of state/local branches/Defence branch and individual member. It shall have the following powers:

a. To conduct business at meetings of the Central Council.

b. To look after the maintenance and administration of the Association library and all other properties.

c. To be responsible for the organization and direction of publications of the association and to decide policies of various publications and starting various new publications.

d. To frame, alter or modify various guidelines.

e. To frame, alter or repeal rules and byelaws of the association by a simple majority vote in the Central Council, subject to the approval of the AGM/EOGM of the Association.

f. To review, revise and recommend membership fees from time to time, subject to approval by the AGM or EOGM.

g. To peruse sub-committees, including the Working Committee, Constitution Committee, the Screening and Scrutinizing Committee and other Committees, appointed by the President, in consultation with the secretary.

h. To appoint any other sub-committees if it considers necessary, subject to the approval of the President.

i. To represent to the Government, public bodies, or any constituent authority, any matter in which the interests of the Association or the dental profession are involved and only secretary shall represent on all official matters including International Associations/Organizations, related Organizations and media, etc. The Office Bearers shall express the views of the Central Council.

j. To consider and take decisions on applications for direct membership and resignation.

k. To take disciplinary action on the removal of any members for want of qualification.

l. To take necessary disciplinary action against any member or branch.

m. To write off the whole or part of the arrears, or any other outstanding sums, against any individual member or a branch, if considered desirable.

n. To delegate all or some of its powers (apart from the power of altering rules and byelaws), to a working committee, if and when required.

o. To appoint or remove salaried employees of the Head Office of the Association.

p. To exercise, in addition to the powers by the rules expressly conferred on it, all such powers and execute all such facts and things as may be done by the Association and which are not hereby or by legislative enactment expressly directed or required to be exercised or done by the Association in the AGM/EOGM meeting.

q. To purchase, take on lease, sell, mortgage, or otherwise buy or dispose of immovable properties of every description, in particular any land, building, etc. and to form a trust as per govt. regulations, for which 2/3rd majority of Central Council is required, from amongst the members who are present and those who cast their votes.

r. To purchase, manage, lend and exchange movable properties or rent any accommodation when deemed necessary in the interest of the association.

s. To buy utensils, books, newspapers, periodicals, instruments, fittings, appliances, apparatus, etc., when deemed necessary, in the interest of the association.

t. To erect, maintain, improve or alter and keep in repair any building for utilization of the association.

u. To borrow or raise money in such a manner as the association may think fit and collect subscriptions and donations for the purposes of the association.

v. To invest any funds of the association, not immediately required, for any of its objectives, in such a manner as may from time to time be determined by the Central Council.

w. To assist, subscribe to, co-operate, affiliate or amalgamate with any other public body, having objectives partially or completely similar to the association, whether that body is registered or incorporated or not.

x. To approve or derecognize the state/local branches, if necessary.

y. To declare null and void elections, held at the state/local branches, in case of a contestant appealing to HO, and questioning the merit of the election, after a detailed enquiry and with a 2/3 majority amongst the members who are present and who cast their vote.

z. To give a directive to a branch or a member on any issue.

aa. To grant the seal of acceptance of the IDA, for oral health products/instruments/dental materials, by 2/3 majority amongst the members who are present and who cast their vote. The power to grant the seal of acceptance is vested only with the Central Council and not with State and Local branch.

bb. To appoint one Conference Secretary, in charge of National Conferences. The Conference Secretary shall be a liaison officer between the Head Office and the Organizing Committee and shall be answerable to the Head Office and Central Council.

cc. The Central Council shall be the authoritative body for any international congress hosted by IDA. The organizing committee, like any other sub-committee, shall work under the guidance of the Head office..

dd. To approve one Chairman; Organizing Committee, Organizing Secretary, Treasurer, Convener; Scientific Sessions and Convener; Trade Exhibitions for national conferences.

ee. To approve proposed delegate fees and budget of National/International Conference.

ff. To nominate 10 members of Central Council to Council of Dental Health (CDH) and 10 members of Central

Council to the Continuing Dental Education (CDE) Committee.

gg. If any member does not possess the requisite qualifications to join as a member but has been admitted by any of these, Head Office, State branch/Local branch, the Central Council has the powers to enquire into the matter and remove the member from the rolls of the Association.

hh. To approve the audited balanced sheet and the proposed budget for the year, before presenting them at the AGM/EOGM.

ii. To represent matters pertaining to the Indian Dentists' Act, 1948 and allied matters.

jj. To frame policies and public statements of IDA.

Term of the Central Council

a. The Central Council shall enter upon its duties at the close of the AGM of Head office, and shall hold office till the end of the next AGM of Head office, or till 28th February, whichever is earlier.

b. The office bearers and members shall function forthwith after election at the close of the AGM of the Head office and shall continue as members till the end of their tenure as mentioned in clause 1.A in this Article Central Council and will automatically cease to be office bearers or Central Council members after their tenure is over.

c. Any member of the Central Council who is absent for three consecutive meetings without assigning a valid, reason/apology in writing shall cease to be a member of the Central Council, automatically. Notice to such members shall not be sent for the next Central Council meeting. Such members shall not be eligible for re-election/re-nomination for that Association year.

Office Bearers Duties and Powers

The President

a. Shall be the Chairman of AGM/EOGM, and all meetings of the Central Council and sub committees appointed by him, and any other committee for which no chairman has been appointed. He shall be a member of all committees.

b. Shall preside at the Annual Conference of Head office.

c. Shall guide and render advice on the activities of the association.

d. Shall regulate the proceedings of meetings and conferences.

e. Shall, in addition to his ordinary vote, have a casting vote. In case of equality of votes, if he fails to give his casting vote, the motion shall be declared invalid.

f. Shall continue as a member of the Central Council for one year, beginning with the end of his tenure of office as President.

g. Shall have the right to attend and take part in any meeting (EC/AGM/EOGM) of state/local branches anywhere in India.

The President—Elect

a. Shall be a member of the Central Council and shall assist the President in the performance of his duties.

b. Shall succeed to the office of the President at the end of the closing ceremony/open session of the conference or at the end of the AGM in case of there being no conference in the year following his election as President Elect.

The Vice President

a. In case of the absence of the President, the senior most Vice-President, shall act as Chairman of the meetings of the Central Council/AGM/EOGM.

b. Any one of the four Vice-Presidents in their order of precedence shall be the Chairman of all sub-committees for which no

Chairman has been appointed even if he is not a member of that committee only in the absence of the President.

c. All Vice Presidents shall help the branches in organizational activities.

The Honorary Secretary General

a. Shall be in charge of the Head Office.

b. Shall be in charge of all correspondence and he shall be the only to correspond or represent an official matters of the Association.

c. Shall oversee general supervision of accounts; pass all bills for payments and sign cheques jointly with the Hon. Treasurer.

d. Shall get prepared by the Honorary Treasurer, an annual statement of accounts, duly audited by the auditor, for presentation before the Central Council and at the AGM/EOGM.

e. Shall prepare a budget and get it passed in the Central Council.

f. Shall organize, arrange and convene meetings, conferences, lecturers and demonstrations.

g. Shall attend meetings of the Central Council and sub-committees and keep records of the proceedings thereof; and be a member of all committees.

h. Shall assist the President in appointing sub-committees.

i. Shall maintain a correct and up-to-date register/computer database of all types of members of the association.

j. Shall promote the IDA with the help of the Honorary Joint Secretary and Honorary Assistant Secretary, by encouraging the establishment of the branches where they do not exist and by creating a general interest in the IDA.

k. Shall maintain a property register.

l. Shall have the right to attend and take part in any meeting (EC/AGM/EOGM), of the state/local/Defence branches, anywhere in India.

m. If the Secretary changes his personal head quarters to any other town, after he is duly elected, the Head office shall not be shifted to his new headquarters without the prior approval of the Central Council and the final approval of the General Body.

n. Only he shall correspond or represent on the all official matters of the association and issue a press release.

The Honorary Joint-Secretary

The Honorary Joint-Secretary shall assist the Secretary in looking after the office, in conducting correspondence and in preparing agendas for meetings statements, etc.

The Honorary Assistant Secretary

The Honorary Assistant Secretary shall assist the Secretary, the Joint Secretary, and the Treasurer.

The Honorary Treasurer

a. Shall receive all funds of the Association and deposit them to the credit of the Association in a bank approved by the Central Council, and operate all accounts and funds jointly along with the Secretary. These funds or a part of them may, if approved by the Central Council, be deposited with a nationalized bank or government/semi government financial body as specified by Income Tax Authority.

b. Shall maintain Head of Account for populations; CDH; CDE and any other office requiring handling of funds and credit it, in that, Head of Account shall issue cheques/DD, whenever the Editor, Chairman CDH, CDE or any other officer demands it and debit it to that Head of Account.

c. Shall be responsible for the collection of subscription from all members of the Association either directly or through branches.

d. Shall dispose off the bills for payments as sanctioned by the HSG and only on his written order.

e. Shall have the right to point out any error or discrepancy in the order of payment of the HSG and refer the order back to him with his remarks. In the event of disagreement still persisting between the HSG and the Honorary Treasurer, the matter shall be referred to the President for a final decision.

f. Shall be responsible for keeping up-to-date, the accounts and account books of the association.

g. Shall get all the accounts audited, by the auditor of the association.

h. Shall prepare an annual statement of accounts and a balance sheet showing the financial position of the association, get it audited by the registered auditor, appointed at the AGM, and put it up for adoption before the Central Council and then before the AGM/EOGM, for adoption through the Secretary.

Editor – Journal

a. Shall be in charge of the Journal of the IDA.

b. Shall, with the help of the Journal Committee, be responsible for raising funds for the publication and management of the journal.

c. Shall be Chairman of the Journal Committee.

d. Shall have the sole discretion of publishing or correcting any of the articles received for publication.

e. Shall prepare and submit the statement of accounts yearly with the help of treasurer to the Central Council.

Chairman—Council on Dental Health (CDH)

a. Shall be the Chairman of all meetings of the CDH and shall guide and control its activities.

b. Shall prepare and submit the statement of accounts yearly with the help of Treasurer to Central Council.

c. Shall nominate an Honorary Secretary of the CDH, to be approved by the Central Council, for a period of two years.

d. The Honorary Chairman shall organize, arrange and convene meetings of the CDH at an All India level, state level and local branch level in various places in consultation with HSG.

Chairman—Council on Dental Education (CDE)

a. The duty of the Chairman is to conduct continuing dental education programs at an All India level, state level and local branch level in various places.

b. Shall be the Chairman of all meetings of the CDE and shall guide and control its activities.

c. Shall prepare and submit the statement of accounts yearly with help of Treasurer to Central Council.

d. Shall nominate as Honorary Secretary to the CDE, to be approved by the Central Council, for a period of two years.

e. The Chairman shall organize, arrange and convene meetings of the CDE in consultation with the Secretary.

Chairman—International Committee

a. The duty of the Chairman is to assist the President and the Secretary to represent IDA at International level with affiliated bodies such as APDF, FDI, CDA.

b. Shall express the views of the association.

c. The Chairman shall organize, arrange and convene meetings of the International committee before the Central Council meetings.

d. Shall attend Central Council meeting for two year, from beginning till the end of his tenure of office as Chairman – International Committee.

Vice Chairman—International Committee

a. Vice Chairman shall assist the President, HSG and Chairman International Committee to represent IDA at International level.

b. Shall attend Central Council meeting for two year, from beginning till the end of his tenure of office as Vice Chairman – International Committee.

Chairman—ICCDE India Division

a. Shall be the Chairman of all meetings of the ICCDE India Division and shall guide and control its activities.
b. Shall draft policies for conduction of ICCDE/Accreditation program.
c. Shall represent India ICCDE Division at the International level.
d. Shall oversee general supervision of ICCDE Programs in India.
e. The Chairman shall organize, arrange and convene meetings of the ICCDE before the Central Council meetings in consultation with the Secretary – ICCDE India Division and Secretary.
f. Shall regulate the proceedings of ICCDE India Division meetings.
g. Shall attend Central Council meeting for two year, from beginning till the end of his tenure of office as Chairman ICCDE India Division.

Secretary– ICCDE India Division

a. Shall assist Chairman.
b. Shall liaison between the International CDE accreditation bodies.
c. Shall assist in drafting policies for conduction of accreditation Program.
d. Shall get prepared draft annual report in consultation with the Chairman for presentation before the Central Council.
e. Shall organize, arrange and convene ICCDE meeting before the Central Council meetings and keep records of the proceedings thereof.
f. Shall attend Central Council meeting for two year, from beginning till the end of his tenure of office as Secretary ICCDE India Division.
g. Shall promote the ICCDE in India.

De-Recognition of Branches

a. In the opinion of the Central Council, if a Branch is not functioning or functioning against the interests of the Association, the Central Council shall direct the HSG to issue a show cause notice as to why the recognition of the branch should not be withdrawn, giving three week's time to reply.
b. If the branch replies, kit shall be placed before the Central Council for consideration.
c. If the branch does not give any reply, the Central Council shall direct the Secretary to call for an EOGM of the members of the branch concerned, giving proper notice. In case of state branch or local branch de-recognition, the President and the Secretary General and the concerned state/local branch President and Secretary shall attend a meeting to redirect the branch to function in accordance with the directive of the Head Office. In case of the matter not being sorted out, a report will be made to the Central Council, which will have the right to withdraw the recognition granted to the state/local branch.

Elections

a. Persons, who are members in good standing only (as per clause no.6.H in the Article Membership), are eligible to contest for all offices of Head Office. Offices shall include all office bearers, and Representatives to Central Council.
b. Nominations shall be received by the HSG, with the name and signature of the proposer, and the seconder and the consent letter of the candidate in case of election for post of President Elect and 4 Vice Presidents. If a candidate/proposer/seconder is not in good standing at the time of filling his/her nomination, the nomination shall become invalid.
c. Only Annual/Silver/Gold and life members whose subscription has reached Head

Office before 31st July shall have the right to attend the AGM/EOGM of the Head Office an of State branch and of Local branch and vote on all resolutions put forward at the meetings and vote for elections of Office Bearers and for other post. Those who have paid the subscription after 31st July can only attend the AGM/EOGM but cannot vote.

d. A person who resigns from his post of an office-bearer before the completion of the tenure of his post is debarred from contesting for any other position of office till the completion of his unfinished tenure of office (HO).

e. Office bearers who do not submit their accounts, within the prescribed time limit at the time of handling over office to successors, are not eligible to contest for any office bearer's post at any level, including representative to Central Council/State or Local Branch Executive Committee, for a period of five years. On this issue the decision of Central Council shall be final.

f. If a member is readmitted, his previous attendance in Central Council and/or Local Branch Executive Committee or State branch Executive Committee will be held valid while considering eligibility criteria while contesting for any post at Local Branch or State Branch or Head Office if he has completed the tenure of the said post. Similarly, any office bearer post held by him previously at Local Branch, State Branch or Head Office will be considered valid while contesting for any office bearer post at Local Branch or State Branch or Head Office if he has completed the tenure of that post.

Qualifications for the nomination and contesting for Office Bearers

a. President Elect:

i. Should have served in the Executive Committee of a state branch for three terms, with at least 50% attendance in each term. The current term's attendance should not be considered.

ii. Should have been President of the state branch with at least 75% attendance in the meetings of the Executive Committee during the said term. The current term's attendance should not be considered.

iii. Should have served in the Central Council for three terms with at least 50% attendance in each term, out of which at least one term should have been within the preceding two terms. The current term's attendance shall not be considered.

iv. Should have served as Vice President of Head Office.

b. Vice President:

i. Should have served in the Executive Committee of a state branch for three terms with at least 50% attendance in each term. The current term's attendance should not be considered.

ii. Should have been President/Vice President of a state branch with at least 75% attendance at the meeting of EC during the said term. The current term's attendance should not be considered.

iii. Should have served in the Central Council for three terms with at least 50% attendance in each term, out of which at least one term should be within the preceding two terms. The current terms' attendance shall not be considered.

c. Hon. Secretary General:

i. Should have served in the Executive Committee of a state branch for three terms with at least 50% attendance in each term. The current term's attendance should not be considered.

ii. Should have served as President/Vice President of state branch with at least 75% attendance at the meeting of the Executive Committee during the said term. The current term's attendance should not be considered.

iii. Should have served in the Central Council for five terms with at least 50% attendance in each term, out of which at least one term should have been within the preceding two terms. The current terms' attendance shall not be considered.

d. **Hon. Joint Secretary:** The Hon. Joint Secretary must reside in the city where the HO is located, must be a member of that local branch and must have served for at least one term in the EC of the branch. The current term's attendance should not be considered.

e. **Hon. Asst. Secretary:** The Hon. Asst. Secretary must reside in the city where the HO is located, must be a member of that local branch and must have served for at least one term in the Executive Committee of the Branch. The current term's attendance should not be considered.

f. **Hon. Treasurer:** The Hon. Treasurer must reside at the city where the HO is located, must be a member of that local branch and must have served for at least one term in the Executive Committee of the Branch. The current term's attendance should not be considered.

g. **Editor Journal**
   i. Should have served in the Executive Committee of the state branch for three terms with at least 50% attendance in each term. The current term's attendance should not be considered.
   ii. Should have served in the Central Council for three terms with at least 50% attendance in each term, out of which at least one term should have within the preceding two terms. The current term's attendance should not be considered.
   iii. Should produce evidence of being Editor of a publication.

h. **Chairman C.D.H.**
   i. Should have served in the Executive Committee of a local or state branch for two terms, with at least 50% attendance in each term. The current term's attendance should not be considered.
   ii. Should have served in the Central Council for three terms with at least 50% attendance in each tem, out of which at least one term should be within the preceding two terms. The current term's attendance should not be considered.
   iii. Should have experience of conducting dental health programs at the state/local level and produce a certificate to that effect from the President or Secretary of the state or local branch.

i. **Chairman C.D.E.**
   i. Should have served in the Executive Committee of a local or state branch for two terms with at least 50% attendance in each term. The current term's attendance should not be considered.
   ii. Should have served in the Central Council for three terms with at least 50% attendance in each tem, out of which at least one term should be within the preceding two terms. The current term's attendance should not be considered.
   iii. Should have experience of conducting scientific programs, as a Convener of state/local branches or a Scientific Convener of annual IDA conferences of local or state branch or HO and produce a certificate to that effect from the President/Secretary/Chairman of the Conference.

j. **Chairman–International Committee:** Should have served as past President/past Hon. Secretary General of the Head Office.

k. **Vice Chairman–International Committee:** Should have served as past President/past Hon. Secretary General of the Head Office.

l. **Chairman – ICCDE India Division:** Should have served as past President/past Hon. Secretary General of the Head Office.

m. **Secretary – ICCDE India Division:** Should have served as past President/past Hon.

Secretary General or Chairman CDE/CDH of the Head Office.

Election Procedure for President—Elect and Vice President

a. The HSG shall on or before 1st May, each year, issue notice to state and local branches to nominate one member of the Association for the office of President-Elect and four members of the Association for the office of four Vice Presidents.

b. The nominations for these offices shall be by the branch Executive Committee, but before the nominations are forwarded to HSG, the Secretary of the branch should ascertain from the persons concerned whether he accepts the nomination and send such letter of acceptance to the HO along with eligibility certificate.

c. No member shall be eligible to stand for or hold two offices in HO during the same term. In such a case, his nomination becomes null and void for all posts. However, he can simultaneously apply for Representative to Central Council' from the State Branch.

d. The nomination should reach the office of the Secretary by 15th June each year. Nominations received after that date shall not be considered.

e. The eligible candidates as declared by the Screening and Scrutinizing Committee shall be intimated after the meeting and also shall be informed of the names of their co-contestants for the post they intend standing for. They shall be given 15 days time for withdrawal of their candidature if they so desire. The candidate or his/her representative can attend the Screening and Scrutinizing Committee meeting. The representative should carry authority letter from the candidate and should be member of IDA.

f. The HSG shall, on or before 15th September, send to all the branches and the direct members, the list of nominations received, requesting them to elect one name for the post of President-Elect and three names for the post of Vice-Presidents, from amongst the names in the list of nominees.

g. The Branch Secretary shall use this list for preparation of ballot papers to be used for voting at the EOGM, especially called for the purpose. The notice of the EOGM shall be forwarded to HO well in advance.

h. The counting of votes shall be done by two scrutinizers appointed by the President, in the presence of the President, Secretary and the candidates, or their representatives, who shall be IDA members and who shall have written authority from the Candidate, if present, at the EOGM of the Branch.

i. The voting by ballot shall be according to the procedure laid down by the Central Council, from time to time.

j. The voting by direct members shall be carried out by post, for which they will be supplied ballot papers from the HO, under postal certificate/Register A.D./speed post/courier, along with the list of nominations. The ballot papers must be sent to the HO by registered post/speed post/courier, before the specified last date.

k. The state branches, which have no local branches, shall conduct elections by calling an EOGM. The state branches having local branches under them should conduct elections by postal ballot for their direct members. They should follow the same procedure as above. The state branches, while sending the ballot papers, shall intimate the last date for receipt of ballot. The Screening and Scrutinizing Committee of the state branch shall meet on a fixed date earlier, tabulate the results, and send them to HO, in the format provided by HO, along with the original ballot papers received before the last date.

l. The election results should reach Secretary not later than 31st October, each year, after which they shall not be considered.

m. There shall be a Screening and Scrutinizing Committee. All the sealed envelopes shall be opened by the Secretary in the meeting of this committee and the committee shall tabulate the results and place the same before the Central Council.

n. The Secretary shall give 15 days clear notice to all candidates informing them about the date, time and place of the Screening and Scrutinizing Committee meeting, to enable them to be present at the meeting, either in person or by proxy, who shall carry an authority letter from candidate and who shall be a member of the association.

o. The person getting the largest number of votes shall be declared elected by the Central Council. In case of equality of votes, the President shall give his casting vote.

p. In the event of there being no nomination either for the posts of one President-Elect or any of the four Vice-Presidents received by the HO by the prescribed date of 15th June, the elections for these posts shall be held at the AGM and the eligibility criteria for the President-Elect and the Vice President shall remain the same. Election will be held by secret vote. The procedure for conducting elections remains the same as followed for the Secretary.

q. The candidate securing the highest number of votes at the election shall be deemed as the first Vice-President. The candidate securing the second highest number of votes shall be deemed as the second Vice-President. The candidate securing third highest number of votes shall be deemed as third Vice-President and the candidate securing forth highest number of votes shall be deemed as fourth Vice President. In case of a tie, the President shall give his casting vote.

r. If nominations are received for the posts of Vice-Presidents only, and if any of the elected Vice-Presidents resign to contest for the election of President-Elect at the AGM or for some other reasons, the order of precedence of the four Vice-Presidents will be determined on the basis of the number of votes polled by each of the remaining candidates, contesting for the election of Vice-President.

Election Procedure for Hon. Secretary General/Joint Secretary/Asst. Secretary/Treasurer/Editor/Chairman CDH/Chairman CDE/Chairman SDHP

a. One Honorary Secretary General, one Honorary Joint Secretary, one Honorary Assistant Secretary, one Honorary Treasurer, one Editor of the Journal, one Chairman-CDH, one Chairman on CDE shall be elected at the AGM of HO.

b. The outgoing Central Council shall have the power to nominate office bearers, whenever such a vacancy arises, with the previous consent of members concerned and recommend them to the Annual General Body.

c. AGM notice shall be posted to Members by Secretary not later than 30th November every year.

d. Nominations shall be called for in the AGM notice of HO for vacant posts with the last date for the receipt of nominations.

e. After getting the eligibility certificate from Branches and HO, the candidate shall send the nomination to the HSG by December 25 duly proposed and seconded to contest for the post. If the candidate, proposer and seconder are not member of good standing at time of filling the nomination, the nomination will be invalidated.

f. One candidate is eligible to contest only for one post. If one applies to contest for more than one post, all the nominations of the member shall become invalid automatically for all the posts. However, he can simultaneously apply for 'Representative to Central Council from the State Branch.

g. Names of eligible contestants as approved by the Central Council shall be announced at the AGM and the election conducted at the AGM by secret ballot.

h. Members, who would like to withdraw their candidature, shall withdraw within the stipulated date if announced in the AGM notice or at the AGM. No fresh nomination shall be received at the AGM unless there is a vacancy. Eligibility criteria to contest for HSG/Chairman CDE and CDH/Editor Journal shall remain same as prescribed under election qualification criteria even if nominations are taken on the floor of the House in case of vacancy. Also condition as mentioned in clause 6.E in this Article will apply. Members whose subscription is received in HO on or before 31st July every year only are eligible to vote in the AGM/EOGM.

Election Procedure for Chairman International Committee, Vice Chairman–International Committee and Chairman–ICCDE India Division, Secretary-ICCDE India Division

a. One Chairman-International Committee, Vice Chairman – International Committee, One Chairman – ICCDE India Division, One Secretary – ICCDE India Division shall be nominated at the Council Office Bearers meeting.
b. If more than one candidate is nominated for the posts then the election will be held through secret ballots in the council office bearers meeting.
c. Council Office bearers are only eligible to vote in such election, if held.
d. In case of a tie, the President shall give his casting vote.

Criteria for election of Representatives to the Central Council from State Branches

State branches shall elect their representatives to the Central Council at their AGM in the following scale, the number shall be on the basis of the total strength (Annual/Silver/Gold/Life membership) of the state branch as on 31st July as per HO records. Two Central Council posts namely that of State President and Secretary shall not be included in the above number:

a. For the first hundred Annual/Silver/Gold/Life Members or part thereof, there shall be three representatives.
b. For every additional two hundred Annual/Silver/Gold/Life Members or part thereof, there shall be one representative.
c. The names of such representatives shall be communicated to the HSG. The number of representatives of the state branches to the Central Council will be on the basis of the annual/Silver/Gold/life membership strength on 31st July. The membership strength will be calculated as per HO records and not the state or branch registers.
d. The election of the representatives to Central Council shall take place at the AGM of the state branch and the results shall be communicated to HO within a week of the election. The elected representatives shall hold office till the completion of their tenure and thereafter shall automatically cease to be representatives to the Central Council.

Removal of Office Bearers

Any office bearer shall be removed from office before completing his/her tenure, only by following the procedure as laid down hereunder, by bringing about a no confidence motion.

a. The changes against any office bearer has to be enunciated in the form of a resolution, signed by not less than 1/4th of the total number of members of the Association, as on 15th January addressed to the President and HSG, who shall circulate the same to all members and convene a special EOGM to discuss the issue, within 60 days from the date of receipt of the resolution. In case they fail to do so, the members signing the resolution can convene a special meeting themselves, after expiry of 60 days, but within a period of two months only for this purpose.

b. The Central Council has the right to enquire into the charges levelled against the office bearer concerned and every opportunity has to be provided to representing his case at any enquiry. Then the whole matter shall be placed before the special EOGM of the Association, giving the office bearer ample opportunity to state his case, after which the resolution shall be moved, to remove him from office.

c. If 2/3 of the members who are eligible to vote and who are present at the meeting and who cast their vote, vote in favour of the resolution it shall be passed with immediate effect.

d. The quorum for the special meeting shall be 1/4th of the total strength of the members as on the list.

e. The voting shall be by secret ballot.

f. Any member of the Central Council who is absent for three consecutive meetings without assigning a valid, reason/apology in writing, shall cease to be a member of the Central Council automatically. Notice to such members shall not be sent for the next Central Council meeting. Such members shall not be eligible for re-election/re-nomination for that Association term. This shall be intimated to the state office.

Casual Vacancies

a. Any vacancy occurring during the year, from amongst office bearers as mentioned in this chapter, except that of the President and Hon. Secretary General shall be filled by the Central Council. Eligibility criteria for any office bearer/Central Council member shall remain the same as prescribed under election qualification criteria.

b. Such office bearers/Central Council members elected from State branches shall hold office for the remaining tenure of that office.

c. In case of elected members from the branches, such as Representative to Central Council, such vacancies shall be filled by the State branch Executive concerned. Such members shall hold office only for the remaining tenure of the office.

d. A representative to the Central Council from states if removed as stated under clause 5.F in this article, shall not be re-nominated for that post again for that current term.

e. The candidate should be present at the Central Council/EOGM/AGM at the time of filling the causal vacancy to give his consent to accept the post or he should have sent his consent letter to HSG prior to the meeting or should send it through some member present at the time of the meeting. No member can suggest the name of any candidate on the floor of the House unless his consent letter has been received by HO.

f. In the event of the post of the President falling vacant due to some contingency such as resignation, demise etc., the first Vice-President shall succeed to the post of President for the remaining tenure of the post and in case of the HSG, the Joint Secretary shall succeed to the post of HSG for the remaining tenure of the post.

Meetings

Council Meetings

a. The Council Office Bearers shall ordinarily meet one hour prior to the Central Council meeting to discuss the matters of the HO, Subcommittees and etc.

Central Council Meeting

a. The Central Council shall ordinarily meet once in every three months. The exact date, time and place shall be fixed by the HSG in consultation with the President/Central Council.

b. The 1st Central Council and last Central Council of the year shall be held along with the HO conference, if one is held.

c. At least 21 days notice of the meeting shall be given to all the Central Council members, giving the place, date and hour of the meeting and the agenda of business to be transacted there-at. The business hours shall be form or between 9.00 am to 5.00 pm.

d. In emergencies, a shorter notice shall be allowed at the discretion of the HSG in consultation with the President. Btu in no case shall it be less than ten days.

e. 15 members shall form the quorum, of whom at least 10 shall be other than office bearers. In the absence of a quorum within 30 minutes of the appointed time, the meeting shall be adjourned. The adjourned meeting shall be held on the same day and place immediately. No quorum shall be required for the transaction of any business at such adjourned meetings.

f. A special meeting of the Central Council shall be called within 4 weeks on receipt of a requisition signed by at least 20 member of the Central Council, stating the business for which the special meeting is required. Notice for such special Central Council meeting shall be given 21 days in advance and quorum shall be 15, out of which 10 members shall be from amongst the requisitionists'. In the absence of a quorum within 30 minutes of the appointed time, the special meeting shall be dissolved.

g. The proceedings of the meeting of the Central Council shall be recorded, later on shall be typed and after confirmation shall be permanently preserved duly signed by President or Vice President or Chairman and HSG. The Central Council minutes shall be sent to all Central Council members, 30 days in advance of the next Central Council. If no correction is received within 10 days before the next Central Council meeting, no correction shall be taken on floor of the House at the time of approval of previous Central Council minutes. This register shall be kept in the HO and shall be open to members of the Central Council for inspection with 15 days prior notice.

The Annual General Body Meeting

The AGM shall be held once every year, ordinarily in the month of December/January (New year). This shall be the ordinary AGM of the Association. The notice of the AGM of HO shall be posted to the members, not later than 30th November every year, mentioning the place, date and time of the meeting and the agenda of the business to be brought up before it. The quorum for the AGM of HO shall be 50. If there is no quorum after 30 minutes of the scheduled time, the meeting shall be adjourned and reconvened immediately at the same venue with the same agenda where quorum will not be necessary.

a. The Agenda of the AGM shall be in the following order:

   i. The election, if necessary, (in the absence of the President and the Vice Presidents) of a Chairman from amongst the members present.

   ii. Welcome address by the President/Chairperson.

   iii. Confirmation of minutes of the previous AGM and E.O.G.M, if any.

   iv. Announcement of the results of the election for President Elect/Vice Presidents.

   v. Adoption of the annual report of HO; Journal Office; CDH Office; for the year ending 31st October.

   vi. Adoption of annual report of Treasurer and audited statement of accounts of the previous year, ending 31st March.

   vii. Any other motion for charge in the order of business.

   viii. Election of the Office-bearers and other elections, if any.

   ix. Appointment of an Auditor.

   x. Appointment of Legal Advisor.

   xi. Resolutions brought forward by the Central Council.

   xii. Resolutions brought forward by the state branches.

xiii. Resolutions brought forward by the local branches.

xiv. Resolutions brought forward by the individual members of the Association.

xv. Any other matter, with the permission of the Chair. (Matters raised under this agenda shall only be discussed and appropriate action shall be taken after discussion in the Central Council/ EOGM at a later date).

xvi. President's concluding remarks.

xvii. Handling over charge to incoming president and office bearers in the absence of closing ceremony.

xviii. Vote of thanks by the HSG.

b. **General rules about the Annual General body meeting**

i. No resolution shall be placed before the AGM that has not been previously considered by the Central Council.

ii. Resolutions to HO/AGM proposed by State EC, Local Branch EC or by individual members, duly signed and seconded by another member, shall be sent to HSG, with a copy to the state and local branches, not later than 1st October.

iii. The branch or the member sending the resolution must be informed immediately after the Central Council meeting in the month of November/ December, whether their resolution has been accepted or rejected by the Central Council.

iv. The HSG/Honorary Secretary shall issue, with the notice of the AGM, the preliminary agenda paper showing the business to be brought before the meeting, the terms of all motions to be moved, of which notice in writing has previously reached him and the name of the mover.

v. A member, who wishes to move a change to any item included in the agenda paper, or ask any question pertaining thereto, shall give notice thereof to the HSG so as to reach him not less than 14 clear days before the date fixed for the meeting.

vi. A notice of a resolution or an amendment shall be invalid unless accompanied by a copy of such motion or amendment.

vii. Any resolution of the Central Council may be considered at the AGM without notice being given.

c. **General rules of procedure at meetings: EOGM/AGM/Central Council**

i. The election, if necessary, (in the absence of the President and the Vice Presidents) of a Chairman from amongst the members present.

ii. Minutes of Central Council meetings shall be circulated by the HSG and shall be confirmed by the President/ Chairman of the meeting.

iii. Minutes of EOGM/AGM meetings shall be read at the respective AGM only and shall confirmed by the President/Chairman of the meeting of AGM.

iv. No resolution adopted or negated at a meeting shall be reconsidered unless either six months have elapsed or 1/5 of the members of the Central Council sign a requisition for such reconsideration.

v. The President/Chairman shall, in case of equality of votes, having a casting vote.

vi. No business shall be transacted at a special meeting/EOGM other than for which the meeting is called.

vii. The proceedings of any meeting shall not be invalid by reasons of there being any vacancy or any invalid appointment or election of any member or accidental omission to give notice of such meeting to any member.

viii. A notice may be served on any member either personally through an employee servant of the association or by post/courier.

d. **Extraordinary General Body Meeting (EOGM) of Head Office:**

i. The Central Council, whenever it thinks fit, or on requisition made in writing by at least 100 Annual/Silver/Gold/Life Members shall call an EOGM of HO.

ii. The members, while requisitioning, should state the objectives of the meeting proposed to be called and sign legibly giving their full name and address to the HSG who in consultation with the President, will call an EOGM within two months of the receipt of the requisition.

iii. If the meeting is not called within 2 months of the date on which notice is received by the HO, the concerned members themselves may convene an EOGM, but such meeting shall not be convened after four months of the date of the notice. After that the requisition notice will be treated as cancelled.

iv. Notice of the EOGM shall be sent to the members at least 21 days before the date fixed for the meeting, giving the place, date and time of the meeting and the agenda of the business to be transacted at such a meeting.

v. The EOGM on requisition shall be convened only at the HO of the Association. In other cases, the Central Council shall decide the venue. The quorum for the EOGM is 50 and in case of a requisitioned meeting it shall be 760, out of which at least 50 must be amongst the requisitionists.

vi. In case of there being no quorum within 30 minutes of an EOGM called by the Central Council, the meeting shall be adjourned and will meet again at the same venue with the same agenda after 30 minutes. In case of an adjourned meeting, no quorum is necessary. In case of requisitioned EOGM, if there is no quorum within 30 minutes, the EOGM shall be dissolved.

vii. Such meeting can be chaired by the President, Vice-Presidents in order of their precedence or Chairman can be elected.

Records

It will maintain the following records:

a. A register/computerized database of members with their membership number, name, qualification, current residence/mailing address, affiliated branch and a record of membership subscription renewals.

b. Account books, ledgers, cash books shall be retained up to a period of eight years, after which they can be destroyed. Audited balance sheets of all years shall be retained.

c. Correspondence beyond five years may be destroyed at the discretion of the HSG.

d. AGM and EOGM minutes, Central Council minutes, attendance registers of Central Council and AGM, membership records and important correspondence shall be retained permanently.

Funds/Finance

A. Branches are independent on their own with regard to finances, purchase of movable and immovable assets and formation of a Trust/Charitable Trust.

The funds of the Association shall be invested in the manner as specified in Section 11(5) of Income Tax Act. This association is an irrecoverable association. However, if the association becomes defunct or dissolved, the assets/funds of the association shall be vested with an association or society with similar objectives. There shall not be any activity of the association with intention of earning any profit. The funds of the Association shall be solely utilized towards the objects and no portion of it will be utilized for payment to its members by way of profit, interest, dividend etc.

The Treasurer shall pay Rs.5,000/10,000 cash as advance to an Office bearer of the above section as approved by Central Council on reimbursement basis on receipt of vouchers.

One copy of the audited and approved statement of accounts shall be forwarded to the HO in case of State branches; HO and State office in case of Local branches every year immediately after the AGM. The accounts of the HO shall be audited and approved by the Central Council and circulated to the members before being placed at the AGM or HO for its final approval.

Income

Funds of the Association irrespective of whatever heads they belong to, i.e., Journal, CDH, CDE, etc., shall be received only by the Treasurer HO and credited in respective heads of account maintained with the Head Office.

The funds or the income of the HO shall be derived from the following sources:

a. Subscription from direct members.
b. Central share of contribution from the branches on account of the members on their rolls.
c. Special contributions or donations raised directly or through the branches.
d. Income derived from the journal and other publications of the Association.
e. Contributions received on account of organizing Indian Dental Conferences.
f. Bequests received through legacies from persons who desire benefit the association.
g. Member's benevolent fund in which the life members subscription as paid by member shall be credited after the death of Life Member.
h. Sponsorship of such other sources as may be authorized by the Central Council.

i. Surplus funds from CDE/CDH programs if any.

Expenditure

a. The Central Council shall out of the funds of the Association debit all ordinary expenses and shall pay rents, salaries, wages and such other charges as may be necessary for carrying out the work of the Association.
b. It shall, further provide for the issue of the journal/publication of the Association and such other publications as may be authorized.
c. It shall be empowered to spend money on scientific investigations, conferences, prizes scholarships and on such other purposes as it may consider advisable in furtherance of the objects of the Association.
d. All major expenses in excess of Rs.50,000/- other than routine administrative expenses shall have to be approved by the Central Council.

Head of Account

a. Only IDA Head Office shall open and operate/handle all accounts/financial matters of Head Office.
b. All receipts pertaining to CDE, CDH, Journal/Publications and any other activity shall be received by IDA Head Office Treasurer and remitted in respective heads.
c. No other office bearer shall operate independent account/s in bank/s.
d. The Hon. Treasurer shall maintain various heads of accounts of income and expenditure.
e. All income shall be payable to Treasurer IDA Head Office and it shall be credited into respective head of accounts.
f. On the expenditure side, the Hon. Treasurer shall debit the expenses on the respective head of account and issue Demand Draft on the advice of Chairman

CDH/CDE, and journal and publication/s Editor and other Conveners if any and debit it in the head of account.

g. In case of Head Office, all funds/all bank accounts and all other accounts will be operated and handled by Hon. Treasurer jointly with the Secretary.

Accounts

The Annual Statement of audited accounts and the Balance Sheet, for the period starting from 1st April and ending 31st March of every year, after auditing, shall be submitted to the Central Council, circulated to members and placed in AGM by the Treasurer and the Secretary.

The IDA Head Office Conference Accounts shall be audited by Head Office auditor and presented separately to Central Council for approval.

Reserve Fund

There shall be a reserve fund of the Association. The reserve fund shall be 50% of the net surplus income of the first year of the branch concerned. In addition, 25% of the net surplus should be credited to this fund every year. This applies to Head Office and branches. The reserve fund shall only be drawn upon by a special resolution of a meeting of the Central Council in case of Head Office, EC in case of branches in which ¾ of the members who are present and who cast their vote, vote in favour of the resolution of withdrawal.

Appointment of an Auditor

a. A Chartered Accountant shall be appointed as auditor at the AGM of the Association every year for auditing the accounts of the Head Office. Similarly an auditor shall be appointed at AGM of State Branch and Local Branch for auditing the accounts of respective branches. One Internal Auditor may be appointed. He should go through

accounts before the auditor certifies the accounts. The guidelines to be framed by the Central Council.

b. Duties of the auditor:
   • Shall audit the accounts at the end of the year, and certify to their correctness.
   • Shall give suggestions for the proper keeping of accounts as required.

Liability

Neither the IDA nor any of its branches shall be liable for any of the debts or liabilities of one another.

STATE BRANCHES

The State Branch is that branch of the association which has its jurisdiction within the stat territory and shall cover all members of the State or Union Territory. It shall be made up of various local branches within the same territory and shall have its office headquarters within the same State/Union Territory where the Hon. State Secretary resides/practices. Every state branch will act as the co-ordinating link between the HO and local branches. It will oversee the functions and activities of its local branches. The state branch shall function under the auspice of the HO and abide by the rules and regulations of the HO who may de-recognize it for breach of rule or condition of the byelaws.

Formation

a. The members residing and practicing in an individual state (if there are no local branches), or the President/Secretaries or members of local branches in a state shall unite to form a state branch on a territorial basis.

b. The members or Presidents/Secretaries of the local branches should sign a written document, proposing to start the branch, mentioning the name, address and membership number. They will elect their office bearers and shall forward the complete proposal to the Head Office for approval. After verification the HSG will put the proposal before the Central Council or final approval. On approval, the HSG will inform the President and Hon. State Secretary to officially commence the functioning of the state branch.

c. There will be only one state branch in a State/Union Territory.

d. The general management of the state branches shall be vested with the EC of the branch, under guidance from Head Office. No one in receipt of salary or honorarium from the funds of the association can be elected as office bearer of the association.

Management

The general management of the state branch as a whole shall be vested with the EC of the branch, under guidance from Head Office. No one in receipt of salary or an honorarium from the funds of the association can be elected as office bearer of the association.

a. Composition:

Staff office bearers	Tenure
1. President	One Term
2. President Elect	One Term
3. Three Vice-Presidents	One Term
4. Honorary State Secretary	Three Terms
5. Honorary Joint Secretary	Three Terms
6. Honorary Assistant Secretary	Three Terms
7. Honorary Treasurer	Three Terms
8. Editor of the Journal (Optional)	Three Terms
9. Chairman – Council on Dental Health	One Term
10. Chairman – Council on Dental Education	One Term
11. Immediate Past President	One Term

b. Members of the EC (Without portfolio) — One Term

(The number shall be on the basis of the total strength of the state branch as on 31st July as per HO records. For every 100 Life/Silver/Gold/Annual Members or part thereof, there shall be one EC member).

c. Representatives from local branch to State Executive — One Term

d. Representatives from state branch to Central Council HO — One Term

The number shall be on the basis of the total strength of the state branch as on 31st July as per Head Office records (for every 100 Life/Silver/Gold/Annual Members or part thereof, there shall be three representatives. For every additional 200 Life/Silver/Gold/Annual members or part thereof there shall be one representative. In addition, State President and Secretary will be the Central Council members from the State). It is optional for state branches to decide whether they should be members of the State EC also or not, in addition to their duties as representative of the Central Council which shall be decided in the AGM of the State branch.

Functions and Powers of the State Executive Committee (EC)

The state branch office will look after all the activities linked to its respective state. It will guide the local branches, which are affiliated to it, in all matters and shall become the medium of communication between local branches and Head Office.

The State Executive Committee shall regulate the general affairs of the association and work within the framework of the Constitution and as per the directive of the Central Council. It will have the following powers and functions:

a. To conduct business at the EC meetings, maintain the Association office, office equipment, properties, etc. and organize scientific deliberations and publications.

b. To peruse sub-committees appointed by the President in consultation with the Hon. State Secretary.

c. To represent the Association to the State Government or to any other public body within the state, in the interests of the dental profession and of the Association.

d. To consider and to take decisions on resignations and applications for direct membership to the state branch, and to recommend any disciplinary action required against members of the state branch, to the Central Council.

e. To write off the whole or part of the arrears against members of the state branch, to the Central Council.

f. To approve the audited balance sheet before presenting it at the AGM/EOGM.

g. To appoint or remove salaried employees of the state branch office.

h. To purchase, take lease or otherwise acquire, to form a trust as per govt. regulations, to manage, lend, exchange, sell, mortgage or otherwise dispose of movable or immovable properties of every description and all rights and privileges necessary or convenient for the purpose of the association within the same limits, if agreed on by a 2/3 majority, amongst the member who are present and those who cast their vote.

i. To build, maintain improve or alter and repair any buildings or premises owned by the state branch of the Association.

j. To borrow or to raise funds in such a manner as the State Executive may think fit and to collect subscriptions and donations for the state branch of the association.

k. To invest funds of the state branch, not immediately required for any of the objectives of the Association, in such manner as may from time to time be determined by the State EC.

l. To recommend the formation of local branches in the state branch territory.

m. To appoint one Conference Secretary for state conferences.

n. To approve one Chairman, Organizing Committee, Organizing Secretary and Treasurer for conducting state conferences.

o. To send the branch's quarterly activity reports to the HO at the end of every quarter of the IDA year.

p. To resolve any disputes at the state level or at the local branch level, within the state.

Term of the Central Council

a. The EC shall enter upon its duties at the close of the AGM of the state branch and shall hold office till the next AGM of the state branch or till 31st December, whichever is earlier.

b. The Office Bearers and members shall function forthwith after election and shall continue as members till the end of their tenure as mentioned in clause 2.A in this Article State Branch, and will automatically cease to be office bearers or EC member after that.

c. Any member of the EC who is absent for three consecutive meetings without assigning a valid, reason/apology in writing shall cease to be a member of the EC, automatically. Notice to such members shall not be sent for the next EC meeting. Such members shall not be eligible for re-election/re-nomination for that Association year.

Office Bearers' Duties and Powers

The President

a. Shall be the Chairman of AGM/EOGM, at all meetings of the EC and sub committees appointed by him, and any other committee for which no chairman has been appointed. He shall be a member of all committees.

b. Shall preside at the Annual Conference of his branch.

c. Shall guide and render advice for the activities of the Association, in his/her branch.

d. Shall regulate the proceedings of the meetings and conferences.

e. Shall, in addition to his ordinary vote, have a casting vote. In case of equality of votes, if he fails to give his casting vote, the motion shall be declared invalid.

f. Shall continue as a member of the state branch EC, as the case may be, for one term, beginning with the end of his tenure of office as President.

g. Shall have the right to attend any meeting EC; AGM; EOGM of any local branch in his/her state.

The President—Elect

a. Shall be a member of the EC and shall assist the President in the performance of his duties.

b. Shall succeed to the office of the President at the end of the AGM of the conference or at the end of the AGM/EOGM if there is no conference in the year following his election as President Elect.

The Vice President

a. Any one of the three Vice-Presidents in their order of precedence shall act as Chairman of the meetings of the EC/AGM/EOGM, in the absence of the President.

b. Any one of the three Vice-Presidents in their order of precedence shall be the Chairman of all sub-committees for which no Chairman has been appointed, even if he is not a member of that committee only in the absence of the President.

c. All Vice Presidents shall help the branches in organizational activities.

The Honorary Secretary General

a. With the help of Hon. Joint Secretary and Hon. Asst. Secretary of his/her branch, the Honorary State Secretary will have the following duties:

b. Shall be in charge of the branch office. Shall conduct all correspondence of his/her branch and shall maintain a proper register of the branch.

c. Shall have general supervision of accounts; pass all bills for payments and sign cheques of his/her branch jointly with the Hon. Treasurer.

d. Shall obtain from the Hon. Branch Treasurer an annual statement of accounts duly audited by the Auditor, for presentation before the EC and AGM of the branch.

e. Shall prepare a budget and present it for approval at the EC meeting of his/her branch after the AGM.

f. Shall organize, arrange and convene meetings, conferences, lectures and demonstrations of his/her branch.

g. Shall attend a meeting of the EC and sub-committees of his/her branch and keep proceedings thereof; and be a member of all committees of his/her branch.

h. Shall assist the President in appointing sub-committees of his/her branch.

i. Shall maintain a correct and up-to-date register/computer database of all members of the branch.

j. Honorary State Secretary shall have the right to attend any meeting of EC/AGM/EOGM of local branches within his/her state.

k. Shall be responsible for sending the share of subscription to HO within 15 days/before due date i.e. 31st January, whichever is earlier along with Names, address, membership no., Local branch name etc., of the members whose share has been sent to him.

l. Shall maintain a property register.
   In case the State Secretary, changes his/her personal head quarters to any other town, after being duly elected, the State Secretary Office shall not be shifted to his/her new head quarters, without the prior approval of the EC of the state branch.

The Honorary Joint-Secretary

a. Shall help the Hon. State Secretary in his/her looking after the office, in conducting correspondence, in preparation of agenda of meetings, in preparing budget etc.
b. Shall act for the Hon. State Secretary, in his/her absence.

The Honorary Assistant Secretary

Shall help the Hon. State Secretary in looking after the office, conducting correspondence, preparation of agenda of meetings and preparing budget, etc.

The Honorary Treasurer

a. Shall receive all funds of his/her branch and deposit them in a bank approved by the EC of the branch, to the credit of the branch and shall operate all funds and all accounts jointly with the Hon. State Secretary.
b. The Hon. Treasurer shall be responsible for the collection of subscriptions from all the members of the branch through the Secretary.
c. Shall dispose off the bills for payment as sanctioned by the Hon. Secretary of the branch and only on his written order.
d. Shall have the right to point out any error or discrepancy in the order of payment of the Hon. State Secretary and refer the order back to him with his remarks. In the event of disagreement still persisting between the Hon. State Secretary and Honorary Treasurer, the matter shall be referred to the President for a final decision.
e. Shall be responsible for keeping up-to-date, the accounts and accounts books of the branch.
f. Shall get all the accounts audited by the auditor of the branch.
g. Shall prepare an annual statement of accounts and a balance sheet showing the financial position of the branch, get it audited by the registered auditor, appointed at the AGM of his branch and put it for adoption before the AGM through the Hon. State Secretary of the branch.

Editor—Journal

a. Shall be in charge of the Journal of the state branch.
b. Shall, with the help of the Journal Committee of the branch, be responsible for publication and management of the journal.
c. Shall be Chairman of the Journal Committee of the Branch.
d. Shall have the sole discretion of publishing or correcting any of the articles received for publication in the journal of the branch.
e. Shall submit the yearly statement of accounts to the EC of the branch.

Chairman—Council on Dental Health

Shall coordinate/liaison with Chairman CDH of HO in conducting CDH activities of HO at the state level.

J. Chairman – Council on Dental Education

Shall coordinate/liaison with Chairman CDE of HO in conducting CDE programs of HO at the state branch level.

Elections

General Rules for Election of Office-bearers

a. Persons, who are members in good standing (membership [new/renewed] subscription received at HO by 31st January) only, are eligible to stand for office of the State Branch. This includes all office bearers and Representatives to the Central Council and EC members without portfolio.
b. Nominations shall be received by on. State Branch Secretary with the name and signature of the proposer and seconder, along with the written consent of the candidate (only in case of election for the post of President Elect and 3 Vice Presidents if State Branch elect them as per HO procedure. If the President Elect and VP's are elected at the AGM they have to apply

themselves individually and their consent is not necessary) and copies of the relevant eligibility documents. If a candidate/proposer/seconder is not in good standing at the time of filling his/her nomination, the nomination shall become invalid.

c. Only those members who subscription is received at the HO by 31st July every year are eligible to vote for elections of President Elect and Vice Presidents of the State Branch.

d. Only Annual/Silver/Gold and life members whose subscription has reached HO before 31st July shall have the right to attend the AGM/EOGM of the HO and of State branch and of Local branch and vote on all resolutions put forward at the meetings and vote for elections of Office Bearers and for other post. Those who have paid the subscription after 31st July can only attend the AGM/EOGM but cannot vote in elections or on any resolution.

e. A person who resigns from his post of an office-bearer before the completion of the tenure of his/her post, to contest for any other office bearer's post during his/her unfinished tenure is debarred from contesting for any other office till the completion of his/her unfinished tenure of office in state branch.

f. Office bearers who do not submit accounts of their office on time or at the time of handling over office to successors, conference accounts within the prescribed time limit are not eligible to contest for any office bearer's post at Head Office, State Branch or Local Branch including representative to Central Council/EC for a period of five years. On this issue the decision of Central Council shall be final.

g. The candidate securing the highest number of votes at the election shall be deemed as the first Vice-President. The candidate securing the second highest number of votes shall be deemed as the Second Vice-President and the candidate securing the third highest number of votes shall be

deemed as the third Vice-President. In case of a tie, President shall give his casting vote.

h. If a member is readmitted, his previous attendance in Central Council and/or Local Branch EC or State branch EC will be held valid while considering eligibility criteria while contesting for any post at Local Branch or State Branch or HO if he has completed the tenure of the said post. Similarly, any office bearer post held by him previously at Local Branch, State Branch, HO will be considered valid while contesting for any office bearer post at the Local Branch or State Branch or HO if he has completed the tenure of that post.

Qualifications required to contest for Office Bearer posts

a. **President Elect**
   i. Should have served as President of a local branch with at least 75% attendance in the meetings of the EC during the said term. The current term's attendance should not be considered.
   ii. Should have served in the EC of the state branch for five terms with 50% attendance in each term, out of which one term should be within the preceding two terms. The current term's attendance should not be considered.

b. **Vice Presidents**
   i. Should have served as President/Vice President of a local branch with at least 75% attendance in the meeting of the EC. The current term's attendance should not be considered.
   ii. Should have served in the EC of the state branch for three terms with at least 50% attendance in each term, out of which one term should be within the preceding two terms. The current terms' attendance should not be considered.

c. **Hon. Secretary General**
   i. Should have served as Hon. Secretary of a local branch with at least 75% attendance in the meeting of the EC during

the said term. The current term's attendance should not be considered.

ii. Should have served in the Executive Committee of the state branch for three terms with at least 50% attendance in each term, out of which one term should be within the preceding two terms. The current terms' attendance shall not be considered.

d. **Hon. Joint Secretary:** Should have served in Local Branch Executive Committee for one term with at least 50% attendance and must reside in the same place/town where the Hon. State Secretary resides/practices. The current term's attendance should not be considered.

e. **Hon. Asst. Secretary:** Should have served in Local Branch Executive Committee for one term with at least 50% attendance and must reside in the same place/town where the Hon. State Secretary resides/practices. The current term's attendance should not be considered.

f. **Hon. Treasurer:** Should have served in Local Branch Executive Committee for one term with at least 50% attendance and must reside in the same place/town where the Hon. State Secretary resides/practices. The current term's attendance should not be considered.

g. **Editor Journal**

i. Should have served in the Executive Committee of the state branch for three terms with at least 50% attendance in each term. The current term's attendance should not be considered.

ii. Should produce evidence of being associated with any Committee of Scientific Publication, or at least Chairman, Co-Chairman of the Scientific Session of any state or local branch conference.

h. **Chairman – Council on Dental Health:** Should have served in the State EC for two terms with 50% attendance in each term. The current term's attendance should not be considered.

i. **Chairman = Council on Dental Education:** Should have served in the state EC for two terms with 50% attendance in each term. The current term's attendance should not be considered.

j. **For EC members (without portfolio) no special qualification is required.**

k. **Representatives to the Central Council from State Branch**

(Kindly refer to Article – State Branch clause No.C.7 also)

i. President/Secretary category-Category 1 State branch President and State branch Secretary shall be Central Council members.

ii. Existing Central Council Members category – Category 2

Out of total Central Council seats, 60% seats are reserved for existing Central Council members as follows:

1. *Category 2-A:* 30% seats are reserved for existing Central Council member who have attended 75% of Central Council meetings till 31st October of the current ongoing term.

2. *Category 2-B:* 30% seats are reserved for existing Central Council member who have attended 50% of Central Council meetings till 31st October of the current ongoing term.

iii. New Central Council Member's category – Category-3

1. Existing Central Council members not eligible to contest under Category-2.

2. Life/Silver/Gold/Annual member who was a member of Central Council/ EC in a state or local branch for two terms, with at least 50% attendance in each term. The current term's attendance should not be considered.

3. Those members who contested in Category-2 and lost.

The names of all office bearers, Central Council members, other state representative shall be communicated to the HO within a week of the election. The Central Council representatives elected from State shall hold office till the completion of his/her tenure of office and thereafter shall automatically cease to be a representative to the Central Council.

Election Procedures

1. **President and Vice Presidents:** The state branch has no option of conducting these elections either as per the procedure laid down for HO President Elect and Vice President election or at the state AGM.

    Those branch who wish to conduct elections as per HO should follow the following procedure. If they prefer to follow this procedure only those members whose subscription is received at HO by 31st July are eligible to vote.

    a. The Hon. State Secretary shall, on or before 1st of July each year, invite local branches to nominate one member for the office of President-Elect and three members for the office of three Vice Presidents.

    b. The nominations for these offices shall be by the local branch Executive Committee.

    c. The nomination should reach the office of the Hon. Secretary not later than 15th August each year. Nominations received after that date shall not be considered.

    d. The eligible candidates as declared by the Screening and Scrutinizing Committee shall be intimated after the meeting and also shall be informed of the names of their co-contestants for the post they intend to contest for. They shall be given 15 days for withdrawal of their candidature if they desire to do so. The candidate on his/her representative, who shall be a member of the Association and who shall carry authority letter from the candidate, may attend the screening and scrutinizing committee meeting.

    e. The Hon. State Secretary shall, on or before 30th September, send the election notice to all the local branches and the Direct Members along with the list of nominations received, requesting them to elect one candidate for the post of President-Elect and 3 candidates for the post of Vice-Presidents from amongst the candidates in the list of nominees.

    f. The local Branch Secretary shall use this list for preparation of ballot papers to be used for voting at the EOGM, especially called for the purpose and a copy of notice of EOGM shall be posted so as to reach State Office one week in advance.

    g. The counting of the votes shall be done by two scrutinisers recommended by the President and approved by the EOGM, in the presence of the candidates, or their representatives, if present, at the EOGM of the Branch.

    h. The voting shall be done according to the procedure laid down by the Central Council from time to time.

    i. The voting by direct members shall be by post for which they will be supplied ballot papers from the state office under postal certificate/Register AD/Speed Post/Courier, along with the list of candidates. The ballot papers must be sent to the State Office by Registered/Speed Post/Courier before the last date.

    j. The election results should reach the Hon. State Secretary not later than 31st October each year if elections are held at the local branch AGM/EOGM after which they shall not be considered.

    k. There shall be a Scrutinizing Committee. All the sealed envelopes shall be opened by the Hon. State Secretary during the meeting of the Scrutinizing Committee and the committee shall tabulate the results and place the same before the EC.

    l. The Hon. State Secretary shall give 15 days clear notice to all the candidates informing them about the date, time and place of the Scrutinizing Committee meeting to enable them to be present at the meeting, either in person or by proxy, who shall be a member of the association and who shall carry a letter of authority from candidate.

m. The person getting the highest number of votes shall be declared elected as president Elect by the Executive Committee. In case of equality of votes, the President shall give his casting vote.

n. For the post of Vice-President, the candidate securing the highest number of votes at the election shall be deemed as the first Vice-President. The candidate securing the second highest number of votes shall be deemed as the second Vice-President and the candidate securing the third highest number of votes shall be deemed as the third Vice-President. In case of a time, the President shall give his casting vote.

o. In the event of there being no nomination received by the state office, by the prescribed date of 15th August, either for the post of one President-elect or any one of the three Vice-Presidents, the elections for these posts shall be held at the AGM and the eligibility criteria for the President-Elect and the Vice-President shall remain the same. Election will be held by secret ballot. The procedure for conducting elections remains the same as followed for the HSS.

p. If nominations are received for the posts of Vice-President only, and if any of the elected Vice-Presidents resign to contest for the election of President-Elect at the AGM, or for some other reasons, the order of precedence of the three Vice-Presidents will be determined on the basis of the number and votes polled by each of the remaining candidates contesting for the election of the Vice-President.

q. In the event of the post of the President falling vacant due to some contingency such as resignation, demise etc., the first Vice-President shall succeed to the post of President and act as President for the remaining tenure of the office. In such a case the same person will get attendance certificate as Vice President only for the same tenure and not as President.

The state branches shall elect the Hon. State Secretary, Hon. Joint Secretary, Hon. Assistant Secretary, Hon. Treasurer, Editor (if any), Chairman CDH, Chairman CDE and representatives to the Central Council and EC members (without portfolio) (and President Elect and Vice Presidents as per the option exercised by the State Branch) at the AGM.

2. **Representatives to the Central Council:** The state branches shall elect their representatives to the Central Council at their AGM in the following scale:

a. State President and Secretary shall be Central Council members.

b. The number of representatives of the state branches to the Central Council will be on the basis of the Annual/Silver/Gold/life membership strength of the branch as on 31st July as per the HO records. While calculating the number of Central Council members from State, the President and Secretary seats will not be included in that number.

c. For the first 100 Annual/Silver/Gold/Life members, 3 representatives.

d. For every additional 200 Annual/Silver/Gold/Life Members or part thereof, 1 representative. The names of such representatives shall be communicated to the Hon. Secretary General for information.

e. The election of the representatives to Central Council shall take place at the AGM of the State branch and the results shall be communicated to HO within a week of the election.

f. The elected representatives shall hold office till the completion of their tenure of office and thereafter shall automatically cease to be representatives to the Central Council.

g. Out of total number of Central Council representatives from state branch 30% sets are reserved for category 2-A of existing Central Council members with 75% attendance, 30% seats are reserved for category 2-B of existing Central Council members with 50% attendance and 40% seats are reserved for category 3 of new Central Council members. In case there are more candidates than the posts available in category 2 (A & B) of existing Central Council members, elections within these candidates should be carried out. In case there is a vacancy/ies in this category it will be passed on to category 3 of New Central Council members.

3. **Representatives to the State Executive Committee from Local Branches**

   a. The local branches shall elect representatives to the State EC during their AGM on the basis of membership strength as on 31st July, as per HO records. For the first 100 Annual/Silver/Gold/Life members there shall be 3 representatives out of whom one shall be Local Branch President or Secretary. Over and above this, for every additional slab of 100 or part thereof, there shall be one representative.

4. **Election procedure for Hon. State Secretary/Joint Secretary/Treasurer/Editor/Chairman CDH/Chairman CDE/Central Council members/EC members (without portfolio) and President Elect and three Vice President if applicable to be conducted at the AGM**

   a. The state branch shall conduct elections at the AGM as per the procedure hereinafter laid down for all post of office bearers; Members of EC and Representatives of State Branch to the Central Council.

   b. The Hon. State Secretary shall invite nominations from members of the branch for the election of office bearers and President Elect and three Vice Presidents if applicable (in case election of President Elect and Vice Presidents held at AGM, the candidates shall directly send their nominations to HSS and they shall not be nominated by Branches) Members of the EC and Representative to Central Council on or before 30th September every year.

   c. These nominations from the candidates duly proposed and seconded by members in good standing shall reach the Hon. State Secretary by 25th October.

   d. Candidates who would like to withdraw their candidature shall withdraw before the last date, announced in the AGM notice or at the AGM.

   e. No fresh nominations shall be received at the AGM unless there is a vacancy.

   f. No member shall stand for two state offices simultaneously. If he/she does so, his/her candidature shall become null and void for all posts. However, the candidate may simultaneously apply for EC member without portfolio and/or Representative to Central Council from State Branch.

   g. A state EC shall be called for before the AGM to consider the eligibility of the candidates.

   h. The contestants found eligible to contest, received from amongst the members of the branch shall be put to vote at the AGM of the state branch.

   i. Two Scrutinisers shall be appointed at the AGM.

   j. The office bearers/Members of EC/Representative to Central Council shall be elected at the AGM of the branch.

   k. Should there be more than the allotted number of candidates for any office the voting shall be carried out by secret ballot.

   l. In case of a tie, the President shall cast his casting vote.

5. Mode of exercising options of State Branch

  a. State and local branches are given certain options in this Constitution to be decided. Such options shall be decided at the AGM or EOGM of the branch concerned and intimated to the HO accordingly.

6. Casual Vacancies

  a. Any vacancy occurring during the year, from amongst office bearers as mentioned in this chapter, except that of the President and Hon. State Secretary shall be filled by the State EC. Eligibility criteria for any office bearer/EC members shall remain the same as prescribed under election qualification criteria.

  b. Such office bearers/EC members elected from Local branches shall hold office for the remaining tenure of that office.

  c. In case of EC members elected from the Local Branches, any vacancies arising shall be filled by the Local Branch Executive concerned. Such members shall hold office only for the remaining tenure of the office.

  d. A representative to the EC from Local Branches if removed as stated under Clause C.7.f in this Article shall not be re-nominated for this post again for that current term.

  e. The candidate should be present at the State EC/EOGM/AGM at the time of filling the causal vacancy to give his consent to accept the post or he should have sent his consent letter to the Hon. State Secretary prior to the meeting or should send it through some member presents at the time of the meeting. No member can suggest the name of any candidate on the floor of the House unless his consent letter has been received by State Office.

  f. In the event of the post of the President falling vacant due to some contingency such as resignation, demise etc., the first Vice-President shall succeed to the post of President for the remaining tenure of the post and in case of Hon. State Secretary, the Joint Secretary shall succeed to the post of Hon. State Secretary for the remaining tenure of the post.

7. Removal of Office Bearers: Any office bearer can be removed from office before completing his/her tenure, only by following the procedure as laid down here under, for bringing a no confidence motion.

  a. The charges against any office bearer have to be enunciated in the form of a resolution signed by not less than 1/4th of the total number of members of the branch as on 1st November, to the President and Honorary State Secretary who shall circulate the same to all the members and convene a special EOGM to discuss the issue, within 60 days from the date of receipt. In case they fail to do so, the members signing the resolution can convene a special meeting themselves, after expiry of 60 days within a period of 2 months only for this purpose.

  b. The EC has the right to enquire into the charges levelled against the office bearer concerned and every opportunity has to be provided to him/her to appear or to represent his case at any enquiry.

  c. The whole matter shall then be placed before the special EOGM of the State branch, giving ample opportunity to the office bearer to state his case, after which the resolution shall be moved, to remove him from Office and if 2/3 of the members present at the meeting and who are eligible to vote and who cast their vote, vote in favour of the resolution, it shall be passed with immediate effect.

  d. The voting shall be by secret ballot.

  e. The quorum for the special meeting shall be 1/4th of the total membership strength of the branch as on 31st October as per HO records.

f. Any member of the EC (without portfolio directly elected or representatives from local branch to State EC) of branches who is absent for three consecutive meetings, without assigning a valid, reason/apology in writing, shall cease to be a member of the EC automatically. Notice to such members shall not be sent for the next EC meeting. Such members shall not be eligible for re-election/re-nomination for that Association term. This shall be intimated to local branch.

8. Meetings

A. *Executive committee meeting of state branch*

a. The State EC shall ordinarily meet at least once in three months. The last EC shall be held one day prior to the State conference or the AGM, if the conference is not held. A notice of 14 days shall be given to members. However, in case of urgent meetings, the notice shall be of seven days. The exact date and time (between 9.00 am to 5.00 pm only), shall be fixed by the Hon. State Secretary in consultation with state president. 10 members of the EC, of whom at least 5 shall be other than office bearers, shall form the quorum. In the absence of a quorum within 30 minutes of the appointed time, the meeting shall be adjourned. The adjourned meeting shall be held immediately at the same venue with the same agenda where quorum will not be necessary.

b. A special requisition meeting of the EC shall be called within 4 weeks on receipt of the requisition signed by at least 10 members of the EC, stating the business for which a special meeting is required. Notice for such a meeting shall be given 14 days in advance and quorum shall be 10 members of the EC, out of which at least 5 members shall be from amongst the requisitionists'. In the absence of a quorum, within 30 minutes of the appointed time, the special requisition meeting shall be dissolved.

c. Proceedings of the meeting of the EC shall be recorded in the form of typed minutes and after confirmation shall be permanently preserved. The Executive Committee minutes shall be sent to all the state Executive Committee members along with the notice and agenda for the next Executive Committee meeting. Any correction by state executive members should reach Hon. State Secretary at least three days prior to the date of the Executive Committee Meeting. If no correction is received by the State Secretary, at least three days before the next EC, either by register post/courier/email, no correction shall be permitted at the EC meeting unless approved by the President. This register shall be kept in the State Secretary's Office and shall be open to members of the State Executive Committee for inspection.

B. *The annual general body meeting:* It is compulsory for all the branches to conduct their AGM between 1st November and 31st December every year and make known the election results to HO. If a state branch does not conduct its AGM and election by 31st December, the President Elect of the branch shall assume office automatically as President on 1st January. He shall then issue a notice of the AGM and elections of office bearers, whose tenure is over by that time and he shall be the returning officer for the Election.

The President Elect who assumes charges as a President has the right to intimate the bank, informing names of the newly elected office bearers who are authorized to operate branch accounts henceforth. Outgoing office bearers cease to operate the bank accounts with immediate effect. He shall inform the election result to HO and to all members of the branch. The notice of AGM shall be sent at least 14 days in advance. The quorum required for the state branch AGM is 30. In the absence of a quorum within 30 minutes of the appointed time, the meeting shall be adjourned. The adjourned meeting shall be held immediately at the same venue with the same agenda where quorum shall not be necessary.

a. *The agenda of the AGM shall be in the following order:*

    i. The election, if necessary, (in the absence of the President and the Vice Presidents) of a Chairman.

    ii. Welcome address by the President/ Chairperson.

    ii. Confirmation of minutes of the previous Annual General Body/ EOGM.

    iii. Announcement of election results of President Elect/Vice President, if any.

    iv. Adoption of the annual report of the branch.

    v. Adoption of the annual report of the Treasurer and audited statement of accounts of the previous year ending 31st March.

    vi. Any other motion for charge in the order of business.

    vii. Election of the Office-bearers and representatives to Central Council.

    viii. Election of members of EC.

    ix. Appointment of an Auditor.

    x. Resolutions brought forward by the EC.

    xi. Resolutions brought forward by the local branches.

    xii. Resolutions brought forward by the individual members of the Association.

    xiii. Any other matter, with the permission of the Chair (Matters raised under this agenda shall only be discussed and appropriate action shall be taken after discussion in EC/EOGM).

    xiv. President's concluding remarks.

    xv. Taking over of office by President-Elect along with his new team.

    xvi. Vote of thanks by the Honorary State Secretary.

b. *General rules about the annual general body meeting:*

    i. No resolution shall be placed before the AGM that has not been previously considered by the EC.

    ii. Resolutions to state AGM, proposed by the individual members, duly signed and seconded by another member, shall be sent to the Honorary State Secretary, with a copy to the local branches, not later than 15th October.

    iii. Notice of resolutions to be moved at the AGM proposed by the EC of a local branch shall reach the Honorary State Secretary not later than 15th October.

    iv. The branch or the member sending the resolution has to be informed immediately after the EC meeting held for the same, whether their resolution has been accounted or rejected by the EC.

    v. The Honorary State Secretary shall issue, with the notice of the AGM, the preliminary agenda showing the business to be brought before the meeting, the terms of all motions to be moved, of which notice in writing has previously reached him along with the names of the mover.

    vi. A member, who wishes to move an amendment to any item included in the agenda paper, or ask any question pertaining thereto shall give notice thereof to the Honorary State Secretary so as to reach him not less than 7 clear days before the date fixed for the meeting. Members shall, however, have the right to propose amendments to any motion when it is before the house.

vii. The Honorary State Secretary shall make available to all members attending the meeting, a list of all amendments of which notice had been given.

viii. A notice of a resolution or an amendment shall be invalid unless accompanied by a copy of such motion or amendment.

ix. Any resolution of the EC of the State Branch may be considered at the AGM without notice being given.

c. *General rules of procedure EC/AGM/EOGM*

i. Proceedings at the meetings of the Annual General Body shall be recorded in the form of typed minutes and after confirmation by the President/Chairman, at the next AGM, shall be permanently preserved.

ii. No resolution adopted or negated at a meeting shall be reconsidered unless, either six months have elapsed or 1/5 of the members of the EC, in case of branches, sign a requisition for such reconsideration.

iii. The President/Chairman shall, in case of equality of votes, having a casting vote.

iv. No business shall be transacted at a special meeting/EOGM other than for which the meeting is called.

v. The proceedings of any meeting shall not be invalid by reason of there being a vacancy/vacancies or any invalid appointment or election of any member or accidental omission to give notice of such meeting to any member.

vi. A notice may be served on any member either personally through an employee of the Association or by post/courier/email etc.

C. *Extraordinary general body meeting (EOGM) of head office*

a. The EC, whenever it thinks fit or on requisition made in writing by at least 100 Annual/Silver/Gold/Life Members shall call an EOGM of state office.

b. The members, while requisitioning, should state the objects of the meeting proposed to be called and sign legibly giving their full name and address to the HSS, who in consultation with the President, will call an EOGM within two months of the receipt of the requisition. If the meeting is not called within 2 months of the date on which notice is received by the Hon. State Secretary/State Branch, the concerned members themselves may convene a meeting of the EOGM, but such a meeting shall not be convened after four months of the requisition notice and after that the requisition notice will be treated as cancelled.

c. Notice of the EOGM shall be sent to the members at least 14 days before the date fixed for the meeting, giving the place, date and time of the meeting and the agenda of the business to be transacted at such a meeting.

d. The EOGM, if on requisition, shall be convened only at the staff office of the Association.

e. The quorum for the requisitioned EOGM shall be 60, out of which at least 50 must be amongst the requisitionists. If there is no quorum at the given time the meeting shall stand dissolved.

f. If the EC decided to convene an EOGM, the venue shall be decided by the EC.

g. The quorum for the EOGM called by the EC, shall be at least 30 Annual/Silver/Gold/Life members or 50% of the total strength of the state branch, whichever is less.

h. If there is no quorum at an EOGM called by the EC, within 30 minutes, it shall be adjourned and will be reconvened immediately at the same venue with the same agenda where quorum will not be necessary.

9. **Funds/Finance**

a. The state branch is independent on its own with regard to finance, purchase of movable and/or immovable assets and formation of a Trust/Charitable Trust.

b. If a state branch closes down or suspends its activities or is de-recognized, its funds including cash securities, fixed deposit certificates etc., shall forthwith be transferred to the HO, to be kept in a Trust. It will not be annexed or clubbed with any funds of the HO.

c. The accounts of the state branch shall be scrutinized, audited and approved by its EC and circulated to members before being placed at the respective AGM of the state branch. One copy of the audited and approved statement of accounts shall be forwarded to the HO every year after the AGM.

d. The funds of the state branch shall be invested in the manner as specified in Section 11(5) of Income Tax Act. This association is an irrecoverable association. However, if the association becomes defunct or dissolved, the assets/funds of the association shall be vested with an association or society with similar objectives. There shall not be any activity of the state branch with intention of earning any profit. The funds of the state branch/Association shall be solely utilized towards the objectives and no portion of it will be utilized for payment to its members by way of profit, interest, dividend etc.

e. Funds of the state branch/association, irrespective of whatever head they come under CDH, CDE, Journal, etc, shall be received only by the Treasurer and credited to respective heads of the A/c maintained with the state branch. He may pay cash as advance to an Office bearer of the above sections as approved by EC or on reimbursement basis on receipt of vouchers.

f. Funds and all bank accounts and other accounts shall be operated and handled by the Treasurer jointly with the State Secretary of the state branch.

A. *Income:* The funds or the income of the state branch shall be derived from the following sources:

a. State share of subscription from the local branches on account of the members on their rolls.

b. Special contributions or donations raised by the state branch.

c. Income derived from the journal and other publications of the Association.

d. Contributions received on account of organizing state conferences or IDC.

e. Bequests received by legacies from persons who desire to assist the association.

f. Sponsorships and such other sources as may be authorized by EC.

g. Surplus from conferences, if any.

h. Surplus funds from CDE/CDH programs if any.

B. *Reserve fund:* There shall be a reserve fund of the state branch. The reserve fund shall be 50% of the net surplus income of the first year of the branch concerned. In addition, 25% of the net surplus should be credited to this fund every year. The reserve fund shall only be drawn upon by a special resolution of a meeting of the EC, in which ¾ of the member's present and who cast their vote, vote in favour of the resolution of withdrawal.

C. *Head of accounts:* All accounts/financial matters of the state branch shall be handled only by the state office. All receipts pertaining to CDE, CDH, Journal and any other activity shall be received by the IDA state office Treasurer and remitted under respective heads. No other office bearer except Conference Accounts (optional, to be decided the state EC) shall operate independent accounts in a bank. The Hon. Treasurer shall maintain various heads of accounts of income and expenditure. All income shall be payable to Treasurer IDA State Office and it shall be credited into respective head of accounts. Similarly on the expenditure side, the Hon. Treasurer shall debit the expenses on the respective head of account and issue a Demand Draft on the advice of Convener CDH/CDE, Editor etc., and other Conveners, if any, and debit it to the head of Account. In case of HO, all funds, all bank accounts and all other accounts shall be handled and be operated by the respective Treasurer of the branch, jointly with the Hon. State Secretary of the branch.

D. *Expenditure:* The EC, in case of state branches shall out of the funds of the Association/branch debit all ordinary expenses and shall pay rents, salaries, wages and such other charges as may be necessary for carrying out the work of the Association. It shall, further provide for the issue of the journal of the Association and shall be empowered to spend money on scientific investigations, seminars, conferences, prizes scholarships and on such other purposes as it may consider advisable in furtherance of the objects of the Association.

All major expenses in excess of Rs. 50,000/ other than routine administrative expenses shall require an approval from the EC.

E. *Audited Accounts*
 a. The annual statement of accounts and the balance sheet, for the period starting 1st April and ending 31st March of every year, after auditing, shall be submitted to the EC and after approval by the EC, shall be circulated to members and placed in the AGM by the Treasurer and the Hon. Secretary.
 b. Similarly state branch conference accounts shall be audited by the state

branch auditor and approved by the respective state EC.

F. *Appointment of an Auditor in a State Branch*
 a. A Chartered Accountant shall be appointed as auditor at the AGM of the state branch every year for auditing the accounts.
 b. Duties of the auditor for the State Branch:
  i. Audit the accounts at the end of the year, and certify that they are accurate and correct.
  ii. Shall assist and give suggestions for proper book keeping of accounts as required.

G. *Liability:* Neither the IDA nor any of its branches shall be liable for any of the debts or liabilities of one another.

10. **Records:** The State Branch will maintain the following records:
 a. A register/computerized database of members with their membership number, name, qualification, current residence/mailing address and the branch they belong to.
 b. Account books, ledgers, cash books shall be retained up to a period of eight years, after which they can be destroyed. Audited balance sheets of all years shall be retained.
 c. Correspondence beyond five years may be destroyed at the discretion of the Hon. State Secretary.
 d. The AGM, EOGM and EC minutes, attendance registers of EC, AGM and EOGM., membership registers and important correspondence shall be retained permanently.

LOCAL BRANCH

The Local Branch is that branch of the IDA, which is demographically located within he boundaries of a town, city, district or municipal corporation.

Formation

The Dental Surgeons of an individual town/city/district/municipal corporation where a minimum of 20 or more members of the IDA or dental surgeons eligible to become Annual/Silver/Gold/Life IDA members are practicing or residing, shall come together and form/constitute a local branch. They will specify the name of their branch, as adopted by their branch members and declare their area of operation.

a. The members require to sign a written proposal, stating their intention of starting a branch, mentioning therein the serial no., membership no., if any, name, address and their existing branch, if any. They will elect their office bearers and shall forward the complete proposal to the CC for approval, through the state branch with an advance copy to the HO.

b. More than one local branch can be formed in an area, provided that the parent local branch has more than 500 annual/life members and the members practicing within the stipulated area agree to form another local branch.

c. In case a state branch is not functioning, local branches within the state shall be permitted by the CC to function directly under the HO.

d. If the local branch strength reduces to less than the minimum prescribed after recognition, the branch shall be permitted to continue as a local branch.

Composition of Executive Committee (EC)

A. Local Office Bearers	Tenure
1. President	One Term
2. President Elect	One Term
3. Two Vice President	One Term
4. Hon. Branch Secretary	Two Terms
5. Hon. Joint Secretary	Two Terms
6. Hon. Asst. Secretary (Optional)	Two Terms
7. Hon. Treasurer	Two Terms
8. Representative to Council on Dental Health	One Term
9. Representative to Council on Dental Education	One Term
10. Editor Journal/ Newsletter (Optional)	Two Terms
11. Immediate Past President	One Term
B. EC Members: Three members of EC for strength of first 100 Life/Gold/Silver/ Annual Members or part thereof; For every additional 100 Life/ Gold/Silver/Annual Members or part thereof; there shall be one EC Member for membership strength of branch as on 31st July as per HO records	One Term
C. Representative from local branches to State Executive	One Term

For 100 Annual/Gold/Silver/Life Members or part thereof, there shall be three representatives out of which one will be either President or Secretary. For every additional slab of 100 or part thereof, there shall be one representative for membership strength of branch as on 31st July as per HO records. It is optional for local branch AGM/EOGM to decide whether they should be member of Local EC also, or not, in addition to their duties as representative to State EC.

The functions and powers of office bearers of local branch are the same as for state branches. The only difference is:

- The term of Secretary/Joint Secretary/Asst. Secretary/Treasurer/Editor Journal is for **two** years in local branch whereas **three** years in state branches.
- The number of Vice Presidents is **two** in local branches and **three** in state branches.
- From local branches representatives are chosen for state executive committee whereas from state branches Central Council members are chosen for Head Office.

The President and Secretary of IDA Head Office for the last ten years:

Year	President	Secretary
2001	Dr. Krishna Nayak	Dr. V.M. Veerabahu
2002	Dr. C. Krishnarjun Rao	Dr. Ashok Dhoble
2003	Dr. V.M. Veerabahu	Dr. Ashok Dhoble
2004	Dr. B. Subhash Chandra Shetty	Dr. Ashok Dhoble
2005	Dr. Bhagwant Singh	Dr. Ashok Dhoble
2006	Dr. S.G. Damble	Dr. Ashok Dhoble
2007	Dr. M.C. Mohan	Dr. Ashok Dhoble
2008	Dr. Deepak Kamdar	Dr. Ashok Dhoble
2009	Lt. Gen. (Dr.) Paramjit Singh	Dr. Ashok Dhoble
2010	Dr. L. Krishna Prasad	Dr. Ashok Dhoble

Glossary

Agent: Anything living or non-living, the presence or relative absence of which may initiate or perpetuate disease process.

Amphixenosis: A zoonosis maintained in nature by man and lower animals, certain streptococci and staphylococci and can be transmitted in either direction.

Analytical Epidemiology: Observational studies designed specifically to examine the hypothesis developed as a result of descriptive study.

Analytical survey: is an explanatory survey that studies a determinative process to explain the particular situation, for example, 'why that disease occurred in those persons?'

Anthropology: It is the study of teeth in a perspective beyond the clinical science. It includes the study of dental growth, theories of dental origin, primate dentition and population variation.

Anthropozoonosis: A zoonosis maintained in nature by lower vertebrates, for example, rabies, brucellosis, etc.

Asymptomatic infection: See inapparent infection.

Arithmetic Mean: Simplest measure of central tendency obtained by summing up of all observations divided by number of those observations.

Asymptomatic Disease Carrier: A person or an organism infected with an infectious agent without displaying any symptoms.

Atraumatic Restorative Treatment (ART): A minimal intervention, minimal invasion procedure based on removing carious tooth structure by using hand instruments alone and restoring the cavity with adhesive restorative material.

Attack rate or Case rate: The number of cases of a disease occurring in a specified population during a specified interval. It is a proportion measuring cumulative incidence often used for particular groups, observed for limited periods and under special circumstances, as in an epidemic; it is usually expressed as percent (cases per 100 in the group).

Attributable Risk: The difference in the incidence rates of disease between exposed group and non-exposed group.

Auxiliary Worker: One who has less than full professional qualification in a particular field and is supervised by a professional worker (WHO).

Auxiliary: Technical worker in any field with less than full professional training—WHO.

Basic Health Service: A network of co-ordinated peripheral and intermediate health units capable of performing essential functions by assuring the availability of competent professional and auxiliary personnel to perform those functions (WHO/UNICEF; 1965).

Behaviour management: It means the techniques by which the dental health team effectively and efficiently performs the treatment and instills a positive dental attitude.

Berkson's bias: It is a type of selection bias which may occur in the case control studies which are based entirely on hospital records. It arises because of different rates of admission to hospitals for people with different disease.

Bias: A term used to describe the tendency or preference towards a particular perspective, ideology or result; especially when the tendency interferes with the ability to be impartial, unprejudiced or objective.

Bimodal Distribution: A distribution having two scores occurring with greatest frequency, i.e. it has two modes.

Biological Environment: The universe of living things which surrounds the man, including the man himself.

Biostatistics: It is the application of statistics to a wide range of biology.

Caries Activity Tests: These are the laboratory tests designed to evaluate the susceptibility of the individual towards caries.

Caries Susceptibility: The inherent tendency of the tooth to be affected by the caries.

Carrier: A person or animal that harbours a specific infectious agent without discernible clinical disease and serves as a potential source of infection. The carrier state may exist in an individual with an infection that is inapparent throughout its course (commonly known as healthy or asymptomatic carrier), or during the incubation period, convalescence and post convalescence of an individual with a clinically recognizable disease (commonly known as an incubatory or convalescent carrier). The carrier state may be of short or long duration (temporary/transient carrier, or chronic carrier).

Case Control Study: An investigation employing an epidemiological approach in which previously existing incidents of a medical condition are used in lieu of gathering information from a randomized population. Control is obtained by comparing known cases of medical condition with the group of persons who have not developed that medical problem.

Case Fatality Rate: The ratio of deaths within a designated population of people with particular condition over a certain period of time. It is usually expressed as the percentage of persons diagnosed as having a specified disease who die as a result of that illness within a given period. This term is most frequently applied to a specific outbreak of acute disease in which all patients have been followed for an adequate period of time to include all attributable deaths.

Case: A person in the population or study group identified as having the particular disease, health disorder or condition under investigation.

Census: An official, usually periodic enumeration of population, often including a collection of related demographic information. It is the collection of information from all the individuals of population.

Chemoprophylaxis: The administration of a chemical, including antibiotics, to prevent the development of an infection or the progression of an infection to active disease; or to eliminate the carriage of a specific infectious agent so as to prevent transmission of disease in others.

Child Mortality Rate: Number of deaths within the age of 1–4 years in a given year per 1000 children in that age group at the mid point of the year (usually till June-July).

Circumstance: Any factor present in the environment that might be suspected of causing the disease.

Cleaning: The removal by scrubbing and washing (may be with hot water, soap, detergent or by vacuum cleaning) of infectious agents and of organic matter from surfaces on/in which infectious agents may find favourable conditions for surviving or multiplying.

Co-efficient of Variation: A relative measure of dispersion used to compare two or more series of data with either different units of measurement or either marked differences in their mean.

Cohort Study: A longitudinal study of the same group of people (the cohort) over time. It is a study in which particular outcome, such as death from the heart attack, is compared in groups of people who are alike in most ways but differ by a certain characteristics, such as smoking.

Cohort: In a clinical study, a well-defined group of subjects or patients, who have had a common experience or exposure and are then followed up for the incidence of new disease or events.

Colorado Stain: A term used by McKay, for mottled enamel, characterized by minute white flecks, or yellow or brown spots on areas, scattered irregularly or streaked over the surface of tooth; or it may be a condition where the entire tooth surface has the appearance of dead paper.

Communicable Disease: An illness due to specific infectious agent or its toxic products which occurs through transmission of that agent or its products from an infected person, animal or inanimate reservoir to a susceptible host; either directly or indirectly through an intermediate plant or animal host, vector or the inanimate environment.

Communicable Period: The time during which an infectious agent may be transferred directly or indirectly from an infected person to another person; from an infected animal to human, or from infected persons to animals; including arthropods.

Community Dental Health: A field of dental public health, which is involved in the assessment of dental health needs and improvement of dental health of populations rather than individuals.

Community Dentistry: A branch of dentistry that deals with the community and its aggregate dental or oral health rather than of an individual patient.

Community Diagnosis: The identification and quantification of health problems in a community as a whole in terms of mortality and morbidity rates and ratios; and identification of their correlates for the purpose of defining those at risk or those in need of health care.

Community Health: A field of public health; includes all the personal health and environmental services in any human community, irrespective of whether such services were private or public ones.

Community Medicine: It provides the solution to health or disease problems not only in the setting of a clinic or hospital but also in the community setting, with an active community participation.

Comprehensive Dental Care: A process of providing preventive, therapeutic and maintenance care necessary for function, aesthetics and integrity of oral tissues with balanced consideration of patient's physical, social, economical and psychosomatic status.

Concurrent disinfection: It is the application of disinfective measures as soon as possible after the discharge of infectious material from the body of an infected person, or after the soiling of articles with such infectious discharges; all personal contact with such discharges or articles should be minimized period to such disinfection.

Confidence Interval: It is about the mean and range of values within which that mean probably falls.

Confounding factor (*confounding variable or lurking variable*)**:** It is an extraneous variable in a statistical model that correlates (positively or negatively) with both dependent and independent variables. It may even mask an actual association or falsely demonstrate an apparent association between the study variables where no real association exists between them.

Contact: A person or animal that has been in association with an infected person, animal or a contaminated environment so as to have an opportunity to acquire the infection.

Contamination: The presence of an infectious agent on a body surface, in clothes, bedding, toys, surgical instruments, dressings, or any other inanimate articles or substances including water and food.

Continuous Data: The variable that can take any value in a given range (decimal or fractional) is termed as continuous data; for example, temperature, arch length, mesio-distal width of erupted teeth, etc.

Cross-sectional Study: The study of population at a single point in time. It is useful for studying the association and correlation between variables at individual level rather than at aggregate level and thus avoiding ecological fallacy.

Crude Death Rate: The number of deaths per 1000 population per year in a given community.

Crude mortality rate: See mortality rate.

Cumulative Indices: Indices that measure all the evidences of past and present conditions, for example, DMF, PMA index.

Data: Collection of facts from which conclusions can be drawn.

Defluoridation of water: The process of removal of excess of fluoride salts from the potable water.

Dental Auxiliary: The person who is given responsibility by the dentist so that he or she can help the dentist to render dental care but who is not himself or herself qualified with a dental degree.

Dental Ethics: The moral obligation to render to the patient the best possible quality of dental services and to maintain the honest relationship with other members of profession.

Dental floss: An inter-dental cleansing aid in the form of a thread that is used to remove plaque from inter-proximal surfaces.

Dental Fluorosis: A condition of enamel hypoplasia or hypo-mineralization characterized by white chalky spots, brown staining or pitting of teeth due to increased level of fluoride in drinking water affecting enamel matrix formation and calcification, because of impairment of ameloblastic function during tooth development.

Dental Health Education: Education that aims to persuade people to adopt and sustain healthy dental practices, to use judiciously and wisely dental health services available to them and to take their own decisions both individually and collectively so as to improve their oral health status. It is an integral part of general health education.

Dental Health: It is the state of complete normality and functional efficiency of the teeth and their supporting structures, surrounding parts of oral cavity and of the various structures related to mastication and maxillofacial complex.

Dental Hygienist: A person who is trained and given licence to clean teeth, take dental x-rays and provides related dental services usually under the supervision of the dentist.

Dental Laboratory Technician: A person who makes dental prostheses and orthodontic appliances as prescribed by the dentist.

Dental plaque: It is specific but highly variable structure entity resulting from colonization of microorganismss on tooth surfaces, restorations and other parts of oral cavity. It consists of salivary components like mucin, desquamated epithelial cells, debris and microorganisms embedded in a gelatinous extracellular matrix.

Dental Practice Management: It is defined as the process of obtaining and allocating inputs (human and economic resources) by planning, organizing, staffing and directing and controlling for the purpose of outputs (dental services) defined by patients, so that practice objectives are achieved.

Dental Public Health: The science and art of preventing and controlling dental disease and promoting dental health through organized community efforts – American Board of Dental Public Health.

Dentifrices: Any substance, especially paste or powder that is used for cleaning of teeth.

Dentist: A person licenced to practice dentistry under the laws of the appropriate state or nation. To become licenced, a prospective person must undergo specified training and learning as prescribed by Dental Council of India.

Dentistry: The evaluation, diagnosis, prevention and/or treatment of diseases; disorders and or conditions of the oral cavity, maxillofacial area and/ or the adjacent and associated structures and their impact on the human body.

Denturist: Those laboratory technicians, who can fabricate dentures directly for patients without dentist's prescription.

Dependent variable (Behavioural measure): Any measurable behavioural variable in a psychological investigation is called a dependent variable.

Descriptive Epidemiology: The distribution of disease, with the comparison of its frequency in different populations and in different segments of same population.

Descriptive survey: The survey that describes a particular situation; for example, distribution of a disease in a population in relation to age, sex, caste, etc.

Disability: Any restriction or lack of ability (resulting from an impairment) to perform an activity in a manner or range considered normal for a human being (WHO).

Disease specific mortality rate: See mortality rate.

Discrete Data/Discontinuous Data: When the variable under the observation takes only fixed values like whole numbers, e.g. pulse, B.P, DMF teeth (always occur as 1, 2, 3….. not as 1.1, 1.5, 2.6, etc.)

Disease control: The measures taken to reduce the incidence, duration, risk of transmission, and

development of complications due to any particular disease and thus reducing the burden on the community.

Disease Elimination: The reduction of infectious disease prevalence to zero in regional population; or the reduction of the global prevalence of a disease to negligible amount.

Disease prevalence: All the current cases, i.e. old and new existing in a given population at a given point of time or in a period of time.

Disease: A pathological condition of part, organ or system of an organism resulting from various causes such as infection, genetic defect or environmental stress and characterized by identifiable group of signs or symptoms.

Disinfection: Killing of infectious agents outside the body by direct exposure to chemical or physical agents.

Double blind trials: The trial is so planned that neither doctor nor the participants know which groups are study ones and which are controls.

Early detection of health impairment: The detection of disturbances of homeostatic and compensating mechanism when biochemical, morphological and functional changes are still reversible.

Ecological association: The ecological association is the association between two characteristics both measured at an aggregate level rather than at individual level. It has nothing to do with ecology.

Endemic: Prevalent in a particular region.

Endemic disease: The presence of a disease within a given geographic area at all times but in low frequency, for example, fluorosis, typhoid, etc.

Enzootic: Occurring endemically among animals.

Epidemic: The occurrence of cases of illness in a community or region with an excess frequency than expected. The number of cases indicating presence of an epidemic will vary according to the infectious agent, size and type of population exposed, previous experience or lack of exposure to the disease, and time and place of occurrence; epidemicity is thus relative to usual frequency of the disease in the same area, among the specified population, at the same season of the year.

Epidemiological Triad: The occurrence and manifestations of any disease, whether communicable or non-communicable are determined by interactions between three factors – the host, agent and environment; which together constitute epidemiological triad.

Epidemiology: The study of occurrence and distribution of disease. The 'pattern' and the 'dynamics' of any disease is also involved in epidemiology process. The pattern implies variables such as age, sex, occupation and social characteristics, etc; and dynamics implies trends and timing of the concerned disease.

Epizoology (veterinary epidemiology): The study of epidemic diseases among animals.

Epizootic: An epidemic disease occurring among animals.

Ethics: The science of moral obligation; a system of moral principles, quality or practice.

Evaluation: The process of making judgement about selected objectives and events by comparing them with specified value standards for the purpose of deciding alternative course of action.

Exotic: Disease that is imported into the country (of foreign origin).

Experimental Epidemiology: Experimental studies on the human populations conducted to test in a stringent manner; or those hypothesis that stand the test of observational and analytical studies.

External Environment: All that is external to the individual host, constitutes external environment.

Family: The primary unit of society, which includes a group of individuals who are biologically related, live together and eat in a common kitchen.

Fluoride Varnish: A sticky yellowish fluoride salt solution in the resin base which can be painted over tooth surface to prevent decay and decrease sensitivity.

Fluorine: A trace element, most electronegative and reactive of all elements; a member of halogen family with relative atomic weight of 19 and atomic number 9.

Fluorosis: An endemic disease in geographical areas where the content of fluoride ions in drinking water exceeds 2 ppm.

F-ratio: A ratio of variance between the means of group to the variance within the groups; it determines if the observed difference among the sample means is significant.

Genetic Disease Carrier: A person, or an organism that has inherited a genetic trait or mutation, but is not displaying symptoms.

Geriatric Dentistry: The branch of dentistry that deals with the special knowledge, attitudes and technical skills, required in provision of oral health care to older adults. The term older adults has no specific chronological boundary, rather it refers to the adults who are affected by physical, social, psychological, physiological and/or biological changes associated with aging, with or without concomitant disease – ADA.

Gerodontology: Multidisciplinary study of the process of aging in the orofacial tissues and its relation to the surroundings.

Goal: Ultimate desired state towards which objectives and resources are directed.

Good Samaritan Law: The laws or acts protecting from liability, those who choose to aid others who are injured or ill.

Habit: Acquired tendency to respond in an identical way to a situation or stimulus.

Handicap: The disadvantage for a given individual resulting from an impairment or disability that limits or prevents the fulfillment of a role (depending on age, sex, social and cultural factors) for the individual (WHO).

Handicapped Person: Any individual who is prevented from participating in the normal activities of his age due to physical/mental abnormality.

Health Appraisal: The process of determining the total status through history taking, teacher's and nurse's observation, screening tests and mental, dental and psychological examination.

Health Care: Multitude of services rendered at individual, family or community level by the agents of the health services or professions for the purpose of promoting, monitoring or restoring health.

Health Development: The process of continuous progressive improvement of health status of a population (WHO).

Health Education: 'Health education, like general education, is concerned with changes in knowledge, feelings and behavior of people. In its most usual forms, it concentrates on developing such health practices as are believed to bring about the best possible state of well-being' (WHO).

Health for All: Organized application of local, state, national or international resources to achieve health for all, i.e. attainment by all the people of world by the year 2003 a level of health that will permit them to lead a socially and economically productive life.

Health Indicators: Variables used for assessment of community health. OR variables, which help to measure changes in the health status (WHO).

Health Information System: Mechanism for the collection processing, analysis and transmission of information required for organizing and operating health services and training (WHO).

Health Man-Power Planning: The process of estimating the number of persons and the kind of knowledge, skills and attitudes required to achieve predetermined health targets and ultimately health status objectives.

Health Promotion: It is a process of enabling individuals to improve their health through personal choice and social responsibility.

Health Protection: The provision of conditions for the normal mental and physical functioning of the human being individually and in the group. It includes the promotion of health, the prevention of sickness and curative and restorative medicine in all its aspects (WHO).

Health Services Research: The systematic study of means by which biomedical and other relevant knowledge is brought to bear on the health of individuals and communities under a given set of conditions (WHO).

Health Team: Group of person who share a common health goal and objectives, determined by the community needs and towards the achievement of which each member of the team contributes in accordance with his/her competence and skills, and respecting the functions of the other (WHO).

Health: A state of complete physical, mental and social well-being and not merely absence of disease or infirmity (WHO).

Hospital: A residential establishment which provides short term or long term medical care, consisting of observational, diagnostic, therapeutic or rehabilitative services to persons suffering or suspected to be suffering from a disease. It may or may not provide services to ambulatory patients.

Host: A person or other living animal, including birds and arthropods, that affords subsistence of lodgment to an infectious agent under natural (as opposed to experimental) conditions.

  i. Definitive host: hosts in which the parasite attains maturity or passes its sexual stage are primary.

  ii. Secondary host: those in which the parasite is in a larval or asexual state are secondary or intermediate hosts.

  iii. Transport host: is a carrier in which the organism remains alive but does not undergo development.

Hyper-endemic: A high level of infection beginning early in the life and affecting most of the child population, leading to a state of equilibrium, such that the adult population shows evidence of the disease much less commonly than do children.

Hypothesis: A supposition arrived at from an observation or reflection.

Iatrogenic: Any adverse or untoward consequence of a preventive, diagnostic or therapeutic procedure that causes impairment, handicap, disability or death resulting from health professional activity.

Immune individual: A person or animal that has specific protective antibodies and/or cellular immunity as a result of previous infection or immunization, or is so conditioned by such previous specific experience as to respond in such a way that prevents the development of infection and/or clinical illness following re-exposure to the specific infectious agent.

Immunity: The resistance usually associated with the presence of antibodies or cells having a specific action on the microorganism concerned with a particular infectious disease or on its toxin. Effective immunity includes both cellular immunity, which is conferred by T-lymphocyte sensitization, and/or humoral immunity, which is based on B-lymphocyte response.

Impairment: Any loss or abnormality of psychological, physiological or anatomical structure or function.

Inapparent infection: The presence of infection in a host without recognizable clinical signs or symptoms. Inapparent infections are identifiable only by laboratory means such as a blood test or by the development of positive reactivity to specific skin tests. (Synonyms: asymptomatic, subclinical, occult infection)

Incidence rate: The number of new cases of a specified disease diagnosed or reported during a defined period of time, divided by the number of persons in a stated population in which the cases occurred. This is usually expressed as cases per 1,000 or 100,000 per annum.

Incremental Dental Care: Treatment of children at the earliest stage available and providing maintenance care through further periodic treatments.

Incubation period: The time interval between initial contact with an infectious agent and the first appearance of symptoms associated with the infection.

i. Extrinsic incubation period: It is the time between entrance of an organism into the vector and the time when that vector can transmit the infection. See extrinsic incubation period.

ii. Latent period: The period in between the time of exposure to a parasite and the time when the parasite can be detected in blood or stool.

Independent variable: Any variable which can be manipulated by the experimenter either directly or through selection in order to determine its effects on behavior measures or dependent variable.

Index: A numerical value, describing the relative status of population on a graduate scale with definite upper and lower limits, which is designed to permit and facilitate comparison with other populations, classified by same criteria and methods (Russell).

Infected individual: A person or animal that harbours an infectious agent and either manifest disease or inapparent infection (see carrier). An infectious person or animal is one from whom the infectious agent can be naturally acquired.

Infection: The entry, development (of many parasites) or multiplication of an infectious agent in the body of persons or animals. Infection is not synonymous with infectious disease; the result may be inapparent (see Inapparent infection). The presence of living infectious agents on exterior surfaces of the body, or on articles of apparel or soiled articles, is not infection, but represents contamination of such surfaces and articles (see Infestation and Contamination).

Infection rate: It is a proportion that expresses the incidence of all identified infections.

Infectious agent: An organism (virus, bacteria, fungus, protozoan) that is capable of producing infection or infectious disease.

Infectiousness: It indicates the relative ease with which a disease is transmitted to other hosts.

Infectious Disease: A clinically manifested disease of humans or animals resulting from an infection.

Infectivity: It expresses the ability of the disease agent to enter, survive and multiply in the host.

Infestation: The lodgement, development and reproduction of arthropods on the surface of the body or in the clothing. Infested articles or premises are those that harbor to give shelter to animal forms, especially arthropods and rodents.

Informed consent: It is a legal procedure to ensure that the patient or client knows all the risks and costs involved in treatment. Its elements include informing the client about the nature of the treatment, possible alternative treatments and the potential risks and benefits of the treatment.

Insecticide: Any chemical substance used for the destruction of insects, whether applied as powder, liquid, atomized liquid, aerosol or "paint" spray; residual action is usual.

Internal Environment: Each and every component, tissue, organ and their harmonious functioning within the system constitutes internal environment.

Intervention: Any attempt to intervene or interrupt the usual sequence in development of disease in man.

Isolation: Separation for the period of communicability of infected person or animals from healthy ones at such places and under such conditions so as to prevent or limit the direct or indirect transmission of infectious agents from infected persons to those who are healthy or susceptible.

Jurisprudence: It is the philosophy of law; science that deals with study of law and legal relations.

Licensure: The process by which an agency of government grants permission to those meeting the predetermined qualifications to engage in a given occupation and use a particular title or by which it grants permission to institutions to perform specified functions.

Median: The middle value in distribution such that one half of the units in the distribution have smaller or equal value than median; and other half has value higher or equal to the median.

Medical Statistics: It is specialty of biostatistics that represents the mathematical facts and data related to health, preventive medicine and disease.

Mode: The value occurring with the greatest frequency in a series of observations.

Morbidity: Any departure, subjective or objective from a state of physiological well being.

Mortality Rate: The number of deaths due to a disease in a general population or in a community. An incidence rate is used to include all persons in the population under consideration who become clinically ill during the period of time stated. The population may be limited to a specific gender or age group, or to those with certain other characteristics.

Multimodal Distribution: A distribution having more than two scores occurring with greatest frequency.

Nalgonda Technique: A technique of water defluoridation, developed in India by National

Environmental Engineering Research Institute (NEERI) at Nagpur in 1961; involves the sequential use of sodium aluminate or lime, bleaching powder and filter alum to water followed by flocculation, sedimentation and filtration.

National Health Planning: The orderly process of defining community health problems, identifying unmet needs and surveying the resources to meet them, establishing priority goals that are realistic and feasible and projecting administrative action to accomplish the purpose of proposed program.

National Health Policy: An expression of goals for improving the health situation, the priorities among those goals, and the main directions for attaining them formed by a country.

National pathfinder survey: Type of pathfinder survey that incorporates all the important subgroups of a population that may have differing disease levels or treatment needs and at least three of the index age groups.

Negative predictive value: The probability of absence of disease in a person who receives a negative test result.

Nosocomial: Pertaining to hospital.

Nosocomial Infection (Hospital acquired infection): An infection occurring in a patient, in a hospital or other healthcare facility in whom it was not present or incubating at the time of admission; or the residual of an infection acquired during a previous admission. It includes infections acquired in the hospital but appearing after discharge.

Null Hypothesis: A type of hypothesis used in statistics that proposed that no statistical significance exists in a set of given observations.

Objective: It is the pre use, planned and point of all the activities.

Odds Ratio: Indirect method of measuring relative risk used for case control studies; is a measure of strength of association between risk factor and outcome.

Opportunistic Infection: An infection by an organism who takes an opportunity provided by any defect in host's defence mechanisms so as to infect the host and hence cause the disease in him.

Oral Health Survey: The survey to collect basic information about the oral disease status and treatment needs that is required for planning or monitoring oral health programs (WHO).

Outbreak: An epidemic usually affecting a large proportion of population occurring over a wide geographical area such as section of nation, entire nation, a continent or world.

Pandemic: Occurring over a wide geographical area affecting an exceptionally high proportion of the population, for example, influenza, cholera, etc.

Panel Study: A longitudinal study in which variables are measured on the same units over time; for example—Indian Election Panel studies have interviewed respondents after one election, again after the following elections and sometimes at various points in between.

Parameter: The characteristic of a population is known as parameter, e.g. average age of all the dental patients in a particular year.

Pathfinder survey: This survey assesses the 0.1% or 1% of the population by 5 specific groups of different ages, i.e. 5 years (for primary teeth); 12 years; 15 years; 35–44 years and 65–74 years with each group containing 25–50 subjects.

Pathogenicity: The property of an infectious agent that determines the extent to which an overt disease is produced in an infected population; or the power of an organism to produce disease.

Period prevalence: The total number of existing cases (old and new) known to have existed at some time during a specified time period.

Physical Environment: Non-living things and physical factors (like air, water, soil, housing, climate, etc.) with which human beings are in constant interaction.

Physician: A person, who have been regularly admitted to a medical school duly recognized in a country, has successfully completed the prescribed courses of studies in medicine and has acquired the required qualification to be legally licensed to practice medicine (comprising prevention, diagnosis, treatment and rehabilitation), using his independent judgements to promote community and individual health (WHO).

Pilot survey: Type of pathfinder survey that includes only the most important subgroups in the population of only 1 or 2 index age groups.

Pit and fissure sealants: Agents used to occlude dental enamel pits and fissures or prevention of dental caries.

Plan: A plan is a decision about a course of action. It serves as a blue print of action to be taken.

Plaque control: Removal of microbial plaque and prevention of its accumulation on teeth and adjacent gingival tissues by use of mechanical and chemical means, which also prevents the formation of calculus.

Point prevalence: See prevalence.

Pollution: It is distinct from contamination and implies the presence of offensive, but not necessarily infectious, matter in the environment.

Positive Health: A state beyond the mere absence of disease and is measurable. Positive health is a combination of excellent status on biological, subjective and functional measures.

Positive predictive value: It is the probability of disease among those who received a positive test result.

Prevalence: The total number of diseased persons suffering from or portraying a certain condition in a state population at a particular time. (point prevalence), or during a period of time (period prevalence), divided by the population at risk of having the disease or condition at the point in time or midway through the period in which they occurred.

Preventive Dentistry: Procedure employed in practice of dentistry and community dental health programs which prevent occurrence of oral disease and oral abnormalities.

Preventive Medicine: The organized activities of community to prevent occurrence as well as progression of a disease, mental or physical disability and timely application of all means to promote the health of individual and community as a whole; including prophylaxis, health education and similar work done by a good doctor in looking after individuals and families.

Primary Health Care: Essential health care based on practical, scientifically sound and socially acceptable methods and technology made universally accessible to the individual and families in the community through their full participation and at a cost that the community and the country can afford to maintain at every stage of their development in the spirit of self determination (WHO).

Primary Prevention: Concept of positive health; actions taken prior to the onset of disease, which remove or reduce the possibility of occurrence of that disease, for example, use of fluorides, caries activity tests, etc.

Primordial Prevention: It is the prevention of emergence of risk factors in a population groups in which they have not appeared yet.

Profession: A profession is a vocation founded upon specialized educational training.

Program: It is a sequence of activities designed to implement policies and accomplish objectives.

Proportion: The relation between things (or part of things) with respect to their quantity, magnitude or degree.

Prosodemic: Type of epidemic disease that spreads by person to person contact, for example, cerebrospinal fever.

Psychological Environment: Those psychological factors which affect personal health, health care and community well being that stem from psychosocial makeup of individuals and the structure and functions of social groups.

Public Health Dentistry: Public Health Dentistry is that branch of dentistry, which concerned with the diagnosis, prevention and control of dental diseases and the promotion of oral health through organized community efforts

Public Health: The art and science of preventing disease, prolonging life and prolonging physical and mental efficiency, through an organized community efforts, for the sanitation of environment, the control of communicable infections, the education of an individual in personal hygiene, the organization of medical and nursing services. For the early diagnosis and preventive treatment of disease and the development of the social machinery to ensure everyone a standard of living adequate for maintenance of health, organize these benefits so as to enable every citizen to realize his birthright of health and longevity.

Qualitative Data: That is collected or categorized on the basis of attributes or qualities like caste, creed, colour, sex and has no numerical basis.

Quality of Life: The condition of life resulting from the combination of the effects of complete range of factors such as those determining health, happiness (including comfort in physical environment and a satisfying occupation), education, social and intellectual attainments, freedom of action, justice and freedom of expression—WHO.

Quantiles: It is family of values each of which divides distribution in equal parts. The different types of quantiles are:

a. *Centiles:* Divides distribution in 100 equal parts.

b. *Quartiles:* Divide the distribution into 4 equal parts. They are further divided as:

1st quartile: Divides the distribution in the ratio of 1:3.

2nd quartile: Divides the distribution in the ratio of 2:2.

3rd quartile: Divides the distribution in the ratio of 3:1.

Quantitative Data (Numerical data): The data measured or identified on a numerical scale that can be analyzed using statistical methods.

Quarantine: The limitation of freedom of movement of persons or domestic animals exposed to communicable diseases; but without manifestation of the disease, for a time not longer than the usual incubation period of that disease, so as to prevent effective contact. It is of following types:

a. *Absolute or complete quarantine:* The limitation of freedom of movement of those exposed to a communicable disease for a period of time not longer than the longest incubation period of that disease, so as to prevent effective contact.

b. *Modified quarantine:* A selective partial limitation from freedom of movement of contacts, commonly on the basis of known or presumed differences in susceptibility and related to the danger of disease transmission. It may be designed to accommodate particular situations, for example, exclusion of children from school, exemption of immune persons from provisions applicable to susceptible persons, or restriction of military populations to the post or to quarters.

Questionnaire: A list of questions pertaining to a particular survey.

Random Sampling: It is a sampling procedure in which every element in the population has an equal and independent chance of being selected in a sample.

Range: The difference between the value of largest and smallest item.

Rate: A magnitude or frequency relative to time unit.

Ratio: The relative magnitudes of two quantities (usually expressed as a quotient).

Registration: An attribute or exposure that is significantly associated with the development of disease.

Rehabilitation: The combined and coordinated use of medical, social, educational and vocational measure for training and retraining the individual to highest possible level of functional ability (WHO).

Relative Risk: The ratio of rate (incidence/mortality) of disease among those exposed to risk factors to the rate among those not exposed to the risk factors.

Reservoir: Any person, animal, arthropod, plant, soil or substance (or combination of these) in which an infectious agent normally lives and multiplies, on which it depends primarily for survival, and where it reproduces itself in such manner that it can be transmitted to a susceptible host.

Resistance: The sum total of body mechanisms that interpose barriers to the invasion or multiplication of infectious agents, or to damage by their toxic products.

Inherent resistance: An ability to resist disease independent of immunity or of specifically developed tissue responses; it commonly resides in anatomic or physiologic characteristics of the host and may be genetic or acquired, permanent or temporary (Synonym: Non-specific immunity).

Resource: Anything that can be used for support or help.

Risk Factor: Determinant that can be modified by intervention, thereby reducing the possibility of occurrence of disease or other specified outcomes.

Risk Ratio (RR): Ratio between incidence of disease among persons exposed to risk factor to the ratio of incidence of disease among persons not exposed to risk factor.

Root mean square deviation: See standard deviation.

Sample: Group of individuals who are actually available for investigation.

Sampling Frame: List of sampling units is also known as sampling frame.

Sampling Unit: The individual entity that is considered as focus of the study.

Screening/Case Detection: The presumptive identification of unrecognized disease in a patient.

Secondary attack rate: It is the number of cases among familial or institutional contacts occurring within the accepted incubation period following exposure to a primary case, in relation to the total of exposed contacts; the denominator may be restricted to susceptible contacts when determinable.

Secondary Prevention: Actions taken which halt the progress of disease at its incipient stage and prevent the development of complications; for example, preventive resin restorations, oral prophylaxis, etc.

Segregation: Separation of a group of persons from others to facilitate the control of communicable diseases.

Sensitivity: 'True positive rate', is the probability of correctly identifying a case of disease after screening tests.

Sentinel Surveillance: Monitoring of rate of occurrence of specific conditions to assess the stability or change in health levels of a population.

Serologic surveillance: It identifies patterns of current and past infection using serologic tests.

Single blind trials: The trial is so planned that the participants are not aware of that whether they belong to study or control group.

Social Integration: The active participation of disabled and handicapped people in the mainstream of community life.

Society: A group of individuals who have organized themselves to follow a particular way of life.

Source of infection: The person, animal, or substance from which an infectious agent passes to a host. Source of infection should be clearly distinguished from source of contamination; such as overflow of a tank contaminating a water supply, or an infected cook contaminating the salad.

Specificity: It is the ability to identify the persons who are actually not suffering from disease. It thus identifies the 'true negative cases'.

Sporadic: Scattered incidence of disease.

Standard Deviation: It is a summary measure of differences of each observation from the mean of all the observations.

Standard of Living: Income and occupation, standards of housing, sanitation and nutrition, the level of provision of health, educational, recreational and other services; may all be used individually as a measure of socio-economic status and collectively as an index of standard of living (WHO).

Statistic Value: A value obtained from a sample that estimates the value of parameters, for example, average age of 50 patients selected from all dental patients of OPD.

Statistics: It is the science of compiling, classifying and tabulating numerical data and expressing the results in mathematical or graphical form.

Sterilization: A process by which an article surface or medium is made free from all the microorganisms, either in active or resting (spore) state. It involves destruction of all forms of life by heat, irradiation, gas (ethylene oxide or formaldehyde) or chemical treatment.

Surveillance of disease: It the continuous scrutiny of all aspects of occurrence and spread of a disease. It includes the systemic collection and evaluation of morbidity and mortality reports, special reports of field investigations of epidemics, isolation and identification of infectious agents by laboratories, data concerning the availability, use and untoward effects of vaccines and toxoids, immune globulins, insecticides and other substances used. It also provides information regarding immunity levels of the population; and other relevant epidemiologic data.

Survey: A non-experimental investigation in which information is collected systematically without the active intervention by investigators.

Susceptible: A person or animal not possessing sufficient resistance against a particular pathogenic agent to prevent contracting infection or disease when exposed to the agent.

Suspect: In infectious disease control, illness in a person whose history and symptoms suggest that he or she may have or be developed a communicable disease.

Terminal disinfection: It is the application of disinfective measures after the patient has been shifted to a hospital, or has ceased to be a source of infection.

Tertiary Prevention: When the disease process has advanced beyond its early stages, it is still possible to accomplish prevention by tertiary level of prevention, i.e. intervention in the late stage of disease, for example, dentures, implants, periodontal surgery, etc.

Tooth Fatality: It is determined by dividing number of missing teeth by total number of decayed and missing teeth.

Tooth Mortality: It is determined by dividing number of lost teeth divided by total number of teeth possible in that individual or group.

Tooth brush: The cleansing aid that is designed primarily to promote cleanliness of teeth and oral cavity.

Transmission of infectious agents: Any mechanism by which an infectious agent is spread from a source to a person. These mechanisms are as follows:

1. *Direct transmission:* The direct and immediate transfer of infectious agents to a receptive is called direct transmission. This may be by direct contact such as touching, biting, kissing or sexual intercourse, or by the direct spray of droplets onto the conjunctiva or mucous membranes of the eye, nose or mouth during sneezing, coughing, spitting, singing or talking (usually the distance is less than one meter).

2. *Indirect transmission*
   a. *Vehicle-borne:* Contaminated objects such as toys, handkerchiefs, clothes, cooking or eating

utensils, surgical instruments of dressings; and biological products including blood, serum, plasma, tissues or organs; or any substance serving as an intermediate means by which an infectious agent is transported and introduced into a susceptible host. The agent may or may not have multiplied or developed before being transmitted.

b. *Vector-borne*

   i. *Mechanical:* It includes mechanical carriage by a crawling or flying insect through soiling of its feet, or by passage of organisms through its gastrointestinal tract. This does not require multiplication or development of the organism.

   ii. *Biological:* The propagation, cyclic development, or a combination of these is required before the arthropod can transmit the infective form of the agent to humans. An incubation period is required following infection. The infectious agent may be passed vertically to succeeding generations.

3. *Airborne:* Microbial aerosols are suspensions of particles in the air consisting partially or wholly of microorganisms. The dissemination of microbial aerosols to the respiratory tract is airborne transmission. Aerosols may remain suspended in the air for longer periods. Minute particles are easily drawn into the alveoli of the lungs. The droplets and other large particles are not considered as airborne.

a. *Droplet nuclei:* These are the small residues that result from evaporation of fluid from droplets emitted by an infected host. They may also be created purposely, or accidentally as in microbiology laboratories. They usually remain suspended in the air for longer periods.

b. *Dust:* The small particles of widely varying size that may arise from soil (e.g. spores, etc. separated from soil by wind or mechanical agitation), clothes, bedding or contaminated floors.

Triple blind trials: In this trial, the participant, investigator and person analyzing the data are not aware of the division of the groups for investigation.

Utilization of services: It is expressed as the proportion of people who are in need of service to those who actually receive it in a given time period - usually a year.

Vaccine: Microbial preparations of killed or modified microorganisms that can stimulate an immune response in the body to prevent future infection with similar microorganisms.

Value (correlation value): It indicates the degree of correlation between two variables with range from -1 to $+1$.

Variable: A condition, occurrence or effect that can assume different value.

Variate: Any piece of information referring to patient or patient's disease.

Vector: Commonly used for arthropods which transmit infectious agents from human to human or from animal to human.

Virulence: The degree of pathogenicity of an infectious agent, indicated by case-fatality rates and/ or the ability of the agent to invade and damage tissues of the host.

Water Fluoridation: Controlled adjustment of the concentration of fluoride in a communal water supply so as to achieve maximum caries reduction and clinically insignificant level of fluorosis.

Zoonosis: Any disease transmitted from vertebrate animals to humans. It may be enzootic or epizootic (see Endemic and Epidemic).

Index

533